Books should be returned to the SDH Library on or before
the date stamped above unless a renewal has been arranged

Salisbury District Hospital Library
Telephone: Salisbury (01722) 336262 extn. 4481 / 33
Out of hours answer machine in operation

Contents

Foreword   vii
by Boyd E Metzger
Preface   ix
Contributors   xi
Abbreviations used   xix

Chapter 1   1
History of diabetic pregnancy
David R Hadden

Chapter 2   13
The Priscilla White legacy
John W Hare

Chapter 3   23
The Pedersen legacy
Lars Mølsted-Pedersen

Chapter 4   30
The Freinkel legacy
Boyd E Metzger

Chapter 5   39
Pathogenesis of gestational diabetes
mellitus
*Yariv Yogev, Avi Ben-Haroush,
Moshe Hod*

Chapter 6   50
Maternal metabolic adaptation to
pregnancy
Patrick M Catalano

Chapter 7   64
Epidemiology of gestational diabetes
mellitus
*Avi Ben-Haroush, Yariv Yogev,
Moshe Hod*

Chapter 8   90
Pregnancy in diabetic animals
Eleazar Shafrir, Gernot Desoye

Chapter 9   113
Immunology of gestational diabetes
mellitus
*Alberto de Leiva, Dídac Mauricio,
Rosa Corcoy*

Chapter 10   126
The placenta in diabetic pregnancy
*Gernot Desoye, Sylvie Hauguel-de
Mouzon, Eleazar Shafrir*

Chapter 11   148
Amniotic fluid in non-diabetic and
diabetic pregnancies
Marshall W Carpenter

Chapter 12   158
Classification of diabetic pregnancy
Yasue Omori

Chapter 13   168
Detection and diagnostic strategies for gestational diabetes mellitus
Boyd E Metzger, Yoo Lee Kim

Chapter 14   183
Gestational diabetes in developing countries
Liliana S Voto, Matías Uranga Imaz, Miguel Margulies

Chapter 15   191
Diabetes following gestational diabetes mellitus
Peter Damm, Jeannet Lauenborg, Lars Mølsted-Pedersen

Chapter 16   201
Nutrient delivery and metabolism in the fetus
William W Hay

Chapter 17   222
Regulation of fetal growth
David J Hill

Chapter 18   240
Pre-implantation embryopathy and maternal diabetes
René De Hertogh, Amaya Leunda Casi, Laurence Hinck

Chapter 19   253
Fetal oxygenation and mineral metabolism in diabetic pregnancy
Francis B Mimouni, Galit Sheffer-Mimouni

Chapter 20   262
Clinical and experimental advances in the understanding of diabetic embryopathy
Ulf J Eriksson, Parri Wentzel, Moshe Hod

Chapter 21   276
Fetal maturity
Antonio Cutuli, Gian Carlo Di Renzo

Chapter 22   289
Short-term implications: the neonate
Paul Merlob, Moshe Hod

Chapter 23   305
Long-term implications: child and adult
Dana Dabelea, David J Pettitt

Chapter 24   317
Growth and neurodevelopment of children born to diabetic mothers and to mothers with gestational diabetes mellitus
Asher Ornoy

Chapter 25   330
Management of gestational diabetes mellitus
Massimo Massi-Benedetti, Marco Orsini Federici, Gian Carlo Di Renzo

Chapter 26   340
Nutritional management in diabetic pregnancy: a time for reason not dogma
Anne Dornhorst, Gary Frost

Chapter 27   359
Insulin therapy in pregnancy
John L Kitzmiller, Lois Jovanovic

Chapter 28 379
Use of oral hypoglycemic agents in pregnancy
Oded Langer

Chapter 29 394
Continuous glucose monitoring during pregnancies complicated by diabetes mellitus
Lois Jovanovic, Yariv Yogev, Moshe Hod

Chapter 30 404
Prenatal ultrasound assessment of the diabetic patient
Israel Meizner, Reuven Mashiach

Chapter 31 418
Monitoring in labor
Roberto Luzietti, Karl G Rosén

Chapter 32 430
Timing and mode of delivery
Jeremy JN Oats, Oded Langer

Chapter 33 442
Prevention of fetal macrosomia
Giorgio Mello, Elena Parretti, Federico Mecacci, Moshe Hod

Chapter 34 447
Timing and delivery of the macrosomic infant: induction versus conservative management
David A Sacks

Chapter 35 455
Management of the macrosomic fetus
Gerard HA Visser, Inge M Evers, Giorgio Mello

Chapter 36 460
Hypertensive disorders and diabetic pregnancy
Jacob Bar, Michael Kupferminc, Moshe Hod

Chapter 37 475
Diabetic retinopathy
Tamar Perri, Nino Loya, Moshe Hod

Chapter 38 486
Diabetic vascular complications in pregnancy: nephropathy
Barak M Rosenn, Menachem Miodovnik

Chapter 39 495
Diabetic ketoacidosis in pregnancy
Yariv Yogev, Avi Ben-Haroush, Moshe Hod

Chapter 40 502
Diabetes and multiple pregnancies
Yenon Hazan, Isaac Blickstein

Chapter 41 508
Evidence-based medicine and diabetic pregnancy
Pauline Green, Zarko Alfirevic

Chapter 42 519
Databases: a tool for quality management of diabetic pregnancies
Dina Pfeifer, Rony Chen, Moshe Hod

Chapter 43   **529**
Cost analysis of diabetes and pregnancy
Michael Brandle, William H Herman

Chapter 44   **539**
Quality of care for the woman with
diabetes in pregnancy
*Alberto de Leiva, Rosa Corcoy,
Eulalia Brugués*

Chapter 45   **554**
Ethical issues in management of
pregnancy complicated by diabetes
*Frank A Chervenak,
Laurence B McCullough*

Chapter 46   **563**
Legal aspects of diabetic pregnancy
Kevin J Dalton

Chapter 47   **578**
Diabetologic education in pregnancy
Luis Cabero Roura

Chapter 48   **589**
Optimal contraception for the diabetic
woman
Siri L Kjos

Chapter 49   **597**
Hormone replacement therapy and
diabetes
*Bari Kaplan, Michael Hirsch,
Dov Feldberg*

Chapter 50   **606**
Diabetes and infertility
*Avi Ben-Haroush, Raoul Orvieto,
Benjamin Fisch*

Index   622

Foreword

Publication of the first edition of a new textbook on diabetes and pregnancy a well-established topic of clinical activity and research, is likely to raise questions about its need or the educational role that it is expected to fill. In my view, this is not simply another text on the same topic and in the following few paragraphs, I will give the reasons for this perspective.

For more than half a century, advances in knowledge and in the clinical management of the pregnant diabetic have come from a truly international base. In past years, there have been numerous forums for presentation, discussion of new research findings related to both pregestational and gestational diabetes mellitus. There is a true sense of collegiality among leaders in the field. The philosophy embodied in the organization of this volume seeks to provide a similar venue for the presentation of the educational material of a textbook.

The prospects for success appear bright. The editor, Moshe Hod is from Israel and he has assembled a team of co-editors with members from the USA, Italy and Spain. The more than 60 additional contributing authors come from equally diverse backgrounds and fields of expertise, as well as institutional and national affiliations. Likewise, the content of the volume is comprehensive and promises great depth in coverage of the field.

I am pleased that this, the first edition of what hopefully will be a recurring publication, leads off with a historical perspective that features the contributions of several pioneers that played major roles in the advancement of knowledge and in establishing the international flavor that characterizes the field and is captured in the contributors and the contributions to this text. I recommend it for all clinicians and investigators in the field of diabetes and pregnancy.

Boyd E Metzger MD
Tom D Spies Professor
Department of Medicine
Northwestern University Feinberg School of Medicine
Chicago, IL, USA

Preface

The field of diabetes and pregnancy has come of age. From the conception of the terminology 'gestational diabetes' and 'diabetes in pregnancy' to the creation of an entire subspecialty, this textbook documents the 'gestation' of the field. Now we have even subdivided the field and have created subspecialists in gestational diabetes, and pregestational or diabetes in pregnancy, Type 1 and Type 2. In fact we have created our own internal debating groups as to the correct terminology for each type of diabetes and its impact on pregnancy and the pregnancy's impact on the type of diabetes. It is a great honor to be on the team of editors who have sought out the most creative and progressive of scientists, and learned from them the latest techniques and opinions as to the optimal management of all types of diabetes in pregnancy.

This textbook not only documents the past 80 years of progress in the field of diabetes and pregnancy, but also presents the most up-to-date tools, techniques and management protocols to ensure the optimal outcome of pregnancies complicated by diabetes. In addition, the areas that remain controversial are discussed in detail to enable the reader to come to an opinion while waiting for the evidence to validate many of the expert opinions presented in this book. A scan of the table of contents shows that every area in the field of diabetes and pregnancy has been covered. After a retrospective and historical perspective this textbook covers both gestational diabetes and the Type 1 and Type 2 diabetic woman who becomes pregnant. There are four chapters devoted to the history written by giants in the field who have had the opportunity to sit at the feet of the pioneers in our field: the great Drs Pricilla White, Norbert Freinkel, John O'Sullivan and Jørgen Pedersen. The authors of each of the subsequent chapters are world renowned. Thus if there is not the highest level of evidence-based literature to substantiate an opinion, the expert presents the data upon which a decision can be made about optimal care.

The most controversial topic today in the field of diabetes and pregnancy is in the area of screening and diagnosis. Here the evidence to date is presented and the justification for a multi-national, multi-center clinical trial to elucidate the optimal methods for screening and diagnosis are presented. In addition, the pure physiology of normal metabolism in pregnancy and the pathophysiology of diabetes in pregnancy are discussed in detail. These chapters set the stage for deriving the optimal therapy for the pregnant diabetic women and creating the algorithms that most closely mimic the normal physiology and metabolism of pregnancy.

The chapters devoted to malformations, placental pathology and defects of growth and development of the fetus are the strongest discussions to date in our understanding of diabetic fetopathy and teratogenesis. Based on this literature the reader will be motivated to learn the difficult protocols to achieve and maintain normoglycemia before, during, and in-between all pregnancies complicated by diabetes.

The *Textbook of Diabetes and Pregnancy* also includes the latest theories and literature on the immunology of Type 1 diabetes and gives us hope that the near future holds the answers to prevention of this disease. Perhaps the solutions to the enigma may lead us to a cure of Type 1 diabetes. However, until there is a cure for diabetes, we must continually take on the burden of astutely diagnosing diabetes and treating all pregnant women who are at risk of an untoward outcome of pregnancy. Understanding and diagnosing all the metabolic abnormalities associated with pregnancy and providing the best management protocols to ensure a normal outcome of pregnancy is the objective. This textbook not only fulfills this objective, but also provides the answers for the clinician to help her/him to deliver optimal care of all pregnancies complicated by diabetes while we wait for the cure.

Moshe Hod
Lois Jovanovic
Gian Carlo Di Renzo
Alberto de Leiva
Oded Langer

Contributors

Zarko Alfirevic
Consultant and Senior Lecturer in
Feto-Maternal Medicine
University Department
Liverpool Women's Hospital
Liverpool
UK

Jacob Bar MD
Perinatal Division and WHO Collaborating
Center for Perinatal Care
Women's Comprehensive Health Care Center
Rabin Medical Center – Beilinson Campus
Sackler Faculty of Medicine
Tel Aviv University
Petah Tiqva
Israel

Avi Ben-Haroush MD
Perinatal Division and WHO Collaborating
Center
Women's Comprehensive Health Care Center
Rabin Medical Center – Beilinson Campus
Sackler Faculty of Medicine
Infertility and IVF Unit
Tel Aviv University
Petah Tiqva
Israel

Isaac Blickstein MD
Department of Obstetrics and Gynecology
Kaplan Medical Center, Rehovot
Hadassah-Hebrew University
School of Medicine
Jerusalem
Israel

Michael Brandle MD
Postdoctoral Research Fellow
Division of Endocrinology and Metabolism
Department of Internal Medicine
University of Michigan Medical Center
Ann Arbor, MI
USA

Eulalia Brugués MSc
Department of Endocrinology and Nutrition
Hospital de Santa Creu I Sant Pau
Assistant Professor;
Universitat Autònoma
Barcelona
Spain

Luis Cabero Roura
Passeio Vall d'Hebron, 125
Barcelona
Spain

Marshall W Carpenter MD
Maternal Fetal Medicine
Women and Infants Hospital
Providence, RI
USA

Patrick M Catalano MD
Chair, Department of Obstetrics and
Gynecology
Professor, Reproductive Biology
Case Western Reserve University
Cleveland, OH
USA

Rony Chen MD
Perinatal Division and WHO Collaborating
Center for Perinatal Care
Women's Comprehensive Health Care Center
Rabin Medical Center – Beilinson Campus
Sackler Faculty of Medicine
Tel Aviv University
Petah Tiqva
Israel

Frank A Chervenak MD
Department of Obstetrics and Gynecology
New York Presbyterian Hospital
Weill Medical College of Cornell University
New York, NY
USA

Rosa Corcoy MD PhD
Attending Physician
Department of Endocrinology and Nutrition
Hospital de Santa Creu I Sant Pau
Assistant Professor,
Universitat Autònoma
Barcelona
Spain

Antonio Cutuli MD
Centre of Perinatal and Reproductive Medicine
University of Perugia
Perugia
Italy

Dana Dabelea MD PhD
Assistant Professor
Preventive Medicine and Biometrics
University of Colorado
Health Sciences Center
Denver, CO
USA

Kevin J Dalton DFMS LLM PhD FRCOG FCLM
Consultant in Obstetrics and Gynaecology
and in Legal Medicine
Department of Obstetrics and Gynaecology
University of Cambridge
Addenbrooke's Hospital
Cambridge
UK

Peter Damm MD DMSc
Consultant in Obstetrics and Gynecology
Department of Obstetrics and Gynecology
Copenhagen University Hospital
Rigshospitalet
Copenhagen
Denmark

René De Hertogh MD PhD
Professor of Endocrinology and Diabetology
Physiology of Human Reproduction Research Unit
University of Louvain-La-Neuve
School of Medicine, UCL
Brussels
Belgium

Alberto de Leiva MD PhD DMSc MHE
Professor of Medicine and Director
Department of Endocrinology and Nutrition
Hospital de la Santa Creu i Sant Pau
Universitat Autònoma
Barcelona
Spain

Gernot Desoye PhD
Professor of Biochemistry
Clinic of Obstetrics and Gynecology
Karl-Franzens-University
Graz
Austria

Gian Carlo Di Renzo MD PhD
Director
Centre of Perinatal and Reproductive Medicine
University Hospital Monteluce
Departments of Gynaecology, Obstetrics and
Paediatrics
Perugia
Italy

Anne Dornhorst DM FRCP MRCPath
Senior Lecturer
Department of Metabolic Medicine
Imperial College School of Medicine
Hammersmith Hospital
London
UK

Ulf J Eriksson MD PhD
Professor
Department of Medical Cell Biology
Uppsala University
Biomedical Center
Uppsala
Sweden

Inge M Evers
Department of Obstetrics, Neonatology
and Gynecology
University Hospitals
Utrecht
The Netherlands

Dov Feldberg MD
Women's Comprehensive Health Care Center
Rabin Medical Center – Beilinson Campus
Sackler Faculty of Medicine
Tel Aviv University
Petah Tiqva
Israel

Benjamin Fisch
Perinatal Division and WHO Collaborating Center
Women's Comprehensive Health Care Center
Rabin Medical Center – Beilinson Campus
Sackler Faculty of Medicine
Infertility and IVF Unit
Tel Aviv University
Petah Tiqva
Israel

Gary Frost PhD
Head of the Departments of Nutrition
and Dietetics; and Nutrition and Dietetic
Research Group
Reader, Imperial College School of Medicine
Hammersmith Hospital
London
UK

Pauline Green
Consultant Obstetrician
Arrowe Park Hospital
Wirral
UK

David R Hadden MD FRCP
Professor
Royal Maternity Hospital and Royal Victoria
Hospital
Belfast
Northern Ireland
UK

John W Hare MD
Senior Physician, Associate Clinical Professor
of Medicine
Joslin Diabetes Center
Harvard Medical School
Boston, MA
USA

Sylvie Hauguel-de Mouzon PhD
UPRESA 2396-Université Paris 6
CHU Sainte Antoine
Paris
France

William W Hay MD
Department of Pediatrics
Section of Neonatology and Division of
Perinatal Medicine
University of Colorado School of Medicine
Denver, CO
USA

Yenon Hazan
Department of Obstetrics and Gynecology
Kaplan Medical Center
Rehovot; and the Hadassah-Hebrew University
School of Medicine
Jerusalem
Israel

William H Herman MD MPH
Professor of Internal Medicine and Epidemiology
Division of Endocrinology and Metabolism
Department of Internal Medicine
University of Michigan Medical Center
Ann Arbor, MI
USA

David J Hill DPhil
Scientific Director
MRC Group in Fetal and Neonatal Health and
Development Lawson Research Institute
St Joseph's Health Centre
Departments of Medicine, Paediatrics
and Physiology
University of Western Ontario
London, Ontario
Canada

Laurence Hinck PhD
Research Assistant
Physiology of Human Reproduction Research
Unit
University of Louvain-La-Neuve
School of Medicine, UCL
Brussels
Belgium

Michael Hirsch MD
Women's Comprehensive Health Care Center
Rabin Medical Center – Beilinson Campus
Sackler Faculty of Medicine
Tel Aviv University
Petah Tiqva
Israel

Moshe Hod MD
Director of Perinatal Division
WHO Collaborating Center for Perinatal Care
Women's Comprehensive Health Care Center
Rabin Medical Center – Beilinson Campus
Sackler Faculty of Medicine
Tel Aviv University
Petah Tiqva
Israel

Lois Jovanovic MD
Clinical Professor of Medicine
University of Southern California;
Adjunct Professor of Biomolecular Science
and Engineering
University of California – Santa Barbera;
Director and Chief Scientific Officer
Sansum Medical Research Institute
Santa Barbara, CA
USA

Bari Kaplan MD
Women's Comprehensive Health Care Center
Rabin Medical Center – Beilinson Campus
Sackler Faculty of Medicine
Tel Aviv University
Petah Tiqva
Israel

Yoo Lee Kim MD
Department of Internal Medicine
College of Medicine
Pochon CHA University
Seoul
Korea

John L Kitzmiller MD
Division of Maternal–Fetal Medicine
Good Samaritan Hospital
San Jose, CA; Sansum Medical Research Institute
Santa Barbara, CA
USA

Siri L Kjos MD
Professor and Chief, Division of Women's Health
Obstetrics and Gynecology
University of Southern California Keck School of
Medicine
Los Angeles, CA
USA

Michael Kupferminc
The Liss Tel Aviv Medical Center
Sackler Faculty of Medicine
Tel Aviv University
Israel

Oded Langer MD
Babcock Professor and Chairman
Department of Obstetrics and Gynecology
St Luke's – Roosevelt Hospital Center
University Hospital of Columbia
New York, NY
USA

Jeannet Lauenborg
Department of Obstetrics and Gynecology
Copenhagen University Hospital
Rigshospitalet
Copenhagen
Denmark

Amaya Leunda Casi PhD
Research Assistant
Physiology of Human Reproduction Research Unit
University of Louvain-La-Neuve
School of Medicine, UCL
Brussels
Belgium

Nino Loya MD
Department of Ophthalmology
Rabin Medical Center
Petah Tiqva
Israel

Roberto Luzietti MD PhD
Centre of Perinatal and Reproductive Medicine
University of Perugia
Perugia
Italy

Miguel Margulies MD
Emeritus Professor of Obstetrics
Juan A Fernández Hospital and
Miguel Margulies Foundation
University of Buenos Aires
Argentina

Reuven Mashiach
Ultrasound Department
Women's Health Center
Rabin Medical Center
Petah-Tiqva; and Sackler Faculty of Medicine
Tel Aviv
Israel

Massimo Massi-Benedetti
Department of Internal Medicine
University of Perugia
Perugia
Italy

Dídac Mauricio MD PhD
Chief, Section of Endocrinology and Nutrition
Hospital Parc Tauli
Sabadell
Barcelona
Spain

Laurence B McCullough
Department of Obstetrics and Gynecology
New York Presbyterian Hospital
Weill Medical College of Cornell University
New York, NY
USA

Federico Mecacci MD
Careggi University Hospital
Department of Gynecology, Perinatology and
Human Reproduction
University of Florence
Italy

Israel Meizner MD
Head, Ultrasound Department
Women's Health Center
Rabin Medical Center
Petah-Tiqva; and Sackler Faculty of Medicine
Tel Aviv
Israel

Giorgio Mello MD
Associate Professor of Maternal–Fetal Medicine
Department of Gynecology, Perinatology and
Human Reproduction
University of Florence
Italy

Paul Merlob MD
Department of Neonatology
Rabin Medical Center
Beilinson Campus
Petah Tiqva
Israel

Boyd E Metzger MD
Tom D Spies Professor
Division of Endocrinology, Metabolism and
Molecular Medicine
Department of Medicine
Northwestern University Feinberg School
of Medicine
Chicago, IL
USA

Francis B Mimouni MD FACN FAAP
Professor and Chairman,
Department of Neonatology
The Sackler School of Medicine;
Director of Neonatology,
The Lis Maternity Hospital;
Tel Aviv Sourasky Medical Center
Tel Aviv
Israel

Menachem Miodovnik MD
Professor and Vice Chair
Department of Obstetrics and Gynecology
St Luke's Roosevelt Health Center
University Hospital of Columbia University
College of Physicians and Surgeons
New York, NY
USA

Lars Mølsted-Pedersen
Department of Obstetrics and Gynaecology
The Juliane Marie Centre
Rigshospitalet
University of Copenhagen
Copenhagen
Denmark

Jeremy JN Oats MD
Clinical Director of Women's Services;
Adjunct Professor, School of Public Health
La Trobe University
Carlton, Victoria
Australia

Yasue Omori MD
Director, Diabetes Center
Eastern Japan Medical Center
Kanagawa-pref
Japan

Asher Ornoy
Developmental Pediatrician and Clinical
Teratologist; Professor of Anatomy, Embryology
and Teratology
Hebrew University Hadassah Medical School
Jerusalem
Israel

Marco Orsini Federici
Department of Internal Medicine
University of Perugia
Italy

Raoul Orvieto
Perinatal Division and WHO Collaborating Center
Women's Comprehensive Health Care Center
Rabin Medical Center – Beilinson Campus
Sackler Faculty of Medicine
Tel Aviv University
Infertility and IVF Unit
Petah Tiqva
Israel

Elena Parretti MD PhD
Researcher
Department of Gynecology, Perinatology
and Human Reproduction
University of Florence
Italy

Tamar Perri MD
Perinatal Division and WHO Collaborating
Center for Perinatal Care
Women's Comprehensive Health Care Center
Rabin Medical Center – Beilinson Campus
Sackler Faculty of Medicine
Tel Aviv University
Petah Tiqva
Israel

David J Pettitt MD PhD
Senior Scientist
Sansum Medical Research Institute
Santa Barbara, CA
USA

Dina Pfeifer
Department of Obstetrics and Gynecology
Medical School University of Zagreb
Zagreb
Croatia

Karl G Rosén
Plymouth Postgraduate Medical School
University of Plymouth
UK; and Neoventa Medical
Gothenburg
Sweden

Barak M Rosenn MD
Associate Professor, Director of Obstetrics and
Maternal Fetal Medicine
Department of Obstetrics and Gynecology
St Luke's Roosevelt Health Center
University Hospital College of Physicians
and Surgeons
New York, NY
USA

David A Sacks MD
Director, Division of Maternal-Fetal Medicine
Department of Obstetrics and Gynecology
Kaiser Foundation Hospital
Bellflower, CA; Clinical Professor
Department of Obstetrics and Gynecology
Keck School of Medicine
University of Southern California
Los Angeles, CA
USA

Eleazar Shafrir
Department of Biochemistry
Haddassah University
Kiryat Hadassah
Jerusalem
Israel

Galit Sheffer-Mimouni MD
The Departments of Neonatology and
Gynecology and Obstetrics
The Lis Maternity Hospital
The Tel Aviv Sourasky Medical Center and
The Sackler School of Medicine
Tel Aviv
Israel

Matías Uranga Imaz MD
Assistant Professor of Obstetrics
Juan A Fernández Hospital and Miguel
Margulies Foundation
University of Buenos Aires
Argentina

Gerald HA Visser
Professor of Obstetrics; Chairman,
Department of Perinatology and Gynecology
University Medical Center
Utrecht
The Netherlands

Liliana S Voto MD PhD
President of Exercise
Juan A Fernández Hospital and Miguel
Margulies Foundation
University of Buenos Aires
Argentina

Parri Wentzel PhD
Associate Professor
Department of Medical Cell Biology
Uppsala University
Biomedical Center
Uppsala
Sweden

Yariv Yogev MD
Perinatal Division and WHO Collaborating
Center for Perinatal Care
Women's Comprehensive Health Care Center
Rabin Medical Center – Beilinson Campus
Sackler Faculty of Medicine
Tel Aviv University
Petah Tiqva
Israel

Abbreviations used

AA	autoantibodies	ELISA	enzyme-linked immunosorbent assay
AACC	American Association of Clinical Chemists	ESIMS	electrospray ionization mass spectrometry
ACE	angiotensin-converting enzyme	ETSI	European Telecommunications Standard Institute
ACOG	American College of Obstetrics and Gynecology	FAD	flavin adenine dinucleotide
ADA	American Diabetes Association	FBS	fetal blood sampling
ADD	attention deficit disorder	FDA	Food and Drug Administration
AGA	appropriate for gestational age	FDR	first-degree relative
AGE	advanced glycation endproducts	FFA	free fatty acid
AMP	adenosine monophosphate	FGF	fibroblast growth factor
ARI	aldose reductase inhibitor	FGFR	fibroblast growth factor receptor
ATP	adensine triphosphate	FHR	fetal heart rate
AUGC	area under the glucose curve	FI	finger identification
BMD	bone mineral density	FPG	fasting plasma glucose
BMI	body mass index	FVW	flow velocity waveforms
BP	blood pressure	GAD	glutamic acid decarboxylase
BPD	biparietal diameter	GAMA	gamma-aminobutyric acid
BPS	biophysical score	GCT	glucose challenge test
CAD	coronary artery disease	GDM	gestational diabetes mellitus
CDAPP	California Diabetes and Pregnancy Program	GFR	glomerular filtration rate
CEA	cost-effectiveness analysis	GIGT	gestational impaired glucose tolerance
CEE	conjugated equine estrogen	GLIMA	glycosylated islet cell membrane-associated antigen
CGM	continuous glucose monitoring		
CHD	coronary heart disease	GLUT	glucose transporter
CI	confidence interval	GSH	growth stimulating hormone
CM	congenital malformation	GUR	glucose utilization rate
CMS	Continuous Monitoring System	HAPO Study	Hyperglycaemia and Adverse Pregnancy Outcome study
CNS	central nervous system		
CoA	coenzyme A	HbA1c	glycosylated haemoglobin
CPR	C-peptide response	HCG	human chorionic gonadotropin
CRL	crown—rump length	hCS	human chorionic somatomammotropin
CRP	C-reactive protein	HDL	high-density lipoprotein
CS	Cesarean Section	HERS	Heart and Estrogen/progestin Replacement Study
CSII	continuous subcutaneous insulin infusion		
CT	computerized tomography	HGF	hepatocyte growth factor
CTG	cardiotocography	HLA	human leucocyte antigen
DAG	diacylglycerol	HPL	human placental lactogen
DCCT	Diabetes Control and Complications Trial	HPLC	high-performance liquid chromatography
DiabCare BIS	DiabCare basic information sheet	HRT	hormone replacement therapy
DIEP Study	Diabetes in Early Pregnancy Study	HVR	hypervariable region
DKA	diabetic ketoacidosis	IA	insulin antibodies
DM	diabetes mellitus	IAA	insulin autoantibodies
DPP	Diabetes Prevention Program	ICA	islet cell autoanitibodies
DPSG	Diabetic Pregnancy Study Group	IDDM	insulin-dependent diabetes mellitus
DR	diabetic retinopathy	IDF	International Diabetes Federation
DZ	dizygotic	IDM	infants of diabetic mothers
EAR	estimated average requirements	IFCC	International Federation of Clinical Chemistry
ECG	electrocardiogram		
EFM	electronic fetal monitoring	IFG	impaired fasting glucose

IGDM	infants of gestational diabetic mothers	PBSP	prognostically bad signs during pregnancy
IGF	insulin-like growth factor	PC	plasma cell membrane glycoprotein
IGFBP	insulin-like growth factor binding proteins	PCO	polycystic ovary
IGFR	insulin-like growth factor receptor	PCOS	polycystic ovary syndrome
IGT	impaired glucose tolerance	per os	bucal administration
IL	interleukin	PET	pre-eclampsia toxemia
IM	intra-muscular	PG	phosphatidylglycerol
iNOS	inducible nitric oxide synthase	PGDM	pregestational diabetes mellitus
IP	intraperitoneal	PGE_2	prostaglandin E_2
IQ	intelligence quotients	PGF	placental growth factor
IR	insulin receptor	PGH_2	prostaglandin H_2
IRMA	intra-retinal microaneurysms	PI	phosphatidylinositol
IRP	iron-regulatory proteins	PID	pelvic inflammatory disease
IRS	insulin receptor substrate	PIH	pregnancy-induced hypertension
ISO	International Standard Organization	PKB	protein kinase B
IT	information technology	PKC	protein kinase C
IUD	intrauterine device	PPG	postprandial plasma glucose
IUFD	intrauterine fetal deaths	PPV	positive predictive value
IUGR	intrauterine growth restriction	PreAGT	previous abnormality of glucose tolerance
IV	intravenous	PROM	premature rupture of membranes
IVGTT	intravenous glucose tolerance test	PTCA	percutaneous transluminal coronary balloon angioplasty
JDF	Juvenile Diabetes Foundation		
JNC	Joint National Committee	PTH	parathyroid hormone
LADA	latent autoimmune diabetes of adulthood	PUFA	polyunsaturated fatty acid
LBW	low birthweight	RCT	randomized controlled trial
LDL	low-density lipoprotein	RDS	respiratory distress syndrome
LGA	large for gestational age	REM	rapid eye movement
LS	lecithin-sphingomyelin	RIA	radioimmunoassay
LTS	localization of tactile stimuli	ROC	receiver-operating curve
MA	microalbuminuria	ROS	reactive oxygen species
MAP	mitogen-activated protein	RR	relative risk
MAPK	mitogen-activated protein kinase	SAP	surfactant-associated protein
MDA	malonyldialdehyde	SBGM	self-blood glucose monitoring
MFI	manual form perception	SCBU	special care baby unit
MFPR	multifetal pregnancy reduction	SCF	stem cell factor
MGH	mild gestational hyperglycemia	SD	standard deviation
MNT	medical nutrition therapy	S/D	systolic/diastolic
MODY	maturity onset diabetes of the young	SES	socio-economic status
MPA	medroxyprogesterone acetate	SF	saturated fat
MRI	magnetic resonance imaging	SGA	small for gestational age
mRNA	messenger ribonucleic acid	SHR	spontaneously hypertensive rats
MSAFP	maternal serum alpha-fetoprotein	SHS	Strong Heart Study
MUFA	monosaturated fatty acid	SOD	superoxide dismutase
MZ	monozygotic	STZ	streptozotocin
NAC	N-acetylcysteine	TG	triglyceride
NADH	reduced nicotinamide adenine dinucleotide	TK	tyrosine kinase
NDDG	National Diabetes Data Group	TLC	thin layer chromatography
NETA	norethisterone acetate	TNF	tumour necrosis factor
NHC	neonatal hypocalcemia	TRH	thyroprophin-releasing hormone
NIDDM	non-insulin-dependent diabetes mellitus	UKPDS	United Kingdom Prospective Diabetes Study
NIH	National Institute of Health	VEGF	vascular endothelial growth factors
NTD	neural tube defects	VLBW	very low birthweight
OBSQID	OBStetrical Quality Indicators and Data	VLDL	very-low-density lipoprotein
ODFD	operative deliveries for fetal distress	VNTR	variable number tandem repeat
OGTT	oral glucose tolerance test	WHI	Women's Health Initiative
OR	odds ratio	WHO	World Health Organization
PAD	perinatal aggregated data	WISC-R	Wechsler Intelligence Scales for Children Revised
PAI	plasminogen activator inhibitor		

1

History of diabetic pregnancy
David R Hadden

Introduction

One hundred years ago the medical literature on diabetic pregnancy was very limited. Pregnancy itself was no less frequent, but the outcome was affected by so many other major problems that the influence of a medical disorder of a chronic nature was both unrecognized and disregarded. Diabetes mellitus was also less prevalent, due both to demographic differences in the age of the population and to epidemiological factors – mainly the absence of any effective treatment so that young people with diabetes had a life expectancy of only a few years. The diagnosis of diabetes depended on the demonstration of sugar in the urine and the well-known symptoms of thirst, polyuria and weight loss, but there was no accurate measurement to assess severity, and the distinction between what are now known as Type 1 and Type 2 diabetes was only anecdotal. There was no documentation of the specific long-term complications of hyperglycaemia in the eyes, nerves, heart, kidneys or blood vessels.

Early history of diabetes

Diabetes was well recognized as a medical disorder > 2000 years ago, and some well-known references are worth quoting. The ancient Egyptian Ebers papyrus, dating to 1500 BC records abnormal polyuria; the Greek father of medicine Hippocrates (466–377 BC) mentioned 'making water too often' and Aristotle also referred to 'wasting of the body'. Aretaeus of Cappodocia (AD 30–90) in Asia Minor (now Turkey) is credited with first using the name diabetes, which is Greek for a siphon, meaning water passing through the body: 'diabetes is a wasting of the flesh and limbs into urine – the nature of the disease is chronic, but the patient is short lived … thirst unquenchable, the mouth parched and the body dry …'. The famous Arabian physician Avicenna (AD 980–1027) recorded further important observations that maintained and extended the previous Greek knowledge through what became known in Europe as the Dark Ages: he described the irregular appetite, mental exhaustion, loss of sexual function, carbuncles and other complications. There are also references to diabetes in ancient Hindu texts (AD 500) as a 'disease of the rich, brought about by gluttony or over-indulgence in flour and sugar', and in early Chinese and Japanese writings 'the urine of diabetics was very large in amount and so sweet that it attracted dogs'.[1,2]

After the European Renaissance the first physician to rediscover and record the sweetness of the urine in diabetes was Thomas Willis in London (1679), 'The diabetes or pissing evil

... in our age given to good fellowship and guzzling down of unalloyed wine', and Mathew Dobson 100 years later in Liverpool first demonstrated chemically the presence of sugar in the urine of diabetic patients. The demonstration by Oscar Minkowski (1889) that removal of the pancreas in a dog unexpectedly resulted in uncontrolled polyuria – the urine sugar attracted flies in the laboratory to the puddles on the floor – was the significant observation that eventually led to the extraction of insulin from the pancreatic islets in Toronto in 1922.[3] The story of the discovery of insulin is a remarkable record of disappointment: it was almost discovered in 1906 by Zuelzer in Berlin, and then in 1912 by Scott in Chicago, but was actually extracted by Paulesco in Romania in 1920. However, the world recognizes the story of the Toronto group – including Banting, Best, Collip and Macleod – as the definitive discovery and in 1923 the Nobel prize for medicine and physiology was awarded to two of them, Frederick Banting and JJR Macleod.[4]

Up until then the only effective treatment for diabetes had been dietary, and it was well known that restriction of food would ameliorate the symptoms. John Rollo had demonstrated this with his patient Captain Meredith in the army in Ireland in 1797, who obeyed his doctor's advice, documented the reduction in urine volume and subsequent weight loss, and even extracted sugar from the urine by evaporation. The dietary approach was carried to its logical extreme by the overenthusiastic approach of FM Allen in New York (1919), whose starvation therapy often temporarily returned the blood glucose to normal, but only succeeded in extending life for a year or so in the severe juvenile cases, all of whom became skeletally thin. Dr Elliott Joslin is remembered as the Boston physician who bridged the period immediately before insulin's discovery and the

exciting clinical demonstration of its effectiveness in the following decade.[5] In London, Dr Robin Laurence, diabetic himself, on dietary therapy only in his early twenties, recorded how his life was saved in 1923 by a telegram from his doctor in Kings College Hospital, 'I've got insulin, and it works – come back quick': he survived for many years and became the leading diabetes specialist in England.[6]

These two doctors, Joslin in Boston and Laurence in London, became the leaders of the revolution which would take place in both the opportunity for and the outcome of pregnancy in diabetic women.

Pregnancy and diabetes before the discovery of insulin

A full historical review of fertility and of the outcome of pregnancy in different parts of the world is beyond the scope of this chapter, but there are a number of aspects that are of particular relevance to the story of diabetes. Medical history in particular is constrained by publication bias, and there is much more available data regarding Europe and North America than in other parts of the world. The geographical and ethnic differences in the distribution, development and management of diabetes in different places at different times would be of great interest to review, but as the data are patchy and both diabetic and obstetric treatments often poorly defined, it may be that: 'History followed different courses for different peoples, because of differences among peoples' environments, not because of biological differences among peoples themselves'.[7] There are certainly both environmental and genetic reasons for the differing prevalence and incidence of diabetes in different countries, as much as for the different outcomes of pregnancy, but the international historical study of these factors is still in its infancy.

The collection of vital statistics first became available at varying times in the developed Western countries. The Scandinavian countries were first (Sweden 1749, Denmark 1801), England and Wales followed (1838) and then Russia (1867); although the process was initiated in the USA in 1880 it did not become complete until 1933.[8] Fertility rates have varied as much as death rates and migration in different countries, so that population dynamics will have a considerable effect on reported statistics for a single condition such as diabetes in pregnancy. The classical Malthusian checks on death rate – disease, famine and war – and the effects of celibacy and restraint on birth rate, will have more effect on the overall outcome statistics of pregnancy in diabetic mothers than the diabetes itself. The general fertility rate for England and Wales was about 130 live births per 1000 women between the ages of 15 and 44 in 1840, but is now only half that rate. At present the total fertility rate (average number of children born per woman) varies from 2.1 in Western Europe to 6.7 in West Africa.[9] However, there is no doubt that untreated diabetes must have been virtually incompatible with successful pregnancy before about 1850. In 1856 Blott in Paris wrote that 'True diabetes was inconsistent with conception', and certainly the then short life expectancy of a young woman with what we now call Type 1 diabetes before the discovery of insulin would support that statement. Recent speculation on the possible nutritional causes of the present-day epidemic of Type 2 diabetes in older patients mean that any data on diabetes successfully treated by diet only (which was probably Type 2, rather than Type 1) is of considerable theoretical interest, but it is perhaps important that these cases were not often reported in the literature and may well have been missed due to not even testing the urine for sugar.

In the pre-insulin days, and for sometime after, death of the mother during or soon after pregnancy from uncontrolled diabetes was the major risk. But maternal mortality was high for many reasons unrelated to diabetes, and retrospective analysis of data from England and Wales between 1850 and 1937 shows that poor interventional obstetric care with increased risk of puerperal sepsis was more important than social or economic deprivation.[10] The maternal mortality rates for Scandinavian countries were much lower, and it is now clear that this was due to better overall obstetric management in the prevention of sepsis; in the USA maternal mortality between 1921 and 1924 was 6.8 per 1000 births, in England and Wales 3.9 per 1000 births and in The Netherlands only 2.5 per 1000 births.[8] These differences at national level have been widely discussed, but must be borne in mind when considering the isolated effect of maternal diabetes over those years.

Overall perinatal mortality (death of the fetus after 28 weeks or within 7 days of delivery) has shown a more consistent fall over the same period of time in all Western countries. Most of the decline was in postneonatal mortality related to rising standards of living and nutrition, but also to improved public health measures – broadly speaking, the predominant form of infant mortality in Western countries was postneonatal in the nineteenth century and neonatal in the twentieth. There was not a close link between neonatal and maternal mortality, but there were very considerable differences in each of these measures between countries at the time of discovery of insulin (Table 1.1). The overall infant mortality rates in Scandinavian countries were persistently lower than in England and Wales, or Belgium, between 1920 and 1965, although all countries

	Maternal deaths 1921–1924 per 1000 births	Infant deaths 1924 per 1000 births	Neonatal deaths 1924 per 1000 births
The Netherlands	2.5	67.3	18.6
Japan	3.3	166.4	67.5
England/Wales	3.9	75.1	33.1
Australia	4.5	57.1	29.8
USA	6.8	70.8	38.6

Table 1.1. *Overall maternal mortality and infant and neonatal mortality for selected countries at the time of discovery of insulin (from Loudon[8]).*

show a steady exponential decline.[8] As perinatal mortality is now used as a main comparator for the outcome of diabetic pregnancy, it is important to bear these long-standing historical trends in mind.

Congenital malformations are also an important comparator for obstetrical results but the recognition of a possible link with maternal diabetes is much more recent: anecdotal accounts in small series in the 1940s were not supported until the report by the UK Medical Research Council in 1955[11] and the larger series from Copenhagen in 1964.[12] Historical records on the frequency of congenital malformations are very incomplete and it was not until the International Clearinghouse for Birth Defects began to operate after 1974 that any baseline data on the prevalence of congenital malformations became possible.[13] It is still difficult to compare results for specifically identified diabetic pregnancies with overall national malformation rates where the collection of cases is much less detailed.[14] Other obstetrical complications such as pre-eclampsia appear today to be more common in diabetic pregnancy but it is difficult to trace this possible interrelationship back to the days before organized antenatal care. Some of the cases where maternal death occurred in a diabetic pregnancy may have been due to eclampsia rather than diabetic coma.

Gestational diabetes

The concept of gestational diabetes, actually meaning hyperglycaemia due to the pregnancy itself but in practice defined as 'carbohydrate intolerance of varying severity with onset or first recognition during pregnancy', is also recent.[15] In the very first recorded case Bennewitz, in 1823, considered that the diabetes was actually a symptom of the pregnancy, and as the symptoms and the glycosuria disappeared after at least two successive pregnancies he had some evidence to support his views.[16] That lesser degrees of maternal hyperglycaemia were also a risk to pregnancy outcome dates back to studies in the 1940s in the USA[17,18] and Scotland,[19] which showed increased perinatal mortality some years before the recognition of clinical diabetes mellitus. This led to the term prediabetes in pregnancy, and to poorly defined concepts of temporary and latent diabetes. The first prospective study of carbohydrate metabolism in pregnancy was established in Boston in 1954, using a 50 gram 1 hour screening test, which has subsequently been widely adopted in the USA.[20] O'Sullivan[21] first used the name gestational diabetes in 1961, following the term metagestational diabetes used by Dr JP Hoet in 1954 after his early studies in Louvain Belgium.[22] At that time the US emphasis was on establishing criteria for the 100 gram oral glucose tolerance test in pregnancy as an index of the subsequent risk of the mother developing established diabetes, and the well-known O'Sullivan criteria were derived on this basis.[23] At about the same time, Mestman in southern California, began to identify the very considerably increased perinatal mortality associated with abnormal oral glucose tolerance in the obstetric population of Los Angeles County Hospital, which then comprised > 60% Latino mothers with the rest African-American and only a few Caucasian.[24] Subsequent studies in many parts of the world have extended the recognition of what has now become, in some places, an epidemic of hyperglycaemia in pregnancy. Jorgen Pedersen also used the term gestational diabetes in his monograph in 1967, but preferred to so classify a mother only after delivery, when he had demonstrated that her abnormal glucose tolerance in pregnancy had actually returned to normal postpartum; this rigorous definition has proved too difficult to achieve in practice.[25,26] The true definition of hyperglycaemia in pregnancy judged by the internationally acceptable 75 gram oral glucose tolerance test awaits the results of the large Hyperglycaemia and Adverse Pregnancy Outcome (HAPO) study.[27] The enthusiasm of the team at Northwestern University, Chicago, led by Norbert Freinkel and subsequently by Boyd Metzger has ensured that the concept of gestational diabetes is now firmly imprinted on the obstetric mind, as well as having established a major place as an epidemiological tool to study not only the immediate outcome of pregnancy but also the long-term effects on

both mother and baby of the relatively short phase of hyperglycaemia during the latter part of the pregnancy.

Important early publications

The historical development of understanding in obstetric, metabolic and paediatric disciplines over the past 100 years is perhaps best illustrated by several more extensive quotations and commentaries on seminal papers from the early literature.

HG Bennewitz: Diabetes mellitus – a symptom of pregnancy, *MD Thesis, University of Berlin, 1824 [translated from Latin]*[28]

This is the first reference to diabetes in pregnancy. Although the patient was young the clearly described onset of her symptoms during the pregnancy would now classify this as gestational diabetes. Is it possible that she only survived because she was a milder case who responded to diet, while all the more severe Type 1 diabetic patients died?

Henry Gottleib Bennewitz publicly defended his thesis for the degree of Doctor of Medicine at the University of Berlin on 24 June 1824 (Fig. 1.1). It is a simple case report and review of the literature on the causes and treatments of diabetes known at that time. His Greek derivation of the word diabetes and his one-line definition of the symptoms are unchanged today: '*Urine differing in quality and quantity from the normal ... accompanied by unquenchable thirst and eventual wasting.*' Before giving the case history, he summarized his belief that the diabetic condition was in some way a symptom of the pregnancy, or due to the pregnancy. He noted that: '*Other*

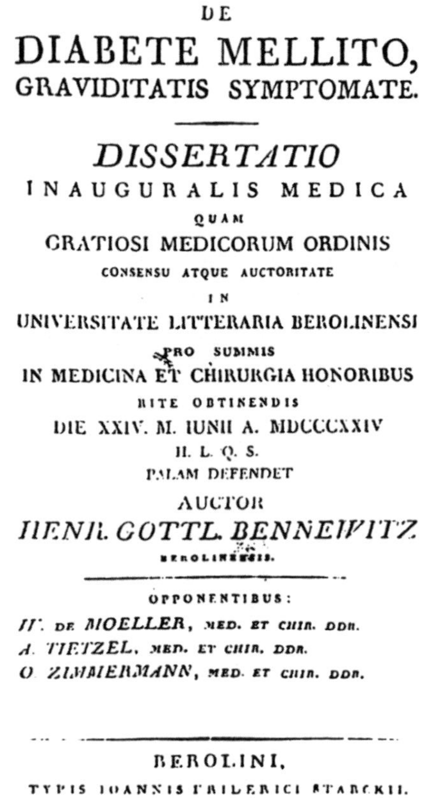

DE
DIABETE MELLITO,
GRAVIDITATIS SYMPTOMATE.

———

DISSERTATIO
INAUGURALIS MEDICA
QUAM
GRATIOSI MEDICORUM ORDINIS
CONSENSU ATQUE AUCTORITATE
IN
UNIVERSITATE LITTERARIA BEROLINENSI
PRO SUMMIS
IN MEDICINA ET CHIRURGIA HONORIBUS
RITE OBTINENDIS
DIE XXIV. M. IUNII A. MDCCCXXIV
H. L. Q. S.
PALAM DEFENDET
AUCTOR
HENR. GOTTL. BENNEWITZ
BEROLINENSIS.

————————

OPPONENTIBUS:
W. DE *MOELLER*, MED. ET CHIR. DDR.
A. TIETZEL, MED. ET CHIR. DDR.
O. ZIMMERMANN, MED. ET CHIR. DDR.

—— ———— —— ——

BEROLINI,
TYPIS IOANNIS FRIDERICI STARCKII.

DIABETES MELLITUS: A SYMPTOM OF PREGNANCY

An inaugural dissertation in medicine in which
its author
Heinrich Gottleib Bennewitz
of Berlin
will defend publicly with the consent and on the authority of the distinguished order of doctors in the University of Letters of Berlin to obtain in due order the highest honours in medicine and surgery, on the 24th day of the month of June in the year 1824.

HLQS.

The opponents being
W. de Moeller, Doctor of Medicine and Surgery
A. Tietzel, Doctor of Medicine and Surgery
O. Zimmermann, Doctor of Medicine and Surgery

Berlin, at the press of Johann Friederich Starck

Figure 1.1. *The title page of Dr Bennewitz's thesis* De diabete mellito, graviditatis symptomate,[28] *with translation into English.*

disorders ... began to break out as the pregnancy matured ... the little fires which had hidden beneath the smouldering deceiving ashes broke forth and devoured again the woman's condition in the most wretched manner.' He was convinced that: *'The disease appeared along with pregnancy, and at the very same time ...; when pregnancy appeared, it appeared; while pregnancy lasted, it lasted; it terminated soon after the pregnancy.'* He showed a degree of humility when he remarked that his patient must be something of a rare bird.

The case history commences on 13 November 1823, when Frederica Pape, aged 22, was admitted at 7 months in her fifth pregnancy to the Berlin Infirmary. The first three pregnancies appear to have been unremarkable, but in the fourth in 1822 she had an onset of thirst and polyuria which had resolved spontaneously after delivery. These symptoms returned at an unspecified time in her fifth pregnancy: she had *'a really unquenchable thirst – she consumed more than six Berlin measures of beer or spring water, although the quantity of urine greatly exceeded the amount of liquid consumed, and the urine itself smelt like stale beer. Her voice was weak, skin dry, face cold and she complained of a dragging pain in her back.'*

Treatment was more a matter of belief than of understanding, but apart from having withdrawn 360 ml of venous blood all at once (the equivalent of 36 10 ml routine blood tests today) and taking a high-protein diet, probably deficient in vitamins, she must have benefited from the rest and care. The measurement of 2 oz of sugar in 16 lb (224 oz) of urine, which is equivalent to about 1% glycosuria, was Bennewitz's only biochemical evidence of diabetes mellitus. From about 32 to 36 weeks the patient had a recurrent sore throat and increased abdominal distension such that twins were suspected. When examined on 28 December 1823 the cervix was dilating and the fetal head already partially descended. On 29 December she had an obstructed labour, and the child died intrapartum, probably due to delay in the second stage. Bennewitz remarks that the baby was of *'such robust and healthy character whom you would have thought Hercules had begotten.'* The infant weighed 12 lb, a fact witnessed carefully. Postpartum, in spite of continued dieting, sweating and purging, and the application of eight leeches, the patient's strength improved daily, and sugar disappeared from her urine. 'With nature to preserve and treat her, we dismissed our patient cured' (Fig. 1.2).

Unfortunately there is no record of the woman's subsequent health, perhaps because Dr Bennewitz presented his thesis within 6 months and having been successful in obtaining his doctorate, dropped out of academic medicine. This pregnancy would certainly qualify as 'carbohydrate intolerance of varying severity with onset or first recognition during pregnancy' – which was the definition agreed for gestational diabetes at the first workshop–conference in Chicago in 1980.

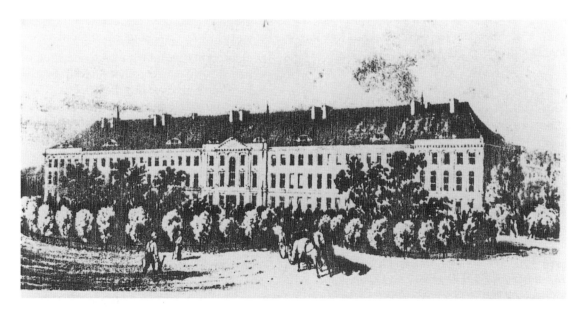

Figure 1.2. *Die Charite in Berlin (1785–1800) from a lithograph by von C Koppen (from Murken AH, Vom Armenhospital zum Grossklinikum die Geschichte des Krankenhauses, Vom 18. Jahrhundert biszur Gegenwart Koln, Durmont, 1988, 39).*

JM Duncan: On puerperal diabetes, *Trans Obstet Soc London* 1882; 24:256–85[29]

Matthews Duncan graduated in Aberdeen and became one of the leading obstetricians of his day (Fig. 1.3). This compilation of cases from the literature, from anecdotal reports and from his own experience first identified the serious problem of diabetes to the obstetrical world. He recorded at least 22 pregnancies in 15 mothers between the ages of 21 and 38 (the data are confused in places): the mother survived the pregnancy for long enough to become pregnant again in nine instances, in five she

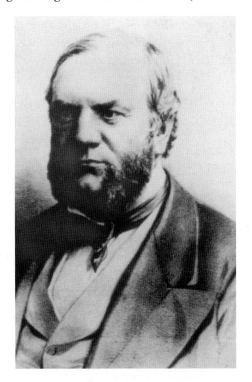

Figure 1.3. *J Matthews Duncan MD: born in 1826, and educated in Aberdeen and Edinburgh. He studied obstetrics under Sir James Simpson and was closely involved in the discovery of chloroform. He moved to London in 1877 and had a large practice based at St Bartholomew's Hospital (courtesy of Dr DWM Pearson, Aberdeen).*

died at the delivery and in six within a few months. The cause of maternal death was usually diabetic coma, although it is not possible to exclude eclampsia, and some must also have developed puerperal sepsis and one died from exacerbation of tuberculosis. Twelve of the 22 babies died, usually *in utero*, and they were usually of a large size: at least 10 survived and only three miscarriages are recorded: another 20 pregnancies seem to have occurred before the recorded cases, so some of these mothers must represent late-onset Type 2 or gestational diabetes, and these seemed to have a better prognosis for both mother and child.

'So far as is known, all, with one exception, were multipara, the pregnancy of highest number being the tenth. They cannot be read without giving a strong impression of the great gravity of the complication, but they are not sufficiently numerous to justify any statistical argument based on the number of occurrences.

The histories further show that:
- diabetes may come on during the pregnancy;
- diabetes may occur only during pregnancy, being absent at other times;
- diabetes may cease with the termination of the pregnancy, recurring some time afterwards;
- pregnancy may occur during diabetes;
- pregnancy and parturition may be apparently unaffected in its healthy progress by diabetes;
- pregnancy is very liable to be interrupted in its course; and probably always by the death of the foetus.'

JW Williams: The clinical significance of glycosuria in pregnant women, *Am J Med Sci* 1909; 137:1–26[30]

Whitfield Williams was Professor of Obstetrics at the Johns Hopkins University and wrote the first major American textbook on obstetrics, which still survives today in the eighteenth edition. He was concerned that the demonstration of sugar in the urine in pregnancy would be overinterpreted. *'I know of no complication of pregnancy the significance of which is more variously interpreted than the presence of sugar in the urine of pregnant women.'* Williams blamed Matthews Duncan for concluding that the detection of sugar in the urine constituted one of the most serious complications of pregnancy, as Duncan's views were accepted without question, although they were based on a small series of 22 pregnancies in 16 women collected from the then medical literature over 60 years, and his own small experience in Aberdeen. Williams presented six case reports to illustrate the various conditions in which sugar may be observed in the urine of pregnant women: simple lactosuria, transient glycosuria (two cases), alimentary glycosuria, recurrent glycosuria and mild diabetes. All resulted in a normal pregnancy outcome (although all the recorded birthweights were > 8 lb). He then analysed the urinary records of 3000 consecutive patients in the obstetrical department of the Johns Hopkins Hospital, in 167 of whom sugar had been demonstrated by Fehling's solution. He concluded that 137 of these represented definite postpartum lactosuria, being recognized only during lactation, and that almost all the others who had been recognized in late pregnancy were similar. He was able accurately to distinguish glucose from lactose in a few cases and found only two of the 167 cases had definite glycosuria, and could thus be considered to have mild diabetes complicating pregnancy. This may be the first evidence of screening for gestational diabetes, suggesting a rather low prevalence in hospital practice in Baltimore, USA, nearly 100 years ago.

The major difficulty in the bedside measurement of reducing sugars by Fehling's test is no longer apparent, as all test strips now use a glucose oxidase system and recognize only glucosuria (lactosuria will still occur but no longer causes medical concern). Whitfield Williams then tabulated all reported cases (81) of diabetes complicating pregnancy from 1826 to 1907: he considered 15 cases to be doubtful, as glycosuria disappeared after delivery (including the famous patient first reported by Bennewitz in 1826, although he had not read the full case report in the original Latin). He calculated an overall immediate maternal mortality of 27%, with an additional 23% of mothers dying within the following 2 years. He concluded: *'Pregnancy may occur in diabetic women, or diabetes may become manifest during pregnancy; either is a serious complication, although the prognosis is not so alarming as is frequently stated.'*

EP Joslin: Pregnancy and diabetes mellitus, *Boston Med Surg J 1915; 173:841–9*[31]

Joslin was the first internist to specialize in diabetes and wrote the first textbook on the subject. In 1915, 6 years before the discovery of insulin, he was able to describe seven personal cases of moderate or severe diabetes associated with pregnancy. He wished to take a more hopeful view, but admitted that little progress had been made. Of his seven cases, four were dead – one by suicide, one with uraemic manifestations (? eclampsia), one of diabetic coma while under the care of a clairvoyant, and the fourth having survived one pregnancy with a healthy child died of pulmonary tuberculosis 2 months after losing her second child. But he was pleased that of the three remaining cases, one was in exceptionally good health, free from sugar and had a normal child, another in a tolerable condition having been pregnant three times but with only one child now living, and the remaining case alive although severely ill with diabetes 6 years after confinement. He closed his paper with an optimistic comment: '*It is certainly true that with the improvements in the treatment of diabetic patients* [he meant strict diet], *diabetic women will be less likely to avoid pregnancy.*'

E Brandstrup and H Okkels: Pregnancy complicated with diabetes, *Acta Obstet Gynecol Scand 1938; 18:136–63*[32]

The immediate post-insulin period was marked by some euphoria by both patients and their doctors, but it took a long time for the very considerable fear of pregnancy to diminish, and to some extent that fear remains to the present day. A careful retrospective assessment of those early years of insulin at the Rikshospital in Copenhagen from 1926 to 1938 showed that although there had been no maternal deaths in 22 pregnancies in 19 diabetic women mostly treated with insulin (probably the more severe and often referred cases), the perinatal mortality was still 57%.[32] The 13 perinatal deaths included six stillbirths, two intrapartum deaths and five early neonatal deaths; of the 10 living children three were asphyxiated at birth, one weighed only 1500 grams and one was 5250 grams. Histological examination of the pancreas in two full-weight fetuses showed a pronounced increase in the size and number of the islets of Langerhans. Dr Brandstrup, who was in charge of these mothers' care during that time, set the scene for the future advances made by his successor Dr Jorgen Pedersen after the war.

Brandstrup noted that most of his patients had been considered to be well adjusted with insulin treatment, but that they still had high levels of blood sugar for the greater part of the day. He had previously undertaken physiological studies in pregnant rabbits on the passage of carbohydrates across the placenta after intravenous injection, and had shown that while glucose and the pentoses passed across by a process of slow diffusion, the placental membrane was almost impermeable to disaccharides, including saccharose and lactose.[33] He described one case treated in 1927, illustrated by a 24 hour curve for blood sugar, who had been treated with two doses of insulin daily, felt well and was looked upon as treated adequately but he was unhappy with the level of control achieved (Fig. 1.4). '*The blood sugar is seen to keep at very high levels through a great part of the day. This feature is typical of the severe cases of diabetes under treatment with insulin, and it explains why the children are subject to intrauterine obesity through excessive supply of sugar also now in the epoch of insulin therapy. But these children are not only fat: they are large too. They present a condition of universal macrosomia ... it seems probable that it is the maternal hyperglycaemia alone that brings about the pathologic–anatomical changes in the child.*'

Conclusion

Further historical development of the management of diabetes in pregnancy will be considered in the next three chapters, which will focus on the work of Dr Jorgen Pedersen in Copenhagen, Dr Norbert Freinkel in Chicago and Dr Pricilla White in Boston. There is no doubt that had insulin not been discovered in 1922 then the present-day outlook for successful pregnancy in a diabetic mother would still remain very poor because of the continued maternal hyperglycaemia, in spite of the enormous improvements in social, medical and obstetrical care which has occurred in the intervening years.

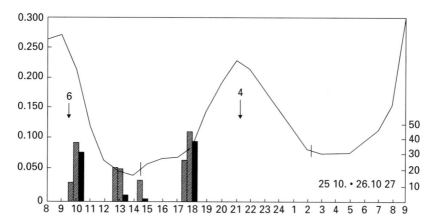

Figure 1.4. *Blood sugar curve for a pregnant diabetic treated at the Rikshospital in Copenhagen in 1927, with two doses of insulin (6 units at 09.30 and 4 units at 21.00). Units are grams per cent blood sugar (0.100 g% = 100 mg/dl). Food intake is shown as histograms, with unidentified units on the right side (From Brandstrup and Okkels.[32])*

References

1. Peel J. A historical review of diabetes and pregnancy. *Obstet Gynaecol Br Comm* 1972; **79**:385–95.
2. Reece EA. The history of diabetes mellitus. In: (Reece EA, Coustan DR, eds) *Diabetes Mellitus in Pregnancy*, 2nd edn. (Churchill Livingstone: New York, 1995) 1–10.
3. Banting FG, Best CH. The internal secretion of the pancreas. *J Lab Clin Med* 1922; **7**:256–71.
4. Bliss M. *The Discovery of Insulin*. (Paul Harris Publishing: Edinburgh, 1983) 20–58.
5. Joslin EP. Pregnancy and diabetes mellitus. *Boston Med Surg J* 1915; **173**:841–9.
6. Laurence RD, Oakley WG. Diabetic pregnancy. *Q J Med* 1942; **11**:45–54.
7. Diamond J. *Guns, Germs and Steel: The Fates of Human Societies*. (Norton & Co.: New York, 1997) 25.
8. Loudon I. *Death in Childbirth: An International Study of Maternal Care and Maternal Mortality 1800–1950*. (Clarendon Press: Oxford, 1992) 1–622.
9. Chamberlain G. Birth rates. In: (Turnbull A, Chamberlain G, eds) *Obstetrics*. (Churchill Livingstone: Edinburgh, 1989) 1105–10.
10. Turnbull A. Maternal Mortality In: (Turnbull A, Chamberlain G, eds) *Obstetrics*. (Churchill Livingstone: Edinburgh, 1989) 1121–32.
11. Medical Research Council Conference on Diabetes and Pregnancy. The use of hormones in the management of pregnancy in diabetes. *Lancet* 1955; **ii**:833–6.
12. Molsted-Pedersen L, Tygstrup I, Pederson J. Congenital malformations in newborn infants of diabetic women. *Lancet* 1964; **i**:1124–6.
13. International Clearinghouse for Birth Defects Monitoring Systems. *Congenital Malformations Worldwide*. (Elsevier: Amsterdam, 1991) 1–8.
14. Kalter H. *Of Diabetic Mothers and their Babies: An Examination of Maternal Diabetes on Offspring, Perinatal Development and Survival*. (Harwood Academic Publishers: Amsterdam, 2000) 95–111.
15. Freinkel N. Of pregnancy and progeny. The Banting Lecture 1980. *Diabetes* 1980; **29**:1023–35.
16. Hadden DR. The development of diabetes and its relation to pregnancy: the long-term and short-term historical viewpoint. In: (Sutherland HW, Stowers JM, Pearson DWM, eds) *Carbohydrate Metabolism in Pregnancy and the Newborn II*. (Springer-Verlag: London, 1989) 1–8.
17. Miller HC. The effect of the prediabetic state on the survival of the fetus and the birthweight of the newborn infant. *N Engl J Med* 1945; **233**:376–8.
18. Hurwitz D, Jensen D. Carbohydrate metabolism in normal pregnancy. *N Engl J Med* 1946; **234**: 327–9.
19. Gilbert JAL, Dunlop DM. Diabetic fertility, maternal mortality and foetal loss rate. *Br Med J* 1949; **i**: 48–51.
20. Wilkerson HLC, Remein QR. Studies of abnormal carbohydrate metabolism in pregnancy. *Diabetes* 1957; **6**:324–9.
21. O'Sullivan JB. Gestational diabetes. Unsuspected, asymptomatic diabetes in pregnancy. *N Engl J Med* 1961; **264**:1082–5.
22. Hoet JP. Carbohydrate metabolism during pregnancy. *Diabetes* 1954; **3**:1–12.
23. O'Sullivan JB, Mahan C. Criteria for the oral glucose tolerance test in pregnancy. *Diabetes* 1964; **13**:278–85.

24. Mestman JH, Anderson GU, Barton P. Carbohydrate metabolism in pregnancy. *Am J Obstet Gynecol* 1971; **109**:41–5.

25. Pederson J. Diabetes og gravid: En introduktion. *Ugeskr Laeger* 1951; **113**:1771–7.

26. Pedersen J. *The Pregnant Diabetic and her Newborn. Problems and management.* (Munksgaard: Copenhagen, 1967) 46.

27. HAPO Study Cooperative Research Group. The Hyperglycemia and Adverse Pregnancy Outcome (HAPO) study. *Int J Gynecol Obstet* 2002; **78**:69–77.

28. Bennetwitz HG. *De diabete mellito, gravidatatis symptomate.* MD Thesis, University of Berlin, 1824 [translated into English, deposited at the Wellcome Museum of the History of Medicine, Euston Road, London, 1987].

29. Duncan JM. On puerperal diabetes. *Trans Obstet Soc London* 1882; **24**:256–85.

30. Williams JW. The clinical significance of glycosuria in pregnant women. *Am J Med Sci* 1909; **137**:1–26.

31. Joslin EP. Pregnancy and diabetes mellitus. *Boston Med Surg J* 1915; **173**:841–9.

32. Brandstrup E, Okkels H. Pregnancy complicated with diabetes. *Acta Obstet Gynecol Scand* 1938; **18**:136–63.

33. Brandstrup E. On the passage of some substances from mother to fetus in the last part of pregnancy. *Acta Obstet Gynecol Scand* 1930; **10**:251–87.

2

The Priscilla White legacy

John W Hare

Introduction

Priscilla White was a pure clinician who devoted her entire professional career to the treatment of diabetic patients. In particular, she had an interest in Type 1 diabetes in women and in youths. This interest led her to the treatment of diabetes in pregnancy, now a formal discipline which her life's work did much to create.

Priscilla White was born in 1900 and attended Radcliffe College (now merged with Harvard College). Since Harvard Medical School did not enroll women until just after World War II, she attended Tufts College Medical School. She was an intern at the Worcester (MA) Memorial Hospital because Boston hospitals did not accept women as house officers. She had worked as a medical student with Elliott Joslin, already well known in the field of diabetes, whose first textbook was published in 1916, six years before the availability of insulin. Elliott Joslin was greatly impressed with '... this early-rising, young medical student ...' and invited her to join his staff in 1924. Legend has it that when she started her career at the Joslin Clinic she was given the task of treating young women with diabetes. Over time they grew up and began to have children, creating her lifelong interest in pregnancy. However, she wrote a chapter entitled Diabetes in Pregnancy in the 1928 edition of the Joslin-edited textbook *The Treatment of Diabetes Mellitus*.[1] This was too short a period for her young charges to have gone through puberty (often late in those days), married and conceived. Thus, her interest in pregnancy must have been manifest and acted upon from the very beginning.

Elliott Joslin was her mentor and a father figure until his death in 1962. Her association with him as a student came just at the exciting time when insulin became available, first given in Boston by Dr Joslin's assistant, Howard Root, in August 1922. It is hard to imagine what the times must have been like for those with diabetes and their doctors. Most diabetes diagnosed in the early twentieth century was symptomatic Type 1. Patients who survived were often severely cachectic as a result of both therapeutic design and pathophysiology. Their absence of fat precluded ketogenesis and thus allowed survival. In some way, the practice of diabetes in 1920 must have been like specializing in the treatment of HIV/AIDS today. Early insulin preparations – crude and cumbersome, consisting of 10 units/ml of crystalline insulin – required frequent and painful injections. It stopped the high proportion of deaths from ketoacidosis but permitted the subsequent expression of the vascular complications of diabetes with which there is now so much concern. These points are relevant to the treatment of diabetes and pregnancy. Many women who became pregnant without the benefit of insulin treatment either died or lost the fetus because of ketoacidosis. Insulin therapy permitted an immediate and marked improvement in the survival of both mother and fetus. Over the next several decades it also permitted women with diabetes to survive and to develop vascular complications. The development of vascular complications, particularly microvascular, became the principal determinant of pregnancy outcomes. The significance of these complications was quickly perceived by Priscilla White and underlies the now famous White Classification. Any subsequent or modern evaluation of diabetes and pregnancy must still adhere to this principle so perceptively noted by her.

An important dimension of White's character and personality was her ability to relate in the warmest way to her patients. She gave them enormous time and energy. A letter from a patient in 1998, in a monograph by Donald M Barnett, MD (*Elliott P Joslin, MD: A Centennial Portrait*) is illustrative:

> Yes, I feel that I know Dr. White very well. I had first come to the Joslin Clinic in 1935 with newly discovered diabetes. ... Dr. White's presence was such a help. Naturally she would chart and guide our medical therapy including the problematic Protamine Zinc Insulin in use at the time. She was endearingly optimistic and happy with each of us individually. She was a naturally beautiful woman and could easily engage in what I felt to be a genuine interest in fashion and feminine things that interest young women. I remember that Dr. White drove me from the Deaconess Hospital to the Faulkner Hospital in a terrible rainstorm as my due date neared.

White never married and had no children. Her great passion was her career and her small passion was her dogs. I have my own experiences with her love of dogs and her capacity for personal relationships. When I was a Junior Assistant Resident at the New England Deaconess Hospital in 1966, my first assignment was to Priscilla White's service. I would meet her early in the morning at the Boston Lying-in Hospital for rounds. Her secretary would afterwards drive us to the Joslin Clinic – where I would find my house officer's whites covered with dark daschund hairs. During this rotation, I told her a story about a boyhood birthday. Eight years later, when I joined the senior staff, she was near retirement and immediately recalled the story. That year was her fiftieth anniversary at the Joslin Clinic. Soon thereafter she began a gradual retirement and only occasionally appeared in our Pregnancy Clinic that she had begun over 50 years before. I subsequently inherited a number of her patients who expected me to give them as much time she did, and to write them a letter after each and every visit – something the time pressure of modern medicine no longer permitted.

White's mental acuity began to decline in the late 1970s and her remarkable mind failed her completely in the last years before her death in 1989. Her last paper, published in 1980, was co-authored with me and fittingly enough was her last revision of her world famous White Classification. These revisions had been done from time to time over 30 years as data and experience dictated, e.g. adding Class T for women who became pregnant after renal transplantation. The 1980 refinement removed gestational diabetes from the standard lettered taxonomy.

The early years

Priscilla White's first chapter in the Joslin-edited textbook *The Treatment of Diabetes*

Mellitus appeared in 1928.[1] In it she reviewed the Joslin Clinic experience with 89 pregnancies. She made the then spectacular and hopeful statement that '... diabetes is no longer a contraindication to pregnancy'. To say such a thing makes clear that for diabetic women before insulin, pregnancy was considered hopeless. Hope is the sentiment that has sustained thousands of diabetic women since, and permitted them to undergo the therapeutic demands and discomforts of pregnancy. This hope was made real and underpinned by the gathering of clinical evidence that documented the likelihood of a successful outcome. White's chapters were typical of those in early Joslin texts, and were largely, if not entirely, case reports and clinical series. In fact, much of her extensive bibliography is comprised of book chapters, clinical series and reviews reporting her collected experience as opposed to peer-reviewed publications of original research.

The dismal reproductive capacity of women in this era is easily inferred by reading White's somewhat optimistic statements in the obverse. For example, 'Insulin, it is true, has decreased the frequency of sterility among diabetic women, but the return to normalcy is slow', meaning sterility had been and still remained a problem. In writing about success she said, 'Fourteen stillbirths, or 25 per cent, occurred among our 59 pregnancies coming to term.' She felt the 25% figure was an improvement because it represented a halving of the 50% risk for fetal death in the pre-insulin era. Sometimes the severity of the reality was obscure. A table summarized the outcomes of the 89 pregnancies: eight outcomes were unknown and four were 'undelivered'. I had to ask a colleague why this category was included, given all the other expected outcomes, such as stillbirths and miscarriage, were listed. It meant that the mother died. If not death in pregnancy, there was death thereafter. Another table in

White's first chapter indicates that of 58 cases, 42 were still alive in June 1926, indicating an eventual mortality of 28% after pregnancy. Even more striking, 10 of the 16 women had developed their diabetes in 1922 or later, meaning that they died despite having short-term diabetes and being insulin treated from the onset. One of the women had survived 23 years postpartum and another 15 years, i.e. they had diabetes in the pre-insulin era.

Some concepts now taken for granted began to emerge. For example, though gestational diabetes was not labeled as such, it was recognized: 'Pregnancy contracted during diabetes is less frequent than diabetes contracted during pregnancy.' The phenomenon of heightened insulin sensitivity postpartum was noted, though incorrectly ascribed to '... the passage of sugar from the blood to the breasts at lactation'. It was in this chapter that White made the prescient statement 'Controlled diabetes is essential to fetal welfare', which has become the bedrock of modern management.

White was not the first to write about diabetes in pregnancy, but this chapter represents the beginning of a systematic clinical analysis of an astounding series of over 2200 cases (most of whom were insulin dependent) that made her famous, and allowed maternity for her patients and countless others all over the world.

Her chapter published in the sixth edition of the Joslin et al-edited textbook *The Treatment of Diabetes Mellitus* represents continued progress in understanding the natural history of diabetes in pregnancy and how to modify it.[2] She noted that the lack of fertility in diabetes women '... has been corrected in great measure in proportion to the extent of control of the disease'. White once again, to some degree by intuition and to some degree supported by data, hit the nail on the head by observing that '... the degree of hyperglycemia appears to be directly related to the frequency of spontaneous miscarriage or abortion'. She found that the abortion rate was 33% in controlled cases and only 2% in those well treated, which seems too low. All this was, of course, without benefit of anything more precise to assess control other than urine tests and occasional blood glucose levels done at the time of clinic visits.

However, one could not expect White to have understood all that is known today about the biology of diabetic pregnancy, and she did not. She admitted, 'The cause of overgrowth of the fetus of the diabetic is not known', although she certainly recognized the problem. Fifty-six percent of Joslin patients' infants had birthweights > 8 lb, compared with 9% of a control series [presumably 8 lb, or *c.* 3600 grams, represented infants large for gestational age (LGA) or the nineteith centile). She noted that 'The greatest growth of the embryo occurs in the last two months, at a time when the blood sugar is often normal', which it surely wasn't. Another statement, now known to be wide off the mark, was 'Congenital defects are beyond our therapeutic control and are, we believe, related to a disease which is genetic in origin.' She later revised her opinion and in 1958 said that 'The 3 percent mortality due to congenital anomalies can perhaps be lowered by avoiding such causes of anoxia as acidosis and hypoglycemia'.[3] This sentence attributing anomalies to metabolic changes presaged by 20 years the notion of hyper- and hypoglycemia as causes of malformations. These hypotheses could not be tested until self-blood-glucose monitoring and glycohemoglobin tests became available. She also felt that some malformations were '... due to chronic vascular insufficiency ...', but she was not alone in having to speculate as to the cause of fetal anomalies.

It is in the paper published in 1937 that White's most important contribution begins to germinate; namely that duration (and its relation to vascular disease) adversely affects outcome.[4] Although over a decade away from publishing her classification, one can see a hint of the concept emerging. She said that 'Long duration of diabetes decreases the number of living births', but by long duration she meant > 1 year. In her discussion of toxemia (which must have included pregnancy-induced hypertension of all types) she noted that mothers over 30 years of age had a higher loss rate and more toxemia. Her most seriously erroneous construct is also mentioned here. She believed that toxemia, a major cause of fetal death, was caused by or related to hormonal imbalance. In particular, she believed prolan [human chorionic gonadotropin (hCG)] excess and estrin deficiency were related to toxemia. To support this thesis she cited both human and animal data derived from urine or bioassays which were immeasurably cruder than today's assays measured in picomoles. She said, 'Estrin therapy seems to be the logical method of treatment.' This belief would lead to the treatment of her pregnant women with sex steroids starting in 1938, and it was a therapy she refused to relinquish. Not until after her retirement was the practice stopped in 1975. The original basis for White's staunch belief in hormonal therapy was the paper published with Smith, Smith and Joslin in 1937.[4] The hypothesis was that prolan (hCG) was utilized in the placental production of estrogen, both by oxidation (early) and metabolism (late). She wrote: 'The damaged vascular tree of the diabetic may interfere with the blood supply to the uterus and placenta and with the normal production of its hormones.'[5] Her insistence on parental sex steroid therapy is often overlooked in view of the more familiar linking of her name to her eponymous classification. When the White Classification first appeared hormonal dysfunction was also a modality of classification, as well as the familiar alphabetized one based upon age, duration and complications. In fact, it occupied as much space in her discussion as did Classes A–F. White firmly believed that this regimen improved fetal survival and increased the hormone doses from Class A to Class F. By the time her last *Joslin's Diabetes Mellitus* chapter appeared in the 11th edition of this textbook in 1971,[6] hormonal therapy was no longer given in increasing doses by class. Class A (abnormal glucose tolerance, treated with diet alone) was excepted from treatment as it always had been.

In the 1980s, the Joslin Clinic formally surveyed the mothers known to have been treated with these hormones. No cases of gynecological cancer in their daughters or genitourinary abnormalities in their sons were reported other than cryptorchidism, which is common and may not have been related. However, anecdotal accounts of daughters having difficulty with habitual abortion and incompetent cervices have been received.

Finally, White also believed that diuretic therapy prevented hydramnios, edema and pre-eclampsia toxemia(PET), the latter having always been a major cause of fetal loss. Thus, at first encapsulated ammonium chloride, then injected mercurial diuretics and finally oral diuretics, thiazides in particular, were routinely used from the 1940s until 1975. Of course, diuretic therapy may have aggravated PET, the very condition it was meant to prevent.

The White Classification

In 1949, White published the first version of the classification system which was to be the single most remembered thing about her work, and has been of immense clinical value to practictioners all over the world.[7] Part of the success of this classification was no doubt rooted in its rationale and utility, but part must have also been that the world leader in the field of diabetic pregnancy espoused it. She was almost precisely at the mid-point in her career and had been on the Joslin Clinic staff for 25 years. She was already well known and her eminence would have been helpful in facilitating its adoption. By way of historical perspective, in 1949 her great European clinical counterpart, Jørgen Pedersen, was just making his debut on the word stage of diabetes and pregnancy, and Norbert Freinkel had just received his medical degree.

Reading papers published by White only a year or two before the appearance of her classification so soon after is somewhat of a surprise. Although she had long recognized the importance of duration of diabetes as a risk factor for vascular disease, she did not particularly link it to pregnancy outcome and certainly not in a graded form, even shortly before 1949. In her 1946 chapter in the eighth edition of Joslin et al-edited book *The Treatment of Diabetes Mellitus* she wrote about how quickly diabetes could cause vascular disease, noting that it was present in 70% of non-pregnant 20 year survivors of diabetes, i.e. not all patients with Type 1 diabetes lived 20 years.[8] By vascular disease she meant both macro- and microvascular, e.g. coronary heart disease and retinopathy. However, she did not discuss the implications of this observation for pregnant women. Despite the generally poor prognosis it is notable that only one maternal death had occurred in 271 pregnancies between January 1936 and March 1946. The one death was due to infectious hepatitis and occurred 8 weeks postpartum. Thus, the striking maternal mortality of the pre-insulin era was gone. Also of interest is her notation that congenital anomalies occurred in 12% of the infants as compared with 1.8% in the non-diabetic population – almost exactly what would be reported 35 years later when Joslin data were published that clearly and quantitatively linked periconceptual control to congenital anomalies by using first trimester glycohemoglobin levels.[9] In the patients studied in that paper, the overall anomaly rate was 12.9% and the non-diabetic rate in the USA was *c.* 2%.

In a 1947 paper entitled Pregnancy Complicating Diabetes of More Than Twenty Years Duration, White rather tediously reviewed 10 cases, but stopped short of systematically linking duration and complications to outcome.[10] However, all the data that she collected and used in her classic 1949 paper[7] must have already been under review. Two years later the original classification appeared and had only six classes, though it was later to have as many as 10 (Box 2.1).

Another important point emerged in this paper.[7] White noted that 68% of stillbirths occurred after the 35th week of gestation. This was the rationale for early delivery of all patients, usually by Cesarean section. By 1953 the schema had been refined: Class A was permitted to go to term, Classes B and C were carried to 38 weeks, and Classes D–F were delivered in the 35th week.[5] White reasoned that prematurity and atelectasis (respiratory distress) were a lesser risk than stillbirth in the more severe classes.

The White Classification underwent several revisions. In her 1971 chapter in *Joslin's Diabetes Mellitus*, which was her last, Class E, pelvic vascular calcification, was no longer used.[6] This category had either been actively sought or incidentally diagnosed when X-ray pelvimetry was used. It was thought that pelvic or uterine arterial calcification caused fetoplacental hypoxia and that this was important information. However, the recognition of the danger of X-rays to the fetus resulted in elimination of the category. Class G had been added some years before: this was a rather vague class and included 'multiple failures in pregnancy'. Class R had been added, and women with both retinopathy and renal disease were placed in a combined class termed Class FR. Class H, women with coronary heart disease, and Class T, women with prior renal transplantation, had yet to be added.

At the 1979 American Diabetes Association Symposium on Gestational Diabetes, the first of the series begun by Norbert Freinkel, the confusing issue of Class A and gestational diabetes was raised. Implicit in raising the issue was the recognition that nearly everyone used the White Classification. Class A was meant to include women treated with diet alone but was

---

Class A: Abnormal glucose tolerance test, treated with diet alone
Class B: Onset before the age of 20, duration < 10 years, no vascular disease
Class C: Onset between the ages of 10 and 19, duration 10 –19 years or minimal vascular disease, including retinal arteriosclerosis or calcifications of lower extremity arteries*
Class D: Onset before the age of 10, duration > 20 years or retinitis, hypertension or albuminuria
Class E: Pelvic vascular calcification, iliac or uterine
Class F: All patients with nephritis (more than just albuminuria).

---

*Background retinopathy and lower extremity calcification were included in Class D in later classifications.

Box 2.1. Priscilla White's first classification.

never synonymous with gestational diabetes; however, in common parlance it often came to be. The Joslin Clinic has traditionally had few patients with gestational diabetes, so the White Classification never really needed to address the issue. At the Joslin Clinic women with gestational diabetes who required insulin were called gestational Bs as opposed to true Bs, meaning women with either pregestational diabetes or the onset of Type 1 diabetes in pregnancy. At the request of the symposium, I revised the classification and separated gestational diabetes from the traditional alphabetic list.[11] Priscilla White was invited to co-author the alteration with me in order to lend it credence, to which she readily agreed. As it turned out, this revision of the White Classification was also her last publication (Box 2.2).

The basic soundness of White's clinical observations that duration and vascular disease were the major determinants of outcome became even clearer to me when I tried to revise the White Classification for the 13th edition of *Joslin's Diabetes Mellitus* in 1994, in order to reflect most recent experience and to try to make it less confusing.[12] Class A had essentially disappeared; it didn't include gestational diabetes and increasingly stringent standards of control meant that no one with pregestational diabetes went through pregnancy without insulin. Duration or onset in women with no complications made no difference to outcome, so women in Classes B and C, as well as those in uncomplicated Class D, did not need to be separated. Classes E and G were obsolete. In my chapter, I ended up with three classifications! First, one specifically for gestational diabetes; second, the 1980 version of the White Classification; and third, one just as cumbersome, which was based on the presence or absence of complications. Each category was identified by a specific complication rather than by using the more non-specific onset or duration. It did make sense to be specific about what the complication was, e.g. autonomic neuropathy or background retinopathy, and it did correlate with outcomes, but it was still cumbersome.

Most of the attention in diabetes complicating pregnancy today is not focused on Type 1

Gestational diabetes:
           Abnormal glucose tolerance test, euglycemia maintained by diet alone
           Diet alone insufficient, insulin required
Class A: Diet alone insufficient, any duration or onset age
Class B: Onset at the age of 20 or older, duration < 10 years
Class C: Onset between the ages of 10 and 19, or duration 10–19 years
Class D: Onset before the age of 10, duration > 20 years, background retinopathy or
           hypertension (not pre-eclampsia)
Class R: Proliferative retinopathy or vitreous hemorrhage
Class F: Nephropathy with > 500 mg/day proteinuria
Class RF: Criteria for both Classes R and F coexist
Class H: Arteriosclerotic heart disease clinically evident
Class T: Prior renal transplantation

All classes following Class A require insulin therapy. Classes R, F, RF, H and T have no onset/duration criteria but usually occur in long-term diabetes. The development of a complication moves the patient to a lower class.

Box 2.2. Priscilla White's last classification.

diabetes but the far more common gestational diabetes, and in particular on fetal outcome in gestational diabetes. (This is curious, because the standard O'Sullivan and Mahan criteria,[13] since revised to reflect refinements in laboratory methodology, are based on a maternal outcome – the subsequent risk of developing diabetes.) I believe that there is an understandable difference in viewpoint between obstetricians who worry mainly about fetal outcome as opposed to physicians who have to treat the mothers for many years to come after delivery. I think it is for that reason, and because of the overwhelming predominance of Type 1 diabetes at the Joslin Clinic, that the White Classification always took into account both maternal and fetal risk. For example, retinopathy (Class R) poses no fetal risk but if aggravated by pregnancy it can cause maternal blindness.

The later years

By the mid-point in her career, Priscilla White was undeniably the doyenne of diabetic pregnancy. She continued to publish reviews and papers which extended and refined her experience. Jørgen Pedersen, who became well established as a student of and expert in diabetic pregnancy in the 1950s and 1960s, used her classification in a modified form. It was included in *The Pregnant Diabetic and Her Newborn*, his classic treatise published in 1967. Although he did adopt and modify White's classification, Pedersen also stated flatly that 'This department has never used hormone therapy'.[14] In fact, by this time few if any centers believed that estrogen and progesterone supplementation made any difference, and White was the only real advocate of its use. This became more of a bone of contention in

the 1960s and 1970s, even within the Joslin Clinic.

White was an invited lecturer all over the world. She was asked to present her data on diabetes complicated by vascular disease at the International Federation of Gynecology and Obstetrics in Mexico City in 1976. However, she was troubled by thromboembolic venous disease and could not travel long distances. She asked me to present her paper for her. At the congress I met Jørgen Pedersen. He was interested in her data and, of course, knew her personally and inquired about her health. He also told me that he thought she should have discouraged her patients with renal disease from becoming pregnant, given the still poor prognosis for this subgroup. In retrospect, I see the differences in their viewpoints as reflecting his realism and her optimism. Patients with nephropathy clearly had the lowest expectation of success of any class, but she started her career when no one had much expectation of success. Having been an effector of triumph over adversity no doubt influenced her optimistic view.

Upon my return to Boston, I suggested that these data be published. She agreed and told me to go ahead. This resulted in a brief but remarkable summation of her experience entitled Pregnancy in Diabetes Complicated by Vascular Disease.[15] Not only were 416 pregnancies with vascular disease (Classes R, F, RF, E, H and T) presented but also summarized was a half century of her experience with over 2200 cases of diabetic pregnancy in which the fetal survival rates rose from only 54% at the beginning of her career to 94% by the end.

She was twice honored by the American Diabetes Association at its annual meeting. In 1960 she received the Banting Medal for Distinguished Scientific Achievement and delivered a lecture entitled Childhood Diabetes: Its

Course and Influences on the Second and Third Generations. In 1978 she was the Outstanding Physician Clinician in Diabetes but this award, after her retirement, in reality recognized her as an *Eminence grise*.

It is of interest that her two contemporaries and colleagues at the Joslin Clinic, Howard Root and Alexander Marble, were both presidents of the American Diabetes Association. Howard Root became a Medical Director of the Clinic and a President of the Joslin Diabetes Center. Alexander Marble was a Research Director and President of the Joslin Diabetes Center. Priscilla White never acheived such high office within or without the Joslin Diabetes Center. She was made head of the Youth Division, created in the 1960s, which reflected her interest not only in pregnancy but also her long-term interest in the Joslin Camps for boys and girls. It may have been that this division was created, at least in part, to make up for her lack of a major title at the Joslin Diabetes Center. Root and Marble had academic appointments in medicine at Harvard; her appointment was in pediatrics at Tufts, her alma mater. She never sought a Harvard appointment because they wouldn't admit her (or any other woman before 1945) to their medical school. To what degree her lack of official recognition, when compared to her peers Root and Marble, reflected intrinsic choices that led her down a different career path or extrinsic forces of latent sexism, or the interplay of both, is an open question.

Her legacies are direct and indirect. She can arguably be personally credited with creating the discipline of diabetes in pregnancy. Others were active in the field, but none were as single-mindedly devoted and as well known before 1950. Special interest groups for diabetic pregnancy now exist within multiple professional societies. Hundreds, if not thousands, of physicians and obstetricians have developed clinical and investigative interests in the field. There are thousands of direct legatees – her patients who became mothers and had children, grandchildren, and now great grandchildren – generations that would not have come into being had it not been for her. Also directly affected were residents and fellows who learned from her how to treat diabetic patients for the rest of their careers. Her indirect legatees are untold numbers of diabetic women all over the world whose doctors enabled them to bear children because she led the way.

References

1. White P. Diabetes in pregnancy. In: (Joslin EP, ed) *The Treatment of Diabetes Mellitus*, 4th edn. (Lea & Febiger: Philadelphia, 1928) 861–72.
2. White P. Pregnancy complicating diabetes. In: (Joslin EP, Root HF, White P, Marble A, eds) *The Treatment of Diabetes Mellitus*, 6th edn. (Lea & Febiger: Philadelphia, 1937) 618–37.
3. White P. Pregnancy and diabetes (editorial). *Diabetes* 1958; 7:494–5.
4. Smith OW, Smith GvS, Joslin EP, White P. Prolan and estrin in the serum and urine of diabetic and nondiabetic women during pregnancy, with especial reference to pregnancy toxemia. *Am J Obstet Gynecol* 1937; 3:365–79.
5. White P, Koshy P, Duckers J. The management of pregnancy complicating diabetes and of children of diabetic mothers. *Med Clin N Am* 1953; 37:1481–96.
6. White P. Pregnancy and diabetes. In: (Marble A, White P, Bradley RF, Krall LP, eds) *Joslin's Diabetes Mellitus*, 11th edn. (Lea & Febiger: Philadelphia, 1971) 581–98.
7. White P. Pregnancy complicating diabetes. *Am J Med* 1949; 5:609–16.
8. White P. Pregnancy complicating diabetes. In: (Joslin EP, Root HF, White P et al, eds) *The Treatment of Diabetes Mellitus*, 8th edn. (Lea & Febiger: Philadelphia, 1946) 769–84.
9. Miller E, Hare JW, Cloherty J et al. Elevated maternal hemoglobin A1c in early pregnancy and major congenital anomalies in infants of diabetic mothers. *N Engl J Med* 1981; 304:1331–4.
10. White P. Pregnancy complicating diabetes of more than twenty years' duration. *Med Clin N Am* 1947; **March**; 395–405.

11. Hare JW, White P. Gestational diabetes and the White Classification. *Diabetes Care* 1980; 3:394.

12. Hare JW. Diabetes and pregnancy. In: (Kahn CR, Weir GC, eds) *Joslin's Diabetes Mellitus*, 13th edn. (Lea & Febiger: Philadelphia, 1994) 889–99.

13. O'Sullivan JM, Mahan CM. Criteria for the oral glucose tolerance test in pregnancy. *Diabetes* 1964; 13:278–85.

14. Pedersen J. *The Pregnant Diabetic and Her Newborn.* (Williams & Wilkins: Baltimore, 1967) 112–18, 142.

15. Hare JW, White P. Pregnancy in diabetes complicated by vascular disease. *Diabetes* 1977; 26:953–5.

3

The Pedersen legacy

Lars Mølsted-Pedersen

Introduction

As an introduction to this chapter it is appropriate to give a brief outline of the founder of the Copenhagen Centre for Pregnant Diabetics, my teacher, chief and during the years 1962–1978 also my personal good friend, the late Professor Jørgen Pedersen.

After his graduation as MD in 1938 he had a thorough training in Copenhagen hospitals and during his term as an assistant physician to HC Hagedorn at the Steno Memorial Hospital from 1943 to 1945 he became fascinated with the problems of diabetes and pregnancy. From 1945 to 1946 he held an appointment as registrar in the Obstetric Department, Rigshospital, University of Copenhagen, where, from 1946 to 1954, he worked as a voluntary consultant and from 1954 until his death in November 1978 as an appointed consultant for pregnant diabetics. Jørgen Pedersen was a very active teacher throughout his long career and from 1970 he held the chair of Professor of Internal Medicine at the University of Copenhagen.

As early as 1945, Jørgen Pedersen started his work on diabetes and pregnancy. He managed to build up a centre for pregnant women with diabetes, a centre which over the years has become well-known worldwide as The Copenhagen Centre for Pregnant Diabetics. His paramount aim was to diminish perinatal mortality through strict control of diabetes and special obstetric management. These efforts were widely successful, as the perinatal mortality during his leadership decreased from nearly 40 to 4%.

However, in connection with his clinical work a very comprehensive continuous research has been performed to elucidate the manifold and intricate pathogenetic problems around the diabetic mother and her conceptus. Some of the papers from the Copehagen Centre are collected in three volumes from 1954, 1961 and 1966, and a fourth was sent out in January 1974 as a memorial volume by Pedersen's co-workers in honour of his 60th birthday.

A survey is given in Pederson's book entitled *The Pregnant Diabetic and Her Newborn*, which came out in its first edition in 1967 and in a greatly revised second edition in 1977. This monograph not only deals with the treatment and prognosis of mother and child, but also with pathogenic, pathoanatomical, metabolic, endocrine and many other problems, largely based on investigations in the Copenhagen Centre.

A few characteristics of Jørgen Pedersen's working methods were: a repeated meticulous control to problems from varying aspects to confirm or weaken results; an ability to differerentiate a large inhomogeneous material in groups to be individually evaluated; and a certain artistic ability to see new problems connected with the old ones, often linked with new discoveries and new techniques. These intellectual faculties combined with an unflagging perfectionism made him a highly admired leader of a multi-disciplinary research team.

It is well known that Jørgen Pedersen was one of the founders of the European Diabetic Pregnancy Study Group (DPSG). During its first 3 years he was a board member and from then until his death he was a highly esteemed and very active member of the group. In 1979, the board of the DPSG decided that a lecture in memory of Jørgen Pedersen should be given at the group's yearly meeting and since 1980 a Jørgen Pedersen memorial lecture has been given every year by a distinguished scientist within the field of diabetes and pregnancy.

Diabetes and pregnancy: 1940–1980

In 1946 it was decided, with Professor Brandstrup at the Rigshospital, University of Copenhagen, to centralize the management and study of diabetes and pregnancy to the Obstetrical Department of Professor Brandstrup, who previously had interest in the problems involved.[1,2]

The first study from the Copenhagen Centre was designed to find possible characteristics of the course of diabetes during pregnancy, to contribute to a quantitative elucidation of the incidence of alterations occurring and to set up rules for the supervision of pregnant diabetics.[3] Two typical periods in diabetic alterations took place, reaching a peak at about the second to third month and at about the seventh month. During the former period, an improvement in tolerance, lasting for an average of 2–3 months, was commonly observed. The

manifestation of this improvement was insulin coma, or other insulin reactions, or an improvement in the degree of compensation. During the latter period there is often a decreased tolerance, manifesting itself as a diabetic precoma, acute acidosis or a necessity for raising the insulin dosage. The duration of this reduction in tolerance averaged 2 months.[3]

A treatment policy was described as follows:[3,4] referral to a diabetes centre as early as possible in pregnancy; outpatient control every 2–3 weeks until the fifth gestational month and weekly thereafter. About 8 weeks before calculated term the patient was hospitalized for prophylactic purposes and remained as an inpatient until delivery, which was usually induced c. 3 weeks before term. This applied to uncomplicated cases. On the whole, the patients were hospitalized in the presence of any complications that failed to yield immediately to ambulatory measures. Perinatal mortality fell from c. 40 to 25% in the period from 1946 to 1952 and for the group with long-term control perinatal mortality was as low as 12%. However, in the period from 1956 to 1965 the total perinatal mortality was still as high as 18.5% and the focus was now on the high incidence of severe congenital malformations (CM), a subject which was still under debate in the 1950s and 1960s. In a paper from 1964, Mølsted-Pedersen et al[5] showed in a convincing way that the incidence of severe CM were significantly higher in newborns of diabetic mothers and, furthermore, that fatal and multiple CM were five times higher in this group, and there was a significant correlation to the severity of the maternal diabetes. Based on these results, it was proposed that CM in infants of diabetic mothers were due in particular to the presence of maternal vascular complications with an insufficient blood supply to the uterus and placenta.

During the 1970s this view was changed in favour of the metabolic hypothesis, i.e. incomplete metabolic compensation at nidation and during the first trimester might be important. In a study from the late 1970s, a series comprising 949 newborn infants of diabetic mothers were treated at the Copenhagen Centre during pregnancy and delivery in the period from 1966 to 1977. The malformation rate was 8.2%.[6] By analysing the series it was found that the rate of CM in White classes B–F was significantly reduced from 14.1 to 7.4% in infants whose mothers preconceptionally attended two hospitals which specialized in the treatment and ambulatory control of diabetes. The observation demonstrated the importance of procuring constant care for diabetic women outside pregnancy in order to decrease the malformation rate.

During the first half of the 1980s the rate of severe CM decreased significantly at the Copenhagen Centre. The explanation for this significant decline is not a simple one and the cause may be non-specific, but some points of possible relevance were reported.[7] Firstly from *c.* 1980, diabetologists in Denmark had intensified their treatment of diabetics,

especially that of the young. Secondly, in 1976 an outpatient clinic for instructions in contraception and planning for future pregnancies in diabetic women was organized at the Copenhagen Centre. A few years after the opening of this clinic a significant increase – from 35 to 70% – in the frequency of planned pregnancies was seen. Thirdly, some induced abortions were performed due to elevated levels of alpha-fetoprotein (ultrasound examination verified severe neural tube defects) and in a few diabetic women from classes D and F who had poorly regulated diabetic metabolism during conception and during the first gestational weeks, and moreover whose fetuses had a significant ultrasound-verified growth delay in early pregnancy, thereby having a significantly increased risk of severe CM (see below).[8]

The impact of preconceptional care has been strongly underlined by the Copenhagen Centre's later clinical experience (Table 3.1).[9] In unplanned pregnancies in Type 1 diabetic women, the rate of pregnancy complications and preterm deliveries are doubled compared to insulin-dependent diabetes mellitus (IDDM) women who preconceptionally planned their pregnancy. Furthermore, the incidence of severe

	Pregnancies		
	Planned (%) (n = 133)	Unplanned (%) (n = 67)	P-value
Pregnancy complications	27.0	52.0	< 0.001
Preterm delivery (< 37 completed weeks)	19.0	39.0	< 0.005
Major congenital malformations	1.5	11.9	< 0.010
Perinatal mortality	0.8	5.9	< 0.100

Table 3.1. *Major clinical differences in planned and unplanned pregnancies in pregestational Type 1 diabetic women – Copenhagen Series 1989–1992.*

CM and the perinatal mortality were markedly increased in the unplanned group.

In his thesis from 1952, Jørgen Pedersen[10] mentioned the hyperglycaemia (maternal) – hyperinsulinism (fetal) hypothesis, but at that time direct measurements of plasma insulin were not possible. In the second edition of his book *The Pregnant Diabetic and Her Newborn*,[11] the hypothesis ran as follows: maternal hyperglycaemia results in fetal hyperglycaemia and, hence, in hypertrophy of fetal islet tissue with insulin hypersecretion. The hyperinsulinism in the presence of more than adequate supplies of glucose, abruptly eliminated at birth, explains several of the characteristic features observed in the offspring. Over the years the theory, its consequences and explanatory powers have been intensively discussed, especially in papers from the Copenhagen Centre.[12-15] The results of many pathoanatomical, clinical, physiological and biochemical investigations have adducted a nearly common agreement of the theory, which is now, more than 20 years after Pedersen's death, simply called the Pedersen theory.

White's[16] widely used classification of pregnant diabetes is based on factors present in the mother before pregnancy, particularly with regard to the severity of her diabetes and vascular complications. This classification indicates groups of pregnant women with a different basic fetal mortality risk and a different proneness to complications, and hence fetal mortality. However, a more individual prognosis was required.

In order to improve the possibilities of predicting the outcome of pregnancies in diabetics, a consecutive series of 304 pregnancies from the Copenhagen Centre in the 5-year period from 1959 to 1963 was analysed. Patients with a poor prognosis were divided into four groups: pregnant women who developed (a) hyperpyretic pyelitis, (b) precoma or severe acidosis, (c) toxaemia or (d) could be designated as 'neglectors'.[17] These four groups are designated as PBSP (prognostically bad signs during pregnancy) and concern complications which become evident during the actual pregnancy. Although the classification may not be perfect, the inherent concept of the White classification, i.e. that the chance of a successful pregnancy is not the same for all pregnant diabetics, is fundamentally correct.[18] The simultaneous combined use of the two complementary classifications is recommended until more precise classifications are available.

Diabetes and pregnancy: 1980–present

In 1976 the Copenhagen Centre started to perform consecutively an ultrasound examination in the first trimester in all diabetic pregnancies to confirm the gestational age. Quite unexpectedly, it was observed that some fetuses in early diabetic pregnancy were smaller by ultrasound measurements than expected from the menstrual history and the term early growth delay was used to describe this phenomenon.[19] When assessing gestational age from a crown–rump length (CRL) measurement, the 95% confidence interval (CI) is +4–5 days. Therefore, significant early growth delay defines an ultrasound age that is at least 6 days less than the menstrual age.[20] There is a significant association between early growth delay and the quality of the diabetes regulation as assessed from the HbAlc concentration.[21] Correspondingly, there has been a significant decrease in the average early growth delay over the past 20 years, from 5.5 to 2.0 days, which is ascribed to the efforts made to improve diabetes regulation around the time of conception and during early pregnancy.

In 1981, it was reported that significant early growth delay predicted an increased risk of CM.[8] To examine whether this was still so, the series was divided at 1980, so that 1976–1979 roughly corresponds to an earlier report. The alarming high rate of malformations in the delay group (18%) fortunately has decreased (4%), and although early growth still may involve a higher risk of malformation the difference does not reach statistical significance. Again, it is believed that this is a result of an improved diabetes regulation around conception and in early pregnancy.

When looking at severe CM, spontaneous abortions and successful outcomes in the whole series of 376 pregnancies (Table 3.2), it is obvious that the too-small fetuses not only had a higher rate of CM [10 of 110 (9.1%) versus 6 of 266 (2.3%)] but also a higher rate of spontaneous abortions [6 of 110 (5.5%) versus 1 of 266 (0.4%)]. The chance of a successful outcome of pregnancy, i.e. delivery of a live, non-malformed baby, was significantly lower in the delay group [93 of 110 (85%) versus 252 of 266 (94%)]. These highly significant differences show that the early growth delay is a real phenomenon and not a result of inaccurate estimation of ovulation.[22]

In order to study postnatal development, the infants of the Copehagen Centre's 1981 report, together with a group of control infants, underwent a pediatric follow-up examination at the age of four. The Denver Development Screening Test showed that the infants in the diabetes group had a slightly poorer psychomotor development than the control infants, only 83% had a normal score as opposed to 88% in the control group.[23] When the diabetes group was divided according to early growth delay, it appeared that only 69% of infants in the delay group had a normal score, thereby differing significantly from the non-delay infants (88%), who performed remarkably similarly to the control infants. In other words, in this series it was the delay infants alone that were responsible for the poorer performance in the diabetic group.

	Delay	No delay
Included in the study	110	266
Spontaneous abortions < 16 weeks	6	1
Spontaneous abortions > 16 weeks	0	3
Induced abortions and intrauterine fetal death	0	8
Delivery of live infant	104	254
Severe malformation	10	3
Trisomi 21	1	0
Successful outcome*	93 (85%)	251 (94%)

* $P = 0.0053$ (Fisher's exact probability test).

Table 3.2. Analyses of early growth delay in 376 singleton pregnancies in Type 1 diabetic mothers – Copenhagen Series 1976–1995

Summary on early growth delay

Some fetuses in early diabetic pregnancy are smaller than normal, i.e. exhibiting early growth delay. This is related to the quality of the diabetes regulation and gives a marked increase in the risk of fetal malformations, and predicts a poorer psychomotor development. A first trimester ultrasound study is mandatory and patient management should be guided by the ultrasound age.

Since the foundation of the Diabetes Centre at the Obstetric Department of the Rigshospital, 13 theses for the DMSc degree at the University of Copenhagen have been published, all of them dealing with the topic diabetes and pregnancy in every possible way. In 1977, the Diabetes Centre got its own laboratory, where it was possible to carry out hormone assay, glucose tolerance tests, etc.

The interest and activity in the field of gestational diabetes mellitus (GDM) has increased since the foundation of the centre and within the following two decades four DMSc theses dealing with GDM have been published. The most well known, and one often quoted in the medical literature, was written by the internist diabetologist Claus Kuhl: Serum insulin and plasma glucagon in human pregnancy – on the pathogenesis of gestational diabetes.[24] After the death of Jørgen Pedersen, Claus Kuhl was appointed consultant for pregnant diabetics at the Copenhagen Centre for the next decade.

Another important work on GDM was done by the present leader of the Diabetes Centre, Peter Damm.[25] His DMSc was entitled: Gestational diabetes mellitus and subsequent development of overt diabetes mellitus – a clinical, metabolic and epidemiological study. He investigated the prognosis of women with previous GDM with respect to subsequent development of diabetes and also the identification of predictive factors for the development of overt diabetes in these women. He also evaluated insulin sensitivity in glucose-tolerant non-obese women with previous GDM and controls. A decreased insulin sensitivity due to a decreased non-oxidative glucose metabolism in skeletal muscle was found in women with previous GDM. The same group of previous GDM women had a relatively reduced insulin secretion evaluated by IVGTT (Intravenous glucose tolerance test). A longitudinal study of 91 GDM women showed a relatively reduced insulin secretion to oral glucose in pregnancy, postpartum and 5–11 years later.

Damm's study showed that even non-obese glucose-tolerant women with previous GDM are charaterized by the metabolic profile of Type 2 diabetics, i.e. insulin resistance and impaired insulin secretion. Hence, the combination of this finding together with the significantly increased risk for development of diabetes indicates that all women with previous GDM should have a regular assessment of their glucose tolerance in the years after pregnancy.

Finally, it should be mentioned that the rigid outline for treatment of the pregnant diabetics described in one of the first publications from the Copehagen Centre has been changed since the mid-1980s. The treatment is now much more individualized and, in uncomplicated diabetic pregnancies, all contact with the pregnant women takes place in the outpatient clinic and a planned delivery happens, on average, in gestational week 39.

The Copenhagen Centre for Pregnant Diabetics is still well functioning, with its own laboratory and a staff of obstetricians (led by Peter Damm) and diabetologists (led by Elisabeth Mathiesen) collaborating with the well-known neonatal department in Rigshospital. Several research projects are in progress with young research fellows working well with the Pedersen legacy.

References

1. Brandstrup E, Okkels H. Pregnancy complicated with diabetes. *Acta Obstet Gyncol Scand* 1938; **18**:136–41.

2. Okkels H, Brandstrup E. Studies on the thyroid gland X. Pancreas, hypophysis and thyroid in children of diabetic mothers. *Acta Pathol Microbiol Scand* 1938; **15**:245–68.

3. Pedersen J. Course of diabetes during pregnancy. *Acta Endocr* 1952; **9**:342–64.

4. Pedersen J, Brandstrup E. Foetal mortality in pregnant diabetics. *Lancet* 1956; **1**:607–11.

5. Mølsted-Pedersen L, Tygstrup I, Pedersen J. Congenital malformation in newborn infants of diabetic women. *Lancet* 1964; **1**:1124–7.

6. Pedersen J, Mølsted-Pedersen L. Congenital malformations: the posible role of diabetes care outside pregnancy. In: *Ciba Foundation Symposium 63*. (Excerpta Medica: Amsterdam, 1979) 265–71.

7. Mølsted-Pedersen L. Significant decrease in severe congenital malformations and perinatal mortality in newborns of diabetic mothers. Paper presened at The Scandinavian Society for the Study of Diabetes, Copenhagen, Denmark, 25 May 1986.

8. Pedersen JF, Mølsted-Pedersen L. Early fetal growth delay detected by ultrasound marks increased risk of congenital malformation in diabetic pregnancy. *Br Med J* 1981; **283**:269–71.

9. Mølsted-Pedersen L, Damm P. How to organize care for pregnant diabetic patients. In: (Mogensen CE, Standl E, eds) *Concepts for the Ideal Diabetes Clinic*. (deGruyter: Berlin, 1993) 199–214.

10. Pedersen J. *Diabetes and Pregnancy – Blood Sugar of Newborn Infants*. (Danish Science Press Ltd: Copenhagen, 1952) [thesis].

11. Pedersen J. *The Pregnant Diabetic and Her Newborn*, 2nd edn. (Munksgaard: Copenhagen and Williams and Wilkins Co: Baltimore, 1977) 211.

12. Pedersen J, Osler M. Hyerglycemia as the cause of charactristic features of the foetus of newborns of diabetic mothers. *Danish Med Bull* 1961; **8**:78–82.

13. Pedersen J, Mølsted-Pedersen L. The hyperglycemia–hyperinsulinism theory and the weight of the newborn baby. In: (Rodrigues RR, Wallance-Owen J, eds) *Diabetes*. (Excerpta Medica: Amsterdam, 1971) 678–82.

14. Mølsted-Pedersen L. *Studies on carbohydrate metabolism in newborn infants of diabetic mothers*. Thesis, University of Copenhagen, 1974.

15. Pedersen J. Fetal macrosomia. In: (Sutherland HV, Stowers JM, eds) *Carbohydrate Metabolism in Pregnancy and the Newborn*. (Churchill Livngstone: Edinburgh, 1975) 127–39.

16. White P. Pregnancy and diabetes, medical aspects. *Med Clin N Am* 1965; **49**:1015–21.

17. Pedersen J, Mølsted-Pedersen L. Prognosis of the outcome of pregnancies in diabetics. A new classification. *Acta Encocr* 1965; **50**:70–7.

18. Pedersen J, Mølsted-Pedersen L, Andersen B. Assessors of fetal perinatal mortality in diabetic pregnancy. Analysis of 1332 pregnancies in the Copenhagen Series, 1946–1972. *Diabetes* 1974; **23**:302–6.

19. Pedersen JF, Mølsted-Pedersen L. Early growth retardation in diabetic pregnancy. *Br Med J* 1979; **1**:18–19.

20. Pedersen JF. Ultrasound studies on fetal crown–rump length in early normal and diabetic pregnancy. *Danish Med Bull* 1986; **33**:296–304.

21. Pedersen JF, Mølsted-Pedersen L, Mortensen HB. Fetal growth delay and maternal hemoglobin A1C in early diabetic pregnancy. *Obstet Gynecol* 1984; **64**:351–2.

22. Pedersen JF. Early fetal growth delay in diabetic pregnancy. Paper presented at the FIGO congress, Copenhagen, Denmark, 1997.

23. Petersen MB, Pedersen SA, Greisen G et al. Early growth delay in diabetic pregnancy: relation to psychomotor development at age 4. *Br Med J* 1988; **26**:598–600.

24. Kuhl C. *Serum insulin and plasma glucagon in human pregnancy – on the pathogenesis of gestational diabetes.* Thesis, University of Copenhagen, 1978.

25. Damm P. *Gestational diabetes mellitus and subsequent development of overt diabetes mellitus – a clinical, metabolic and epidemiological study.* Thesis, University of Copenhagen, 1998.

4

The Freinkel legacy
Boyd E Metzger

Introduction

Professor Norbert (Norbie) Freinkel (Fig. 4.1) was a renowned scholar, investigator and teacher. Although it is now more than a decade since his sudden untimely death, Norbie's influence in the field of pregnancy and diabetes remains profound. What accounts for this enduring legacy? Norbie was a brilliant, intense, dedicated and insightful investigator. He was a gifted and prolific writer, and used language with great skill and flair. Norbert Freinkel was a member of prestigious academic societies, including the American Society of Clinical Investigation and the Association of American Professors, and held important professional leadership positions, including the presidency of both the Endocrine Society and the American Diabetes Association.

However, in the present authors' estimation, an enduring legacy is built more on people who during their career have benefited from exposure to research and intellectual environments and on the concepts that have been promoted rather than on affiliations with prestigious organizations and recognition in 'high places'. Strong evidence of this is seen in the way that Norbert Freinkel's influence continues to be felt in the broad areas of nutrition and metabolism during pregnancy. In the short treatise that follows, the present authors' perspective on some of the people and concepts that best convey the life and legacy of Norbert Freinkel have been summarized. This perspective can be compared and contrasted with the one that was offered a decade ago, 2 years after Norbie's death.[1]

Northwestern University's Diabetes in Pregnancy Center: vehicle of the legacy

After making major contributions to insights into thyroid hormone metabolism[2–4] and to

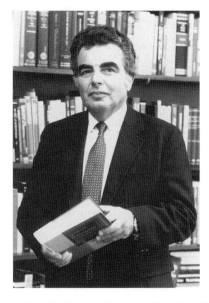

Figure 4.1. *Professor Norbert (Norbie) Freinkel.*

other areas of endocrinology early in his career, Norbert Freinkel turned his interests and talents to the study of intermediary metabolism in normal and diabetic pregnancy in the 1960s.[4-7] By the early 1970s, he had established a Diabetes in Pregnancy Center (DPC) at Northwestern University and had attracted research collaborations globally. Over the next two decades, a virtual who's who of the world's leading established and future investigators of intermediary metabolism in normal and diabetic pregnancy (basic and clinical) could be compiled from those who spent time as visiting scientists at Northwestern University's DPC. Several sources of objective support for this contention are cited below.

Following Norbie's death,[8] the American Diabetes Association established the Norbert Freinkel Lecture through the support and encouragement of many colleagues, friends and patients. The Freinkel Lectureship is held under the auspices of the Diabetes in Pregnancy Council. On a triennial basis, it is integrated into the program of the International Diabetes Federation (IDF) Congress. A review of the names of the Freinkel lecturers chosen to date and the topics chosen for their lectures (Table 4.1) provides a vignette of the Freinkel legacy.

The Diabetic Pregnancy Study Group (DPSG), an affiliate of the European Association for the Study of Diabetes, held its first meeting in 1969. Norbie, then on sabbatical leave at Cambridge University, was invited to be the keynote speaker at that inaugural DPSG event. The annual Jørgen Pedersen Lecture that was established by the DPSG in

Lecturer	Year	Title of lecture
John Bell	1991–IDF	Genetic susceptibility to IDDM
Lars Mølsted-Pedersen	1992	Management of chronic hypertension in the pregnant diabetic woman
Boyd Metzger	1993	Diabetes begets diabetes: the last tenet of the Freinkel hypothesis
John O'Sullivan	1994	The birth of gestational diabetes
Ulf Eriksson	1995	Intracellular mediators of diabetic embryopathy: is there a common pathway?
John Kitzmiller	1996	Pregnancy planning and care for women with chronic diabetic complications
Donald Coustan	1997–IDF	Gestational diabetes: 33 years without consensus
David Pettitt	1998	Long-term impact on the offspring: the Pima experience
Thomas Buchanan	1999	Fetal and maternal risks in GDM: sorting wheat from chaff
Patrick Catalano	2000–IDF	Insulin resistance in pregnancy and gestational diabetes: implications for mother and fetus
Lois Jovanovic	2001	Glucose mediated macrosomia: the over-fed fetus and the future
Jorge Mestman	2002	History of diabetes and pregnancy: lessons from the past

Table 4.1. *Norbert Freinkel lectures. IDF, International Diabetes Federation.*

1980 honors individuals who have made major contributions to the field. Norbie was an early Jørgen Pedersen lecturer, and the depth of his impact on diabetes and pregnancy is reflected in the fact that, eight of the first 20 lecturers between 1980 and 2001 had ties with Norbie through collaboration with, or by time spent at, Northwestern University's DPC. Another measure of his lasting legacy is illustrated by the fact that in the year 2002, > 20% of the 55 members and honorary members of the DPSG had this kind of linkage with Norbert Freinkel.

The last illustration of the enduring human dimensions of the Freinkel legacy is proved through the composition of the editorship and authorship of this text. The lead editor and at least 15 contributing authors have associations with Norbie (first or second generation) by way of their collaboration with or training at Northwestern University's DPC.

Freinkel concepts of metabolic regulation in pregnancy

From his earliest studies of metabolic changes during pregnancy, Norbert Freinkel directed his interests to the mutual interplay between mother and fetus. He regarded these changes as adaptations to facilitate optimal development of the fetus. Norbie had the ability to synthesize diverse observations into cohesive concepts with clinical application. Some examples are summarized briefly below.

Accelerated starvation

In Freinkel's laboratory, and others, it was demonstrated that the transition from a basal or overnight fasting metabolic status to the pattern that is characteristic of the prolonged fasted state, or starvation, is exaggerated in

pregnancy.[7] Since the exaggerated changes differed in both temporal and absolute dimensions, Norbie characterized this pattern as **accelerated starvation**.[9] A number of clinical and epidemiological studies suggest that greater than normal levels of ketonemia/ketonuria during pregnancy may have adverse effects on fetal development and, subsequently, adverse neurological consequences.[10–12] Thus, it is common clinical practice to avoid dietary manipulations during pregnancy that might enhance ketogenesis such as marked restriction of calorie or carbohydrate intake. However, since the demonstration of accelerated starvation was initially documented in animal models and in women that were subjected to prolonged starvation prior to having termination of pregnancy in early or mid-gestation, the relevance of accelerated starvation to the clinical management of normal, healthy pregnancies was uncertain until the report entitled *'Accelerated starvation' and the skipped breakfast in late normal pregnancy*[13] was published in 1982. As noted in Fig. 4.2, this study illustrated that even the common practice of delaying or skipping breakfast until lunchtime is sufficient to provoke early metabolic changes [a fall in the concentration of plasma glucose, and increases in free fatty acids (FFA) and β-hydroxybutyrate], which if continued even for a relatively short interval could result in the full metabolic profile of accelerated starvation.

Facilitated anabolism

The metabolic changes that can be observed during the disposition of food intake are numerous. Many aspects of a characteristic diurnal metabolic profile of pregnancy were described in reports from the Northwestern University group. The mediation of the these changes and the implications for normal

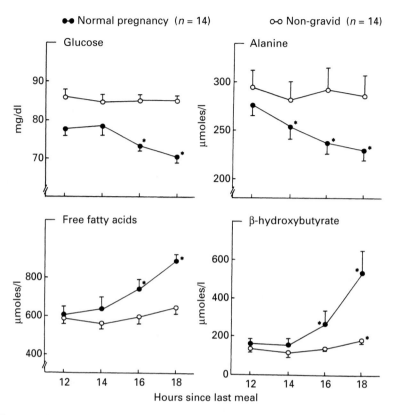

Figure 4.2. *Changes in plasma concentration of glucose, alanine, free fatty acids and β-hydroxybutyrate in non-pregnant and pregnant women between 12 hours fasting and 18 hours fasting during the third trimester. *Denotes significant change from 12 hours. (Adapted from Metger et al,[13] Figure 1.)*

pregnancy, as well as the states of altered nutrition or metabolism (obesity, diabetes, malnutrition), are not fully defined and continue to be of great interest to investigators. Norbie interpreted the perturbations that were observed in normal pregnancy as adaptations to assure an adequate delivery of nutrients to the fetus and coined the phrase **facilitated anabolism**[14] to convey the aggregate changes. In his view, the insulin resistance of pregnancy plays a key role in bringing about the changes in carbohydrate, lipid and amino acid metabolism that **facilitate anabolism.** Thus, during an oral glucose tolerance test (OGTT) in normal pregnant women, the net area under the glucose curve (AUGC)

was found to correlate with the overnight fasting concentration of FFA (Fig. 4.3), and the decline in FFA after a glucose load was delayed despite the increasing glucose and insulin concentrations.[14] Though the postulated mechanisms differ from those originally proposed by Randle and others, the role of FFA metabolism as a concomitant and potentially mediating factor in insulin resistance is presently receiving renewed attention.[15] In the studies mentioned above, correlations were also found between triglycerides and the AUGC, and between basal and stimulated insulin and the AUGC. The strong interrelationships between glycemia, aminoacidemia, lipids, and insulin

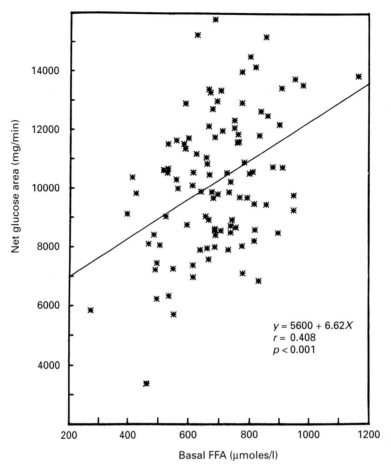

$$y = 5600 + 6.62X$$
$$r = 0.408$$
$$p < 0.001$$

Figure 4.3. *The relationship between the glycemic response to a 100 gram glucose load during pregnancy and fasting FFA concentration. The regression equation was derived to relate fasting FFA at the time of glucose ingestion to the integrated changes in plasma glucose (net glucose area) during the subsequent 3 hours. Subjects were normal women at weeks 30–40 of pregnancy. (Adapted from Freinkel et al,[14] Figure 2.)*

sensitivity and secretion must be considered when trying to interpret correlations between triglycerides and birthweight or fetal body composition, or between birthweight and maternal insulin sensitivity during and outside of pregnancy.[16]

Metabolic change as teratogens

In the late 1970s and early 1980s, Freinkel and his group extended their focus beyond the factors that mediate insulin secretion in the fetus, the insulin-dependent fetal growth and other manifestations of third trimester fetal hyperinsulinism to consider the consequences of an altered intrauterine metabolic environment throughout gestation. Describing pregnancy as 'a tissue culture experience'[17] put this concept into sharp relief, and Norbert Freinkel's 1980 Banting Lecture[18] was a masterful blend of an overview and integration of previous work in concert with a prescient grasp

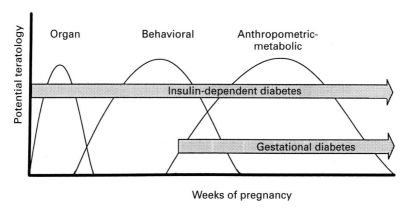

Figure 4.4. *Potential long-range effects upon the fetus of chronic alterations in concentrations of maternal fuels during pregnancy. Fuel-mediated teratogenesis as the basis for long-range anatomic and functional changes. (Reproduced with permission from Freinkel,[18] Figure 12.)*

of the lifelong implications of exposure to the intrauterine environment of diabetes mellitus. He illustrated clearly (Fig. 4.4) that the consequences of metabolic disturbances at various times during gestation are different, and that the implications of altered metabolism in gestational diabetes mellitus (GDM) and pregestational diabetes are also different.

Through work in his laboratory at the DPC,[19–21] as well as through the subsequent and still ongoing work of those initially trained in embryo culture techniques at Northwestern University, Norbert Freinkel was the driving force in demonstrating that at specific, finite times during gestation, the metabolic changes of diabetes, and metabolic changes that can occur through other mechanisms, can be primary factors in teratogenesis. The capacity to define precisely the time and nature of specific metabolic insults led to the realization that the metabolic insults of diabetes mellitus (DM) on fetal development are probably multifactorial, and that recovery from the metabolic perturbation lags behind simple rectification of the altered concentration of metabolites. Though the specific mechanisms and molecular mediators that lead to dysmorphogenesis are

not yet clear, these insights have stimulated efforts to establish optimal metabolic control before conception. Such efforts are highly successful when they are achieved, though good control of DM before pregnancy is far from universal.[22]

Long-term consequences of intrauterine exposures

Testing the hypotheses that the consequences of alterations in intrauterine metabolic insult are conditioned by when in gestation that the exposure occurred, and that important outcomes may have latency before appearing much later in development, required a long-term perspective. At Northwestern University's DPC, that was implemented through a National Institutes of Health (NIH) funded Prospective, Long Term Follow-up Study of Offspring of Diabetic Mothers that has continued for more than two decades. It was initiated between 1978 and 1983 and focused on neurobehavioral and adipose tissue developments, obesity, beta-cell function and glucose homeostasis. However, the majority of the studies that confirmed the initial hypotheses that lifelong functions of these tissues are vulnerable to intrauterine insult were not concluded until after Norbie's death. For the purpose of this chapter, the commentary has been limited to several reports of Silverman and co-workers.[23–26] These indicate that risks of both obesity and altered glucose homeostasis (impaired glucose tolerance and Type 2 diabetes) in late childhood and adolescence are increased by exposure to the intrauterine environment of DM in mid- and/or late gestation. The mechanisms by which adipose tissue development and glucose homeostasis are influenced in later life in offspring of diabetic mothers are not clear. However, in Northwestern University's DPC study, the risks were strongly associated with markers of fetal hyperinsulinism (primarily amniotic fluid insulin concentration measured at the time of third trimester amniocentesis).

Concurrently, the epidemiological studies in the Pima Indian population of Arizona by Pettitt and co-workers have provided very complementary findings.[27–29] However, in this population, with the world's highest prevalence of Type 2 DM, direct information about fetal or neonatal insulin secretion is not available and large size at birth has served as the marker for infants that have been exposed to the intrauterine environment of DM.

The data from Northwestern University's DPC and from the Pima study, along with support animal models, provide convincing evidence that diabetes begets diabetes through the intrauterine environment and is contributing significantly to the epidemic of Type 2 DM in adolescents and young adults, including a rising prevalence of GDM. It remains to be determined if the vicious cycle can be effectively interrupted by more timely diagnosis and effective therapy of diabetes antedating pregnancy, pregestational diabetes and of GDM.

The Freinkel legacy and the future

This brief overview provides evidence that the legacy of Norbert Freinkel is being strongly sustained more than a decade after his death. How this legacy will help shape the future directions of research and stimulate new clinical approaches is uncertain. However, the trail will not be difficult to follow. One area that will continue to reflect Norbie's concepts is future developments in GDM. Norbert Freinkel initiated and chaired the first two International Workshop Conferences on GDM. The third was in an early stage of planning at his death. Studies of GDM were initiated at Northwestern University's DPC for two reasons. The first objective was to learn more about the pathogenesis of GDM and progression to DM among women in this high-risk population. Women with previous GDM have participated successfully in efforts to develop pharmacologic and lifestyle strategies to prevent or delay the onset of Type 2 DM among high-risk subjects. Secondly, GDM was looked upon as a good model to determine how much alteration of nutrient metabolism was required to have adverse effects on the offspring. The Hyperglycemia and Adverse Pregnancy Outcome (HAPO) Study[30] should provide an answer to that dilemma and foster the adoption of criteria for GDM that are based on the level of glycemia that is associated with clinically significant risk.

Acknowledgements

BEM had the extraordinary opportunity to know Norbie Freinkel as a friend and close professional mentor, advisor and colleague for more than 22 years. Now, more than a decade has elapsed since his death and early reviews of his legacy. In this short report, the author has concentrated on the extraordinary impact that Norbie's work and vision continue to exert on clinical and research aspects of pregnancy complicated by diabetes mellitus. This author is convinced that in another decade we will still be harvesting the rewards of that vision. In the course of this review, the work of many others has been alluded to but has not been cited by specific literature reference. This was done to maintain the focus on the specific contributions of Norbert Freinkel and for the sake of brevity.

Work that was cited from Northwestern University's DPC was supported by Research Grants DK 10699, HD 19070, HD 62903 and HD/DK 34243; GCRC Grant RR48; and Training Grant DK 07169.

References

1. Metzger BE. The legacy of Norbert Freinkel: maternal metabolism and its impact on the offspring, from embryo to adult. Diabetes in pregnancy. Norbert Freinkel Memorial Issue. *Israel J Med Sci* 1991; 27:425–31.
2. Ingbar SH, Freinkel N, Hoeprich PD, Tthens FW. The concentration and significance of the butanol-extractable I^{131} of serum in patients with diverse states of thyroidal function. *J Clin Invest* 1954; 33:388–99.
3. Ingbar SH, Freinkel N. Simultaneous estimation of rates of thyroxine degradation and peripheral metabolism of thyroxine. *J Clin Invest* 1955; 34:808–19.
4. Dowling JT, Freinkel N, Ingbar SH. Thyroxine-binding by sera of pregnant women, new-born infants and women with spontaneous abortion. *J Clin Invest* 1956; 35:1263–76.
5. Goodner CJ, Freinkel N. Carbohydrate metabolism in pregnancy: the turnover of I^{131} insulin in the pregnant rat. *Endocrinology* 1960; 67:862–72.
6. Bleicher SJ, O'Sullivan JB, Freinkel N. Carbohydrate metabolism in pregnancy. V. The interrelations of glucose, insulin and free fatty acids in late pregnancy and post partum. *N Engl J Med* 1964; 271:866–72.
7. Herrera E, Knopp RH, Freinkel N. Carbohydrate metabolism in pregnancy. VI. Plasma fuels, insulin liver composition, gluconeogenesis and nitrogen metabolism during late gestation in the fed and fasted rat. *J Clin Invest* 1969; 48:2260–72.
8. Obituary, Norbert Freinkel. *Diabetes* 1990; 39:1990.
9. Freinkel N. Effects of the conceptus on maternal metabolism during pregnancy. In: (Leibel BS, Wrenshall GA, eds.) *On the Nature and Treatment of Diabetes.* (Excerpta Medical Foundation; Amsterdam, 1965) 679–91.
10. Churchill JA, Berendes HW, Nemore J. Neuropsychological deficits in children of diabetic mothers. *Am J Obstet Gynecol* 1969; 105:257–68.
11. Stebbens JA, Baker GL, Kitchell M. Outcome at ages 1, 3 and 5 years of children born to diabetic women. *Am J Obstet Gynecol* 1977; 127:408–13.
12. Rizzo T, Metzger BE, Burns WJ, Burns KC. Correlations between antepartum maternal metabolism and child intelligence. *N Engl J Med* 1991; 325:911–16.
13. Metzger BE, Ravnikar V, Vileisis RA, Freinkel N. 'Accelerated starvation' and the skipped breakfast in late normal pregnancy. *Lancet* 1982; 1:588–92.
14. Freinkel N, Metzger BE, Nitzan M et al. Facilitated anabolism in late pregnancy: some novel maternal compensations for accelerated starvation. Paper presented at the Proceedings of the VIII Congress of the International Diabetes Federation, Brussels, Belgium, July 1973. (Excerpta Medical International Congress Series; Amsterdam, 1974) 312:474–88.
15. Boden G. Role of free fatty acids in the pathogenesis of insulin resistance and NIDDM. *Diabetes* 1997; 46: 3–10.
16. Catalano PM, Thomas AJ, Huston L, Fung CM. Effect of maternal metabolism on fetal growth and body composition. *Diabetes Care* 1998; 21 (Suppl 2):85B–90B.
17. Freinkel N, Metzger BE. Pregnancy as a tissue culture experience: the critical implications of maternal metabolism for fetal development. In: *Pregnancy Metabolism, Diabetes and the Fetus, Ciba Foundation Symposium 63.* (Excerpta Medica: Amsterdam, 1979) 3–28.
18. Freinkel N. The Banting Lecture 1980: of pregnancy and progeny. *Diabetes* 1980; 29:1023–35.
19. Freinkel N, Lewis NJ, Akazawa S et al. The honeybee syndrome: implications of the teratogenicity of mannose in rat-embryo culture. *N Engl J Med* 1984; 310:223–30.
20. Eriksson UJ, Lewis NJ, Freinkel N. Growth retardation during early organogenesis in embryos of experimentally diabetic rats. *Diabetes* 1984; 33:281–4.
21. Freinkel N, Cockroft DL, Lewis NJ et al. The 1986 McCollum Award Lecture. Fuel-mediated teratogenesis during early organogenesis: the effects of increased concentrations of glucose, ketones, or somatomedin inhibitor during rat embryo culture. *Am J Clin Nutr* 1986; 44:986–95.
22. Metzger BE, Buchanan TA. From research to practice. Diabetes and birth defects: insights from the 1980s, prevention in the 1990s. Conclusions. *Diabetes Spectrum* 1990; 3:181–4.
23. Metzger BE, Silverman B, Freinkel N et al. Amniotic fluid insulin concentration as a predictor of obesity. *Arch Dis Child* 1990; 65:1050–2.

24. Silverman BL, Landsberg L, Metzger BE. Fetal hyper-insulinism in offspring of diabetic mothers: association with the subsequent development of childhood obesity. In: (Williams CL, Kimm SYS, eds) *Prevention and Treatment of Childhood Obesity. Volume 699.* (New York Academy of Sciences: New York, 1993) 36–45.

25. Silverman BL, Metzger BE, Cho NH, Loeb CA. Impaired glucose tolerance in adolescent offspring of diabetic mothers: relationship to fetal hyperinsulinism. *Diabetes Care* 1995; **18**:611–17.

26. Silverman BL, Rizzo TA, Cho NH, Metzger BE. Long-term effects of the intrauterine environment. *Diabetes Care* 1998; **21 (Suppl 2)**:142–9.

27. Pettitt DJ, Baird HR, Aleck KA. Excessive obesity in off-spring of Pima Indian women with diabetes during pregnancy. *N Engl J Med* 1983; **308**:242–5.

28. Pettitt DJ, Aleck KA, Baird HR et al. Congenital susceptibility to NIDDM: role of intrauterine environment. *Diabetes* 1988; **37**:622–8.

29. Dabelea D, Pettitt DJ, Hanson RL et al. Birth weight, Type 2 diabetes, and insulin resistance in Pima Indian children and young adults. *Diabetes Care* 1999; **22**: 944–50.

30. HAPO Study Cooperative Research Group. The Hyperglycemia and Adverse Pregnancy Outcome (HAPO) Study. *Int J Gynecol Obstet* 2002; **78**:69–77.

5

Pathogenesis of gestational diabetes mellitus

Yariv Yogev, Avi Ben-Haroush, Moshe Hod

Introduction

Gestational diabetes mellitus (GDM) is characterized by carbohydrate intolerance of variable severity, with onset or first recognition during pregnancy. This definition applies whether or not there is a need for insulin and whether or not it disappears after the pregnancy. It does not apply to gravid patients with previously diagnosed diabetes.[1]

Although pregnancy is a carbohydrate-intolerant state, only a small proportion of pregnant women (3–5%) develop GDM. As pregnancy advances, the increasing tissue resistance to insulin creates a demand for more insulin. In the great majority of women, insulin requirements are readily met, so the balance between insulin resistance and insulin supply is maintained. However, if resistance becomes dominant due to impaired insulin secretion, hyperglycemia develops. In the majority of such cases, it develops in the last half of pregnancy, with insulin resistance increasing progressively until delivery, when, in most cases, it rapidly disappears.

Controversy still exists about the screening and diagnosis of GDM. In the majority of cases, carbohydrate intolerance is asymptomatic and can be detected only by routine screening challenge tests. A detailed discussion of variations in the diagnostic criteria is beyond the scope of this chapter, but the main issue is that the diagnosis of GDM is based on the screening of a large number of apparently healthy young women.

As in non-insulin-dependent diabetes mellitus (NIDDM), GDM is associated with both insulin resistance and impaired insulin secretion.[2–4] The two disorders also share the same risk factors, have a corresponding prevalence within a given population and have the same genetic susceptibility; therefore, they are assumed to be etiologically indistinct, with one preceding the other.

In this chapter, the development of insulin resistance during pregnancy, hormones and newly discovered factors associated with insulin resistance and secretion, the insulin-signaling system during normal and diabetic pregnancy, and metabolic predictors of diabetes will be discussed.

Insulin sensitivity and resistance in pregnancy

The cellular mechanisms underlying insulin resistance in normal and diabetic pregnancy are still unknown. The measurement of fasting insulin concentrations and the calculation of fasting insulin:glucose ratios can provide a qualitative but not a quantitative estimation of insulin sensitivity. In non-pregnant patients, hyperinsulinemic–euglycemic clamps[5] and minimal-model analysis of intravenous glucose tolerance tests (IVGTT)[6,7] have been used to obtain quantitative data about insulin action. The IVGTT model provides data on the glucose infusion that is required to maintain euglycemia during constant insulin infusion. However, its use in pregnancy is limited owing to the change in the relationship between common measures of body size, such as total body weight and body surface area. Catalano et al[8,9] were the first to conduct a prospective longitudinal study using the hyperinsulinemic–euglycemic clamp model in obese and non-obese gravid women with normal glucose tolerance tests. They found a 47% decrease in insulin sensitivity in obese gravid women and a 56% decrease in lean gravid women.

The development of resistance to the glucose-lowering effects of insulin is a normal phenomenon of pregnancy. In a pioneer study, Burt[10] demonstrated that pregnant women experience fewer hypoglycemic events in response to insulin infusion than non-gravid women. Accordingly, later research found women with normal pregnancies had progressively exaggerated insulin responses to ingested glucose, together with a slightly decreased glucose tolerance.[11,12] Using the IVGTT model, Buchanan et al[13] and Cousins et al[14] demonstrated a significant (70%) reduction in insulin sensitivity during the second trimester of normal pregnancy, with a return to normal values shortly after delivery.

Ryan et al[2] were the first to report quantitative differences in insulin sensitivity between normal and diabetic pregnancies. Other researchers noted that insulin sensitivity was lower in patients with GDM than in patients with normal pregnancies at 12–14 weeks of gestation, before the point of maximal physiological insulin resistance however, the difference was not statistically significant. By the third trimester, insulin resistance was similar in the two groups.[8,14]

Much effort has been invested to identify the tissues that contribute to the insulin resistance of pregnancy. Findings, in animal models indicate a 40% reduction in insulin-mediated glucose utilization by skeletal muscle, and a similar effect in cardiac muscle and fat cells.[15,16]

It remains unclear whether hepatic insulin sensitivity is altered during gestation. Kalhan et al[17] and Cowett et al[18] noted no significant differences in basal glucose production in pregnant women at term compared to non-pregnant control subjects when the data were expressed per kilogram of body weight; however, expression of the data in relation to pregravid weight yielded an increase in hepatic glucose production in late pregnancy.[19] Furthermore, in hyperinsulinemic–euglycemic clamp studies, hepatic glucose production was significantly less suppressed in lean and obese patients with GDM than in the control group.[8,9]

Hormonal effect in normal and diabetic pregnancy

Reproductive hormones tend to increase during pregnancy, most of them contribute to insulin resistance and altered beta-cell function.

Estrogen and progesterone

In early pregnancy, both progesterone and estrogen rise but their effects on insulin activity are counterbalanced. Progesterone causes insulin resistance whereas estrogen is protective.[20] An IVGTT test given to estrogen-treated rats showed a significant decrease in glucose concentrations and a twofold increase in insulin concentration;[21] the addition of progesterone was associated with a 70% increase in the insulin response to a glucose challenge test, but there were no alterations in glucose tolerance.[22] In cultured rat adipocyte tissue treated with estrogen, there was no effect on glucose transport, but maximum insulin binding was increased. However, progesterone decreased both maximum glucose transport and insulin binding.[20–21]

Recently, Gonzalez et al[23] evaluated the role played by progesterone and/or 17 beta-estradiol on sensitivity to insulin action that took place during pregnancy. Ovariectomized rats were treated with different doses of progesterone and/or 17 beta-estradiol in order to simulate the plasma levels in normal pregnancy rats. A hyperinsulinemic–euglycemic clamp was used to measure insulin sensitivity. The results suggested that the absence of female steroid hormones leads to decreased insulin sensitivity. Thus, the rise in insulin sensitivity during early pregnancy, when plasma concentrations of 17 beta-estradiol and progesterone are low could be due to 17 beta-estradiol. However, during late pregnancy, when both plasma concentrations of 17 beta-estradiol and progesterone are high, the role of 17 beta-estradiol may serve to antagonize the effect of progesterone, diminishing insulin sensitivity.[23]

Cortisol

Cortisol levels increase as pregnancy advances and by the end of pregnancy concentrations are threefold higher than in the non-pregnant state.[24] Rizza et al,[25] in a clamp study, demonstrated that under infusion of high amounts of cortisol, hepatic glucose production increased and insulin sensitivity decreased. Findings in a skeletal muscle model showed that an excess of glucocorticoid is characterized by decreased total tyrosine phosphorylation of the insulin

receptor; therefore, it seems logical that glucocorticoid-induced insulin resistance is related to a postreceptor mechanism. In a study by Ahmed and Shalayel,[26] 30 pregnant women with GDM and 30 pregnant women with impaired glucose tolerance (IGT) were compared with 30 pregnant women with normal glucose tolerance. The GDM and IGT groups were found to have significantly higher levels of serum cortisol than the control group.

Prolactin

During pregnancy, maternal prolactin levels increase seven- to tenfold. Gustafson et al[27] reported that the basal insulin concentration, and postchallenge glucose and insulin responses were greater in women with hyperprolactinemia than in healthy controls. These findings were supported by studies showing that the culture of pancreatic islet cells with prolactin induces an increase in insulin secretion.[28] Skouby et al[29] investigated the relationship between the deterioration in glucose tolerance and plasma prolactin levels in patients with normal and diabetic pregnancies. Oral glucose tolerance tests (OGTT) were performed in late pregnancy and postpartum. In late pregnancy, the GDM group had significantly elevated fasting glucose levels compared to the controls and, after glucose challenge, their insulin responses were significantly diminished and the suppression of glucagon less pronounced. These differences in glucose metab-olism were markedly reduced in the early postpartum period. There was no difference in basal prolactin concentrations between the two groups at either time point. The prolactin levels were also not altered during the OGTT tolerance tests, and there was no correlation between the deterioration in glucose tolerance and the prolactin concentrations in either group. Thus, abnormal prolactin levels are not of pathophysiologic importance in the development of GDM.

Human placental lactogen

Human placental lactogen (hPL) levels rise at the beginning of the second trimester, causing a decrease in phosphorylation of insulin receptor substrate (IRS)-1 and profound insulin resistance.[20]

Beck and Daughday[30] demonstrated that overnight infusion of hPL results in abnormal glucose tolerance, and increased insulin and glucose concentration in response to an oral glucose challenge. Accordingly, Brelje et al[31] found that in islet cell culture, hPL directly stimulates insulin secretion. This may indicate that hPL directly regulates islet cell function and is probably the principal hormone responsible for the increase in islet function observed during normal pregnancy.[31]

Leptin

Leptin is a 16 kDa protein encoded by the *ob/ob* (obesity) gene secreted by adipocyte tissue. It can modulate energy expenditure by direct action on the hypothalamus. Fasting insulin and leptin concentrations correlate closely with body fat, making leptin a good marker of obesity and insulin resistance. As receptors to leptin are found in skeletal muscle, the liver, the pancreas, adipocyte tissue, the uterus and the placenta, it may be responsible for both peripheral and central insulin resistance.

In animal models, using hyperinsulinemic–euglycemic clamp studies, infusion of leptin was found to increase the glucose infusion rate.[32] Leptin levels are significantly higher in pregnancy than in the non-pregnant state, especially during the second and third trimesters.[33–35]

Yamashita et al[36] suggested that an alteration in leptin action might play a role in GDM and fetal overgrowth weight gain. They found that pregnant mice treated with leptin had markedly lower glucose levels than controls during glucose and insulin challenge tests. However, despite the reduced energy intake and improved glucose tolerance, fetal overgrowth was not reduced. Results provide evidence that leptin administration during late gestation can reduce adiposity and improve glucose tolerance in the model of spontaneous GDM. These data suggest that alterations in placental leptin levels may contribute to the regulation of fetal growth independently of maternal glucose levels.

Kautzky-Willer et al[37] measured plasma concentrations of leptin and beta-cell hormones during fasting and after an oral glucose load (OGTT of 75 grams) in pregnant women with GDM and normal glucose tolerance at 28 weeks gestation, and in women who were not pregnant. Plasma leptin was higher in the women with GDM than in the women with normal glucose tolerance, and higher in both these groups than in the non-pregnant controls. No change in plasma leptin concentrations was induced by OGTT in any group. Basal insulin release was higher in women with GDM than in the women with normal glucose tolerance. The authors concluded that women with GDM and no change in plasma leptin on oral glucose loading have increased plasma leptin concentrations during and after pregnancy. Vitoratos et al[38] investigated the changes in leptin levels and the relationship between leptin substance and insulin and glucose in pregnant women with GDM. Plasma leptin levels were measured in peripheral vein blood samples from healthy and diabetic women at 29 and 33 weeks gestation. Results showed a correlation of plasma leptin levels with fasting plasma insulin levels and plasma glucose levels measured 1 hour after oral administration of 50 grams of glucose. Serum leptin levels were significantly higher in the women with GDM than in the women with uncomplicated pregnancies. The GDM group also showed a significant, positive correlation of serum leptin levels with glycosylated hemoglobin levels, fasting serum insulin levels and plasma glucose levels measured 1 hour after administration of 50 grams of glucose. Thus, levels of leptin are elevated in women with GDM, and leptin metabolism depends on insulin levels and the severity of the diabetes. Wiznitzer et al[39] reported that umbilical cord leptin concentration was an independent risk factor for fetal macrosomia in non-diabetic pregnant women.

Other factors affecting gestational diabetes mellitus

Tumor necrosis factor-alpha

Tumor necrosis factor-alpha (TNF-α) has been implicated in the pathogenesis of insulin resistance in Type 2 diabetes mellitus, but only limited data are available with regard to GDM. Coughlan et al[40] investigated the effect of exogenous glucose on the release of TNF-α from placental and adipose tissue obtained from normal and diabetic pregnant women. They found significantly greater TNF-α release under conditions of high glucose concentrations in the GDM group. As TNF-α has been implicated in the regulation of glucose and lipid metabolism, and in insulin resistance, these data are consistent with the hypothesis that TNF-α is involved in the pathogenesis and/or progression of GDM.

Catalano et al[41] reported that changes in insulin sensitivity from early to late pregnancy correlated with a gradual increase in TNF-α

levels, which in turn correlated with the percentage change in body weight.

Adrenomedullin

Adrenomedullin is a newly discovered hypotensive peptide involved in the insulin regulatory system and it may play a rule in modifying diabetes in pregnancy. Di Iorio et al[42] studied its correlation to GDM. Adrenomedullin concentrations were measured in maternal and fetal plasma, and in amniotic fluid in diabetic and non-diabetic pregnancies. Overall amniotic fluid concentration was higher in the pregnant diabetic women (Type 1 or GDM) but there was no between group difference in maternal and fetal plasma levels. These findings suggest that placental adrenomedullin production is upregulated in diabetic pregnancy and that it may be important to prevent excessive vasoconstriction of placental vessels.

Pancreatic beta-cell function in normal pregnancy and gestational diabetes mellitus

Insulin is the main hormone controlling blood glucose concentration. Most commonly, assessment of beta-cell function is made by measuring the fasting insulin concentration or the response to glucose infusion. Fasting plasma insulin increases gradually during pregnancy – by the third trimester levels are twofold higher than before pregnancy. Patients with GDM have fasting insulin levels equal to or higher than those of women with non-diabetic pregnancies, with the highest levels occurring in obese women with GDM.

During normal pregnancy, oral and intravenous glucose tolerance deteriorates only slightly, despite the reduction in insulin sensitivity.[13] The main mechanism responsible for that phenomenon is a gradual increase in insulin secretion by the beta cells. Kual[12] reported a hyperbolic relationship between insulin sensitivity and beta-cell responsiveness to glucose in both pregnant and non-pregnant women, pointing to a role for the beta-cells in pathological states such as GDM and demonstrating the magnitude of the change in insulin secretion that is necessary to maintain glucose tolerance. The mechanism responsible for increase insulin secretion during pregnancy is not well understood. A major contributing factor is the increase in the beta-cell mass, a combination of hyperplasia and hypertrophy.[43] The increased beta-cell mass can contribute to the increased fasting insulin concentration despite normal or lowered fasting glucose concentrations in late pregnancy, and the enhanced insulin response to glucose during pregnancy (two- to threefold above non-pregnant levels).

In GDM, the early insulin response to OGTT (15–30 minutes after glucose ingestion) is reduced compared to non-diabetic pregnant control women, suggesting a defect in the beta-cell response.[44] First-phase beta-cell responses to glucose infusion in GDM patients is also been reported to be reduced. GDM tends to milder in women with a normal beta-cell response and they are at relatively low risk for developing diabetes.[45]

Genetics, immunology and gestational diabetes mellitus

Some GDM patients manifest evidence for autoimmunity towards beta cells (insulin autoantibodies and anti-islet cell antibodies); however, the prevalence of such autoimmunity has been reported to be extremely low (< 10%).[46–47] Mutations in the glucokinase gene occur in no more than 5% of GDM patients.[48] The inheritance of GDM was studied in a group of 100 women with previous GDM.[49] The women were reinvestigated 11 years postpartum and c. 60% were found to have either IGT or Type 2 diabetes. An investigation of their parents showed that a substantial proportion had neither parent affected with IGT or Type 2 diabetes, which suggests a polygenic inheritance or environmental influence rather autosomal dominance inheritance with high penetration rates. In addition, animal studies have shown that prenatal exposure to a diabetic intrauterine milieu increases the risk of GDM.

Harder et al[50] reported that the prevalence of Type 2 diabetes was significantly greater in mothers than in fathers of women with GDM, and there was also significant aggregation of Type 2 diabetes in the maternal–grandmaternal line compared to the paternal–grandpaternal line. Therefore, that may suggest that a history of Type 2 diabetes on the mother's side might be considered as a particular risk factor for GDM.

The possible genetic background of GDM remains unclear. In particular, its association with human leukocyte antigen (HLA) class II polymorphism has been poorly studied and the results are conflicting. In attempt to clarify these discrepancies, Vambergue et al[51] reported that the distribution of HLA class II polymorphism was not significantly different between GDM and IGT samples, and there was no significant variation in DRB1*03 and DRB1*04 allele frequencies. These data provide further evidence that Type 1 or insulin-dependent diabetes mellitus (IDDM) HLA class II susceptibility alleles cannot serve as genetic markers for susceptibility to glucose intolerance during pregnancy.

Ober et al[52] studied the restriction fragment length polymorphisms near 'candidate diabetogenic genes' in order to identify molecular markers for GDM genes. Genotypes for the insulin hypervariable region (HVR), insulin-like growth factor II (IGF2), insulin receptor (IR), and glucose transporter (GLUT1) were studied in GDM and control subjects. The results supported the hypothesis that GDM has heterogeneous phenotypic and genotypic features, and that the risk for GDM in black and Caucasian subjects is not related to obesity *per se* but to interactions between obesity and IR alleles. In Caucasian women, IR and IGF2 alleles interact to confer an additional risk for GDM. Thus, in some women, genes responsible for susceptibility to GDM may be similar to the genes conferring risk of Type 2 diabetes, whereas in others, novel genes may contribute to GDM.

Insulin signaling system in normal pregnancy and in gestational diabetes mellitus

The action of insulin is triggered when it binds to the IR. The IR belongs to the IGF receptor (IGFR) family, which possesses an intrinsic tyrosine kinase (TK) activity. The receptor is composed of two alfa-subunits, each linked to a beta-subunit and to each other by disulfide bonds; only the beta-subunit has enzymatic TK activity. When insulin binds to the receptor, the conformational change activates the beta-subunit and autophosphorylation begins. Thus, activation of the TK enzyme leads to increased tyrosine phosphorylation of cellular substrates. IRS-1, a cytosolic protein, binds to the phosphorylated intracellular substrates, thereby transmitting the insulin signal downstream.

The distribution of the IRS proteins tends to be tissue specific: IRS-2 is more copious in the liver and pancreas, whereas both IRS-1 and IRS-2 are widely expressed in skeletal muscle. Insulin stimulates the activation and binding of the lipid kinase enzyme, phosphatidylinositol (PI)-3-kinase, and its binding to IRS-1. The formation of PI is mandatory for insulin action on glucose transport.

Knockout of the IRS-1 gene causes only a moderate increase in insulin resistance due to increased insulin secretion, but not overt diabetes. In women with GDM, the skeletal muscle contains lower levels of IRS-1 protein and significantly less insulin-stimulated IRS-1 tyrosine phosphorylation, while levels of the IRS-2 protein are increased. These findings suggest that the insulin resistance of GDM may be exerted through a decrease in the insulin resistance cascade at the level of the IRS proteins. The increased IRS-2 level may be a compensation for the reduced IRS-1 level.[53] Glucose uptake by cells is mediated by a family of membrane proteins, GLUT1–GLUT4, which have a significant sequence similarity. GLUT4 is the main insulin-sensitive glucose transport, expressed uniquely in skeletal and cardiac muscles and adipose tissue. Garvey et al[54] reported that in rectus abdominis taken from lean and obese women with GDM, GLUT4 content was similar. In GDM, GLUT4 gene expression is normal in skeletal muscles. To the extent that these muscles are representative of the total muscle mass, insulin resistance in skeletal muscle may involve impaired GLUT4 function or translocation, but not its depletion, as observed in adipose tissue. Garvey et al[55] demonstrated that the insulin-stimulated glucose transport in adipocyte tissue was reduced by 60% at term in women with GDM compared to non-diabetic pregnant women. Moreover, the GLUT4 content in adipocytes was profoundly depleted in *c.* 50% of the GDM group. The whole group exhibited a novel abnormality in GLUT4 subcellular distribution; accumulation of GLUT4 in membranes co-fractionating with plasma membranes and high-density microsomes in basal cells, and absence of translocation in response to insulin. These data suggest that abnormalities in cellular traffic or targeting relegate GLUT4 to a membrane compartment from which insulin cannot recruit transporters to the cell surface. This has important implications for skeletal muscle insulin resistance in GDM. The membrane protein plasma cell membrane glycoprotein-1 (PC-1) has been identified as an inhibitor of insulin receptor TK (IRTK) activity. Shao et al[53] investigated IR function and PC-1 levels in muscle from three groups of obese subjects: women with GDM, pregnant women with normal glucose tolerance and non-pregnant control subjects. No significant differences were found in basal IR tyrosine phosphorylation or IRTK activity among the three groups. After maximal insulin stimulation, IRTK activity increased in all subjects, but was lower in women with GDM by 25 and 39% compared with pregnant and non-pregnant control subjects, respectively. Similarly, IR tyrosine phosphorylation was significantly decreased in the subjects with GDM compared to the other two groups. Treatment of the IR with alkaline phosphatase to dephosphorylate serine/threonine residues significantly increased insulin-stimulated IRTK activity in the pregnant control and GDM subjects, but the rates were still lower than in the non-pregnant controls. PC-1 content in muscle from GDM subjects was increased by 63% compared with pregnant control subjects and by 206% compared with non-pregnant control subjects. PC-1 content was negatively correlated with IR phosphorylation and IRTK. Increased PC-1 content in the pregnant control and GDM groups suggests an excessive phosphorylation of serine/threonine residues in

muscle IR, both of which may contribute to the pregnancy-associated decrease in IRTK activity. In GDM, changes worsened, even when controlling for obesity. These postreceptor defects in insulin signaling may contribute to the pathogenesis of GDM and the increased risk for Type 2 diabetes later in life.

Receptor autophosphorylation has also been reported to be impaired in GDM subjects, a finding consistent with their increased insulin resistance.[54] In addition, overexpression of membrane plasma cell differentiation factor-1 (i.e. PC-1) may play a role in developing insulin resistance by inhibiting the TK activity of the IR.[56] In GDM patients, PC-1 levels were significantly higher in skeletal muscle compared to non-diabetic pregnant women.[57]

Conclusions

GDM is carbohydrate intolerance resulting in hyperglycemia of variable severity with onset or first recognition during pregnancy. The incidence of GDM is 0.15–15%, and it corresponds to the prevalence of Type 2 diabetes and IGT within a given population. The predominant pathogenic factor in GDM could be inadequate insulin secretion. It has been convincingly demonstrated that GDM occurs as a result of a combination of insulin resistance and decreased insulin secretion.

The similar frequencies of HLA-DR2, -DR3 and -DR4 antigens in healthy pregnant women and women with GDM, and the low prevalence of markers for autoimmune destruction of the beta cells in GDM, rule out the possibility that GDM has an autoimmune origin. Pregnancy is associated with profound hormonal changes that have a direct effect on carbohydrate tolerance. In early pregnancy, both progesterone and estrogen levels rise, but their action on insulin is counterbalanced, as progesterone causes insulin resistance and estrogen is protective. In the second trimester, hPL, cortisol and prolactin levels all rise, causing decreased phosphorylation of IRS-1 and profound insulin resistance. In most subjects, pancreatic insulin secretion rise to meet this need, but in those with underlying beta-cell defects, hyperglycemia ensues. In women with GDM, the insulin resistance of pregnancy is exaggerated, especially if fasting hyperglycemia is present, and is related to additional defective tyrosine phosphorylation of the insulin receptor beta-subunit. Recent research suggests that the postreceptor mechanisms that contribute to insulin resistance of pregnancy are multifactorial, but are exerted at the beta-subunit of the IR and at the level of IRS-1. The resistance to insulin-mediated glucose transport appears to be greater in skeletal muscle from GDM subjects than from pregnancy alone. There is also a modest but significant decrease in the maximal IR tyrosine phosphorylation in muscle from obese GDM subjects. Results also suggest that increased IR serine/threonine phosphorylation and PC-1 could underlie the insulin resistance of pregnancy and contribute to the pathogenesis of GDM.

Whether additional defects are exerted further downstream from IRS-1 remains to be investigated. GDM is a predictor of diabetes (mainly Type 2) later in life. The cumulative incidence of Type 2 diabetes is *c.* 50% at 5 years. GDM is also a predictor, or even an early manifestation, of the metabolic (insulin resistance) syndrome. GDM is a cardiovascular risk factor and affected patients should be screened to prevent late complications.

References

1. Metzger BE, Coustan DR. Summary and recommendations of the Fourth International Workshop–Conference on Gestational Diabetes Mellitus. *Diabetes Care* 1998; 21:B161–B167.

2. Ryan EA, O'Sullivan MJ, Skyler JS. Insulin action during pregnancy: studies with the euglycemic clamp technique. *Diabetes* 1985; 34:380–9.

3. Catalano PM, Tyzbir ED, Wolfe RR et al. Carbohydrate metabolism during pregnancy in control subjects and women with gestational diabetes. *Am J Physiol* 1993; 264:E60–E67.

4. Kuhl C. Insulin secretion and insulin resistance in pregnancy and GDM: implications for diagnosis and management. *Diabetes* 1991; 40:18–24.

5. DeFronzo RA, Tobin JD, Andres R. Glucose clamp technique: a method for quantifying insulin secretion and resistance. *Am J Physiol* 1979; 237:E241–E243.

6. Bergman RN, Ider YZ, Bowden CR, Cobelli C. Quantitative estimation of insulin sensitivity. *Am J Physiol* 1979; 236:E667–E677.

7. Bergman RN. The Lilly Lecture 1989. Toward a physiological understanding of glucose tolerance: minimal model approach. *Diabetes* 1989; 38:1512–28.

8. Catalano PM, Tyzbir ED, Roman NM et al. Longitudinal changes in insulin release and insulin resistance in nonobese pregnant women. *Am J Obstet Gynecol* 1991; 165:1667–72.

9. Catalano PM, Huston L, Amini SB, Kalham SC. Longitudinal change in glucose metabolism during pregnancy in obese women with normal glucose tolerance and gestational diabetes mellitus. *Am J Obstet Gynecol* 1999; 180:903–16.

10. Burt RL. Peripheral utilization of glucose in pregnancy. Insulin tolerance. *Obstet Gynecol* 1956; 2:558–664.

11. Spellacy WN, Goetz FC. Plasma insulin in normal late pregnancy. *N Engl J Med* 1963; 268:988–91.

12. Kuhl C. Glucose metabolism during and after pregnancy in normal and gestational diabetic women. *Acta Endocrinol* 1975; 79:709–19.

13. Buchanan TA, Metzger BE, Freinkel N, Bergman RN. Insulin sensitivity and B-cell responsiveness to glucose during late pregnancy in lean and moderately obese women with normal glucose tolerance or mild gestational diabetes. *Am J Obstet Gynecol* 1990; 162:1008–14.

14. Cousins L, Rea C, Crawford M. Longitudinal characterization of insulin sensitivity and body fat in normal and gestational diabetic pregnancies. *Diabetes* 1988; 37:251A (abstract).

15. Hauguel S, Leturque A, Gilbert M, Girard J. Effects of pregnancy and fasting on muscle glucose utilization in the rabbit. *Am J Obstet Gynecol* 1988; 158:1215–18.

16. Leturque A, Ferre P, Burnol AF et al. Glucose utilization rates and insulin sensitivity in vivo in tissues of virgin and pregnant rats. *Diabetes* 1986; 35:172–7.

17. Kalhan SC, D'Angelo LJ, Savin SM, Adan SM. Glucose production in pregnant women at term gestation: sources of glucose for the human fetus. *J Clin Invest* 1979; 63:388–94.

18. Cowett RA, Susa JB, Kahn CB et al. Glucose kinetics in non-diabetic and diabetic women during third

trimester of pregnancy. *Am J Obstet Gynecol* 1983; **146**:773–80.

19. Catalano PM, Ishizika T, Friedman JE. Glucose metabolism in pregnancy. In: *Principles of Perinatal Neonatal Metabolism*, 2nd edn. (Springer-Verlag: New York, 1998) 183–206.

20. Ryan EA, Ennes L. Role of gestational hormones in the induction of insulin resistance. *J Clin Endocrinol Metab* 1988; **67**:341–7.

21. Costrini NV, Kalkhoff RK. Relative effect of pregnancy estradiol and progesterone on plasma insulin and pancreatic islet insulin secretion. *J Clin Invest* 1971; **50**: 992–9.

22. Kalkhoff RK, Jacobson M, Lemper D. Progesterone, pregnancy and the augmented plasma insulin response. *J Clin Endocrinol* 1970; **31**:24–8.

23. Gonzalez C, Alonso A, Alvarez N et al. Role of 17beta-estradiol and/or progesterone on insulin sensitivity in the rat: implications during pregnancy. *J Endocrinol* 2000; **166**:283–9.

24. Gibson M, Tulchinski D. The maternal adrenal In: (Tulchinski D, Ryan KJ, eds) *Maternal-fetal Endocrinology*. (WB Saunders: Philadelphia, 1980) 129–43.

25. Rizza RA, Mandarino LJ, Gerich JE. Cortisol induced insulin resistance in man: impaired suppression of glucose production and stimulation of glucose utilization due to a postreceptor defect of insulin action. *Clin Endocrinol Metab* 1982; **54**: 131–8.

26. Ahmed SA, Shalayel MH. Role of cortisol in the deterioration of glucose tolerance in Sudanese pregnant women. *East Afr Med J* 1999; **76**:465–7.

27. Gustafson AB, Banasiak MF, Kalkhoff RK. Correlation of hyperprolactinemia with altered plasma insulin and glucose: similarity to effects of late human pregnancy. *J Clin Endocrinol Metab* 1980; **51**:242–6.

28. Sorenson RL, Brelje TC, Roth C. Effect of steroid and lactogenic hormones on islet of Langerhans: a new hypothesis for the role of pregnancy steroids in the adaptation of islets to pregnancy. *Endocrinology* 1993; **133**: 2227–33.

29. Skouby SO, Kuhl C, Hornnes PJ, Andersen AN. Prolactin and glucose tolerance in normal and gestational diabetic pregnancy. *Obstet Gynecol* 1986; **67**:17–20.

30. Beck P, Daughday WH. Human placental lactogen: studies of its acute metabolic effects and disposition in normal man. *J Clin Invest* 1967; **46**:103–10.

31. Brelje TC, Scharp DW, Lacy PE et al. Effect of homologous placental lactogens, prolactins, and growth hormones on islet B-cell division and insulin secretion in rat, mouse, and human islets: implication for placental lactogen regulation of islet function during pregnancy. *Endocrinology* 1993; **132**:879–87.

32. Sivitz WI, Walsh SA, Morgan DA et al. Effect of leptin on insulin sensitivity in normal rats. *J Clin Invest* 1997; **138**:3395–401.

33. Henson MC, Swan KF, O'Neil JS. Expression of placental leptin and leptin receptor transcripts in early pregnancy and at term. *Obstet Gynecol* 1998; **92**: 1020–8.

34. Masuzaki H, Ogawa Y, Sagawa N. Nonadipose tissue production of leptin: leptin as a novel placenta-derived hormone in humans. *Nat Med* 1997; **3**:1029–33.

35. Highman TJ, Friedman JE, Huston LP et al. Longitudinal changes in maternal serum leptin concentrations body composition and resting metabolic rate in pregnancy. *Am J Obstet Gynecol* 1999; **178**:1010–15.

36. Yamashita H, Shao J, Ishizuka T et al. Leptin administration prevents spontaneous gestational diabetes in heterozygous Lepr (db/+) mice: effects on placental leptin and fetal growth. *Endocrinology* 2001; **142**:2888–97.

37. Kautzky-Willer A, Pacini G, Tura A et al. Increased plasma leptin in gestational diabetes. *Diabetologia* 2001; **44**:164–72.

38. Vitoratos N, Salamalekis E, Kassanos D et al. Maternal plasma leptin levels and their relationship to insulin and glucose in gestational-onset diabetes. *Gynecol Obstet Invest* 2001; **51**:17–21.

39. Wiznitzer A, Furman B, Zuili I et al. Cord leptin level and fetal macrosomia. *Obstet Gynecol* 2000; **96**:707–13.

40. Coughlan MT, Oliva K, Georgiou HM et al. Glucose-induced release of tumor necrosis factor-alpha from human placental and adipose tissues in gestational diabetes mellitus. *Diabet Med* 2001; **18**:921–7.

41. Catalano P, Highman T, Huston L, Friedman J. Relationship between reproductive hormones/TNF-α and longitudinal changes in insulin sensitivity during gestation. *Diabetes* 1996; **45**:175a.

42. Di Iorio R, Marinoni E, Urban G et al. Fetomaternal adrenomedullin levels in diabetic pregnancy. *Horm Metab Res* 2001; **33**:486–90.

43. Van Assche FA, Aerts L, De Prins F. A morphological study of the endocrine pancreas in human pregnancy. *Br J Obstet Gynecol* 1978; **85**:818–20.

44. Swinn RA, Warham NJ, Gregory R et al. Excessive secretion of insulin precursors characterizes and predicts gestational diabetes. *Diabetes* 1995; **44**:911–15.

45. Kjos SL, Peters RK, Xiang A et al. Predicting future diabetes in Latino women with gestational diabetes: utility of early postpartum glucose tolerance testing. *Diabetes* 1995; **44**:586–91.

46. Damm P, Kuhl C, Buschard K et al. Prevalence and predictive value of women with islet cell antibodies and insulin autoantibodies in women with gestational diabetes. *Diabet Med* 1994; **11**:558–63.

47. Catalano PM, Tyzbir ED, Simms EAH. Incidence and significance of islet cell antibodies in women with previous gestational diabetes. *Diabetes Care* 1990; **113**:478–83.

48. Stoffel M, Bell KL, Blacburn CL et al. Identification of glucokinase mutations in subjects with gestational diabetes mellitus. *Diabetes* 1993; **42**:937–40.

49. McLeallan JAS, Barrow BA, Levy JC et al. Prevalence of diabetes mellitus and impaired glucose tolerance in parents of women with gestational diabetes. *Diabetologia* 1995; **38**:693–8.

50. Harder T, Franke K, Kohlhoff R, Plagemann A. Maternal and paternal family history of diabetes in women with gestational diabetes or insulin-dependent diabetes mellitus type I. *Gynecol Obstet Invest* 2001; **51**:160–4.

51. Vambergue A, Fajardy I, Bianchi F et al. Gestational diabetes mellitus and HLA class II (-DQ, -DR) association: the Digest Study. *Eur J Immunogenet* 1997; **24**:385–94.

52. Ober C, Xiang KS, Thisted RA et al. Increased risk for gestational diabetes mellitus associated with insulin receptor and insulin-like growth factor II restriction fragment length polymorphisms. *Genet Epidemiol* 1989; **5**:559–69.

53. Shao J, Catalano PM, Yamashita H et al. Decreased insulin receptor tyrosine kinase activity and plasma cell membrane glycoprotein-1 overexpression in skeletal muscle from obese women with gestational diabetes mellitus (GDM): evidence for increased serine/threonine phosphorylation in pregnancy and GDM. *Diabetes* 2000; **49**:603–10.

54. Garvey WT, Maianu L, Hancock JA et al. Gene expression of GLUT4 in skeletal muscle from insulin-resistant patients with obesity, IGT, GDM, and NIDDM. *Diabetes* 1992; **41**:465–75.

55. Garvey WT, Maianu L, Zhu J-H et al. Multiple defects in the adipocyte glucose transport system cause cellular insulin resistance in gestational diabetes. *Diabetes* 1993; **42**:1773–85.

56. Goldfine ID, Maddux BA, Youngrem JF et al. Membrane glycoprotein PC-1 and insulin resistance. *J Cell Biochem* 1998; **182**:177–84.

57. Shao J, Catalano PM, Yamashita H et al. Impaired insulin receptor tyrosine kinase activity and overexpression of PC-1 in skeletal muscle from obese women with gestational diabetes mellitus. *Diabetes* 1999; **48**:A53.

6

Maternal metabolic adaptation to pregnancy
Patrick M Catalano

Introduction

There are significant alterations in maternal metabolism during pregnancy that provide for adequate nutritional stores in early gestation in order to meet the increased maternal and fetal demands of late gestation and lactation. In this chapter, maternal glucose metabolism as it relates to pancreatic beta-cell production of insulin and insulin clearance, endogenous, i.e. primarily hepatic, glucose production and suppression with insulin, and peripheral glucose insulin sensitivity will be considered. Also, maternal protein and lipid insulin metabolism will be addressed. Lastly, the impact of these alterations on maternal metabolism will be examined as they relate to maternal energy expenditure, fat accretion and fetal growth.

Carbohydrate metabolism

Normal pregnancy has been characterized as a 'diabetogenic state' because of the progressive increase in postprandial glucose and insulin response in late gestation. However, early gestation can be viewed as an anabolic condition because of the increase in maternal fat stores and the decrease in free fatty acid concentration. Weiss and Hofman[1] have described significant decreases in maternal insulin requirements in early gestation in insulin-dependent women with optimal glucose control prior to conception. The mechanism for this decrease in insulin requirements have been ascribed to various factors, including increased insulin sensitivity, decreased substrate availability secondary to factors such as nausea, the fetus acting as a glucose sink or enhanced maternal insulin secretion. Longitudinal studies in women with normal glucose tolerance have shown significant progressive alterations in all aspects of glucose metabolism as early as the end of the first trimester.[2]

There are progressive increases in insulin secretion in response to an intravenous glucose challenge with advancing gestation (Figs 6.1 and 6.2). The increases in insulin concentration are more pronounced in lean as compared obese women, most probably as a response to the greater decreases in insulin sensitivity in lean women (as will be described later). Data regarding insulin clearance in pregnancy are scant. In separate studies Bellman and Harbman,[3] Lind et al[4] and Burt and Davidson[5] reported no difference in insulin disappearance rate when insulin was infused intravenously in late gestation in comparison with non-gravid subjects. In contrast, Goodner and Freinkel,[6] using a radiolabeled insulin, described a 25% increase in insulin turnover in a pregnant as compared with a non-pregnant rat model. Catalano et al,[7] using the euglycemic clamp

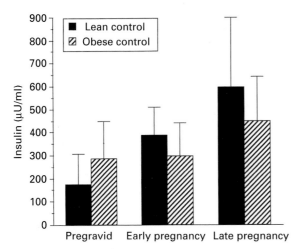

Figure 6.1. *Longitudinal increase in insulin response to an intravenous glucose challenge in lean and obese women with normal glucose tolerance: pregravid, and early and late pregnancy. First phase: area under the curve from 0 to 5 minutes (mean ±SD).*

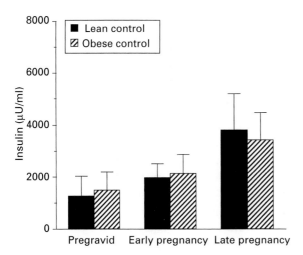

Figure 6.2. *Longitudinal increase in insulin response to an intravenous glucose challenge in lean and obese women with normal glucose tolerance: pregravid, and early and late pregnancy. Second phase: area under the curve from 5 to 60 minutes (mean ±SD).*

model, reported a 20% increase in lean and 30% increase in obese women of insulin clearance by late pregnancy (Fig. 6.3). Although the

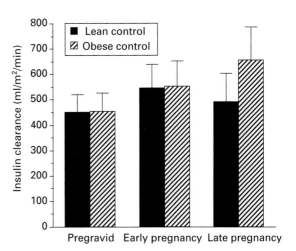

Figure 6.3. *Longitudinal increase in metabolic clearance rate of insulin in lean and obese women with normal glucose tolerance: pregravid, and early and late pregnancy (mean ±SD).*

placenta is rich in insulinase, the exact mechanism for the increased insulin clearance in pregnancy remains speculative.

Although there is a progressive decrease in fasting glucose with advancing gestation (Fig. 6.4), the decrease is most probably a result of the increase in plasma volume in early gestation and the increase in feto-placental glucose utilization in late gestation. Kalhan et al[8] and Cowett et al,[9] using various stable isotope methodologies in cross-sectional study designs, were the first to describe increased fasting hepatic glucose production in late pregnancy. Additionally, Catalano et al,[10] using a stable isotope of glucose in a prospective longitudinal study design, reported a 30% increase in maternal fasting hepatic glucose production with advancing gestation (Fig. 6.5), which remained significant even when adjusted for maternal weight gain. Tissue sensitivity to insulin involves both liver and peripheral tissues, primarily skeletal muscle. The increase in fasting maternal hepatic glucose production occurred despite a significant increase in fasting insulin

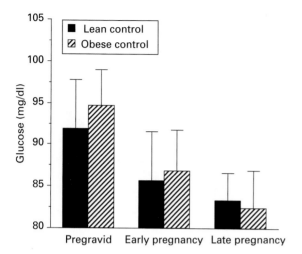

Figure 6.4. *Longitudinal decreases in maternal fasting glucose in lean and obese women with normal glucose tolerance: pregravid, and early and late pregnancy (mean ±SD).*

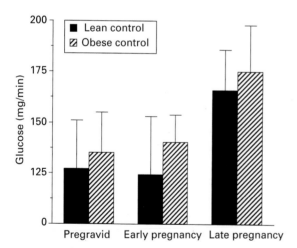

Figure 6.5. *Longitudinal increase in basal endogenous (primarily hepatic) glucose production in lean and obese women with normal glucose tolerance: pregravid, and early and late pregnancy (mean ±SD).*

concentration, thereby indicating a decrease in maternal hepatic glucose sensitivity in women with normal glucose tolerance. Additionally, in obese women there was a decreased ability of infused insulin to suppress hepatic glucose

production in late gestation as compared with pregravid and early pregnancy measurements, thereby indicating a further decrease in hepatic insulin sensitivity in obese women.[11]

Estimates of peripheral insulin sensitivity in pregnancy have included the measurement of insulin response to a fixed oral or intravenous glucose challenge or the ratio of insulin to glucose under a variety of experimental conditions. In recent years, newer methodologies, e.g. the Bergman minimal model[12] and the euglycemic–hyperinsulinemic[13] clamp, have improved the ability to quantify peripheral insulin sensitivity. In lean women in early gestation, Catalano et al[14] reported a 40% decrease in maternal peripheral insulin sensitivity using the euglycemic–hyperinsulinemic clamp. However, when adjusted for changes in insulin concentrations during the clamp and residual hepatic glucose production, i.e. the insulin sensitivity index, insulin sensitivity decreased by only 10% (Fig. 6.6). In contrast, there was a

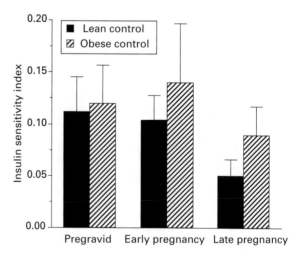

Figure 6.6. *Longitudinal changes in the insulin sensitivity index (glucose infusion rate adjusted for residual endogenous glucose production and insulin concentrations achieved during the glucose clamp) in lean and obese women with normal glucose tolerance: pregravid, and early and late gestation (mean ±SD).*

15% increase in the insulin sensitivity index in obese women in early pregnancy as compared with pregravid estimates.[15] Hence, the decrease in insulin requirements in early gestation observed in some women requiring insulin may be a consequence of a relative increase in insulin sensitivity, particularly in women with decreased insulin sensitivity prior to conception. As compared with the metabolic alterations in early pregnancy there is a uniformity of opinion regarding the decrease in peripheral insulin sensitivity in late gestation. Spellacy et al[16] were among the first investigators to report an increase in insulin response to a glucose challenge in late gestation. Additionally, Burt[17] demonstrated that pregnant women experienced less hypoglycemia in response to exogenous insulin in comparison with non-pregnant subjects. Later research by Fisher et al[18] using a high-dose glucose infusion test, Buchanan et al[19] using the Bergman minimal model, and Ryan et al[20] and Catalano et al[2] using the euglycemic–hyperinsulinemic clamp all have demonstrated a decrease in insulin sensitivity ranging from 33 to 78%. It should be noted, however, that all these quantitative estimates of insulin sensitivity are very likely overestimates due to non-insulin-mediated glucose disposal by the fetus and placenta. Hay et al[21] reported that in the pregnant ewe model, approximately one third of maternal glucose utilization was accounted for by uterine, placental and fetal tissue. Additionally, Marconi et al[22] reported that, based on human fetal blood sampling, fetal glucose concentration was a function of fetal size and gestational age in addition to maternal glucose concentration.

Placental glucose transport is non-energy dependent and takes place through facilitated diffusion. Glucose transport is dependent upon the glucose transporter (GLUT) family. The principal glucose transporter in the placenta is GLUT1, which is located in the syncytiotrophoblast.[23] GLUT1 is located on both the microvillus and basal membranes. Basal membrane GLUT1 may be the rate-limiting step in placental glucose transport. There is a two to threefold increase in the expression of syncytiotrophoblast glucose tranporters with advancing gestation.[24] Although GLUT3 and GLUT4 expression have been identified in placental endothelial cells and intervillous non-trophoblastic cells, respectively, the role they may play in placental glucose transport remains speculative.[25,26]

The mechanisms responsible for the decreases in insulin sensitivity are now just beginning to be understood. Studies in human skeletal muscle and adipose tissue have demonstrated that post receptor defects in the insulin signaling cascade are related to decreased insulin sensitivity in pregnancy. Garvey et al[27] were the first to demonstrate that there were no significant differences in the glucose transporter (GLUT4) responsible for insulin action and skeletal muscle in pregnant as compared with non-pregnant women. Based on the studies of Friedman et al,[28] in both pregnant women with normal glucose tolerance and gestational diabetes compared with weight-matched non-pregnant control subjects, there are defects in the insulin signaling cascade relating to pregnancy. All pregnant women appeared to have a decrease in insulin receptor substrate (IRS)-1 expression as compared with weight-matched non-pregnant controls. The downregulation of the IRS-1 protein closely parallels the decreased ability of insulin to induce additional steps in the insulin signaling cascade in order to result in movement of GLUT4 to the cell-surface membrane in order to facilitate glucose transport into the cell. The downregulation of IRS-1 protein closely parallels the ability of insulin to stimulate 2-deoxyglucose uptake *in vitro*.

The alterations in insulin sensitivity have been ascribed to placental hormone production, human placental lactogen being most often cited, because of the increased concentration in late gestation. However, more recent data implicate the cytokine tumour necrosis factor (TNF)-α as a potential factor affecting IRS-1 function in the signaling cascade.[29]

Amino acid metabolism

Although glucose is the primary source of energy for the fetus and placenta, there are not appreciable amounts of glucose stored as glycogen in the fetus or the placenta. However, accretion of protein is essential for growth of feto-placental tissue. There is increased nitrogen retention in pregnancy in both maternal and fetal compartments. For example, it is estimated that there is c. 0.9 kg accretion of maternal protein by 27 weeks.[30] There is a significant decrease in most fasting maternal amino acid concentrations in early pregnancy prior to the accretion of significant maternal or fetal tissue.[31] These anticipatory changes in fasting amino acid metabolism occur after a shorter period of fasting in comparison with non-pregnant women, and may be another example of the accelerated starvation of pregnancy as described by Freinkel et al.[32] Furthermore, amino acid concentrations, e.g. serine, correlate significantly with fetal growth in both early and late gestation.[33] Maternal amino acid concentrations were significantly decreased in mothers of small-for-gestational-age neonates in comparison with maternal concentrations in appropriately grown neonates.[34]

There is also a significant conservation of nitrogen/protein in late gestation. There is a decrease in maternal plasma urea nitrogen concentrations as well as a decrease in urea nitrogen synthesis and excretion.[35] In evaluating the balance between protein breakdown and resynthesis, estimates of amino acid turnover using stable isotopes of, for example, leucine are useful. Studies by Denne and Kalhan[36] have shown that the rates of basal or fasting proteolysis, or protein turnover, are similar in pregnant and non-pregnant subjects, indicating that there may be no change in fasting amino acid insulin sensitivity in pregnancy. Additionally, there are no published studies evaluating the effects of infused insulin on amino acid turnover during pregnancy in women with normal or abnormal glucose tolerances. Therefore, based on studies of whole-body protein turnover in late gestation, there may be a slight decrease in the rate of protein breakdown during fasting[37] and a small increase in protein turnover during the day.[38] Thus, additional studies are required in order to understand the alterations in amino acid metabolism during pregnancy as related to normal and abnormal maternal and feto-placental protein growth and development.

Amino acids are actively transported across a concentration gradient from the mother to both the fetus and the placenta via energy-requiring amino acid transporters. Amino acid transporters are highly stereospecific, but have low substrate specificity. Additionally, they may vary with location between the microvillus and basal membranes.[39] Decreased amino acid concentrations have been reported in growth-restricted neonates in comparison with appropriately grown neonates. Decreased amino acid transporter activity has been implicated as a possible mechanism. However, the potential role, if any, of placental amino acid transporters in macrosomic infants of women with diabetes is currently unknown.[40]

Lipid metabolism

While there is ample literature regarding the changes in glucose metabolism during gestation, the data regarding the alterations in lipid metabolism are meager by comparison. Knopp et al[41] have reported that there is a two- to fourfold increase in total triglyceride concentration and a 25–50% increase in total cholesterol concentration during gestation. Additionally, there is a 50% increase in low-density lipoprotein (LDL) cholesterol and a 30% increase in high-density lipoprotein (HDL) cholesterol by mid-gestation which decreases slightly in the third trimester. Maternal triglyceride and very-low-density lipoprotein (VLDL) triglyceride levels in late gestation are positively correlated with maternal estriol and insulin concentrations.

Recent studies by Catalano et al[42] have evaluated the longitudinal changes in insulin suppression of using the hyperinsulinemic–euglycemic clamp. There was a significant decrease in the ability of infused insulin to suppress free fatty acid concentration from the time prior to conception through early and late gestation. Hence, there is evidence for decreased maternal lipid insulin sensitivity in late gestation. Similarly, decreases in adipocytes IRS-1 expression may be a factor in the decreased lipid insulin sensitivity in pregnant as compared with non-pregnant subjects.[42]

The increase in maternal lipid concentration in certain free fatty acids in late gestation has been hypothesized as a possible mechanism relating to the decrease in maternal glucose insulin sensitivity in late pregnancy.[43] Free fatty acids have been associated with fetal overgrowth, particularly of fetal adipose tissue. There is a significant difference in the arteriovenous free fatty acid concentration at birth, much as there is with arteriovenous glucose concentration. Knopp et al[44,45] have reported that neonatal birthweight is positively correlated with triglyceride and free fatty acid concentrations, both of which readily cross the placenta in late pregnancy. Similar conclusions were reached by Ogburn et al,[46] who showed, using a pregnant ewe model, that increased fetal insulin concentrations decrease free fatty acid concentrations, inhibit lipolysis and result in increased fat deposition. Lastly, Kleigman et al[47] reported that infants of obese women not only had increased birthweight and skinfold measurements but free fatty acids were also increased in comparison with infants of lean women.

Maternal weight gain and energy expenditure

Estimates of the energy cost of pregnancy range from a cost of 80,000 kcal to a net saving of up to 10,000 kcal.[48] As a result, the recommendations for nutritional intake in pregnancy are diverse and depend upon the population being evaluated. Furthermore, based on more recent data, recommendations for individuals within a population may be more diverse that previously believed, making general guidelines for nutritional intake difficult.[49]

The theoretical energy cost of pregnancy was originally estimated by Hytten and Leitch,[3] using the factorial method. The additional energy cost of pregnancy consisted of the additional maternal and feto-placental tissue accrued during pregnancy, and the additional 'running cost' of pregnancy of, for example, increased cardiac output. In Hytten and Leitch's[3] model the greatest increases in maternal energy expenditure occur between 10 and 30 weeks gestation, primarily because of maternal accretion of adipose tissue – c. 10,000 kcal/kg adipose tissue. However, the mean increases in maternal adipose tissue vary considerably among various ethnic groups. Forsum et al[50] reported a mean increase > 5 kg of adipose tissue in Swedish women, whereas Lawrence et al[51] found no increase in adipose tissue stores in women from the Gambia with their usual nutritional intake.

Basal metabolic rate accounts for 60–70% of total energy expenditure in individuals not engaged in competitive physical activity and correlates well with total energy expenditure. As with the changes in maternal accretion of adipose tissue, there are wide variations in the change in maternal basal metabolic rate during gestation, not only in different populations but also within relatively homogeneous groups. The cumulative energy changes in basal metabolic rate range from a high of 52,000 kcal in Swedish women[52] to a net saving of 10,700 kcal in women from the Gambia[51] without nutritional supplementation. The mean increase in basal metabolic rate in Western women relative to a non-pregnant, non-lactating control group, averages c. 20%.[53] However, the coefficient of variation in basal metabolic rate in these populations during gestation ranges from 93% in women from the UK[54] to > 200% in Swedish women.[52] When assessing energy intake in relation to energy expenditure, however, estimated energy intake remains significantly lower than the estimates of total energy expenditure. These discrepancies have usually been explained by factors such as: (1) increased metabolic efficiency during gestation;[55] (2) decreased maternal activity;[56] and (3) unreliable assessment of food intake.[54]

Data in non-pregnant subjects may help explain some of the wide variations in metabolic parameters measured during human gestation, even within homogeneous populations. Swinburn et al[57] reported that in the Pima Indian population, subjects with decreased insulin sensitivity gained less weight as compared with insulin-sensitive subjects (3.1 versus 7.6 kg) over a period of 4 years. Furthermore, the percentage weight change

per year was highly correlated with glucose disposal as estimated from clamp studies. Catalano et al[58] conducted a prospective longitudinal study in early pregnancy of the changes in maternal accretion of body fat and basal metabolic rate in women with normal glucose tolerance and gestational diabetes in relation to alterations in insulin sensitivity. Women with gestational diabetes had decreased glucose insulin sensitivity in early gestation as compared with the control group, and had significantly smaller increases in body fat than women with normal glucose tolerance. When correlated with the changes in glucose insulin sensitivity, there was a significant inverse correlation between the changes in fat accretion and insulin sensitivity, i.e. women with decreased pregravid insulin sensitivity had less accretion of body fat as compared with women with increased pregravid insulin sensitivity (Fig. 6.7). These results are consistent with a previous report showing that total weight gain in women with gestational diabetes was 2.5 kg less as compared to a weight-matched control group.[59]

In these same subjects there was also a significant inverse correlation between changes in basal metabolic rate and basal hepatic glucose production.[58] In early gestation, there was a 7% increase in basal metabolic rate in women with normal glucose tolerance and only a 2% increase in women with gestational diabetes. As before, there was a significant negative correlation between the changes in basal metabolic rate and estimates of glucose metabolism, in this case basal hepatic glucose production. The results of these studies show that there is a relationship between the changes in maternal insulin sensitivity and the changes in basal metabolic rate and accretion of adipose tissue in early gestation. The ability of women with decreased pregravid glucose insulin sensitivity to conserve energy

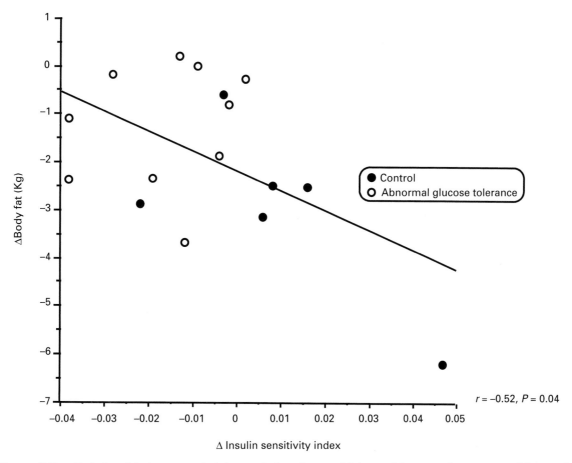

Figure 6.7. *Relationship between the change in insulin sensitivity and fat mass from pregravid to early pregnancy. Increase in fat mass by 12–14 weeks gestation was significantly less in women with decreased pregravid insulin sensitivity compared with subjects with more normal pregravid insulin sensitivity.*

expenditure and accretion of body fat, and make available sufficient nutrients to produce a healthy fetus, supports the hypothesis that decreased maternal insulin sensitivity may have a reproductive metabolic advantage in women when food availability is marginal. In contrast, decreased maternal insulin sensitivity before conception in areas where food is plentiful and a sedentary lifestyle is more common, may manifest itself as gestational diabetes during pregnancy and increase the long-term risk for both diabetes and obesity in the woman and her offspring.

Maternal metabolism and fetal growth

According to the Pedersen hypothesis, maternal hyperglycemia results in fetal hyperglycemia and hyperinsulinemia, resulting in excessive fetal growth. Increased fetal beta-cell mass may be identified as early as the second trimester.[60] Evidence supporting the Pedersen hypothesis has come from studies of amniotic fluid and cord blood insulin, and C-peptide concentrations. Both are increased in the amniotic fluid of insulin-treated women with diabetes at term[61] and correlate with neonatal fat mass.[62] Lipids and amino acids, which are elevated in pregnancies complicated by gestational diabetes, may also play a role in excessive fetal growth by the stimulation of insulin and other growth factors from the fetal pancreatic beta cells and the placenta. Infants of mothers with gestational diabetes have an increase primarily of fat mass as compared with fat-free mass.[63] Additionally, the growth is disproportionate, with chest:head and shoulder:head ratios larger than those of infants of women with normal glucose tolerance, which may contribute to the higher rate of shoulder dystocia and birth trauma observed in these infants.[64]

The results of several clinical series have validated the Pedersen hypothesis inasmuch as tight maternal glycemic control has been associated with a decline in the incidence of macrosomia. In a series of 260 insulin-dependent women achieving fasting plasma glucose concentrations of 109–140 mg/dl, Gabbe et al[65] observed 58 (22%) macrosomic infants. Kitzmiller and Cloherty[66] reported that 11% of 134 women achieving fasting glucose concentrations of 105–121 mg/dl were delivered of an infant with a birthweight > 4000 g. A more dramatic reduction in the rate of macrosomia has been reported when more physiologic control has been achieved. Roversi and Gargiulo[67] instituted a program of 'maximally tolerated' insulin administration and observed macrosomia in only 6% of cases. Jovanovic et al[68] eliminated macrosomia in 52 women who achieved mean glucose levels of 80–87 mg/dl throughout gestation. Landon et al,[69] using daily capillary glucose values obtained during the second and third trimesters in insulin-dependent women, reported a rate of 9% macrosomia when mean values were < 110 mg/dl compared with 34% when less optimal control was achieved. Jovanovic-Peterson et al[70] have suggested that 1 hour

post-prandial glucose measurements correlate best with the frequency of macrosomia. After controlling for other factors, these authors noted that the strongest prediction for birthweight was third trimester non-fasting glucose measurements.

In a series of metabolic studies, Catalano et al[71] estimated body composition in 183 neonates using anthropometry. Fat-free mass, which comprised 86% of mean birthweight, accounted for 83% of the variance in birthweight and fat mass, which comprised only 14% of birthweight, accounted for 46% of the variance in birthweight. There was also a significantly greater fat-free mass in male as compared with female infants. Using independent variables, e.g. maternal height, pregravid weight, weight gain during pregnancy, parity, paternal height and weight, neonatal sex and gestational age, the authors accounted for 29% of the variance in birthweight, 30% of the variance in fat-free mass and 17% of the variance in fat mass (Table 6.1).[72] Including estimates of maternal insulin sensitivity in 16 additional lean subjects, the present author was able to explain 48% of the variance in birthweight, 53% of the variance in fat-free mass and 46% of the variance in fat mass (Table 6.2).[73] Of interest, insulin sensitivity in late gestation had the strongest correlation with birthweight (Fig. 6.8). Studies by Caruso et al[74] corroborated these findings when they reported that women with unexplained fetal growth restriction had greater insulin sensitivity as compared with a control group of women whose infants were of appropriate weight for gestational age. There was a significant positive correlation between weight gain in women with normal glucose tolerance but a negative non-significant correlation in women with gestational diabetes. In women with normal glucose tolerance, the correlation was strongest in women who were lean before conception and became

Dependent and independent variables	R^2	ΔR^2
Birthweight		
Estimated gestational age	0.10	
Maternal weight gain	0.16	0.06
Maternal pregravid weight	0.21	0.05
Neonatal sex	0.25	0.04
Parity	0.29	0.04
Fat-free mass		
Neonatal sex	0.08	
Estimated gestational age	0.17	0.09
Maternal weight gain	0.23	0.06
Maternal pregravid weight	0.27	0.04
Paternal height	0.30	0.03
Fat mass		
Parity	0.08	
Estimated gestational age	0.12	0.04
Pregravid weight	0.14	0.02
Maternal weight gain	0.16	0.02
Neonatal sex	0.17	0.01

Table 6.1.   *Stepwise regression analysis (n = 183).*

Dependent and independent variables	R^2	ΔR^2
Birthweight		
Insulin sensitivity index (late pregnancy)	0.28	
Maternal weight gain	0.48	0.20
Fat-free mass		
Insulin sensitivity index (late pregnancy)	0.33	
Maternal weight gain	0.53	0.20
Fat mass		
Insulin sensitivity index (pregravid)	0.15	
Parity	0.29	0.14
Neonatal sex	0.39	0.07
Placental weight		
Insulin sensitivity index (late pregnancy)	0.28	
Neonatal sex	0.50	0.22
Maternal weight gain	0.58	0.08

Table 6.2.   *Stepwise regression analysis (n = 16).*

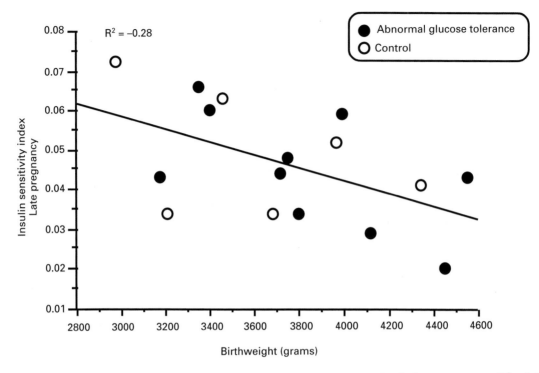

Figure 6.8. *Relationship between birthweight and insulin sensitivity index in late pregnancy (R² = 0.28).*

progressively weaker as pregravid weight for height increased.[59] In women with gestational diabetes, there were no significant correlations between maternal weight gain and birthweight, irrespective of pregravid weight for height. These studies emphasize the role of maternal metabolic environment and fetal growth.

In addition to the perinatal risk associated with fetal macrosomia in the infants of women with abnormal glucose tolerance, there are significant long-term risks. The increase in birthweight of these infants tends to normalize by 1 year of age before increasing again in early childhood.[75] There is an increase in the risk of obesity in these children between the ages of 1 and 9, and in adolescents between the ages of 14 and 16. Silverman et al[75] reported that there is a strong correlation between amniotic fluid insulin levels and increased body mass index

[weight (kg)/height (m)²] in 14–17 year olds, indicating an association between islet cell activation *in utero* and development of childhood obesity. This obesity present in childhood then predisposes to obesity in the adult. Pettitt et al[76] have shown that infants born to Pima Indian women with impaired glucose tolerance were more obese as children than infants of women with normal glucose tolerance, even when they developed diabetes later.[76] These data suggest that there are both *in utero* maternal metabolic factors and genetic factors in the later development of obesity, and possibly Type 2 diabetes.

References

1. Weiss PAM, Hofman H. Intensified conventional insulin therapy for the pregnant diabetic patient. *Obstet Gynecol* 1984; **64**:629–37.

2. Catalano PM, Tyzbir ED, Roman NM et al. Longitudinal changes in insulin release and insulin resistance in non-obese pregnant women. *Am J Obstet Gynecol* 1991; **165**:1667–72.

3. Bellman O, Hartman E. Influence of pregnancy on the kinetics of insulin. *Am J Obstet Gynecol* 1975; **122**:829–33.

4. Lind T, Bell S, Gilmore E. Insulin disappearance rate in pregnant and non-pregnant women and in non-pregnant women given GHRIH. *Eur J Clin Invest* 1977; **7**:47–51.

5. Burt RL, Davidson IWF. Insulin half-life and utilization in normal pregnancy. *Obstet Gynecol* 1974; **43**:161–70.

6. Goodner CJ, Freinkel N. Carbohydrate metabolism in pregnancy: the degredation of insulin by extracts of maternal and fetal structures in the pregnant rat. *Endocrinology* 1959; **65**:957–67.

7. Catalano PM, Drago NM, Amini SB. Longitudinal changes in pancreatic b cell function and metabolic clearance rate of insulin in pregnant women with normal and abnormal glucose tolerance. *Diabetes Care* 1998; **21**:403–8.

8. Kalhan SC, D'Angelo LJ, Savin SM et al. Glucose production in pregnant women at term gestation: sources of glucose for human fetus. *J Clin Invest* 1979; **63**:388–94.

9. Cowett RA, Susa JB, Kahn CB et al. Glucose kinetics in nondiabetic and diabetic women during the third trimester of pregnancy. *Am J Obstet Gynecol* 1983; **146**:773–80.

10. Catalano PM, Tyzbir ED, Wolfe RR et al. Longitudinal changes in basal hepatic glucose production and suppression during insulin infusion in normal pregnant women. *Am J Obstet Gynecol* 1992; **167**:913–19.

11. Sivan E, Chen X, Homko CJ et al. Longitudinal study of carbohydrate metabolism in healthy obese women. *Diabetes Care* 1997; **20**:1470–5.

12. Pacini G, Bergman RN. MINMOD: a computer program to calculate insulin sensitivity and pancreatic responsivity from the frequently sampled intravenous glucose tolerance test. *Comput Meth Prog Biomed* 1986; **23**:113–22.

13. DeFronzo RA, Tobin JD, Andres R. Glucose clamp technique: a method for quantifying insulin secretion and resistance. *Am J Physiol* 1979; **237**:E214–E223.

14. Catalano PM, Tyzbir ED, Wolfe RR et al. Carbohydrate metabolism during pregnancy in control subjects and women with gestational diabetes. *Am J Physiol* 1993; **264**:E60–E67.

15. Catalano PM, Huston L, Amini SB, Kalhan SC. Longitudinal changes in glucose metabolism during pregnancy in obese women with normal glucose tolerance and gestational diabetes. *Am J Obstet Gynecol* 1999; **180**:903–16.

16. Spellacy WN, Goetz FC, Greenberg BZ et al. Plasma insulin in normal 'early' pregnancy. *Obstet Gynecol* 1965; **25**:862–5.

17. Burt RL. Peripheral utilization of glucose in pregnancy. III Insulin intolerance. *Obstet Gynecol* 1956; **2**:558–664.

18. Fisher PM, Sutherland HW, Bewsher PD. The insulin response to glucose infusion in normal human pregnancy. *Diabetologia* 1980; **19**:15–20.

19. Buchanan TZ, Metzger BE, Freinkel N et al. Insulin sensitivity and β-cell responsiveness to glucose during late pregnancy in lean and moderately obese women with normal glucose tolerance or mild gestational diabetes. *Am J Obstet Gynecol* 1990; **162**:1008–14.

20. Ryan EA, O'Sullivan MJ, Skyler JS. Insulin action during pregnancy. Studies with the euglycemic clamp technique. *Diabetes* 1985; **34**:380–9.

21. Hay WW, Sparks JW, Wilkening RB et al. Partition of maternal glucose production between conceptus and maternal tissues in sheep. *Am J Physiol* 1983; **245**:E347–E350.

22. Marconi AM, Paolini C, Buscaglia M et al. The impact of gestational age and fetal growth on the maternal–fetal glucose concentration difference. *Obstet Gynecol* 1996; **87**:937–42.

23. Barros LF, Yudilevich DL, Jarvis SM et al. Quantitation and immunolocalization of glucose transporters in the human placenta. *Placenta* 1995; **16**:623–33.

24. Jansson T, Wennergren M, Illsley NP. Glucose transporter expression and distribution in the human placenta throughout gestation and in intrauterine growth retardation. *J Clin Endocrinol Metab* 1993; **77**:1554–62.

25. Hauguel-de Mouzon S, Challier J, Kacemi A et al. The GLUT3 glucose transporter isoform is differentially expressed within human placental cell types. *J Clin Endocrinol Metab* 1997; **82**:2689–94.

26. Xing A, Cauzac M, Challier J et al. Unexpected expression of GLUT4 glucose transporter in villous stromal cells of human placenta. *J Clin Endocrinol Metab* 1999; **83**:4097–101.

27. Garvey WT, Maianu L, Hancock JA et al. Gene expression of GLUT4 in skeletal muscle from insulin-resistant patients with obesity, IGT, GDM, and NIDDM. *Diabetes* 1992; **41**:465–75.

28. Friedman JE, Ishizuka T, Shao J et al. Impaired glucose transport and insulin receptor tyrosine phosphorylation in skeletal muscle from obese women with gestational diabetes. *Diabetes* 1999; **48**:1807–14.

29. Catalano P, Highman T, Huston L, Friedman J. Relationship between reproductive hormones/TNFa and longitudinal changes in insulin sensitivity during gestation. *Diabetes* 1996; **45**:175A.

30. Hytten FE, Leitch I. The gross composition of the components of weight gain. In: *The Physiology of Human Pregnancy*, 2nd edn. (Blackwell Scientific: London, 1971) 371–87.

31. Metzger BD, Unger RH, Freinkel N. Carbohydrate metabolism in pregnancy. XIV. Relationships between circulation glucagon, insulin, glucose and amino acids in

response to a 'mixed meal' in late pregnancy. *Metabolism* 1977; 26:151–6.

32. Freinkel N, Metzger Be, Nitzan M et al. 'Accelerated starvation' and mechanisms for the conservation of maternal nitrogen during pregnancy. *Israel J Med Sci* 1972; 8:426–39.

33. Kalkhoff RK, Kandaraki E, Morrow PG et al. Relationship between neonatal birth weight and maternal plasma amino acid profiles in lean and obese nondiabetic women and in type 1 diabetic pregnant women. *Metabolism* 1988; 37:234–39.

34. McClain PE, Metcoff J, Crosby WM, Costiloe JP. Relationship of maternal amino acid profiles at 25 weeks of gestation to fetal growth. *Am J Clin Nutr* 1978; 31:401–7.

35. Kalhan SC, Tserng K, Gilfillan C, Dierker LJ. Metabolism of urea and glucose in normal and diabetic pregnancy. *Metabolism* 1982; 31:824–33.

36. Denne SC, Kalhan SC. Leucine metabolism in human newborns. *Am J Physiol* 1987; 253:E608–E615.

37. Debenoist B, Jackson AA, Hall JSE, Persaud C. Whole body protein turnover in Jamaican women during normal pregnancy. *Hum Nutr Clin Nutr* 1985; 39: 167–79.

38. Fitch WL, King JC. Protein turnover and 3-methylhistidine excretion in non-pregnant, pregnant and gestational diabetic women. *Hum Nutr Clin Nutr* 1987; 41C: 327–39.

39. Ogata ES. The small for gestational age neonate. In: (Cowell RM, ed.) *Principles of Perinatal-Neonatal Metabolism*, 2nd edn. (Springer-Verlag: New York, 1998) 1097–104.

40. Liechty EA, Boyle DW. Protein metabolism in the fetal placental unit. In: (Cowett RM, ed.) *Principles of Perinatal–Neonatal Metabolism*, 2nd edn. (Springer-Verlag: New York, 1998) 369–87.

41. Knopp RH, Humphrey J, Irvin S. Biphasic metabolic control of hypertriglyceridemia in pregnancy. *Clin Res* 177; 25:161A.

42. Catalano PM, Nizielski SE, Shao J et al. Down regulation of IRS-1 and PPAR γ in obese women with gestational diabetes: relationship to free fatty acids during pregnancy. *Am J Physiol* 2002; 282:E522–E533.

43. Sivan E, Homko CJ, Chen X et al. Effect of insulin in fat metabolism during and after normal pregnancy. *Diabetes* 1999; 44:384–8.

44. Knopp RH, Magee MS, Walden CE et al. Prediction of infant birth weight by GDM screening tests. *Diabetes Care* 1992; 15:1605–13.

45. Knopp RH, Bergelin RO, Wahl PW, Walden CE. Relationships of infant birth size to maternal lipoproteins, apoproteins, fuels, hormones, clinical chemistries, and body weight at 36 weeks gestation. *Diabetes* 1985; 34:71–7.

46. Ogburn PL, Goldstein M, Walker J, Stonestreet BS. Prolonged hyperinsulinemia reduces plasma fatty acid levels in the major lipid groups in fetal sheep. *Am J Obstet Gynecol* 1989; 161:728–32.

47. Kliegman R, Gross T, Morton S, Dunnington R. Intrauterine growth and postnatal fasting metabolism in infants of obese mothers. *J Pediatr* 1984; 104:601–7.

48. Catalano PM, Hollenbeck C. Energy requirements in pregnancy: a review of OB. *Gynecol Survey* 1992; 47:368–72.

49. Goldberg GR, Prentice AM, Coward WA et al. Longitudinal assessment of energy expenditure in pregnancy by the doubly labeled water method. *Am J Clin Nutr* 1993; 57:494–505.

50. Forsum E, Sadurskis A, Wager J. Resting metabolic rate and body composition of healthy Swedish women during pregnancy. *Am J Clin Nutr* 1988; 47:942–7.

51. Lawrence M, Lawrence F, Coward WA et al. Energy requirements of pregnancy in the Gambia. *Lancet* 1987; ii:1072–6.

52. Forsum E, Kabir N, Sadurskis A, Westerterp K. Total energy expenditure of healthy Swedish women during pregnancy and lactation. *Am J Clin Nutr* 1992; 56:334–42.

53. King JC, Butte NF, Bronstein MN et al. Energy metabolism during pregnancy: influence of maternal energy status. *Am J Clin Nutr* 1994; 59:439S–455.

54. Prentice AM, Poppitt SD, Goldberg GR et al. Energy balance in pregnancy and lactation. In: (Allen L, King J, Lonnerdal B, eds) *Nutrient Regulation During Pregnancy, Lactation and Infant Growth*. (Plenum Press: New York, 1994) 11–26.

55. Prentice AM, Goldberg GR, Davies HL et al. Energy-sparing adaptations in human pregnancy assessed by wholebody calorimetry. *Br J Nutr* 1989; 62:5–22.

56. deGroot LCPGM, Boekholt HA, Spaaij CJK et al. Energy balance of healthy Dutch women before and during pregnancy: limited scope for metabolic adaptations. *Am J Clin Nutr* 1994; 59:827–32.

57. Swinburn BA, Nyomba BC, Saad MF et al. Insulin resistance associated with lower rates of weight gain in PIMA Indians. *J Clin Invest* 1991; 88:168–73.

58. Catalano PM, Roman-Drago N, Amini SB, Sims EAH. Longitudinal changes in body composition and energy balance in lean women with normal and abnormal glucose tolerance during pregnancy. *Am J Obstet Gynecol* 1998; 179:156–65.

59. Catalano PM, Roman NM, Tyzbir ED et al. Weight gain in women with gestational diabetes. *Obstet Gynecol* 1993; 81:523–8.

60. Reiher H, Fuhrmann K, Noack S et al. Age-dependent insulin secretion of the endocrine pancreas in vitro from fetuses of diabetic and nondiabetic patients. *Diabetes Care* 1983; 6:446.

61. Falluca F, Garguilo P, Troili F et al. Amniotic fluid insulin, C-peptide concentrations and fetal morbidity in infants of diabetic mothers. *Am J Obstet Gynecol* 1985; 153:534.

62. Krew MA, Kehl RJ, Thomas A, Catalano PM. Relationship of amniotic fluid C-peptide levels to neonatal body composition. *Obstet Gynecol* 1994; 84:96–100.

63. Brans YW, Shannon DL, Hunter MA et al. Maternal diabetes and neonatal macrosomia, II Neonatal anthropometric measurements. *Early Hum Develop* 1983; **8**:297.

64. Modanlou HD, Komatsu G, Dorchester W et al. Large-for-gestational-age neonates: anthropometric reasons for shoulder dystocia. *Obstet Gynecol* 1982; **60**:417.

65. Gabbe SG, Mestman JH, Freeman RK et al. Management and outcome of pregnancy in diabetes mellitus, class B-R. *Am J Obstet Gynecol* 1977; **129**:723.

66. Kitzmiller JL, Gloherty JP. Diabetic pregnancy and perinatal morbidity. *Am J Obstet Gynecol* 1978; **131**:560.

67. Roversi GD, Gargiulo M. A new approach to the treatment of diabetic pregnant women. *Am J Obstet Gynecol* 1979; **135**:567.

68. Jovanovic L, Druzin M, Peterson CM. Effect of euglycemia on the outcome of pregnancy in insulin-dependent diabetic women as compared with normal control subjects. *Am J Med* 1981; **72**:921.

69. Landon MB, Gabbe SG, Piana R et al. Neonatal morbidity in pregnancy complicated by diabetes mellitus predictive value of maternal glycemic profiles. *Am J Obstet Gynecol* 1987; **156**:1089–95.

70. Jovanovic-Peterson L, Peterson CM, Reed GF et al. Maternal postprandial glucose levels and infant birthweight: the Diabetes in Early Pregnancy Study. *Am J Obstet Gynecol* 1991; **164**:103.

71. Catalano PM, Tyzbir ED, Allen SR et al. Evaluation of fetal growth by estimation of body composition. *Obstet Gynecol* 1992; **79**:46–50.

72. Catalano PM, Drago NM, Amini SB. Factors affecting fetal growth and body composition. *Am J Obstet Gynecol* 1995; **172**:1459–63.

73. Catalano PM, Drago NM, Amini SB. Maternal carbohydrate metabolism and its relationship to fetal growth and body composition. *Am J Obstet Gynecol* 1995; **172**:1464–70.

74. Caruso A, Paradisi G, Ferrazzani S et al. Effect of maternal carbohydrate metabolism in fetal growth. *Obstet Gynecol* 1998; **92**:8–12.

75. Silverman BL, Rizzo TA, Cho NH, Metzger BE. Long-term effects of the intrauterine environment. *Diabetes* 1998; **21**:142–9.

76. Pettitt DJ, Nelson RG, Saad MF et al. Diabetes and obesity in the offspring of Pima Indian women with diabetes during pregnancy. *Diabetes Care* 1993; **16**:310–14.

7

Epidemiology of gestational diabetes mellitus

Avi Ben-Haroush, Yariv Yogev, Moshe Hod

Introduction

Gestational diabetes mellitus (GDM) is defined as carbohydrate intolerance that begins or is first recognized during pregnancy.[1] Although it is a well-known cause of pregnancy complications, its epidemiology has not been studied systematically.[2] One problem is the distinction of GDM, as currently defined, from pre-existing but un-diagnosed diabetes, so that the degree of clinical surveillance may have a major impact on the estimated prevalence of GDM in a given population. This is especially true in high-risk populations in which the onset of non-insulin-dependent diabetes mellitus (NIDDM) occurs at an early age.[2] Furthermore, investigators use different screening programs and diagnostic criteria for GDM, making comparisons among studies difficult.

In this chapter the reported risk factors for GDM, differences in its racial distribution and evidence of a genetic or familial association will be discussed. The close relationship of GDM to polycystic ovary syndrome (PCOS), the question of the possibly greater risk of fetal malformations in GDM pregnancies and the effect of an abnormal glucose challenge screening test (GCT), by itself or together with an impaired glucose tolerance (IGT), on obstetric outcome will also be considered. The risk of hypertensive disorders in diabetic pregnancy and of future NIDDM will also be described.

Racial distribution of gestational diabetes mellitus (GDM)

The prevalence of GDM varies in direct proportion to the prevalence of NIDDM in a given population or ethnic group.[1] The reported prevalence of GDM in the United States (US) ranges from 1 to 14%, with 2–5% being the most common rate.[3] In a study of the prevalence of diabetes and IGT in diverse populations in women between the ages of 20 and 39, the World Health Organization (WHO) Ad Hoc Diabetes Reporting Group[4] noted lower rates of diabetes (< 1%) in Bantu (Tanzania), Chinese, rural Indian, Sri Lankan and some Pacific populations followed (1–3%) by Italian women, and white, black and Hispanic women in the US. Rural Fijian Indian and Aboriginal Australian women had a 7% prevalence; the highest rate was found in Pima/Papago and Nauruan Indians (14–22%). The prevalence of IGT was low (< 3%) in Chinese and Malays, and was > 10% in black and Hispanic women in the US, urban Indian women in Tanzania, Pima and Nauruan Indians, and some other Pacific communities. The combined age-standardized prevalence of diabetes and IGT ranged from 0 to 36%, with a > 10% prevalence in one third of the populations, and a > 30% prevalence in

Pima and Nauruan Indians. Importantly, in some populations more than half of the cases of diabetes were undiagnosed prior to the survey. IGT was mostly overlooked in routine clinical practice. Thus, a substantial proportion of abnormal glucose tolerance in pregnancy will be undetected without screening.

King[2] summarized the work of several research groups who had collected data on the prevalence of diabetes in pregnancy (Table 7.1). Their findings, together with the WHO study, show that for a given population and ethnicity, the risk of diabetes in pregnancy reflects the underlying frequency of NIDDM.

It remains unclear, however, if this marked racial and geographic variation represents true differences in the prevalence of GDM, because of the remarkably variable approaches used across different studies, including different methods of screening, different oral and intravenous glucose loads, and different diagnostic criteria. For example, Dooley et al[5] demonstrated that race as well as maternal age and degree of obesity must be taken into account in comparing the prevalence of GDM in different populations. Their study included 3744 consecutive pregnant women who underwent universal screening. The population was 39.1% white, 37.7% black, 19.8% Hispanic and 3.4% Oriental/other. Black and Hispanic race, maternal age and percentage ideal body weight had a significant independent effect on the prevalence of GDM. The adjusted relative risk (RR) was higher in black [1.81, 95% confidence interval (CI) 1.13–2.89] and Hispanic (2.45, 95% CI 1.48–4.04) women than in white women. The degree of carbohydrate intolerance was similar across racial groups; nevertheless, when the 92 GDM patients under dietary control were analyzed separately, mean birthweight was found to be highest in the Hispanic women, and was lowest in the blacks and Orientals. Hence, race had a significant independent effect on

Population	Prevalence (%)
US	
All ethnicities	4.0
Zuni Indian	14.3
California, US	
Chinese	7.3
Hispanic	4.2
African	1.7
Non-Hispanic white	1.6
Mexico	6.0
Melbourne, Australia	
Australian-born	4.3
Vietnam-born	7.8
Indian-born	15.0
African-born	9.4
Mediterranean-born	7.3
Arabian	7.2
Chinese	13.9
Northern European	5.2
Northern American	4.0
Illawarar, Australia	
All ethnicities	7.2
Asian	11.9
London, UK	
Caucasion	1.2
African	2.7
Asian	5.8
Scandiano, Italy	2.3
Israel	
Jewish	5.7
Bedouin	2.4
Karachi, Pakistan	3.5
South India	0.6
Pietermaritzburg, South Africa	
Predominantly Indian	3.8
Taipei, Taiwan	
Chinese	0.6
Hyogo, Japan	3.1

Table 7.1. *Prevalence of GDM as a percentage of all pregnancies (from King,[2] with permission).*

birthweight, with maternal percentage ideal body weight a significant covariate. These findings are supported by a recent study showing that Asian woman were more likely to have GDM than Caucasian woman (31.7 versus 14%, $P = 0.02$), despite their lower body mass index (BMI).[6]

Risk factors for gestational diabetes mellitus

The traditional and most often reported risk factors for GDM are high maternal age, weight and parity, previous delivery of a macrosomic infant and a family history of diabetes. These and other reported risk factors are summarized in Table 7.2. It is of great importance that the clinician understand and use these characteristics, along with others, such as the racial and geographic attributed risk (discussed above), to improve screening programs and diagnostic accuracy, and perhaps to design better and more cost-effective selective screening and diagnostic tests.

Jang et al[7] examined 3581 consecutive Korean women and found a 2.2% prevalence of GDM. The affected women were older, had higher prepregnancy weights, higher BMI, higher parities and higher frequencies of known diabetes in the family. The risk of diabetes was closely associated with previous obstetric outcome, such as congenital malformation, stillbirth and macrosomia. The number of risk factors present in each individual increased the risk of diabetes, with the prevalence ranging from 0.6% in subjects without any risk factors to 33% in those with four or more. Thus, it is possible that selective screening may be cost-effective in situations where health resources are scarce and where total screening is impossible.[2]

Similar results were reported in a retrospective cohort study of 2574 pregnant women, which suggested that selective screening programs have a high true-positive yield.[8] An age of ≥ 30, a family history of diabetes, obesity (BMI ≥ 27) and previous fetal macrosomia

were the most frequent risk factors. Just over half (54.2%) of the population presented with one or more risk factors. The positive predictive value (PPV) of screening increased with the number of risk factors, from 12% for the women with no risk factors to 40% for those with three or more risk factors.

In another study, Jang et al[9] demonstrated that in the racially homogeneous population of Seoul, Korea, besides prepregnancy BMI, age, weight gain and parental history of diabetes, short stature is an independent risk factor for GDM. Accordingly, Kousta et al[10] reported that European and South Asian women with previous GDM were shorter than control women from the same ethnic groups, perhaps due to a common pathophysiological mechanism underlying GDM and the determination of final adult height. Others have reported similar results.[11]

In a large retrospective cohort study in Canada, Xiong et al[12] evaluated 111,563 pregnancies and detected a 2.5% prevalence of GDM. The risk factors identified were age > 35 years, obesity, history of prior neonatal death and a prior Cesarean section. Interestingly, teenage mothers and women who drank alcohol were less likely to have GDM.

The risk factors mentioned above are mainly of maternal origin. However, cumulative knowledge about the long-term implications of exposure to the diabetic intrauterine environment (see Chapter 23) has led to the addition of the mother's fetal history to the risk factor list. Egeland et al[13] investigated whether the mother's own characteristics at birth could predict her subsequent risk of GDM. Using linked generation data from the Medical Birth Registry of Norway for all women born between 1967 and 1984, who gave birth between 1988 and 1998, the authors identified 498 women aged < 32 years with GDM in one or more singleton pregnancies. They found that the women whose mothers had had diabetes during pregnancy

Risk Factor	Author (reference)	Study and population	Results
Maternal factors			
Older age	Jang et al, 1995 (7)	Universal screening with a 50-gram glucose load at 24–28 weeks gestation of 3581 consecutive Korean women. At 1-hour plasma glucose ≥ 130 mg/dl, they underwent a 3-hour 100-gram OGTT. GDM prevalence was 2.2% (80 cases of GDM versus 3432 normal controls)	Mean age of GDM and normal control groups, 31.7±4.0 and 28.9±3.3 years, respectively ($P < 0.001$)
	Jang et al, 1998 (9)	Same as above in 9005 pregnant women. GDM prevalence was 1.9% (173 GDM, 1735 IGT and 6955 normal controls)	Mean age of GDM and IGT groups versus normal controls, 31.1±4.2, 29.4±3.5 and 28.5±3.4 years, respectively ($P < 0.001$)
	Jimenez-Moleon et al, 2000 (8)	Retrospective cohort study on 2574 pregnant women	Among GDM patients 41.8% were older than 30 years of age, whereas 26.2% were younger than 25 years of age. The PPV of the screen for a single risk factor was 22.9 (95% CI 16.9–29.8)
	Xiong et al, 2001 (12)	Retrospective cohort study on 111,563 deliveries between 1991 and 1997 in 39 hospitals in Canada. Average prevalence of GDM was 2.5% (2755 cases of GDM versus 108,664 normal controls)	Age > 35 years in 22.4% and 10.3% of GDM and normal patients, respectively (adjusted OR = 2.34, 95% CI 2.13–2.58)
	Egeland et al, 2000 (13)	Medical Birth Registry of Norway study of all women born between 1967 and 1984 who gave birth between 1988 and 1998 ($n = 141,107$), excluding 2393 non-singleton pregnancies	GDM prevalence of 2.5%; age > 35
	Bo et al, 2001 (20)	126 pregnant women with GDM, 84 with IGT and 294 with normal glucose tolerance	Prevalence of GDM increased with age, from 1.5 per 1000 deliveries for women aged ≤ 20 to 4.2 for women aged ≥ 30 (OR = 2.8, 95% CI 1.9–4.3)

Table 7.2. Summary of reported risk factors for GDM.

Risk factor	Author (reference)	Study and population	Results
Maternal factors			
	Jolly et al, 2000 (80)	Retrospective analysis of 385,120 singleton pregnancies	Mean age of GDM, IGT and normoglycemic groups, 33.0±4.8, 33.0±4.9 and 31.8±4.4 years, respectively ($P = 0.02$)
	Lao et al, 2001 (81)	Prospective study of 97 GDM patients and 194 matched controls examined at the time of OGTT at 28–31 weeks gestation for serum ferritin, iron and transferrin concentrations. Managing obstetricians blinded to results	Pregnant women aged between 35 and 40 were at increased risk of GDM (OR = 2.63, 99% CI 2.40–2.89)
High parity	Jang et al, 1995 (7)	As described above	Mean parity of GDM and normal control groups, 0.6±0.9 and 0.4±0.5, respectively ($P < 0.05$)
	Jang et al, 1998 (9)	As described above	Parity ≥ 2 in 9.8% of GDM, 4.7% of IGT groups and 2.6% of controls ($P < 0.001$)
	Egeland et al, 2000 (13)	As described above	Age-adjusted OR (95% CI) for women with two, three, four or more deliveries compared with one delivery were 1.5 (1.2–1.9), 1.9 (1.4–2.5), and 3.3 (2.1–5.1), respectively
Pre-pregnancy weight	Jang et al, 1995 (7)	As described above	Mean weight of GDM and normal control groups, 56.4±9.2 and 51.6±6.4 kg, respectively ($P < 0.001$)
	Jang et al, 1998 (9)	As described above	Mean weight of GDM and IGT groups versus normal controls, 56.5±9.5, 52.4±7.2 and 51.6±6.4 kg, respectively ($P < 0.001$)

Table 7.2. Summary of reported risk factors for GDM. (continued)

Risk factor	Author (reference)	Study and population	Results
Maternal factors			
	Jimenez-Moleon et al, 2000 (8)	As described above	BMI > 27 in 12.3% of GDM patients. PPV of the screen for a single risk factor was 32.5 (95% CI 22.4–43.9)
Pregnancy weight	Xiong et al, 2001 (12)	As described above	Obesity ≥ 91 kg detected in 15.8 and 7.3% of GDM and normal groups, respectively (adjusted OR = 2.40, 95% CI 2.06–2.98)
Pregnancy weight gain	Jang et al, 1998 (9)	As described above	Mean weight gain of GDM, IGT and normal control groups, of 8.4±3.9, 8.3±3.3 and 8.1±8.1 kg, respectively (NS)
BMI	Jang et al, 1995 (7)	As described above	Only 1.3% of population was obese, but GDM prevalence increased significantly with increasing BMI. BMI ≥ 27 in 8.8% of GDM and 1.1% of control group (P < 0.001)
	Jang et al, 1998 (9)	As described above	BMI ≥ 27.3 in 9.8% of GDM, 2.4% of IGT and 1.0% of controls (P < 0.001)
	Bo et al, 2001 (20)	As described above	Mean BMI in GDM, IGT and normoglycemic group, 25.4±5.3, 26.0±5.5 and 23.6±4.6, respectively (P = 0.000,02)
	Kousta et al, 2000 (24)	91 previous GDM and 73 normoglycemic control women, a median (interquartile range) of 20 (11–36) and 29 (17–49) months postpartum, respectively	Women with previous GDM had higher BMI [26.4 (22.8–31.4) 31.4 versus 23.8 (21.0–27.5), P = 0.002] and waist:hip ratio [0.82 (0.79–0.88) versus 0.77 (0.73–0.81), P < 0.0001] than controls

Table 7.2. Summary of reported risk factors for GDM. (continued)

Risk factor	Author (reference)	Study and population	Results
Maternal factors			
	Holte et al, 1998 (23)	34 women with GDM 3–5 years before the investigation and 36 controls with uncomplicated pregnancies, selected for similar age, parity and date of delivery	GDM patients had higher BMI than controls (25.2 versus 22.2, $P < 0.001$)
Short stature	Jang et al, 1995 (7)	As described above	Mean height of GDM and normal control groups, 158.1±4.8 and 159.7±4.2 cm, respectively ($P < 0.001$)
	Jang et al, 1998 (9)	As described above	≤157 cm, the OR for GDM was two times greater compared the ≥163 cm group, even after controlling for age and BMI
	Kousta et al, 2000 (10)	346 women with previous GDM and 470 controls with no previous history of GDM	European and South Asian women with previous GDM were shorter than control women from the same ethnic groups (European: 162.9±6.1 versus 165.3±6.8 cm, $P < 0.0001$; South Asian: 155.2±5.4 versus 158.2±6.3 cm, $P = 0.003$, adjusted for age)
	Bo et al, 2001 (20)	As described above	GDM, IGT and normoglycemic groups had a mean height of 1.62±0.06, 1.61±0.006 and 1.63±0.07 cm, respectively ($P = 0.02$)
	Branchtein et al, 2000 (11)	5564 Brazilian women	Height < 150 cm associated with a 60% increase in the odds of GDM, independently of age, obesity, skin color, parity, family history and previous GDM

Table 7.2. Summary of reported risk factors for GDM. (continued)

Risk factor	Author (reference)	Study and population	Results
Maternal factors			
Low birthweight	Egeland et al, 2000 (13)	As described above	Birthweight < 2500 a risk factor for GDM with OR = 9.3, (95% CI 4.1–21.1, P < 0.001), as was weight for gestational age (centiles) < 10 with OR = 1.7, (95% CI 1.2–2.5)
Alpha-thalassemia trait	Lao and Ho, 2001 (21)	Retrospective case-control study: 163 women with alpha-thalassemia trait compared to 163 controls matched for maternal age and parity, following each index case	GDM incidence higher in the study group (62.0 versus 14.7%, P < 0.0001, OR = 11.74, 95% CI 6.37–21.63)
PCOS	Holte et al, 1998 (23)	As described above	Compare with controls, GDM patients showed a higher prevalence of polycystic ovaries [14 of 34 (41%) versus 1 of 36 (3%)]; greater clinical and biochemical evidence of hyperandrogenism and insulin resistance; and a higher prevalence of pregnancy-induced hypertension (50 versus 15%; P < 0.05) during the index pregnancy; 15% developed overt diabetes
	Anttila et al, 1998 (25)	Retrospective comparative ultrasound study of ovaries in 31 women with GDM and 30 healthy controls matched for maternal age and BMI	14 women with GDM (44%) and two controls exhibited PCOS
	Kousta et al, 2000 (24)	As described above	Higher prevalence of PCOS in previous GDM group than controls [47 of 91 (52%) versus 20 of 73 (27%), P = 0.002 overall, OR = 2.7, P = 0.007 by logistic regression allowing for ethnicity]

Table 7.2. Summary of reported risk factors for GDM. (continued)

Risk factor	Author (reference)	Study and population	Results
Maternal factors			
	Mikola et al, 2001 (26)	Retrospective study of 99 pregnancies in women with PCOS compared with an unselected control population	GDM developed in 20% of PCOS patients and 8.9% of controls ($P < 0.001$). BMI > 25 an important predictor of GDM (adjusted OR = 5.1; 95% CI 3.2–8.3), as is PCOS (adjusted OR = 1.9; 95% CI 1.0–3.5)
	Koivunen et al, 2001 (27)	33 women with a history of GDM and 48 controls	Higher prevalence of PCOS in GDM group (39.4% versus 16.7%, $P = 0.03$); also higher serum cortisol, androgens and a greater area under the glucose curve
High intake of saturated fat	Bo et al, 2001 (20)	As described above	Only percentages of saturated fat (OR = 2.0, 95% CI 1.2–3.2) and polyunsaturated fat (OR = 0.85, 95%, CI 0.77–0.92) were associated with gestational hyperglycemia, after adjustment for age, gestational age and BMI
Family history			
Familial history of diabetes	Jang et al, 1995 (7)	As described above	35% of GDM versus 15.4% of normal controls ($P < 0.001$)
	Jang et al, 1998 (9)	As described above	30.1% of GDM, 17.6% of IGT and 13.2% of normal controls ($P < 0.001$)
	Jimenez-Moleon et al, 2000 (8)	As described above	14.8% of GDM patients. PPV of screen for a single risk factor = 25.9 (95% CI 16.8–36.9)

Table 7.2. Summary of reported risk factors for GDM. (continued)

Risk Factor	Author (reference)	Study and population	Results
Family history			
	Bo et al, 2001 (20)	As described above	41% of GDM, 33% of IGT and 28% of normal controls ($P = 0.04$)
	Holte et al, 1998 (23)	As described above	First-degree heredity of NIDDM more prevalent in previous GDM than control group (24 versus 6%, $P < 0.05$)
GDM in subject's mother	Egeland et al, 2000 (13)	As described above	GDM rate 30.6 (per 1000 women) in women whose mother had GDM versus 3.5 in controls (OR = 9.3, 95% CI 4.1–21.1)
Previous obstetric outcome			
Congenital malformation	Jang et al, 1995 (7)	As described above	GDM in 20.7% of patients who had previous malformation versus 2.4% of patients who did not (OR = 22.5, 95% CI 7.15–70.96)
Stillbirth	Jang et al, 1995 (7)	As described above	GDM in 14.3% of patients who had previous stillbirth versus 2.6% of patients who did not (OR = 8.5, 95% CI 2.35–30.78)
	Xiong et al, 2001 (12)	As described above	Previous neonatal death in 1.3% of GDM group versus 0.6% of controls (adjusted OR = 2.09, 95% CI 1.06–1.34)
Macrosomia	Jang et al, 1995 (7)	As described above	GDM in 9.3% of patients who had previous macrosomia versus 2.5% of patients who did not (OR = 5.8, 95% CI 1.98–17.02)

Table 7.2.   Summary of reported risk factors for GDM. *(continued)*

Risk factor	Author (reference)	Study and population	Results
Previous obstetric outcome			
	Jimenez-Moleon et al, 2000 (8)	As described above	OR = 5.8 in patients who had previous macrosomia – 4.9% of GDM patients. The PPV of the screen for a single risk factor was 37.5 (95% CI 21.1–56.3)
Cesarean section	Xiong et al, 2001 (12)	As described above	Previous CS in 14.8% of GDM group and 10.1% of controls (adjusted OR = 1.55, 95% CI 1.11–1.25)
Previous GDM	MacNeill et al, 2001 (44)	A retrospective longitudinal study including 651 women	Recurrence of GDM in 35.6% (95% CI 31.9–39.3%). Infant birthweight in the index pregnancy and maternal prepregnancy weight were predictive of recurrent GDM
	Major et al, 1998 (45)	78 patients with previous GDM	Recurrence rate 69%; more common with parity ≥ 1, BMI ≥ 30. GDM diagnosis at ≤ 24 weeks gestation, insulin requirement, weight gain of ≥ 7 kg (c. 15 pounds) and interval between pregnancies ≤ 24 months
	Spong et al, 1998 (46)	164 Hispanic patients with previous GDM	Recurrence rate 68%; more common with earlier diagnosis of GDM, requirement of insulin and hospital admissions in index pregnancy
	Foster-Powel and Cheung, 1998 (79)	Retrospective review of 540 women	117 women had a subsequent pregnancy with recurrent GDM in 82 (70%). Risk factors were older age, race, BMI and weight gain

Table 7.2. Summary of reported risk factors for GDM.(continued)

Risk factor	Author (reference)	Study and population	Results
Pregnancy factors			
High blood pressure in pregnancy	Ma and Lo, 2001 (14)	Retrospective study of 84 pregnant women with normal and abnormal antenatal OGTT results who delivered in a 12-month period	MAP was increased from 28 weeks until delivery in gestational diabetics (n = 50) as compared with controls (n = 34). The OGTT fasting glucose value significantly correlated with MAP at 32 and 36 weeks gestation
Multiple pregnancy	Sivan et al, 2002 (29)	103 women with consecutive triplet pregnancies, compared to 85 women who elected to undergo fetal reduction to twins	Higher GDM rate in the triplet than the reduction group (22.3 versus 5.8%)
	Schwartz et al, 1999 (30)	Total 29,644 deliveries, 429 twins	GDM increased in twin versus singleton deliveries (7.7 versus 4.1%, $P < 0.05$)
	Hoskins, 1995 (28)	3458 recorded twin live births. Calculated zygocity rate according to sex ratios	Estimated risk for DZ twin pregnancies relative to MZ pregnancies of 8.6 (95% CI 3.5–21.0)
	Wein et al, 1992 (31)	61,914 singleton and 798 twin pregnancies	GDM prevalence of 7.4% in twins versus 5.6% in singletons ($P = 0.025$)
Increased iron stores	Lao et al, 2001 (81)	As described above	Log-transformed ferritin concentration was a significant determinant of OGTT 2-hour glucose value
Protective factors			
Young age	Xiong et al, 2001 (12)	As described above	Age $\leq$ 19 years in 2.6 and 8.5% of GDM and normal patients, respectively (adjusted OR = 0.35, 95% CI 0.27–0.44)

Table 7.2. Summary of reported risk factors for GDM. (continued)

Risk factor	Author (reference)	Study and population	Results
Protective factors			
Alcohol use	Xiong et al, 2001 (12)	As described above	Alcohol use in 0.7 and 2.0% of GDM and normal patients, respectively (adjusted OR = 0.40, 95% CI 0.25–0.76)

BMI, Body mass index; CI, confidence interval; CS, Caesarean section; DZ, dizygotic; GDM, gestational diabetes mellitus; IGT, impaired glucose tolerance; MAP, mean arterial pressure; MZ, monozygotic; NIDDM, non-insulin-dependent diabetes mellitus; NS, non significant; OGTT, oral glucose tolerance test; OR, odds ratio; PPV, positive predictive value.

Table 7.2. Summary of reported risk factors for GDM. (continued)

were at increased risk of GDM themselves. Significant inverse trends in diabetes were noted in relation to birthweight, with an increased risk of GDM of 80, 60 and 40% in women whose birthweights were ≤ 2500, 2500–2999 and 3000–3499 grams, respectively, compared with women in the 4000–4500 grams group. Similar findings were observed for categories of weight for gestational age.

Is GDM a cause or an effect? A retrospective study from Hong Kong[14] in 84 normotensive women showed that progressive glucose intolerance throughout pregnancy is associated with an upward shift in blood pressure in the third trimester. Hence, it is possible that blood pressure changes below the diagnostic threshold for hypertensive disorders of pregnancy may help to identify women at increased risk of GDM.

The relationship between dietary fat and glucose metabolism has been recognized for many years. Epidemiological data in humans suggest that subjects with a higher fat intake are more prone to disturbances in glucose metabolism.[15] Several researchers have hypothesized that polyunsaturated fatty acid plays an essential role in the maintenance of energy balance and, through regulation of gene transcription, may improve insulin resistance.[16–18] A recent small study reported significantly lower cord vein erythrocyte phospholipid fatty acid concentrations in 13 women with GDM compared to 12 women with normal pregnancies.[19] Accordingly, Bo et al[20] investigated the relationship between lifestyle habits and glucose abnormalities in 504 Caucasian women with and without conventional risk factors for GDM. They identified 126 women with GDM and 84 with IGT. These patients were older and shorter than the women with normal pregnancies, and had significantly higher prepregnancy BMI, higher rates of diabetes in first-degree relatives and higher intakes of saturated fat. In a multiple logistic regression model, all of these factors were associated with glucose abnormalities, after adjustment for gestational age. In the patients without conventional risk factors, only the percentages of saturated fats [odds ratio (OR) = 2.0, 95% CI 1.2–3.2) and polyunsaturated fats (OR = 0.85, 95% CI 0.77–0.92) were associated with gestational hyperglycemia, after adjustment for age, gestational age and BMI. Thus, the allegedly independent role of saturated fat in the development of gestational glucose abnormalities takes on greater importance in the absence of conventional risk factors. This suggests that glucose abnormalities could be prevented in some groups of women during pregnancy.

A possible expression of the still unknown genetic linkage in GDM was reported by Lao and Ho,[21] who detected GDM in 62% of 163 women with the alpha-thalassemia trait compared to 14.7% out of 163 controls matched for maternal age and parity.

Polycystic ovary syndrome and gestational diabetes mellitus

PCOS is a heterogeneous disorder affecting 5–10% of women of reproductive age. It is characterized by chronic anovulation with oligo-/amenorrhea, infertility, typical sonographic appearance of the ovaries, and clinical or biochemical hyperandrogenism. Insulin resistance is present in 40–50% of patients, especially in obese women.[22]

Holte et al[23] reported a higher rate of ultrasonographic, clinical and endocrine signs of PCOS in 34 women who had had GDM 3–5 years before, compared to 36 matched controls with uncomplicated pregnancies. Five of the women (15%) with previous GDM had developed manifest diabetes. The authors concluded that women with previous GDM and

PCOS may form a distinct subgroup from women with normal ovaries and previous GDM, who may be more prone to develop features of insulin-resistance syndrome.

Many other researchers reported similar results. Kousta et al[24] found a higher prevalence of PCOS in 91 women with previous GDM compared to 73 normoglycemic control women (52 versus 27%, $P = 0.002$), and Anttila et al[25] reported a 44% prevalence of PCOS in women with GDM, with no differences in BMI before pregnancy or in weight gain during pregnancy compared to controls. They suggested a screening program for GDM for these patients.

Mikola et al[26] retrospectively evaluated 99 pregnancies in women with PCOS compared with an unselected control population. The average BMI and the nulliparity rate were higher in the PCOS group, as was the multiple pregnancy rate (9.1 versus 1.1%). GDM developed in 20% of the patients with PCOS but only in 8.9% of the controls ($P < 0.001$). A BMI > 25 was the best predictor of GDM (adjusted OR = 5.1, 95% CI 3.2–8.3), and PCOS was an additional independent predictor (adjusted OR = 1.9, 95% CI 1.0–3.5).

Koivunen et al[27] found that compared with 48 control women, 33 women with previous GDM more often had significantly abnormal oral glucose tolerance tests (OGTT), higher prevalences of polycystic ovaries (39.4 versus 16.7%, $P = 0.03$), higher serum concentrations of cortisol, dehydroepiandrosterone and dehydroepiandrosterone sulfate, and a greater area under the glucose curve.

Multiple pregnancy and gestational diabetes mellitus

The number of fetuses in multifetal pregnancies is expected to influence the incidence of GDM owing to the increased placental mass and,

thereby, the increase in diabetogenic hormones. However, the reports are somewhat conflicting, probably because of the heterogeneous populations studied.

In an interesting study of the prevalence of GDM in dizygotic (DZ) twin pregnancies with two placentae compared to monozygotic (MZ) twin pregnancies with one placenta, Hoskins[28] evaluated 3458 recorded twin deliveries and found that a higher proportion of different-sex compared with same-sex twin pregnancies were complicated by GDM (3.5 versus 1.6%). The estimated risk for DZ twin pregnancies relative to MZ pregnancies was 8.6 (95% CI 3.5–21.0). The impact of fetal reduction on the incidence of GDM may support this theory. Sivan et al[29] examined 188 consecutive triplet pregnancies of which 85 were reduced to twins. The rate of GDM was significantly higher in the triplet group than in the reduction group (22.3 versus 5.8%).

Similar results were reported by Schwartz et al[30] in a study of 29,644 deliveries. They found that GDM was significantly more frequent in the 429 twin deliveries (7.7 versus 4.1%, $P < 0.05$). However, insulin requirements were not different, suggesting a minor clinical impact. Wein et al[31] compared the prevalence of GDM between 61,914 singleton and 798 twin deliveries performed between 1971 and 1991. The difference was significant only for the earlier decade (5.6 versus 7.4%, $P = 0.025$). However, in a follow-up program there was a trend toward a higher prevalence of overt diabetes in the women who had had a diabetic twin pregnancy (18.5%) compared to those who had had a diabetic singleton pregnancy (7.4%). Whether this represents a true increased risk for diabetes is unknown.

By contrast, using data derived from the Medical Birth Registry of Norway, Egeland and Irgens,[32] controlling for other risk factors such as advanced age, parity, maternal history of diabetes and the woman's own birthweight, found GDM in 6.6 per 1000 multiple pregnancies (n = 9271) and in 5.0 per 1000 singleton pregnancies (n = 640,700) (OR = 1.3, 95% CI 1.0–1.7, P = 0.03). However, analyses stratified by maternal age or parity yielded no elevated risk of GDM. Others have also failed to demonstrate a higher prevalence of GDM in multiple pregnancies.[33,34]

Genetic factors

Animal studies have shown that female fetuses exposed to a diabetic intrauterine milieu have an increased risk of subsequent GDM. In a family history study, Harder et al[35] reported a significantly greater prevalence of diabetes (mainly NIDDM) in the mothers of women with GDM than in their fathers. A significant aggregation of NIDDM was also observed in the maternal-grandmaternal line compared to the paternal-grandpaternal line. However, in patients with IDDM there was no significant difference in the prevalence of any type of diabetes between mothers and fathers. Therefore, a history of NIDDM on the mother's side might be considered as a particular risk factor for GDM via 'intergenerative transmission of NIDDM', which might be prevented by strict avoidance of GDM.

Dorner et al[36] reported a significantly decreased familial diabetes aggregation on the maternal side in children with insulin-dependent diabetes mellitus (IDDM) born between 1974 and 1984 compared to those born between 1960 and 1973. This finding was explained by the improved prevention of hyperglycemia during pregnancy since 1974, and particularly of GDM in women with familial diabetes aggregation. These authors also noted a highly significant predominance of NIDDM in the

great-grandmothers of individuals with infantile-onset diabetes compared to the paternal side. They suggested that GDM, which may represent a risk factor for diabetes transmission on the maternal side, is often followed by 'extra-gestational' NIDDM at a later age. Like Harder et al,[35] these authors suggested that their findings were consistent with the suspected teratogenetic effect of GDM on diabetes susceptibility in the offspring, and that this was preventable by avoiding hyperglycemia in pregnant women and hyperinsulinism in fetuses.

Histocompatibility leukocytic antigen (HLA) studies are one way to establish a genetic linkage in certain diseases. In GDM, conflicting results have been reported. Kuhl[37] described similar frequencies of HLA DR2, DR3 and DR4 antigens in healthy pregnant women and women with GDM, and low prevalences of markers of autoimmune destruction of the beta cells in GDM pregnancies. Likewise, Vambergue et al,[38] in a study of 95 women with GDM, 95 with IGT and 95 control pregnant women, found no significant difference in the distribution of HLA class II polymorphism among the groups. However, the GDM and IGT groups presented some particular HLA patterns, pointing to a genetic heterogeneity of glucose intolerance during pregnancy.

Lapolla et al[39] evaluated 68 women with GDM and matched controls for the frequency of HLA A, B, C and DR antigens; the only significant differences were an increase in Cw7 and a decrease in A10 in the GDM group. Budowle et al[40] reported that the Bf-F allele was found significantly less frequently in non-obese black women with GDM compared to controls, and suggested similar genetic associations in non-obese black women with GDM and with IDDM. Similarly, in another study, women with GDM who required insulin for glycemic control had a lower frequency of the Bf-F phenotype and a higher frequency of the

Bf-f1 phenotype; they also had a lower frequency of the type 2 allele at the polymorphic locus adjacent to the insulin gene.[41]

Freinkel et al[42] evaluated 199 women with GDM and 148 patients with normal pregnancies, and found that the HLA DR3 and DR4 antigens occurred significantly more often in black women with GDM. Ferber et al,[43] in an analysis of 184 women with GDM, did not find an elevation in the frequency of any HLA class II alleles in GDM patients compared with non-diabetic unrelated subjects. However, the DR3 allele was noted significantly more frequently in 43 women with islet autoantibodies and in the 24 women who developed IDDM postpartum. The cumulative risk of developing IDDM within 2 years after pregnancy in the GDM women with DR3 or DR4 was 22%, and in the women without these alleles was 7% ($P = 0.02$). The risk rose to 50% in the DR3- and DR4-positive women who had required insulin during pregnancy ($P = 0.006$). These results indicate that women with GDM who have islet autoantibodies at delivery or develop IDDM postpartum have HLA alleles typical of late-onset Type 1 diabetes, and that both HLA typing and islet antibodies can predict the development of IDDM postpartum.

Recurrence of gestational diabetes mellitus

MacNeill et al[44] conducted a retrospective longitudinal study of 651 women who had had a diabetic pregnancy and at least one other thereafter. They found a 35.6% recurrence rate of GDM. Multivariate regression models showed that infant birthweight in the index pregnancy and maternal weight before the subsequent pregnancy were predictive of recurrent GDM.

Higher recurrence rates (69% of 78 patients) were reported by Major et al.[45] Recurrence was more common when the following variables were present in the index pregnancy: parity ≥ 1 (OR = 3.0), BMI ≥ 30 (OR = 3.6), GDM diagnosis ≤ 24 weeks gestation (OR = 20.4) and insulin requirement (OR = 2.3). A weight gain of ≥ 7 kg (c. 15 pounds) (OR = 2.9) and an interval between pregnancies of ≤ 24 months (OR = 1.6) were also associated with a recurrence of GDM. Spong et al[46] found a similarly high recurrence rate of 68% in 164 women with GDM. Risk factors for recurrence in this study were earlier diagnosis of GDM, insulin requirement and hospital admissions in the index pregnancy.

Impaired glucose tolerance as a risk factor of adverse outcome

The cut-off level of glycemia beyond which the risk of an adverse outcome of pregnancy is increased is of major clinical importance in the management and initiation of therapy. Nasrat et al[47] examined pregnancy outcome in 212 women with IGT and 212 women with normal glucose tolerance. They found a higher mean age and higher parity in the IGT group. The babies in this group also had higher birthweights, lower levels of capillary blood glucose and higher hematocrit. Nevertheless, the proportion of babies with birthweights ≥ 2 standard deviations (SD) above the mean, neonatal capillary blood glucose < 28 mg/dl and hematocrit $\geq 65\%$ was equal in the two groups. Therefore, the authors concluded that IGT does not lead to any adverse outcome. Similar findings were reported by Ramtoola et al,[48] who failed to find an excess perinatal mortality in 267 pregnant women with IGT compared with a background population. The mean birthweight was significantly higher in the babies born to women with GDM and gestational IGT than in the background population, but not in the babies of women with pregestational diabetes. The incidence of macrosomia was highest in the GDM group and it was also significantly increased in the pregestational diabetes group, but not in the IGT group, even though the latter had the highest gestational age at delivery. Both hypoglycemia and hyperbilirubinemia were significantly more common in the infants of women with pregestational and gestational diabetes than in the infants of women with gestational IGT.

By contrast, Moses and Calvert[49] suggested that the clinically optimal level for glycemia during pregnancy should be as near to normal as possible. They studied the proportion of assisted deliveries and the proportion of infants admitted to special care in relation to the range of glucose tolerance, and found an association between glycemia and both outcomes. For assisted deliveries, risk increased only in the higher range (126–142 mg/dl), but for admission to special care there was a linear trend.

Conflicting results were also reported by others. Al-Shawaf et al[50] found that women with gestational IGT were older and more obese, had higher parities and had heavier babies than pregnant women with normal screening plasma glucose. Roberts et al[51] found no significant difference in the incidence of antenatal complications between mothers with normal glucose tolerance and IGT (*n* = 135 each). Although the IGT group had higher rate of induced labor and Cesarean section, there was no between-group difference in fetal outcome or neonatal morbidity. Tan and Yeo,[52] in a retrospective analysis of 944 women with IGT in pregnancy (8.6%) with 10,065 women with normal pregnancies, noted that even when maternal age and obesity were excluded, the IGT group had a significantly higher risk of labor induction (RR = 1.15); Cesarean section (RR: overall = 1.43, elective = 1.72, emergency = 1.31); Cesarean section for dystocia/no progress (RR = 1.60), macrosomia

(RR = 1.69, 1.76 and 1.61 for birthweights ≥ 97th, 95th and 90th percentiles, respectively) and shoulder dystocia (RR = 2.84). The risk of hypertensive disease (RR = 1.22) and Cesarean section for fetal distress/thick meconium-stained amniotic fluid (RR = 1.53) were also higher in the IGT group, but the differences were not statistically significant when maternal age and obesity were excluded. There was no significant difference in the rates of low Apgar scores at 1 and 5 minutes between the two groups.

It is possible that some of the adverse outcomes associated with excess maternal weight were in fact related to GDM. It is also possible that some of the complications attributed to GDM, especially the milder form of IGT, were actually related to excess maternal weight. Jacobson and Cousins[53] reported that good glycemic control did not normalize birthweight percentiles and that maternal weight at delivery was the only significant predictor of birthweight percentile. Thus, IGT diagnosed for the first time in pregnancy might only be a feature of excess maternal weight but not in itself a pathological condition. The clinical significance of IGT has also been disputed.[47,54] Lao and Ho,[55] in a retrospective case–control study, examined the impacts of IGT on the outcome of singleton pregnancies in 128 Chinese women with a high BMI (> 26) and IGT, compared with 128 women with matched high BMI and normal OGTT results. The IGT group was older, with more previous pregnancies, higher incidences of previous GDM, and higher hemoglobin and fasting glucose concentrations. There were no differences in the prepregnancy weight, gestational weight gain or weight or BMI at delivery, and no difference in obstetric complications, mode of delivery, or gestational age or mean infant birthweight. However, the birthweight ratio (relative to mean birthweight for gestation), incidence of large-for-gestational-age (LGA) infants (birthweight > 90th percentile) and macrosomic infants (birthweight ≥ 4000 grams), and events of treated neonatal jaundice were all significantly higher in the IGT group. Thus, some of the complications attributed to GDM are probably related to maternal obesity, but IGT could still affect infant birthweight despite dietary treatment that normalizes maternal gestational weight gain.

In another recent study of 2904 pregnant women the following outcomes measures increased significantly with increasing glucose values on the OGTT: shoulder dystocia, macrosomia, emergency Cesarean section, assisted delivery, hypertension and induction of labor.[56] However, when corrections were made for other risk factors, hypertension and induction of labor were only marginally associated with glucose levels.

Aberg et al[57] conducted a population-based study of maternal and neonatal characteristics and delivery complications in relation to findings for the 75-gram, 2-hour OGTT at 25–30 weeks gestation. The OGTT value was < 140 mg/dl in 4526 women, 140–162 mg/dl in 131 women and ≥ 162 mg/dl in 116 women with GDM. An additional 28 cases of GDM were identified, giving a prevalence of 1.2%. An increased rate of Cesarean section and infant macrosomia was observed in the group with a glucose tolerance of 140–162 mg/dl and in the GDM group. Advanced maternal age and a high BMI were found to be risk factors for increased OGTT values.

Abnormal glucose tolerance test as a risk factor for adverse pregnancy outcome

Is an abnormal GCT alone, without GDM, a risk factor for adverse pregnancy outcome? Using fetal weight and anthropometric characteristics as their parameters, Mello et al[58] evaluated 1615 white women with singleton pregnancies who underwent universal screening for GDM in two periods of pregnancy. They divided the population into three groups according to the GCT results: (1) 172 patients with abnormal GCT in both periods; (2) 391 patients with a normal GCT in the early period and an abnormal GCT in the late period; (3) 1052 patients with a normal GCT in both periods (control group). The incidence of LGA infants was significantly higher in group 1 (40.7%) and group 2 (22.0%) than in the control group (8.3%), and significantly higher in group 1 than in group 2. The newborns of group 1 had higher birthweights than those of group 2 and the control group, and the newborns of the control group had significantly greater lengths and mean cranial circumferences. Group 1 babies had significantly lower ponderal indexes, thoracic circumferences and weight:length ratios than controls, and significantly larger cranial/thoracic circumferences.

Weijers et al[59] defined mild gestational hyperglycemia (MGH) as a positive GCT in the presence of a negative OGTT. Of the 1022 consecutive women evaluated, 813 (79.6%) were healthy, 138 (13.5%) had MGH and 71 (6.9%) had GDM. There was a stepwise significant increase in mean fasting glucose and C-peptide levels among the three diagnostic groups. Maternal age, non-Caucasian ethnicity and prepregnancy BMI were all associated with GDM, whereas only maternal age and prepregnancy BMI were associated with MGH. Therefore, it appears that additional factors promoting the loss of beta-cell function distinguish MGH from GDM. One of these factors is ethnicity.

To determine the predictive value of a negative GCT in subsequent pregnancies, Nahum[60] studied 62 pregnancies of women who had given birth during the past 4 years for whom third-trimester 1-hour, 50-gram glucose screening test results were available for both pregnancies. He found that the GCT results were significantly correlated between the two pregnancies ($r = 0.49$, $P < 0.001$) and concluded that a negative GCT of < 140 mg/dl during pregnancy is strongly predictive of a negative screening result in a succeeding pregnancy within 4 years.

Early gestational diabetes mellitus diagnosis as a risk factor

Early onset of GDM is a high-risk factor. Bartha et al[61] found that among 3986 pregnant women, those with early-onset GDM ($n = 65$) were more likely to be hypertensive (18.46 versus 5.88%, $P = 0.006$), have higher glycemic values and greater needs for insulin therapy (33.85 versus 7.06%, $P < 0.001$) than those in whom diabetes developed later ($n = 170$). All cases of neonatal hypoglycemia ($n = 4$) and all perinatal deaths ($n = 3$) were in this group. The women with early GDM also had an increased risk of postpartum diabetes mellitus, whereas those with late-onset GDM had a minimal risk.[62] The percentages of overt diabetes and abnormal glucose tolerance were significantly higher in the early pregnancy group ($n = 30$) than in the late-pregnancy group ($n = 72$) (26.7 versus 1.4 and 40 versus 5.56%, respectively).

Congenital malformations

Schaefer-Graf et al,[63] in a review of 4180 pregnancies complicated by GDM ($n = 3764$) or NIDDM ($n = 416$), reported that the congenital anomalies in the offspring affected the same organ systems described in pregnancies complicated by IDDM. The risk of anomalies rose with increasing hyperglycemia at diagnosis or presentation for care. However, most other reports had conflicting findings. Bartha et al[61] failed to find an increase in major congenital malformations associated with GDM, as did Kalter[64] in a comprehensive review of the literature. An exception is the recent Swedish Health Registry study covering over 1.2 million births between 1987 and 1997.[65] The authors identified 3864 infants born to women with pre-existing diabetes and 8688 infants born to women with GDM. The total malformation rate in the first group was 9.5% and in the second group 5.7%, similar to the rate in the general population. However, the GDM group was characterized by an excess of certain malformations, suggesting that a subgroup of GDM are at increased risk of diabetic embryopathy, perhaps due to pre-existing but undetected NIDDM.

Martinez-Frias et al[66] analyzed 19,577 consecutive infants with malformations of unknown cause and compared those born to mothers with GDM with those of non-diabetic mothers. Their findings indicated that GDM is a significant risk factor for holoprosencephaly, upper/lower spine/rib anomalies, and renal and urinary system anomalies. However, owing to the heterogeneous nature of GDM, which includes previously unrecognized and newly diagnosed NIDDM, they could not rule out the possibility that the teratogenic effect is related to latent NIDDM. Nevertheless, they concluded that pregnancies complicated by GDM should be considered at risk for congenital anomalies.

By contrast, the relationship between GDM and the development of congenital malformations was examined in another population-based retrospective study using birth certificate data for all live-born children delivered between 1984 and 1991 in Washington State.[67]

The prevalence of congenital malformations was 7.2, 2.8 and 2.1% among the offspring of mothers with established diabetes (n = 8869), GDM (n = 1511) and no diabetes (n = 8934), respectively. That is, the rate of congenital malformations in the GDM group was only slightly higher than in the control group (OR = 1.3, 95% CI 1.0–1.6).

Hypertensive disorders

Pre-eclampsia and gestational hypertension are apparently more frequent in women with GDM. A large study by Xiong et al[12] detected pre-eclampsia in 2.7% of 2755 patients with GDM compared with only 1.1% of 108,664 patients with normal pregnancies (adjusted OR = 1.3, 95% CI 1.20–1.41). Similar results were observed for gestational hypertension. Likewise, Dukler et al[68] studied 380 primiparous women with pre-eclampsia and 385 primiparous control women for a total of 1207 and 1293 deliveries, respectively. When adjusted for confounding variables, GDM was strongly associated with the recurrence of pre-eclampsia in the second pregnancy (OR = 3.72, 95% CI 1.45–9.53).

Go et al,[69] in an 11-year follow-up study of a cross-sectional sample of African-American women with a history of GDM (n = 289), reported one of the highest rates of microalbuminuria (MA) of all ethnic groups. The presence of MA was not associated with insulin resistance, but it was significantly and independently associated with glycosylated hemoglobin (HbAlc) levels and hypertension. Hence, hypertension and glucose intolerance influence MA through different mechanisms, and screening for MA should be considered in this patient population.

Conditions associated with increased insulin resistance, such as GDM, PCOS and obesity, may predispose patients to essential hypertension, hypertensive pregnancy, hyperinsulinemia, hyperlipidemia and high levels of plasminogen activator inhibitor-1, leptin and tumor necrosis factor-alpha. These findings may also be associated with a possible increased risk of cardiovascular complications in these women.[70] Joffe et al[71] provided further support for the role of insulin resistance in the pathogenesis of hypertensive disorders of pregnancy. In a prospective study of 4589 healthy nulliparous women, they found that the women with GDM had an increased relative risk of pre-eclampsia and all hypertensive disorders (RR = 1.67, 95% CI 0.92–3.05 and RR = 1.54, 95% CI 1.28–2.11, respectively). RR were not substantially reduced after further adjustment for race and BMI (OR = 1.41 and 1.48, respectively). Furthermore, even within the normal range, multivariate analysis demonstrated that the level of plasma glucose 1 hour after a 50-gram oral glucose challenge was an important predictor of pre-eclampsia.

Innes et al[72] evaluated 54 normotensive women who developed hypertension in pregnancy and 51 controls with normotensive pregnancies, matched for parity. Mean post-load glucose levels and the total glucose area under the curve were significantly higher in the cases than in the controls, and were positively correlated with peak mean arterial pressure. After adjustment for potential confounders, 2-hour post-load glucose levels remained strongly related to the risk for hypertension and to peak mean arterial blood pressure, as did the total glucose area under the curve. The cases were also more likely to have had one abnormal OGTT. Stratifying analyses by case severity (pre-eclampsia and gestational hypertension) yielded similar results. Among all subjects, more cases than controls were also diagnosed with GDM (31 versus 12%, P = 0.008).

Risk of non-insulin-dependent diabetes mellitus

Women with GDM have a 17–63% risk of NIDDM within 5–16 years.[73] However, the risk varies according to different parameters. For example, Greenberg et al,[74] in a study of 94 patients with GDM, reported that the most significant predictor of 6-weeks postpartum diabetes was insulin requirement, with RR = 17.28 (95% CI 2.46–134.42), followed by poor glycemic control, IGT and a GCT ≥ 200 mg/dl. All of these factors probably represent the magnitude of the insulin resistance, which is the hallmark of future diabetes and of other vascular complications. Similarly, Bian et al[75] reported a diagnosis of diabetes 5–10 years postpartum in 33.3% of patients with previous GDM ($n = 45$), but only 9.7% ($n = 31$) of these with IGT and 2.6% ($n = 39$) of normal controls. Two or more abnormal OGTT values during pregnancy, a blood glucose level exceeding the maximal values at 1 and 2 hours after oral glucose loading, and high pregnancy BMI were all useful predictors of diabetes in later life.

To determine if recurrent episodes of insulin resistance (i.e. another pregnancy) contribute to the decline in beta-cell function that leads to NIDDM in high-risk individuals, Peters et al[76] investigated 666 Latino women with a history of GDM. Among the 87 (13%) who completed an additional pregnancy, the rate ratio of NIDDM increased to 3.34 (95% CI 1.80–6.19), compared with women without an additional pregnancy, after adjustment for other potential diabetes risk factors during the index pregnancy (antepartum oral glucose tolerance, high fasting glucose, gestational age at diagnosis of GDM) and during follow-up (postpartum BMI, glucose tolerance, weight change, breastfeeding and months of contraceptive use). Weight gain was also independently associated with an increased

risk of NIDDM; the rate ratio was 1.95 (95% CI 1.63–2.33) for each 4.5 kg gained during follow-up after adjustment for the additional pregnancy and the other potential risk factors. These data show that a single pregnancy, independent of the well-known effect of weight gain, accelerates the development of NIDDM in women with a high prevalence of pancreatic beta-cell dysfunction.

What about milder, diet-controlled GDM? Damm[77] reported abnormal glucose tolerance in 34.4% of 241 women 2–11 years after a diabetic pregnancy (3.7% IDDM, 13.7% NIDDM, 17% IGT), in contrast to a control group in which none of the women had diabetes and 5.3% had IGT. The independent risk factors for later development of diabetes were high fasting glucose levels at diagnosis of GDM, delivery > 3 weeks before term and abnormal OGTT 2 months postpartum. Low insulin secretion at diagnosis of GDM was also an independent risk factor. Even the non-obese glucose-tolerant women with previous GDM had a metabolic profile of NIDDM, i.e. insulin resistance and impaired insulin secretion. Thus, the first OGTT should probably be performed 2 months postpartum to identify the women who are already diabetic and the women at highest risk of later development of overt diabetes.[77] Interestingly, according to a recent study, both women with a history of GDM as well as their children are at greater risk of progressing to NIDDM.[78] Whether this effect is due to a genetic or an *in utero* influence has yet to be determined.

Summary

The 1997 WHO estimates of the prevalence of diabetes in adults showed an expected total rise of > 120% from 135 million in 1995 to 300 million in 2025.[2] These numbers also include GDM, and should alert physicians to the need to direct special attention to this population, especially in developing countries.

The data presented in this chapter indicate that the epidemiology of GDM is characterized by several features.

- Differences in screening programs and diagnostic criteria make it difficult to compare frequencies of GDM among various populations. Nevertheless, race has been proven to be an independent risk factor for GDM, which varies in prevalence in direct proportion to the prevalence of NIDDM in a given population or ethnic group.
- There are several identifiable predisposing factors for GDM (Table 7.2).
- In the absence of risk factors, the incidence of GDM is low. Therefore, some authors suggest that selective screening may be cost-effective, especially in view the forecasted rise in the burden of GDM.
- PCOS is an important risk factor for GDM, with special similarity in the existence of insulin resistance.
- The genetic diathesis is not well understood.
- The recurrence rate of GDM (35–80%) is influenced by parity, BMI, early diagnosis of GDM, insulin requirement, weight gain and by the interval between pregnancies.
- Pregnant women with IGT and an abnormal GCT may be at increased risk of an adverse outcome relative to woman with a normal glucose tolerance and a normal GCT.
- Women with an early diagnosis of GDM represent a high-risk subgroup, with an increased incidence of obstetric complications, recurrent GDM and development of NIDDM.
- Another subgroup of GDM is characterized by an increased risk of a diabetic embryopathy, perhaps due to pre-existing but undetected NIDDM. This should be considered in all patients with early diagnosis of GDM, accompanied by appropriate patient counseling.
- Hypertensive disorders in pregnancy and afterwards may be more prevalent in women with GDM. One possible mechanism is insulin resistance.
- Women with GDM are at increased risk of developing NIDDM, especially obese patients, those who were diagnosed before 24 weeks gestation and those who required insulin for glycemic control.

References

1. American College of Obstetricians and Gynecologists: *Gestational Diabetes*. Practice Bulletin No. 30, September 2001.
2. King H. Epidemiology of glucose intolerance and gestational diabetes in women of childbearing age. *Diabetes Care* 1998; **21**(Suppl2):B9–B13.
3. Coustan DR. Gestational diabetes. Diabetes in America. In: (National Institutes of Diabetes and Digestive and Kidney Diseases.) 2nd edn, NIH Publication No 95-1468:703–717. (Bethesda, Maryland: NIDDK, 1995.)
4. WHO Ad Hoc Diabetes Reporting Group. Diabetes and impaired glucose tolerance in women aged 20–39 years. *World Health Stat* 1992; **45**:321–7.
5. Dooley SL, Metzger BE, Cho NH. Influence of race on disease prevalence and perinatal outcome in a US population. *Diabetes* 1991; **40**:25–9.
6. Gunton JE, Hitchman R, McElduff A. Effects of ethnicity on glucose tolerance, insulin resistance and beta cell function in 223 women with an abnormal glucose challenge test during pregnancy. *Aust N Z Obstet Gynaecol* 2001; **41**:182–6.
7. Jang HC, Cho NH, Jung KB, Oh KS, Dooley SL, Metzger BE. Screening for gestational diabetes mellitus in Korea. *Int J Gynecol Obstet* 1995; **51**:115–22.
8. Jimenez-Moleon JJ, Bueno-Cavanillas A, Luna-del-Castillo JD, Lardelli-Claret P, Garcia-Martin M, Galvez-Vargas R. Predictive value of a screen for gestational diabetes mellitus: influence of associated risk factors. *Acta Obstet Gynecol Scand* 2000; **79**:991–8.
9. Jang HC, Min HK, Lee HK, Cho NH, Metzger BE. Short stature in Korean women: a contribution to the multifactorial predisposition to gestational diabetes mellitus. *Diabetologia* 1998; **41**:778–3.

10. Kousta E, Lawrence NJ, Penny A et al. Women with a history of gestational diabetes of European and South Asian origin are shorter than women with normal glucose tolerance in pregnancy. *Diabet Med* 2000; **17**:792–7.

11. Branchtein L, Schmidt MI, Matos MC, Yamashita T, Pousada JM, Duncan BB. Short stature and gestational diabetes in Brazil. Brazilian Gestational Diabetes Study Group. *Diabetologia* 2000; **43**:848–51.

12. Xiong X, Saunders LD, Wang FL, Demianczuk NN. Gestational diabetes mellitus: prevalence, risk factors, maternal and infant outcomes. *Int J Gynaecol Obstet* 2001; **75**:221–8.

13. Egeland GM, Skjærven R, Irgens LM. Birth characteristics of women who develop gestational diabetes: population based study. *Br Med J* 2000; **321**:546–7.

14. Ma RM, Lao TT. Maternal mean arterial pressure and oral glucose tolerance test results. Relationship in normotensive women. *J Reprod Med* 2001; **46**:747–51.

15. Lichtenstein AH, Schwab US. Relationship of diatary fat to glucose metabolism. *Atherosclerosis* 2000; **150**:227–43.

16. Clarke SD. Polyunsaturated fatty acid regulation of gene transcription: A mechanism to improve energy balance and insulin resistance. *Br J Nutr* 2000; **83**(Suppl1):s59–s66.

17. Clarke SD. Polyunsaturated fatty acid regulation of gene transcription: A molecular mechanism to improve the metabolic syndrome. *J Nutr* 2001; **131**:1129–32.

18. Rustan AC, Nenseter MS, Drevon CA. Omega-3 and omega-6 fatty acids in the insulin resistance syndrome. Lipid and lipoprotein metabolism and atherosclerosis. *Ann NY Acad Sci* 1997; **827**:310–26.

19. Wijendran V, Bendel RB, Couch SC, Philipson EH, Cheruko S, Lammi-Keefe CJ. Fetal erythrocyte phospholipid polyunsaturated fatty acids are altered in pregnancy complicated with gestational diabetes mellitus. *Lipids* 2000; **35**:927–31.

20. Bo S, Menato G, Lezo A et al. Dietary fat and gestational hyperglycaemia. *Diabetologia* 2001; **44**:972–8.

21. Lao TT, Ho LF. Alpha-thalassaemia trait and gestational diabetes mellitus in Hong Kong. *Diabetologia* 2001; **44**:966–71.

22. Franks S, Gilling-Smith C, Waston H. Insulin action in the normal and polycystic ovary. *Metab Clin North Am* 1999; **28**:361–78.

23. Holte J, Gennarelli G, Wide L, Lithell H, Berne C. High prevalence of polycystic ovaries and associated clinical, endocrine, and metabolic features in women with previous gestational diabetes mellitus. *J Clin Endocrinol Metab* 1998; **83**:1143–50.

24. Kousta E, Cela E, Lawrence N et al. The prevalence of polycystic ovaries in women with a history of gestational diabetes. *Clin Endocrinol (Oxf)* 2000; **53**:501–7.

25. Anttila L, Karjala K, Penttila RA, Ruutiainen K, Ekblad U. Polycystic ovaries in women with gestational diabetes. *Obstet Gynecol* 1998; **92**:13–16.

26. Mikola M, Hiilesmaa V, Halttunen M, Suhonen L, Tiitinen A. Obstetric outcome in women with polycystic ovarian syndrome. *Hum Reprod* 2001; **16**:226–9.

27. Koivunen RM, Juutinen J, Vauhkonen I, Morin-Papunen LC, Ruokonen A, Tapanainen JS. Metabolic and steroidogenic alterations related to increased frequency of polycystic ovaries in women with a history of gestational diabetes. *J Clin Endocrinol Metab* 2001; **86**:2591–9.

28. Hoskins RE. Zygosity as a risk factor for complications and outcomes of twin pregnancy. *Acta Genet Med Gemellol* 1995; **44**:11–23.

29. Sivan E, Maman E, Homko CJ, Lipitz S, Cohen S, Schiff E. Impact of fetal reduction on the incidence of gestational diabetes. *Obstet Gynecol* 2002; **99**:91–4.

30. Schwartz DB, Daoud Y, Zazula P et al. Gestational diabetes mellitus: metabolic and blood glucose parameters in singleton versus twin pregnancies. *Am J Obstet Gynecol* 1999; **181**:912–14.

31. Wein P, Warwick MM, Beischer NA. Gestational diabetes in twin pregnancy: prevalence and long-term implications. *Aust N Z J Obstet Gynaecol* 1992; **32**:325–7.

32. Egeland GM, Irgens LM. Is a multiple birth pregnancy a risk factor for gestational diabetes? *Am J Obstet Gynecol* 2001; **185**:1275–6.

33. Fitzsimmons BP, Bebbington MW, Fluker MR. Perinatal and neonatal outcomes in multiple gestations: assisted reproduction versus spontaneous conception. *Am J Obstet Gynecol* 1998; **179**:1162–7.

34. Henderson CE, Scarpelli S, Larosa D, Divon MY. Assessing the risk of gestational diabetes in twin pregnancies. *J Natl Med Assoc* 1995; **87**:757–8.

35. Harder T, Franke K, Kohlhoff R, Plagemann A. Maternal and paternal family history of diabetes in women with gestational diabetes or insulin-dependent diabetes mellitus type I. *Gynecol Obstet Invest* 2001; **51**:160–4.

36. Dorner G, Plagemann A, Reinagel H. Familial diabetes aggregation in type 2 diabetics: gestational diabetes an apparent risk factor for increased diabetes susceptibility in the offspring. *Exp Clin Endocrinol* 1987; **89**:84–90.

37. Kuhl C. Etiology and pathogenesis of gestational diabetes. *Diabetes Care* 1998; **21**(Suppl2):B19–B26.

38. Vambergue A, Fajardy I, Bianchi F et al. Gestational diabetes mellitus and HLA class II (-DQ, -DR) association: The Digest Study. *Eur J Immunogenet* 1997; **24**:385–94.

39. Lapolla A, Betterle C, Sanzari M et al. An immunological and genetic study of patients with gestational diabetes mellitus. *Acta Diabetol* 1996; **33**:139–44.

40. Budowle B, Huddleston JF, Go RC, Barger BO, Acton RT. Association of HLA-linked factor B with gestational diabetes mellitus in black women. *Am J Obstet Gynecol* 1988; **159**:805–6.

41. Bell DS, Barger BO, Go RC, Goldenberg RL, Perkins LL. Risk factors for gestational diabetes in black population. *Diabetes* 1990; **13**:1196–201.

42. Freinkel N, Metzger BE, Phelps RL et al. Gestational diabetes mellitus: a syndrome with phenotypic and genotypic heterogeneity. *Horm Metab Res* 1986; **18**:427–30.

43. Ferber KM, Keller E, Albert ED, Ziegler AG. Predictive value of human leukocyte antigen class II typing for the development of islet autoantibodies and insulin-dependent diabetes postpartum in women with gestational diabetes. *J Clin Endocrinol Metab* 1999; **84**:2342–8.

44. MacNeill S, Dodds L, Hamilton DC, Armson BA, Vanden Hof M. Rates and risk factors for recurrence of gestational diabetes. *Diabetes Care* 2001; **24**:659–62.

45. Major CA, deVeciana M, Weeks J, Morgan MA. Recurrence of gestational diabetes: Who is at risk? *Am J Obstet Gynecol* 1998; **179**:1038–42.

46. Spong CY, Guillermo L, Kuboshige J, Cabalum T. Recurrence of gestational diabetes mellitus: identification of risk factors. *Am J Perinatol* 1998; **15**:29–33.

47. Nasrat AA, Augnesen K, Abushal M, Shalhoub JT. The outcome of pregnancy following untreated impaired glucose intolerance. *Int J Gynecol Obstet* 1994; **47**:1–6.

48. Ramtoola S, Home P, Damry H, Husnoo A, Ah-Kion S. Gestational impaired glucose tolerance does not increase perinatal mortality in a developing country: cohort study. *Br Med J* 2001; **28**:1025–6.

49. Moses RG, Calvert D. Pregnancy outcomes in women without gestational diabetes mellitus related to the maternal glucose level. *Diabetes Care* 1995; **18**:1527–33.

50. Al-Shawaf T, Moghraby S, Akiel A. Does impaired glucose tolerance imply a risk in pregnancy? *Br J Obstet Gynaecol* 1998; **95**:1036–41.

51. Roberts RN, Moohan JM, Foo RL, Harley JM, Traub AI, Hadden DR. Fetal outcome in mothers with impaired glucose tolerance in pregnancy. *Diabet Med* 1993; **10**:438–43.

52. Tan YY, Yeo GS. Impaired glucose tolerance in pregnancy – is it of consequence? *Aust N Z J Obstet Gynaecol* 1996; **36**:248–55.

53. Jacobson JD, Cousins L. A population-based study of maternal and perinatal outcome in patients with gestational diabetes. *Am J Obstet Gynecol* 1989; **161**:981–6.

54. Li DFH, Wong VCW, O'Hoy KMKY. Is treatment needed for mild impairment of glucose tolerance in pregnancy? A randomized controlled trial. *Br J Obstet Gynaecol* 1987; **94**:851–4.

55. Lao TT, Ho LF. Impaired glucose tolerance and pregnancy outcome in Chinese women with high body mass index. *Hum Reprod* 2000; **8**:1826–9.

56. Jensen DM, Damm P, Sorensen B et al. Clinical impact of mild carbohydrate intolerance in pregnancy: a study of 2904 nondiabetic Danish women with risk factors for gestational diabetes mellitus. *Am J Obstet Gynecol* 2001; **185**:413–19.

57. Aberg A, Rydhstroem H, Frid A. Impaired glucose tolerance associated with adverse pregnancy outcome: a population-based study in southern Sweden. *Am J Obstet Gynecol* 2001; **184**:77–83.

58. Mello G, Parretti E, Mecacci F et al. Anthropometric characteristics of full-term infants: effects of varying degrees of 'normal' glucose metabolism. *J Perinat Med* 1997; **25**:197–204.

59. Weijers RN, Bekedam DJ, Smulders YM. Determinants of mild gestational hyperglycemia and gestational diabetes mellitus in a large Dutch multiethnic cohort. *Diabetes Care* 2002; **25**:72–7.

60. Nahum GG. Correlation between 1-hour 50-gram glucose screening test values in successive pregnancies. *Obstet Gynecol* 2001; **97**(Suppl1):S39–S40.

61. Bartha JL, Martinez-Del-Fresno P, Comino-Delgado R. Gestational diabetes mellitus diagnosed during early pregnancy. *Am J Obstet Gynecol* 2000; **182**:346–50.

62. Bartha JL, Martinez-del-Fresno P, Comino-Delgado R. Postpartum metabolism and autoantibody markers in women with gestational diabetes mellitus diagnosed in early pregnancy. *Am J Obstet Gynecol* 2001; **184**:965–70.

63. Schaefer-Graf UM, Buchanan TA, Songster G, Montoro M, Kjos SL. Patterns of congenital anomalies and relationship to initial maternal fasting glucose levels in pregnancies complicated by type 2 and gestational diabetes. *Am J Obstet Gynecol* 2000; **182**:313–20.

64. Kalter H. The non-teratogenicity of gestational diabetes. *Paediatr Perinat Epidemiol* 1998; **12**:456–8.

65. Aberg A, Westbom L, Kallen B. Congenital malformations among infants whose mothers had gestational diabetes or preexisting diabetes. *Early Human Dev* 2001; **61**:85–95.

66. Martinez-Frias ML, Bermejo E, Rodriguez-Pinilla E, Prieto L, Frias JL. Epidemiological analysis of outcomes of pregnancy in gestational diabetic mothers. *Am J Med Genet* 1998; **78**:140–5.

67. Janssen PA, Rothman I, Schwartz SM. Congenital malformations in newborns of women with established and gestational diabetes in Washington State, 1984–91. *Paediatr Perinat Epidemiol* 1996; **10**:52–63.

68. Dukler D, Porath A, Bashiri A, Erez O, Mazor M. Remote prognosis of primiparous women with preeclampsia. *Eur J Obstet Gynecol Reprod Biol* 2001; **96**:69–74.

69. Go RC, Desmond R, Roseman JM, Bell DS, Vanichanan C, Acton RT. Prevalence and risk factors of microalbuminuria in a cohort of African-American women with gestational diabetes. *Diabetes Care* 2001; **24**:1764–9.

70. Solomon CG, Seely EW. Brief review: hypertension in pregnancy: a manifestation of the insulin resistance syndrome? *Hypertension* 2001; **37**:232–9.

71. Joffe GM, Esterlitz JR, Levine RJ et al. The relationship between abnormal glucose tolerance and hypertensive disorders of pregnancy in healthy nulliparous women. Calcium for Preeclampsia Prevention (CPEP) Study Group. *Am J Obstet Gynecol* 1998; **179**:1032–7.

72. Innes KE, Wimsatt JH, McDuffie R. Relative glucose tolerance and subsequent development of hypertension in pregnancy. *Obstet Gynecol* 2001; **97**:905–10.

73. Kjos SL, Buchanan TA. Gestational diabetes mellitus. *N Engl J Med* 1999; **341**:1749–56.

74. Greenberg LR, Moore TR, Murphy H. Gestational diabetes mellitus: antenatal variables as predictors of post-partum glucose intolerance. *Obstet and Gynecol* 1995; **86**:96–101.

75. Bian X, Gao P, Xiong X, Xu H, Qian M, Liu S. Risk factors for development of diabetes mellitus in women with a history of gestational diabetes mellitus. *Chin Med J (Engl)* 2000; **113**:759–62.

76. Peters RK, Kjos SL, Xiang A, Buchanan TA. Long-term diabetogenic effect of single pregnancy in women with previous gestational diabetes mellitus. *Lancet* 1996; **347**:227–30.

77. Damm P. Gestational diabetes mellitus and subsequent development of overt diabetes mellitus. *Dan Med Bull* 1998; **45**:495–509.

78. Fletcher B, Gulanick M, Lamendola C. Risk factors for type 2 diabetes mellitus. *J Cardiovasc Nurs* 2002; **16**:17–23.

79. Foster-Powel KA, Cheung NW. Recurrence of gestational diabetes. *Aust N Z J Obstet Gynaecol* 1998; **38**:384–7.

80. Jolly M, Sebire N, Harris J, Robinson S, Regan L. The risks associated with pregnancy in woman aged 35 years or older. *Hum Reprod* 2000; **15**:2433–7.

81. Lao TT, Chan PL, Tam KF. Gestational diabetes mellitus in the last trimester – a feature of maternal iron excess? *Diabet Med* 2001; **18**:218–23.

8

Pregnancy in diabetic animals

Eleazar Shafrir, Gernot Desoye

Introduction

It would be expected that pregnancy in many of the animal models of Type 1 or Type 2 diabetes would result in a typical overt diabetes or gestational diabetes mellitus (GDM). However, although this is true in cytotoxin-induced diabetes it is not in most genetically predetermined diabetes in animals. The lepr^{db} mice, lepr^{fa} rats and KK mice are infertile, and heterozygote siblings are used to obtain the homozygote individuals. Most studies of diabetes in pregnancy in animals have therefore been performed in cytotoxin-treated animals, predominantly rodents.

Streptozotocin-induced diabetes

STZ-induced diabetes results from either intravenous (IV) or intraperitoneal (IP) injection of the toxin. Alloxan is also an effective diabetogenic agent but is now rarely used in pregnant animals. The mode of action of STZ and typical observations on the resulting diabetic derangements in various animal species have been extensively described in several reviews.[1–5] A wide range of animals may be used to elicit diabetes in pregnancy by STZ, including rabbits, pigs, sheep and subhuman primates.[6–9]

However, the preferred and most often used experimental models are rodents because of their convenient maintenance, short length of pregnancy, multiparity (enabling studies on multiple fetuses and generations), and lack of special problems in termination of pregnancy and fetus recovery. The need for animal models for research of pathophysiology of diabetic pregnancy, a goal not fully attainable by study of human subjects, was underscored by Baird and Aerts.[10] Useful information on various animals suitable for perinatal metabolic research has been contributed by Susa.[11]

There is a marked difference in the effect of diabetes on the maternal, fetal and placental histopathology and metabolism depending on STZ dosage and time of injection. Rodents rendered diabetic before conception manifest hyperglycemia and hypoinsulinemia during organogenesis. As a result, they experience a high degree of fetal resorption and a high percentage of malformed fetuses.[12–16] Injection of STZ into rats in midgestation between days 5 and 14 of gestation, produces diabetes with a low percentage of fetal malformations, and provides the opportunity to follow the metabolic changes induced by maternal diabetes and to study those effects on the placenta and fetus.[17,18]

STZ injected into the mother does not affect the fetal pancreas. Although STZ crosses the placenta, its maternal half-life is of the order of minutes and the amount reaching the fetal circulation does not damage fetal beta cells, as investigated in rhesus monkeys.[19] Injection of STZ into rodents in the postorganogenesis phase, but before full pancreas development, also does not affect the function of the fetal pancreas, except of beta-cell degranulation secondary to the prevalent hyperglycemia.

Diabetes characteristics in pregnant STZ-induced diabetic rats

STZ-induced diabetes should serve mainly as a model for pregestational diabetes since the hyperglycemia and metabolic derangements are the result of beta-cell destruction, whereas GDM is characterized by insulin resistance and compensatory hyperinsulinemia with possible secondary lesion to beta cells as a result of the strain of oversecretion. Even moderate doses of STZ, which result in mild hyperglycemia, do not represent GDM, since the result is a limited insulin deficiency due to a reduced beta-cell mass.

Glucose and glycogen metabolism in STZ-induced diabetes

The decreased glucose uptake by muscles, the reduction in glucose transporter activity and concentration, and the increased hepatic glucose production in diabetes are well documented and discernible early. The hyperglycemia of diabetes is also a concentration-dependent factor causing increased deposition of glycogen in both rodent and human placentae (Fig. 8.1).[20,21] It is remarkable that glycogen accumulation in the placenta occurs despite the maternal insulin deficiency, while the glycogen content in the typical insulin-sensitive maternal tissues (e.g. adipose tissue,

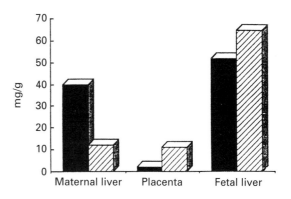

Figure 8.1. *Glycogen content in the placenta and in maternal and fetal liver of control and STZ-induced diabetic rats on day 20 of gestation. Values are means of determinations in 20–26 rats at the mean level of plasma glucose of 6.0 and 24.5 mmol/l in control and diabetic rats, respectively. The insulinopenic STZ-induced diabetes caused a marked decrease in maternal hepatic glycogen content, whereas the placental glycogen content rose about fivefold. Fetal liver glycogen also increased, but this was associated with intrafetal hyperinsulinemia. Data adapted from Barash et al.[23]*

muscle and liver) becomes reduced. Fetal liver glycogen content is increased most probably in response to the fetal hyperglycemia and consequent hyperinsulinemia. The responses of maternal insulin-sensitive tissues in insulinopenic diabetes are well known, entailing glycogen breakdown as regulated by the reciprocal activities of the enzymes glycogen synthase and glycogen phosphorylase. However, in the placenta these enzymes are not sensitive to insulin and the deposition of glycogen is positively correlated with the abundance of glucose. This is accompanied by an increase in the intracellular concentration of glucose-6-phosphate,[22] a potent activator of the phosphorylated (inactive) form of glycogen synthase. Such a mechanism was shown to operate not only in diabetes but in normal pregnant animals rendered hyperglycemic by glucose infusion.[23] Thus, the placenta exhibits a mode of regulation of glycogen metabolism similar to other insulin-insensitive tissues, such as kidneys or intestine, which also accumulate glycogen in insulin-deficient diabetes in response to the augmented hyperglycemic gradient across the cells.[24–27]

Lipid metabolism and transport in STZ-induced diabetic rats

Hypoinsulinemic diabetes is known to result in fat release from adipose tissues, due to the weakened restraint of triglyceride (TG) lipolysis. In non-pregnant animals, this leads to increased hepatic fat oxidation and ketogenesis. However, in pregnant animals, additional tissues take up free fatty acids (FFA) released by lipolysis, namely the placenta and fetus. In STZ diabetic rats, a significant correlation was found between maternal levels of TG, placental TG and fetal TG, all of which were markedly elevated (Fig. 8.2).[18] There was also a marked increase in TG and FFA in the fetal circulation. Fetal weight does not increase, probably due to the short duration of diabetic pregnancy insufficient for appreciable intrafetal fat accretion and also due to rather severe diabetes in these experiments.[18] In another report on diabetes in pigs, fetal obesity was observed.[28] Based on the pattern of distribution of the injected [^{14}C]fatty acid and $^{3}H_2O$ radioactivity, it was shown that the increment in fetal TG in STZ-induced diabetes is derived from the

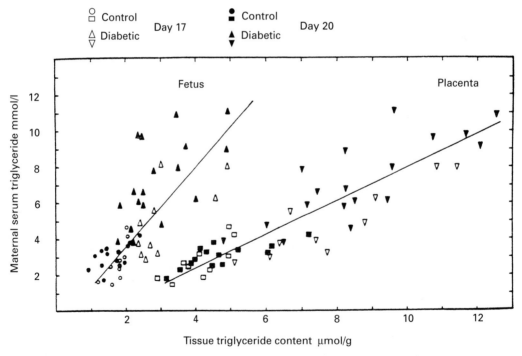

Figure 8.2. *Relationship between the elevated triglyceride (TG) concentration in rat maternal circulation and the TG content in placentae and fetuses towards the end of gestation. Regression lines for placentae: y = –1.1 + 0.9 x; r = 0.88; for fetuses: y = –0.5 + 2.1 x; r = 0.74. Each point is a mean of TG values in five placentae and five fetuses from each of the 52 litters. Adapted from Shafrir and Khassis.[18]*

Injected VLDL*	Placenta	Fetal liver	Fetal carcass
1.23	4.22	5.43	5.88

* VLDL, Very-low-density liproprotein.
Double-labeled VLDL were prepared by the injection of [14C]palmitate and [3H]glycerol into rats followed by exsanguinations 20 minutes later and separation of the VLDL by ultracentrifugation. The isolated VLDL were injected into non-diabetic or STZ-induced diabetic rats (10 mg VLDL TG rat) on day 20 of gestation, and the 3H:14C ratio was measured after 2 hours in the placenta, fetal liver and fetal carcass after extraction of lipids in chloroform:methanol 2:1. (Unpublished data: Shafrir, Barash and Levy.)

Table 8.1. *Free fatty acid:glycerol ratio change during triglyceride (TG) uptake by the placenta and transfer to the fetus.*

transfer of maternal TG and FFA rather than from increased *de novo* intrafetal lipogenesis.[18]

The passage of lipids across the placenta involves an initial uptake of FFA and very-low-density-lipoprotein (VLDL)-borne TG from the circulation. The latter are lipolysed in the process of uptake in proximity to the tissue. The uptake of FFA does not represent a direct transfer to the fetus but a sequential process of intermediate re-esterification to TG and phospholipids within the placental cells, with subsequent lipolysis by an intracellular lipase and release to the fetal side.[29] The presence in the placenta of lipoprotein lipase-like activity was inferred from the change in the FFA:glycerol ratio during TG uptake (Table 8.1). The presence and pH optima of other intracellular lipases have also been reported (Fig. 8.3).[30] The activity of intracellular lipase is linked to the transfer of placental lipids to the fetus and is elevated in diabetes.[31] In the face of an augmented maternal–fetal gradient of FFA and TG, there is an increased flow associated with a substantial amount of intracellular FFA. Thus, the transplacental passage in diabetes may also involve a diffusion of FFA along the membrane lipids of interfacial capillaries.[31]

The increased maternal–fetal transport of fat in STZ-induced diabetes was also demonstrated by an altered distribution of polyunsaturated fatty acids in maternal, placental and fetal tissues near the time of delivery. These fatty acids must be of nutritional origin and therefore derived from the maternal circulation. A pronounced (60%) increase in the relative content of linoleate was recorded in the placental and fetal carcass TG, and as much as *c.* 200% in the fetal liver.[30] This suggests that after placental transfer, the fetal liver is the primary recipient of fatty acid excess from the diabetic mother, but the fetal liver TG are then redistributed to other fetal tissues through the hepatic synthesis of VLDL.

Results similar to those in rodents have been obtained in diabetic pigs. Induction of diabetes in Yorkshire gilts during the third trimester of gestation resulted in a twofold increase in the carcass fat content in the progeny compared with controls injected with either saline or insulin,[29] indicating a direct incorporation of maternal fatty acids into fetal adipocytes. Diabetes decreased the maternal lipogenesis while increasing the *de novo* fetal fat synthesis in pigs.[32]

Enzymes of metabolic pathways in diabetic pregnant animals

STZ-induced and insulin-deficient diabetes have, in general, far-reaching effects on the

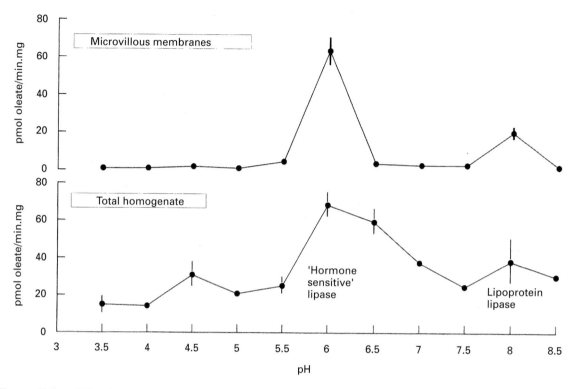

Figure 8.3. *Triacylglycerol (TG) lipases from human placenta characterized by their pH optima. Cytosolic pH 6 lipase is referred to as 'hormone sensitive lipase' and that of pH 8 as 'lipoprotein lipase'. Adapted from Waterman et al.[31]*

synthesis and activity of numerous rate-limiting enzymes in the pathways of carbohydrate, lipid and protein metabolism in both human and animal tissues. These enzymes respond to hormone alterations, which include insulin, glucocorticoids, triiodothyronine, and pregnancy-related hormones such as estrogen and progesterone. This involves both activity responses to changes in concentrations of metabolic effectors as well as translational or transcriptional influences at the DNA or mRNA level. To mention but a few, the regulatory enzymes of carbohydrate metabolism, glucokinase, hexokinase, pyruvate kinase, pyruvate dehydrogenase and glucose-6-phosphate dehydrogenase are severely reduced in the liver or adipose tissue, whereas those regulating gluconeogenesis, PEPCK and glucose-6-phosphatase, increase in activity and concentration. Similarly, lipogenic enzymes, e.g. acetyl coenzyme A (acetyl CoA) carboxylase, are markedly reduced in diabetes, both in concentration and in activity, whereas those responsible for TG lipolysis and FFA oxidation are enhanced. These changes have also been documented in pregnant diabetic animals, as exemplified in the STZ-induced diabetic rats[17] or alloxan-induced diabetic pigs.[33]

The placenta is an exception to these activity changes. The placental enzymes are constitutive, almost devoid of capacity to adapt in activity to diabetes or other hormonal and pathophysiological changes in the maternal organism.[17,34] Treatment of pregnant rats with different hormones or protracted fasting, which has a pronounced effect the activity of maternal hepatic and adipose tissue enzymes, is without appreciable effect on most placental enzymes in the rat[34,35] or rabbit.[36] Fetal liver enzymes do respond, although to a lesser extent than those in the maternal liver.[17,37] These observations suggest that, by maintaining the constancy of enzymatic function, the placenta confers metabolic stability to the fetus, thus shielding the fetus from hormonally induced fluctuations on the maternal side, and attenuating the possible variations in the metabolite flow and substrate availability to the fetus.

Embryopathy in STZ-induced diabetic animals

One of the numerous problems confronted in overt diabetic pregnancy is fetal wastage together with a large percentage of congenital malformations, mainly in neural tissues and skeleton development. Cytotoxin-induced diabetic rodents are therefore preferred models for the study of fetal malformations. As mentioned before, a correlation exists between hyperglycemia in the organogenesis phase and the extent of malformations in the offspring of diabetic rodents.[16,38] Since hyperglycemia is the main culprit, apart from the study of malformations *in vivo*, normal or STZ-induced diabetic animals are often used as a source of embryos for *in vitro* studies after removal at various stages of gestation.[38–40]

As elegantly demonstrated by Strieleman et al[41] and Hod et al,[42,43] myoinositol is vital in preventing malformations. In cultured rat fetuses the teratogenicity of 400 mg/dl glucose was evident by a decrease in the concentration of inositol phosphates and in reduced DNA synthesis. The extent of neural and extraneural malformations rose *c*. 10-fold. Addition, at normal glucose concentrations, of scylloinositol – a non-metabolizable isomer of inositol preventing its intracellular transport – produced a decrease in cellular myoinositol and inositol phosphates, impaired growth with dysmorphogenesis, and malformations similar in extent to high glucose concentrations. Hod et al[42,43] found that sorbinil – an inhibitor of aldose reductase – was ineffective in preventing malformations in cultured fetuses which amounted to > 50 versus 4% at normal glucose concentrations; however, the addition of 1.5 mg/ml of exogenous inositol substantially reduced the malformations.

Extensive investigations of the glucotoxicity of advanced glycation endproducts (AGE) and of the detrimental effect of oxidative radicals were performed by Erickson and associates, and is described in Chapter 20. It is worth emphasizing here that many of these studies were performed in cytotoxin-induced diabetic models or fetuses cultured in diabetic mileu. Ornoy and co-workers[44,45] cultured 10.5 day old normal fetuses in 'diabetic' serum containing 200 mg/dl glucose, 200 mg/dl β-hydroxybutyrate and 1 mg/dl acetoacetate. As determined by cyclic voltametry, a marked drop in natural, protective antioxidative components was noted, along with depletion of vitamins E and C. The malformations could, in large measure, be prevented by raising the antioxidant defences using superoxide dismutase and resupplying vitamins E and C.

The particular contribution of the oxidative stress in the diabetic milieu is not only due to AGE but to the plethora of reducing equivalents emanating from high glucose metabolism. The inflow of reduced nicotinamide adenine dinucleotide (NADH) to mitochondria is not only from the Krebs cycle metabolizing significant loads of glycolysis-derived products but also from the aldose reductase pathway.

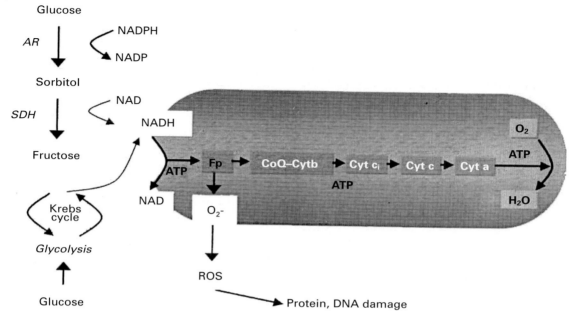

Figure 8.4. *Sources of reduced nicotinamide adenine dinucleotide (NADH) flowing into the mitochondria, the Krebs tricarboxylic acid cycle and NADH derived from aldose reductase initiated dehydrogenation of glucose and the NAD-dependent conversion of sorbitol to fructose. In hyperglycemia, the flow of reducing equivalents is considerably increased, overloading the mitochondrial electron transport chain. The accumulation of reducing equivalents at the stage of flavin adenine dinucleotide (FAD) oxidase results in the production of reactive oxygen species with a detrimental effect on multiple feto-placental systems.*

The mitochondrial electron transport system is overloaded, particularly at the flavin adenine dinucleotide (FAD)-dependent oxidase (flavoprotein) step, which results in extrusion of the reactive oxygen species as illustrated in Fig. 8.4.

Neonatally STZ-administered rats

Among the syndromes resembling mild Type 2 diabetes as a consequence of reduced beta-cell mass are rats which received neonatal STZ injection (nSTZ), either at the time of birth[46] or 2 days after birth.[47,48] It should be stressed, however, that these animals, although non-obese, do not represent a true Type 2 diabetes, but rather a model of limited insulin deficiency with little, if any, peripheral or hepatic insulin resistance.

The IP or IV injection of 90–100 mg/kg STZ into neonatal rats causes a c. 90% destruction of pancreatic beta cells with hyperglycemia that peaks 3–5 days thereafter. This acute diabetes is transient, the beta cells at the neonatal stage are endowed with a remarkable regeneration capacity, although up to 30% of mortality is also occurring. After 3–5 weeks, fasting plasma glucose and insulin levels return to normal, even though the regenerated cells are not completely normal and an impairment in insulin secretion persists, as seen in the response to a glucose load. The inferior performance of the regenerated cells is further exposed by subjecting the young animals to stress. By 8 weeks and thereafter blood glucose is 150–180 mg/dl with impaired glucose tolerance (IGT) and a 50% decrease in pancreatic insulin content with mild hypoinsulinemia. As reviewed by Portha et al,[49] the incompetence of the regenerated beta cells may be due to a reduced GLUT2 content limiting glucose entry and metabolism, and a decreased glucokinase affinity to glucose. More probably there is a reduced mitochondrial oxidation capacity of glucose-derived products, which is evident since leucine oxidation and insulinotropic action is similar to normal, i.e. acetyl CoA from leucine is metabolized without impediment. It has been suggested that the affected site is the FAD glycerol phosphate shuttle slowing the flow of reducing equivalence into the mitochondria. The activity of K^+ adenosine triphosphate (ATP) channels, the rate-limiting step in insulin secretion, may be also affected. The polarization of these channels allows Ca^{2+} entry into the cell, triggering the insulin secretion. However, no defect in K^+ ATP channels has been detected but their function may be slowed due to ATP deficiency.

One form of stress that exposes the latent diabetes in nSTZ rats is pregnancy. The basal plasma glucose concentration is elevated, both during the pregnancy and postpartum, and plasma insulin levels are reduced compared with those of normal pregnant rats. Glucose intolerance was explicit during the response to a glucose load and persisted for 2 months postpartum. As demonstrated by Triadou et al,[50] the secretion defect is particularly evident in the significantly decreased plasma insulin:glucose ratio during the pregnancy and postpartum (Table 8.2). Insufficient information is available on the pregnancy and malformations in the nSTZ model, and should be extensively explored because of the implication that the reduced or incompetent beta-cell mass may be an aggravating factor to human GDM. Complications in various tissues of the nSTZ rats have been reviewed by Schaffer and Mozaffari.[51]

	Body weight (grams)	Plasma glucose (mg/dl)	Plasma insulin (mU/l)	Insulin/glucose at 0–90 minutes
Neonatally STZ-treated rats				
Virgin	153±3*	203±5*	30±3*	4±1*
Pregnant (day 21)	281±11*	128±15*	52±11	5±1*
Postpartum (2 months)	265±9	173±5	47±4	3±1*
Normal rats				
Virgin	174±3	156±6	51±7	19±2
Pregnant (day 21)	330±13	83±3	45±7	29±4
Postpartum (2 months)	272±5	145±3	54±5	10±1

* Significant difference from corresponding control at $P \leq 0.05$.
Data are means ± SE; $n = 7$–9 rats/group. The nSTZ rats were mated at 3–4 months and compared with control rats mated at 2.5–3 months. An IV glucose load (0.5 g/kg) was given during pregnancy and postpartum, and the integrated insulin increment was related to the glucose increment. Adapted from Triadou et al.[50]

Table 8.2. *Pregnancy in normal and neonatal (nSTZ) streptoztocin injected rats.*

It is of interest to mention the results of nSTZ injection into spontaneously hypertensive (SHR) rats. These insulin-resistant rats, which are used as a model of human essential hypertension, are prone to develop hypertensive cerebrocardiovascular disease with aging.[52] Diabetes was induced by IP injection of 75 mg STZ 2 days after birth and the animals were mated with untreated male SHR rats at 4–5 months of age. Hyperglycemia of 20 mmol/l was evident during the pregnancy, with an elevated systolic blood pressure (213 versus 192 mmHg) and albuminuria. The progeny was microsomic. nSTZ treatment of SHR rats decreased the lifespan of male offspring from *c*. 18 to 15 months and raised the systolic blood pressure in correlation with their birthweight.[53,54] Such a model may be useful for the study of combined hypertension and diabetes.

Progeny of STZ-induced diabetic animals

With regard to the progeny of diabetic animals as models of insulin-deficient diabetes, it should be recalled that the intrauterine metabolic fuel milieu is untoward for the fetus.

Fetal pancreatic beta cells are vulnerable to hyperglycemia and to changes in other metabolites. The inflicted injury persists after birth, resulting in mild Type-2-like, insulin-deficient diabetes and is propagated into successive generations.[55] STZ-induced diabetes was produced either by a low (30 mg/kg) or high (50 mg/kg) dose of STZ on day 1 of gestation, and created mild or severe maternal diabetes, respectively, resulting in a reduction in the maternal beta-cell content.[56,57] The characteristics of mild and severe STZ maternal diabetes, and its effect on the fetus, is shown in Table 8.3. Mildly diabetic mothers are moderately hypoinsulinemic and hyperglycemic, whereas severely diabetic mothers are insulin deficient, markedly hyperglycemic and hyperlipidemic, with low body weights.

In the fetal pancreas, beta-cell granulation starts at day 17 of gestation in non-diabetic rats, with a pronounced expansion in islet size, continuing up to the birth. In severely diabetic rats, hypertrophy of islets with poor granulation is observed on day 20 of gestation. The degranulated beta cells in the islets are evident but there is appearently no decrease in the beta-cell number.[57] The degranulation should

	Non-diabetic	Mildly diabetic	Severely diabetic
Fetal weight (grams)	2.0±0.02	2.1±0.05*	1.9±0.02*
Fetal plasma glucose (mg/dl)	54±2	69±3*	317±27*
Fetal plasma insulin (mU/l)	87±7	103±8*	45±4*
Placental weight (grams)	460±20	462±23	560±31*
Placental glycogen (mg/g)	1.7±0.1	1.6±0.1	5.8±0.3*
Offspring weight at 100 days (grams)	209±5	205±3	186±6*
Fasting plasma glucose (mg/dl)	91±2	91±1	94±3
Plasma glucose at day 20 of gestation (mg/dl)	80±3	110±5*	98±4*
Granulated beta cells in islets (%)	66±2	50±3	56±2*

* Significant difference from control values at $P < 0.05$ at least.
Data are means ± SE; n = 19–34 rats/groups. Adapted from Aerts et al[57] and Bihoreau et al.[58]

Table 8.3. *Effect of severe and mild STZ diabetes on mothers and their progeny.*

be attributed to the secretory overtaxation of the newly organized endocrine pancreas, with granule depletion overtaking the usually rapid regranulation. This is striking on the day of birth in severely diabetic rats, showing, in addition to pronounced degranulation, disorganization of the rough endoplasmic reticulum, swelling of mitochondria and glycogen deposits. Insulin stores of the pancreas are correlated with morphological observations: at birth, the fetal insulin content is very low, compared with doubling of insulin stores in fetuses of non-diabetic rats at birth. The response to secretagogues is also concordant with the morphology and insulin content: fetal islets of mildly diabetic mothers are capable of response, whereas those of severely diabetic mothers have a minimal response, indicating a defective stimulus coupling.[58,59] Newborns of severely diabetic mothers exhibit microsomia (even if they are born *c.* 1 day later than those of mildly diabetic mothers) in association with placentomegaly (Table 8.3). Newborns of mildly diabetic mothers are macrosomic, with a postnatal period of hypoglycemia followed by a mild hyperglycemia. At weaning after 1 month, these pups return to fasting normoglycemia, but they exhibit latent diabetes, as seen from the IGT with a low insulin:glucose ratio after a glucose load.

At *c.* 3 months of age, the percentage of granulated cells in pancreatic islets is normal in the progeny of both mildly and severely diabetic mothers; however, the granules of the offspring of the severely diabetic mothers are pale,[55] suggesting insulin depletion. Fasting plasma glucose and insulin levels are normal, but even on slight stress, e.g. anesthesia, glucose and insulin become elevated. At 8 months of age, the situation worsens, basal hyperglycemia, IGT and resistance to insulin action increasing.[60] The half-maximal suppression of hepatic gluconeogenesis requires insulin concentrations *c.* 50% higher than in controls.

The important aspect of the first generation of female offspring of diabetic mothers is their metabolic–endocrine reaction to pregnancy. They develop mild hyperglycemia and IGT during gestation, and their fetuses grow again in hyperglycemic fuel milieu, ensuing in derangements similar to those of the first-generation fetuses. Islet hyperplasia and hypertrophy with beta-cell degranulation and hyperinsulinemia, with loss of insulin stores, are perpetuated in the subsequent female pregnant generations. The non-genetic consequence of the abnormal metabolic milieu gives credence to the concept that 'diabetes begets diabetes' by imprinting of alterations in metabolism in the fetus *in utero*, with a propensity to diabetes and obesity in adult life.[61,62] The hyperglycemia may effect DNA mutagenesis of the reporter *lacI* transgene during embryonic development. In a transgenic mouse a twofold increase in mutation frequency of the *lacI* transgene was observed in fetuses developing in a hyperglycemic milieu.[63] This finding provides evidence for gene toxicity of the diabetic environment, suggested to be due to the effect of AGE, known for their mutagenecity.

It is worthy to note that similar changes in pancreatic function and characteristics of the offspring can be produced in non-diabetic rats by continuous glucose infusion during the last stage of pregnancy, strengthening the contention that the glycemia is mainly responsible for the persistent transgenerational GDM.[64,65] This was demonstrated by maintaining rats on protracted glucose infusion through indwelling catheters during the last third of gestation. Female offspring of the glucose-infused rats exhibited IGT when 3 months old that persisted during their pregnancy. The newborn second generation was hyperglycemic, hyperinsulinemic and macrosomic, quite similar to the second generation of rats born to STZ-induced diabetic mothers, and on adulthood became glucose intolerant with defective insulin secretion.

Mild GDM

A model much sought after is that of mild GDM that reverts to normal after delivery.[66] An attempt to provide such a model was made by transplanting STZ-induced diabetic female rats with isogeneic islets of Langerhans[67] and mating them with non-diabetic partners. The results were promising in that the hyperglycemia in dams transplanted with 700–1000 islets was moderate and no congential anomalies were observed in the offspring.

Fetal hyperinsulinemia as a cause of macrosomia in pregnancy

Diabetes produces major changes in the hormonal and metabolic homeostasis in pregnancy that have divergent effects on maternal and feto-placental tissues. The hyperglycemia in cytotoxin-induced diabetes was considered to cause maternal tissue malfunction on the one hand and to induce the precocious commencement of fetal insulin secretion on the other. The profuse insulin secretion was assumed to promote fetal overgrowth by the excess of glucose, amino acids and other fuels.[68] The fetuses of STZ-induced diabetic rats were shown to have lower tissue DNA contents and DNA polymerase activities than those of normal or mildly diabetic mothers,[69] suggesting that the fetal tissue growth recedes as the severity of maternal diabetes increases. However, numerous observations underscore that the fetal macrosomia is insulin induced. In mild diabetes it comprises obesity as an important

element, in addition to the selective organ overgrowth.

Fetal fat accretion may result from excessive *de novo* lipogenesis along with stimulated tissue growth during the fetal hyperinsulinemia, or from the excess of maternal lipids entering the fetal circulation because of the steep concentration gradient across the placenta in GDM (Fig. 8.3). Fetal fat increment caused by the accelerated maternal transfer is dependent on maternal hypoinsulinemia or insulin resistance and is abetted by the concomitant fetal hyperinsulinemmia. Szabo and Szabo[70] and Skryten et al[71] were among the first to suggest that the diabetes-augmented lipid gradient across the placenta contributes to fetal obesity. As mentioned above, in more recent studies the extent of endogenous fatty acid synthesis was measured by ^3H incorporation, whereas the transfer of maternal fat was monitored with a ^{14}C-labeled fatty acid.[18] In STZ-induced diabetic rats, the endogenous lipogenesis was substantial but was not higher than that in non-diabetic pregnant controls. In contrast, there was a marked increment in the ^{14}C-labeled, maternally derived fat in placental and fetal tissues during the last third of gestation. Thus, both the maternal contribution and the intrafetal fat synthesis appear to contribute to the fetal macrosomia, particularly in mild maternal diabetes, similar to the factors promoting adipose tissue hypertrophy in human gestation.[72]

In rats, the effect of hyperinsulinemia on fetal growth has been investigated by direct intrafetal insulin injection. Rat fetuses receiving 5 units (U) of long-acting insulin on day 18 of gestation had their plasma insulin elevated for 24 hours, with the body mass of fetuses exceeding that of saline-injected controls. At birth, the weight of insulin-injected fetuses rose significantly from 5.5 to 5.9 grams.[73] Fetal hyperinsulinemia enhanced the

Insulin infusion	Plasma insulin (mU/l)	Weight (g)				
		Fetus	Placenta	Liver	Kidney	Heart
None	28±12	372±54	92±12	11±3	2.7±0.5	2.3±0.6
5 U/day	340±208	459±53*	125±40	14±2	3.0±0.8	3.0±0.7*
19 U/day	3625±1700	474±48*	142±51*	17±4	3.4±0.9	3.7±0.9*

* Significant difference between control and insulin-infused fetuses at $P \le 0.05$.
Insulin was infused for 20 days at day 145 of gestation. Data are means ± SE. Adapted from Susa et al.[77]

Table 8.4. *Chronic hyperinsulinemia in fetal rhesus monkeys.*

hepatic and carcass fatty acid synthesis.[74] Fetal hyperinsulinemia, achieved by transuteral injections of insulin on day 19 of gestation, resulted in macrosomia at birth, and in net increases in protein and mRNA synthesis in the brain, heart and liver.[75] However, one should be aware that maternal, in contrast to fetal, hyperinsulinemia, produced by implantation of insulin minipumps on day 14 of gestation, produced the opposite result: i.e. it deprived the fetus of fuels, retarded fetal growth and hepatic glycogen deposition, and delayed the onset of hepatic gluconeogenesis in the newborn by suppressing the PEPCK activity.[76]

Perhaps the most impressive demonstration of the induction of macrosomia by direct intrafetal insulin infusion was made by Susa and colleagues[77-79] in pregnant rhesus monkeys. Insulin infusion for 19 days during the last third of gestation resulted in a 23% increase in fetal weight, accompanied by placentomegaly. Fetal organomegaly was selective, with heart and spleen weights increasing significantly. Skeletal growth, assessed by the crown–heel length and the head circumference, remained unchanged, as did the lung, kidney, adrenal and thymus weights (Table 8.4). The levels of insulin-like growth factors (IGF) I and II rose only in rhesus

monkeys infused with a high dose of insulin. Because the fetal overgrowth was so prominent, even at moderate hyperinsulinemia, it was clear that insulin was the predominant effector of macrosomia.

The activities of fetal hepatic enzymes concerned with glycolysis were not affected by the hyperinsulinemia; gluconeogenic enzymes were suppressed but lipogenic enzymes became enhanced, indicating an increased *de novo* fetal fat synthesis.[79] Additional evidence that diabetic macrosomia entails an enhanced cholesterol and lipoprotein metabolism has recently been provided.[80] Macrosomic pups of mildly hyperglycemic STZ pregnant rats had elevated plasma low-density lipoprotein (LDL) and high-density lipoprotein (HDL) cholesterol associated with increased lecithin–cholesterol acyl transferase activity compared with normal birthweight controls. There was no change in hepatic cholesterol content, but hepatic HMG-CoA reductase and cholesterol 7α-hydroxylase activities were higher in both macrosomic males and females. By 3 months, macrosomic rats had developed hypercholesterolemia with a rise in all lipoproteins. These findings demonstrate that macrosomia throughout adulthood is associated with accentuation of both cholesterol synthesis and metabolism.

Pregnant animals with genetically determined Type 1 diabetes and their heterozygotes

BB rats

BB rats offer a good opportunity to study the interaction of genetics, autoimmunity and environment in the outcome of pregnancy. The attractive features of this spontaneously diabetic animal occur at the *c.* 3-month long prediabetic period prior to the onset of insulin dependency. Because the female BB rat is fertile at *c.* 60 days of age, it is possible to achieve pregnancy in the prediabetic period and to study GDM in an autoimmune animal. Brownscheidle and colleagues[81,82] found a high rate of perinatal mortality, and neural tube and skeletal defects. Intensive treatment with insulin decreased perinatal mortality and reduced the incidence of malformation from *c.* 40 to *c.* 10%, close to the rate in non-diabetic animals. Verhaege et al[83] found a marked degranulation of beta cells in the fetuses of diabetic BB rats, indicating pancreas overstimulation *in utero* similar to that previously described in fetuses of STZ-induced diabetic rats. Baird et al[84] obtained a good pregnancy outcome in their diabetic BB/E rats by individually adjusting insulin dosage by monitoring weight and glucosuria. They found that insulin requirements during pregnancy doubled in comparison with those of non-pregnant diabetic BB rats. There was no significant difference in the size of litters produced by non-diabetic and diabetic treated animals, but the number of pups weaned per litter was significantly lower in diabetic animals and their growth rate fell off from 15 days of age. Stopping the insulin treatment for any 2 days between 2 and 9 days of gestation resulted in loss of maternal weight and ketosis, higher rates of fetus resorption, lower fetal and higher placental weights, and reduced skeletal maturity.[85]

Because BB rats represent a model for the study of perinatal morbidity, microsomia and malformations, attention was directed to early fetal growth processes. Embryo development in BB rats depends on successful trophoblast invasion into the uterine endometrium and protection of the conceptus, which may be antigenic to the maternal immunocompetent cells. Lea et al[86] measured trophoblast proliferation by [³H]thymidine incorporation during incubation with 8.5 day decidual extracts. Decidual supernatants from diabetes-resistant BB/E rats or non-diabetic Wistar rats significantly reduced trophoblast outgrowth relative to non-pregnant rats, as expected. However, decidual supernatants from diabetic BB/E rats did not inhibit the trophoblast cell growth. This finding suggests that BB rat decidual cells secrete a profile of trophoblast reactive factors different to those from non-diabetic rats, and that this increase in the number of trophoblast cells may be related to the subsequent fetal intrauterine growth retardation and congenital malformations.

NOD mice

Among mildly diabetic NOD mice, offspring born before the onset of ketonuria (between 26 and 52 weeks of age) tend to be macrosomic, with a mean increase of 31% in body weight. They show a selective nephromegaly and adiposity compared with non-diabetic controls, but no cardiomegaly (Table 8.5).[87] The macrosomic progeny have a highly elevated pancreatic insulin content but smaller litter sizes. Presence of malformations and subsequent glucose intolerance should be investigated in this model as well as in its heterozygotes.

In further studies with NOD mice, it was observed that the maternal hyperglycemia may not be the only causative factor of macrosomia.[88]

	Maternal glucose (mg/dl)	Fetal weight (grams)	Heart weight (mg/g)	Kidney weight (mg/g)	Pancreas insulin (mg/g)
Control	145±8	1.4±0.1	1.0±1.7	9.6±1.3	0.7±0.0
Mildly diabetic	187±5*	1.8±0.1*	9.0±2.3	10.4±2.3	1.3±0.2*

* Significant difference at $P < 0.05$ at least for 14–19 mice.
Adapted from Formby et al.[87]

Table 8.5. *Macrosomia in the offspring of young, mildly diabetic NOD mice prior to the onset of insulin dependency.*

High parity and age are also associated with increased birthweights. Mild hyperglycemia plays a major role when age, maternal size, duration of gestation and parity are controlled. Pregnant NOD mice that received pancreas transplants from neonatal donors were demonstrated to have lower plasma glucose and glycohemoglobin levels, and their offspring had lower birthweights. Thus, the increased maternal beta-cell mass effectively reduced the macrosomia in the offspring of prediabetic NOD mice.[89]

Placental glucose transporters and hexokinase I were also investigated in diabetic NOD mice.[90] The protein concentrations of these glucose-uptake- and phosphorylation-determining entities were not downregulated so as to protect the feto-placental unit from the maternal hyperglycemia-induced alterations, e.g. placental overgrowth and glycogen accumulation, and fetal hyperglycemia and hyperinsulinemia.

Pregnant animals with genetically determined Type-2-like diabetes

As mentioned before, animals with Type-2-like diabetic syndromes are generally infertile. This appears to be related to insulin resistance impairing the mediobasal hypothalamus–pituitary system, resulting in decreased gonadotropin release.[91,92] Breeding of these animals in most cases involves mating heterozygotes, among whom GDM is often detected.

C57 BlKS lepr[db+] heterozygotes

These mice are highly attractive for the study of GDM. Only a few experimental protocols have been carried out with these animals,[93] but the information gained suggests that they may represent an excellent experimental approach. Heterozygous lepr[db+] mice have a significant glucose intolerance and elevated glycohemoglobin levels during pregnancy, compared with pregnant homozygous non-diabetic siblings. There was no difference in litter size, whereas the mean weight of pups of heterozygous mice was significantly higher, with 19% of them > 95th percentile of the weight of pups from non-diabetic mice. The GDM in lepr[db+] was extensively reviewed by Shao and Friedman.[94] They found that lepr[db+] mice do not develop any diabetic symptoms in the non-pregnant state and have normal body weights, and plasma glucose and fasting insulin levels are similar to those in wild-type mice. During the early stages of pregnancy (days 1–15) there is no IGT, but from day 16 > 98% of lepr[db+] mice have significantly higher glucose levels at 30 minutes and 1 hour during IP glucose tolerance testing (GTT). At the end of day 19 of pregnancy, fasting plasma glucose levels are still in the normal range, despite IGT, and this finding is similar to most human GDM patients who may manifest insulin secretion adequate to compensate for the resistance. However, mice exhibit higher body weights and plasma insulin levels, and fetal macrosomia. After delivery all these parameters revert to normal.

The lepr[db+] pregnant mice are extremely insulin resistant – they almost do not respond to injected insulin with a reduction of plasma glucose (Fig. 8.5). Lepr[db+] mice consume c. 13% more food and gain more weight during pregnancy compared with their non-heterozygous siblings, suggesting that the leptin receptor site is not fully recessive with regard to fat mass, and that heterozygosity at the leptin receptor may play a role in the susceptibility to environmental conditions favoring obesity and insulin resistance. IGT was present despite significantly higher insulin levels,

compared with normal pregnant or non-pregnant lepr[db+] mice, and despite enhanced insulin synthesis and secretion in response to glucose, indicating insufficient compensation of hyperglycemia by insulin oversecretion. The wild-type pups from lepr[db+] mothers return to normal body weights as adults, but +/+ female offspring in particular are more likely to become obese on a high-fat diet compared with the wild-type offspring of normal mothers. GLUT4 activity and translocation in GDM is reduced, but may be improved by transfection of the human *GLUT4* gene.[95] Glucose-stimulated insulin secretion is increased and insulin receptor (IR) and IR substrate (IRS)-1 activity reduced independent of food intake.

C57BL/6J Mice

The non-obese, non-diabetic BL/6J mice, the genomic host of the *ob/ob* mutation, when placed on an affluent fat and sucrose-rich diet

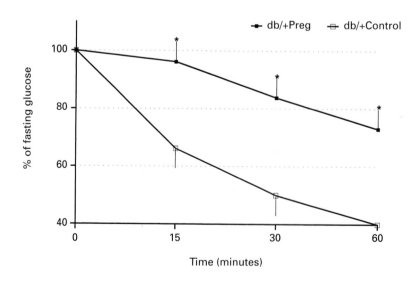

Figure 8.5. *Response to exogenous insulin in pregnant lepr[db+] mice compared with pregnant controls. At day 18 of gestation the mice were fasted for 6 hours and then injected intraperitonealy with 7.5 U/kg insulin. Glucose values are means ±SE. *Significance P < 0.02 at least.*

become hypertensive and insulin resistant with first-phase insulin release disappearing at 6 months of age.[96–98] Abnormalities, characterized by increased outflow from the sympathetic nervous system, deranged beta-cell function and adipocyte metabolism were found to be responsible for the resultant IGT and insulin-resistance syndrome. No hyperphagia or elevation in corticosterone were seen. Thus, inbred laboratory mice, without overt metabolic disturbance, were shown to be susceptible to nutritionally induced diabetes and obesity with marked hyperinsulinemia, hyperlipidemia and polygenic vulnerabilities. The C57/BL/6J mice retain their fertility after developing diabetes and are a potential model of GDM. Pregnancy produced significant hyperinsulinemia beyond the diet alone in BL/6J but not in the control A/J mice. There were differences in the number and weight of pups per litter for either strain or diet groups. There was no fetal loss on a regular diet but a high rate of pup loss in the high-energy diet groups. There was no hyperglycemia, which was most probably compensated by hyperinsulinemia. Maternal mice returned to normal weights and glucose tolerances after birth, and there was no macrosomia in the progeny. These mice might be of interest for the study of GDM and pup loss elicited by high-energy diets.

Goto-Kakizaki rats

Apart from animals with spontaneous alterations leading to inappropriate hyperglycemia, a diabetic line was isolated by repeated breeding of normal animals. The selection was of individuals with minimal deviation from the mean response to a glucose load. This emphasizes the polygenic basis of diabetes within the 'normal' genetic mosaic. A Goto-Kakizaki (GK) diabetic rat line was obtained by breeding Wistar rats for > 35 generations in Japan, using a relative intolerance to a 2 g/kg glucose load as a selection index.[99] The GK rats are non-obese and non-hyperinsulinemic, their diabetes is inheritable but is stable with age. Insulin resistance is present and decreased hepatic insulin receptor numbers were noted with normal tyrosine kinase (TK) activity per receptor.[100] During pregnancy at 15–20 days gestation, GK rats had gained less weight than controls, though the number of fetuses in each litter were similar. The abortive fetal development averaged 40% compared with 6% in controls. A particular finding was the low number of ossification points in the lumbosacral spine, pelvic girdle, and anterior and posterior limbs (Fig. 8.6).[101] These anomalies were not related to lower plasma insulin levels before or during the pregnancy and may be related to the impaired vitamin D metabolism in the GK rats.[102]

Elevated muscle triglyceride content and protein kinase C overexpression

The investigation of lipid abnormalities in diabetic pregnancy merits special attention, since one recent finding was the negative outcome of enhanced lipid deposition in muscles of diabetic subjects. Increased muscle TG content (Table 8.6) and overexpression of PKC isoenzymes were found in several non-pregnant and pregnant diabetic animals, e.g. *Psammomys obesus* (sand rat),[103] animals maintained on fat-rich diets[104] and C57BLKSlepr[db+] mice.[94] Overexpression of PKC isoenzymes leads to a negative feedback of the insulin signaling pathway, since it causes increased serine/threonine phosphorylation of several protein components of insulin signal transduction. This was correlated with the elevated muscle fat and diacylglycerol (DAG) levels.[103] DAG is an intermediate of both FFA esterification to TG and TG breakdown

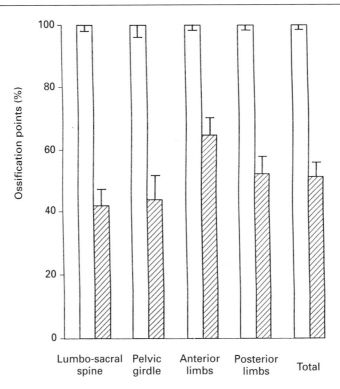

Figure 8.6. *Number of ossification points in fetus as from Goto-Kakizaki rats (hatched bars) versus controls (open bars). Values are means ±SE for 61 GK and 125 control fetuses expressed as a percentage of the control value. From Malaisse-Laege et al.[101]*

	Serum glucose (mmol/l)	Serum TG (mmol/l)	Liver TG (mg/g)	Muscle TG (mg/g)
Control	5.1±0.3	2.4±0.4	0.28±0.3	0.040±0.008
Mild diabetes	11.5±0.7*	3.9±0.6	0.45±0.6*	0.084±0.016[†]
Severe diabetes	22.8±1.6[†]	7.1±0.9[†]	0.83±1.0[†]	0.133±0.022[†]

* Significant difference between mild diabetic and control rats at $P < 0.05$ at least.
[†] Significant difference between mild and severe diabetic rats at $P < 0.02$ at least.
  Values are means ± SE for 10 rats. Unpublished data of ES.

Table 8.6. *Triglyceride (TG) levels in serum, liver and gastrocnemius muscle of control, mildly and severely streptozotocin (STZ)-induced diabetic rats on day 20 of pregnancy.*

during lipolysis to FFA, and glycerol is known to activate PKC. The raised muscle concentrations of DAG result from increased TG turnover in muscle, which occurs in the situation of hyper-insulinemia, hyperglycemia and high plasma FFA levels, related to insulin resistance. A

scheme illustrating the events following PKC overexpression and serine/threonine phosphorylation is presented in Fig. 8.7. Indeed, *in vitro* uptake of saturated FFA was recently reported to raise muscle DAG levels and to lead to PKC activation.[105] FFA infusion to human subjects

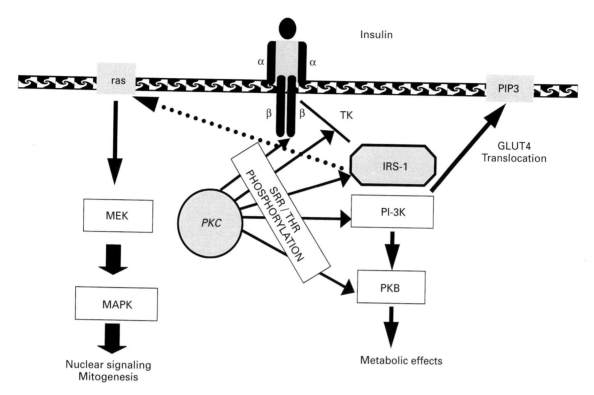

Figure 8.7. *Principles of insulin signaling pathway inhibition by overexpression of protein kinase C (PKC) isoenzymes. The PKC activated serine/threonine phosphorylation affects the β-subunit of the insulin receptor (IR), the IR substrate (IRS), phosphatidylinositol P13-kinase and PKB activities. The latter is responsible for activation of multiple metabolic systems. The mitogenic activity activated by insulin through MAP kinase is not affected by PKC.*

was found to elicit insulin resistance and activation of the θ isoform of PKC.[106]

The accumulation of lipids in intramyocellular muscle is inversely correlated with insulin resistance and delayed glucose disposal in human subjects.[107] This most probably results in reduced glucose uptake by inducing insulin resistance through PKC overexpression. Zierath et al[108] have shown that high-fat feeding impairs the recruitment of GLUT4 and produces a defect in the function of the phosphatidylinositol (PI)-3 kinase in muscle of mice. In lepr[db+] mice with GDM it was found that serine phosphorylation of IRS-1 was was associated with redistribution of PI-3 kinase to the β-subunit of the insulin receptor. This was suggested to result in the inhibition of the receptor TK activity and in the increase of the PKC activity in pregnancy that inhibits IRS serine phosphorylation. These data indicate that a new in-depth approach is needed to assess the insulin resistance in GDM at the molecular level of insulin signal transduction.

Conclusions

The choice of an animal model for the study of diabetes in pregnancy depends very much on the particular pathophysiological alteration exhibited by the animal and its relation to human diabetes, whether pre- or intragestational. It also depends on the specific interest of the investigator. Because of the complexity of human gestation and the variety of its complications, more than one model may be necessary for exploration, since the similarities between diabetic derangements in certain animals and in the diabetic woman may be limited. The endocrine–metabolic aberrations and the histopathological lesions of diabetes in a given animal may either surpass or be constrained in relation to those encountered in human diabetes. Many new models, including a variety of mild and severe STZ-induced diabetes, are now available to fulfil the needs of this approach.

The use of STZ-generated diabetic pregnant animals was predominant until recently. These models represent the condition of absent or limited endogenous insulin presence. The proper approach to GDM is the use of models with normal or excessive endogenous insulin to compensate, or attempt to compensate, the salient insulin resistance of pregnancy. More models of this kind are becoming available, either from a genetic background or from nutritionally induced Type-2-like diabetes (some of them are described in this chapter). Investigators should increasingly turn to these models as well as developing further models of this kind in order to unravel the various complications of insulin-resistant GDM and the associated macrosomia.

If malformations are of primary interest, one can use the preconceptionally induced STZ-induced diabetic animals or embryos cultured in a diabetic milieu, in which severe multiple malformations and fetal wastage are encountered. If malformations accompanying mild diabetes are the target, than the progeny of STZ-induced diabetic animals or neonatally STZ injected newborns should be selected. The nSTZ animals and the offspring of diabetic mothers are eminently suitable for the investigation of GDM with moderate insulin insufficiency. Effects on the fetal pancreas,

particularly those governing beta-cell replication, are good research targets in these models. Much remains to be done on pancreas morphology and the possibility of stimulation of beta-cell replication *in vivo*.

However, insulin resistance most probably represents the main cause of GDM, with limitation of secretion appearing afterwards, unless there is a precondition affecting the efficiency of insulin secretion. Therefore, the emphasis should be placed on factors causing insulin resistance in pregnancy, leading to macrosomia and fetal obesity, including the increased fetal lipogenesis in this condition. The heterozygote animals in a prediabetic stage introduce new facets of etiology of GDM on a range of backgrounds, spanning from pancreatic cell lability to peripheral and hepatic insulin resistance. Both hormonal alterations inducing insulin resistance in pregnancy and enhancing muscle lipid deposition, which induces the accumulation of diacylglycerol and activation of PKC, should be actively explored together with possible effects on the insulin signaling pathway in pregnancy.

Another aspect which should not be omitted is the research which may lead to the active use of oral antidiabetic modalities, e.g. metformin or thiazolidinediones, to increase insulin sensitivity in pregnancy, counteracting hyperglycemia as the main culprit of pregnancy complications.

References

1. Cooperstein SJ, Watkins D. Action of toxic drugs on islet cells. In: (Cooperstein SJ, Watkins D, eds). *The Islets of Langerhans.* (Academic Press: New York, 1981) 387–425.
2. Shafrir E. Contribution to the understanding of diabetes by its etiopathology in animal models. In: (Porte Jr D, Sherwin R, Baron A, eds). *Diabetes Mellitus* (McGraw-Hill: New York, 2000).
3. Okamoto H. The molecular basis of experimental diabetes. In: (Okamoto H, ed.) *Molecular Biology of the Islets of Langerhans.* (Cambridge University Press: Cambridge, UK, 1990) 209–31.

4. Boquist L. Aspects of the diabetogenecity of alloxan and streptozotocin with special regard to a 'mitochondrial hypothesis.' In: (Shafrir E, ed.) *Lessons from Animal Diabetes*, Volume 4. (Smith-Gordin: London, 1992) 1–16.

5. McNeill JH (Ed.). *The Streptozotocin-induced Diabetic Rat. Section I. Experimental Models of Diabetes.* (CRC Press: Boca Raton, 1999).

6. Dickinson JE, Meyer BA, Chmielowiec S, Palmer SM. Streptozotocin induced diabetes mellitus in the pregnant ewe. *Am J Obstet Gynecol* 1991; 165:1673–7.

7. Hay Jr WW, Meznarich HK. Use of fetal streptozotocin injection to determine the role of normal levels of fetal insulin in regulating uteroplacental and umbilical glucose exchange. *Pediatr Res* 1988; 24:312–17.

8. Peterson CM, Jovanovic-Peterson L, Bevier W, Formby B. Animal models of diabetic pregnancy. *Adv Diabetol* 1992; 5 (Suppl 1):11–16.

9. Mintz DH, Chez RA, Hutchinson DL. Subhuman primate pregnancy complicated by streptozotocin-induced diabetes mellitus. *J Clin Invest* 1972; 51:837–47.

10. Baird JD, Aerts L. Research priorities in diabetic pregnancy today: the role of animal models. *Biol Neonate* 1987; 51:119–27.

11. Susa JB. Methodology for the study of metabolism: animal models. In: (Cowett R, ed.) *Principles of Perinatal-Neonatal Metabolism.* (Springer-Verlag: New York, 1991) 48–60.

12. Sybulski S, Maughan GB. Use of streptozotocin as diabetic agent in pregnant rats. *Endocrinology* 1974; 94:1247–53.

13. Pitkin RM, Van Oren DE. Fetal effects of maternal streptozotin-diabetes. *Endocrinology* 1974; 94:1247–53.

14. Golob EK, Rishi S, Becker KL, Moore C. Streptozotocin diabetes in pregnant and nonpregnant rats. *Metabolism* 1970; 19:1014–19.

15. Prager R, Abramovici A, Liban E, Laron Z. Histopathological changes in the placenta of streptozotocin induced diabetes rats. *Diabetologia* 1974; 10:89–91.

16. Eriksson UJ. Congenital malformations in animal models. *Diabetes Res* 1984; 1:57–66.

17. Diamant YZ, Shafrir E. Placental enzymes of glycolysis, gluconeogenesis and lipogenesis in the diabetic rat and in starvation: comparison with maternal and fetal liver. *Diabetologia* 1978; 15:481–591.

18. Shafrir E, Khassis S. Maternal–fetal transport versus new fat synthesis in the pregnant diabetic rat. *Diabetologia* 1982; 22:111–17.

19. Reynolds WA, Chez RA, Bhuyan BK, Neil GL. Placental transfer of streptozotocin in the Rhesus monkey. *Diabetes* 1971; 23:777–82.

20. Shafrir E, Barash V. Placental glycogen metabolism in diabetic pregnancy. *Israel J Med Sci* 1991; 27:449–61.

21. Diamant YZ, Metzger BE, Freinkel N, Shafrir E. Placental lipid and glycogen content in human and experiment diabetes mellitus. *Am J Obstet Gynecol* 1982; 144:5–11.

22. Barash V, Gutman A, Shafrir E. Mechanism of placental glycogen deposition in diabetes in the rat. *Diabetologia* 1983; 24:63–8.

23. Barash V, Gimmon Z, Shafrir E. Placental glycogen accumulation and maternal-fed metabolic responses in hyperglycaemic non-diabetic rats. *Diabetes Res* 1986; 3:97–101.

24. Sochor M, Baquer N, McLean P. Glucose overutilization in diabetes: evidence from studies on the changes in hexokinase, the pentose phosphate pathway, and glucuronate–xylulose pathway in rat kidney cortex in diabetes. *Biochem Biophys Res Commun* 1979; 86:32–9.

25. Khandelwal RL, Zinman M, Knull HR. The effect of streptozotocin-induced diabetes on glycogen metabolism in rat kidney and its relationship to the liver system. *Arch Biochem Biophys* 1979; 197:310–16.

26. Delaval E, Moreau E, Adriamanantsara S, Geloso JP. Renal glycogen content and hormonal control of enzymes involved in renal glycogen metablism. *Pediatr Res* 1983; 17:766–9.

27. Anderson W, Jones AL. Biochemical and ultrastructural study of glycogen in jejunal mucosa of diabetic rats. *Proc Soc Exp Biol Med* 1984; 145:268–72.

28. Ezekwe MO, Martin RJ. The effects of maternal alloxan diabetes on body composition, liver enzymes and metabolism and serum metabolites and hormones of fetal pigs. *Hormone Metab Res* 1980; 12:136–9.

29. Shafrir E, Barash V. Placental function in maternal–fetal fat transport in diabetes. *Biol Neonate* 1987; 51:102–12.

30. Goldstein R, Levy E, Shafrir E. Increased maternal–fetal transport of fat in diabetes assessed by polyunsaturated fatty acid content in fetal lipids. *Biol Neonate* 1985; 47:343–49.

31. Waterman IJ, Emmison N, Dutta-Roy AK. Characterisation of triacylglycerol hydrolase activities in human placenta. *Biochim Biophys Acta* 1997; 1394:169–76.

32. Kasser TR, Martin RJ, Allen CE. Effect of gestational alloxan diabetes and fasting on fetal lipogenesis and lipid deposition in pigs. *Biol Neonate* 1981; 40:105–12.

33. Martin RJ, Makula A, Kasser TR. Placental metabolism and enzyme activities in diabetic pigs. *Proc Soc Exp Biol Med* 1980; 165:39–43.

34. Shafrir E, Barash V, Zederman R et al. Modulation of fetal and placental metabolic pathways in response to maternal thyroid and glucocorticoid hormone excess. *Israel J Med Sci* 1994; 30:32–41.

35. Diamant YZ, Neuman S, Shafrir E. Effect of chorionic gonadotropin, triamcinolone, progesterone and

estrogen on enzymes of placenta and liver in rats. *Biochim Biophys Acta* 1975; **385**:257–67.

36. Haguel A, Leturque A, Gilbert M et al. Glucose utilization by the placenta and fetal tissues in fed and fasted pregnant rabbits. *Pediatr Res* 1988; **23**:480–3.

37. Singh M, Feigelson M. Effects of maternal diabetes on the development of carbohydrate metabolizing enzymes in fetal rat liver. *Arch Biochem Biophys* 1981; **209**:655–67.

38. Styrud J, Thunberg L, Nybacka O, Eriksson UJ. Correlations between maternal metabolism and deranged development in the offspring of normal and diabetic rats. *Pediatr Res* 1995; **37**:343–53.

39. Chernicky CL, Redline RW, Tan HQ et al. Expression of insulin-like growth factor-I and factor-II in conceptuses from normal and diabetic mice. *Moles Reprod Dev* 1994; **37**:382–90.

40. Sadler TW. Effects of maternal diabetes on early embryogenesis. I. The teratogenic potential of diabetic serum. *Teratology* 1980; **21**:339–47.

41. Strieleman J, Connors MA, Metzger BE. Phosphoinositide metabolism in the developing conceptus. Effects of hyperglycemia and scyllo-inositol on rat embryo culture. *Diabetes* 1992; **41**:989–97.

42. Hod M, Star S, Passonneau JV et al. Effect of hyperglycemia on sorbitol and myo-inositol content of cultured rat conceptuses: failure of aldose reductase inhibitors to modify myo-inositol depletion and dysmorphogenesis. *Biochem Biophys Res Commun* 1986; **140**:974–80.

43. Hod M, Star S, Passonneau J et al. Glucose-induced dysmorphogenesis in the cultured rat conceptus: prevention by supplementation with myo-inositol. *Israel J Med Sci* 1990; **26**:541–4.

44. Zaken V, Kohen R, Ornoy A. Vitamins C and E improve rat embryonic antioxidant defense mechanism in diabetic culture medium. *Teratology* 2001; **64**: 33–44.

45. Ornoy A, Zaken V, Kohen R. Role of reactive oxygen species (ROS) in the diabetes-induced anomalies in rat embryos in vitro: reduction in antioxidant enzymes and low-molecular weight antioxidants (LMWA) may be the causative factor for increased anomalies. *Teratology* 1999; **60**:1–11.

46. Portha B, Picon L, Rosselin G. Chemical diabetes in the adult rat as the spontaneous evolution of neonatal diabetes. *Diabetologia* 1979; **17**:371–7.

47. Bonner-Weir S, Trent DF, Honey RN, Weir GC. Responses of neonatal rat islets to streptozotocin: limited B-cell regeneration and hyperglycemia. *Diabetes* 1981; **30**:64–9.

48. Bonner-Weir S, Leahy JL, Weir GC. Induced rat models of noninsulin-dependent diabetes. In: (Renold AE, Shafrir E, eds). *Lessons from Animal Diabetes, Volume 2.* (Libby: London, 1988) 295–300.

49. Portha B, Giroix MH, Serradas P et al. The neonatally streptozotocin-induced (n-STZ) diabetic rats, a family of NIDDM models. In: (Sima AAF, Shafrir E, eds) *Animal Models of Diabetes. A Primer.* (Harwood Academic Publishers: 2001) 247–71.

50. Triadou N, Portha B, Picon L, Rosselin G. Experimental chemical diabetes and pregnancy in the rat: evolution of glucose tolerance and insulin response. *Diabetes* 1982; **31**:75–9.

51. Schaffer SW, Mozaffari M. The neonatal STZ model of diabetes in experimental models of diabetes. In: (McNeill JH, ed.) *Experimental Models of Diabetes.* (CRC Press: Boca Raton, 1999) 231–56.

52. Iwase M, Wada M, Shinohara N et al. Effect of maternal diabetes on longevity in offspring of spontaneously hypertensive rats. *Gerontology* 1995; **41**:181–6.

53. Wada M, Iwase M, Wakisaka M et al. A new model of diabetic pregnancy with genetic hypertension: pregnancy in spontaneously hypertensive rats with neonatal streptozotocin-induced diabetes. *Am J Obstet Gynecol* 1995; **172**:626–30.

54. Iwase M, Wada M, Wakisaka M et al. Effects of maternal diabetes on blood pressure and glucose tolerance in offspring of spontaneously hypertensive rats: relation to birth weight. *Clin Sci* 1995; **89**:255–60.

55. Aerts L, Holeman K, Van Assche FA. Maternal diabetes during pregnancy: consequences for the offspring. *Diabetes Metabolic Rev* 1990; **6**:147–67.

56. Van Assche FA, Gepts W, Aerts L. Immunocytochemical study of the endocrine pancreas in the rat during normal pregnancy and during experimental diabetic pregnancy. *Diabetologia* 1980; **18**:487–91.

57. Aerts L, Van Assche FA. Endocrine pancreas in the offspring of rats with experimentally induced diabetes. *J Endocrinol* 1981; **88**:81–8.

58. Bihoreau Mth, Ktorza A, Picon L. Gestational hyperglycemia and insulin release by the fetal rat pancreas in vitro: effect of amino-acids and glyceraldehydes. *Diabetologia* 1986; **29**:434–9.

59. Aerts L, Holeman K, Van Assche FA. Impaired insulin response and action in offspring of severely diabetic rats. In: (Shafrir E, ed.) *Lessons from Animal Diabetes, Volume 3.* (Smith Gordon: London, 1990), 561–6.

60. Holemans K, Van Bree R, Verhaeghe J et al. In vivo glucose utilization by individual tissues in virgin and pregnant offspring of severely diabetic rats. *Diabetes* 1993; **42**:530–6.

61. Gauguier D, Bihoreau MT, Ktorza A et al. Inheritance of diabetes mellitus as consequence of gestational hyperglycemia in rats. *Diabetes* 1990; **39**:734–9.

62. Zhong S, Dunbar JC, Jen K-LC. Postnatal development in rat offspring delivered of dams with gestational hyperglycemia. *Am J Obstet Gynecol* 1994; **171**: 753–63.

63. Lee At, Plump A, DeSimone C et al. A role for DNA mutations in diabetes-associated teratogenesis in transgenic embryos. *Diabetes* 1995; 44:20–4.

64. Bihoreau MT, Ktorza A, Kinebanyau MF, Picon L. Impaired glucose homeostasis in adult rats from hyperglycemic mothers. *Diabetes* 1986; 35:979–84.

65. Ktorza A, Gauguier D, Bihoreau MT et al. Long-term effects of gestational hyperglycemia: a non-genetic transmission of diabetes in the rat. *Diabetologia* 1988; 31:510A.

66. Hellerstrom C, Swenne I, Eriksson UJ. Is there an animal model for gestational diabetes? *Diabetes* 1985; 34:28–31.

67. Ryan EA, Tobin BW, Tang J, Finegood DT. A new model for the study of mild diabetes during pregnancy: syngeneic islet-transplanted STZ-induced diabetic rats. *Diabetes* 1993; 42:316–23.

68. Freinkel N. Banting Lecutre 1980: Of pregnancy and progeny. *Diabetes* 1980; 29:1023–35.

69. Kim YS, Jatoi I, Kim Y. Neonatal macrosomia in maternal diabetes. *Diabetologia* 1980; 18:407–11.

70. Szabo AJ, Szabo O. Placental free fatty acid transfer and fetal adipose tissue development: an explanation of fetal adiposity in infants of diabetic mothers. *Lancet* 1974; 2:498–9.

71. Skryten A, Johnson P, Samsioe G, Gustafson A. Studies in diabetic pregnancy I. Serum lipids. *Acta Obstet Gynecol Scand* 1976; 55:211–15.

72. Enzi G, Inelmen EM, Caretta F et al. Adipose tissue development 'in utero': relationships between some nutritional and hormonal factors and body fat mass enlargement in newborns. *Diabetologia* 1980; 18:135–40.

73. Ogata ES, Collins Jr JW, Finley S. Insulin injection in the fetal rat: accelerated intrauterine growth and altered fetal and neonatal glucose homeostasis. *Metabolism* 1988; 37:649–55.

74. Catlin EA, Cha C-JM, Oh W. Postnatal growth and fatty acid synthesis in overgrown rat pups induced by fetal hyperinsulinemia. *Metabolism* 1985; 34:1110–14.

75. Johnson JD, Dunham T, Wogenrich FJ et al. Fetal hyperinsulinemia and protein turnover in fetal rat tissues. *Diabetes* 1990; 39:541–8.

76. Ogata ES, Paul RI, Finley SL. Limited maternal fuel availability due to hyperinsulinemia retards fetal growth and development in the rat. *Pediatr Res* 1987; 22:432–7.

77. Susa JB, Neave C, Sehgal P et al. Chronic hyperinsulinemia in the fetal rhesus monkey. *Diabetes* 1984; 33:656–60.

78. Susa JB, Schwartz R. Effects of hyperinsulinemia in the primate fetus. *Diabetes* 1985; 34:36–41.

79. McCormick KL, Susa JB, Widness JA et al. Chronic hyperinsulinemia in the fetal rhesus monkey: effects on hepatic enzymes active in lipogenesis and carbohydrate metabolism. *Diabetes* 1979; 28:1064–8.

80. Merzouk H, Madani S, Boualga A et al. Age-related changes in cholesterol metabolism in macrosomic offspring of rats with streptozotocin-induced diabetes. *J Lipd Res* 2001; 42:1152–9.

81. Brownscheidle CM, Davis DL. Diabetes in pregnancy: a preliminary study of the pancreas, placenta and malformations in the BB Wistar rat. *Placenta Suppl* 1989; 3:203–16.

82. Brownscheidle CM, Wooten V, Mathieu MH et al. The effects of maternal diabetes on fetal maturation and neonatal health. *Metabolism* 1983; 32:148–55.

83. Verhaege J, Peeters TL, Vandeputte M et al. Maternal and fetal endocrine pancreas in the spontaneously diabetic BB rat. *Biol Neonate* 1989; 55:298–308.

84. Baird JD, Bone AJ, Eriksson UF. The BB rat: a model for insulin-dependent diabetic pregnancy. In: (Renold AE, Shafrir E, eds) *Lessons From Animal Diabetes*, Volume 2. (Libby: London, 1988), 412–17.

85. Eriksson UJ, Bone AJ, Turnbull DM, Baird JD. Timed interruption of insulin therapy in diabetic BB/E rat pregnancy: effect on maternal metabolism and fetal outcome. *Acta Endocrinol* 1989; 120:800–10.

86. Leae RG, McIntyre S, Smith W, Baird JD. The effects of diabetes on peri-implantation phase decidual-trophoblast interaction: studies on the pregnant diabetes prone BB/Edinburgh rat. *Abstracts of the Annual DPSG Meeting*, Porto Carras, Cheldiki, Greece, 1993.

87. Formby B, Schmid-Formby F, Jovanovic L, Peterson CM. The offspring of the female diabetic 'nonobese diabetic' (NOD) mouse are large for gestational age and have elevated pancreatic insulin content: a new animal model of human diabetic pregnancy. *Proc Soc Exp Biol Med* 1987; 184:291–4.

88. Bevier WC, Jovanovic-Peterson L, Formby B, Peterson CM. Maternal hyperglycemia is not the only cause of macrosomia: lessons learned from the nonobese diabetic mouse. *Am J Perinatol* 1994; 1:51–6.

89. Chen H-M, Jovanovic-Peterson L, Desai TA, Peterson DM. Lessons learned from the non-obese diabetic mouse II: amelioration of pancreatic autoimmune isograft rejection during pregnancy. *Am J Perinatol* 1966; 13:249–54.

90. Devaskar SU, Devaskar UP, Schroeder RE et al. Expression of genes involved in placental glucose uptake and transport in the nonobese diabetic mouse pregnancy. *Am J Obstet Gynecol* 1994; 171:1316–23.

91. Bestetti GE, Rossi GL. Effects of diabetes on functional and morphological complications in the hypothalamo-pituitary system of diabetic rodent models. A pathogenesis overview. In: (Shafrir E, ed.) *Lessons from Animal Diabetes*, Volume 3. (Smith Gordon: London, 1988) 466–70.

92. Rossi GL, Bestetti GE. In vitro assessment of functional and morphological complications in the hypothalamo-pituitary system of diabetic rodent models. In: (Shafrir

E, ed.) *Lessons from Animal Diabetes, Volume 3.* (Smith Gordon: London, 1988) 471–4.

93. Kaufmann RC, Amankwah KS, Dunaway G et al. An animal model of gestational diabetes. *Am J Obstet Gynecol* 1981; **141**:479–82.

94. Shao J, Friedman JE. Spontaneous gestational diabetes in the heterozygous C57BLKS/Jlepr[db/+] mouse: a unique model for understanding maternal diabetes and its impact on the fetus. In: (Hansen B, Shafrir E, eds) *Insulin Resistance and Insulin Resistance Syndrome,* (Taylor & Francis, London, 2002) 21–34.

95. Ishizuka T, Klepcyk P, Liu S et al. Effects of overexpression of human GLUT4 gene on maternal diabetes and fetal growth in spontaneous gestational diabetic C57BLKS/J Lepr (db/+) mice. *Diabetes* 1999; **48**:1061–9.

96. Livingston EG, Feinglos MN, Kuhn CM et al. Hyperinsulinemia in the pregnant C57BL/6J mouse. *Hormone Metab Res* 1994; **26**:307.

97. Martin-Dixon T, Collins S, Surwit RS. The C57BL/6J mouse as a model of insulin resistance and hypertension. In: (Hansen B, Shafrir E, eds) *Insulin Resistance and Insulin Resistance Syndrome.* (Taylor & Francis, London, 2002) in press.

98. Petro AE, Surwit RS. The C57BL/6J mouse as a model of diet induced type 2 diabetes and obesity. In: (Sima AAF, Shafrir E, ed.) *Animal Models of Diabetes. A Primer.* (Harwood Academic Press, London, 2000) 337–50.

99. Ostenson CG. The Goto-Kakizaki rat. In: (Sima AAF, Shafrir E, eds.) *Animal Models of Diabetes. A Primer.* (Harwood Academic Press: Australia, 2000) 197–212.

100. Shafrir E. Diabetes in animals. In: (Sherwin E, Baron Ad, eds). *Diabetes Mellitus* (McGraw Hill Publishers, New York, 2002) 231–56.

101. Malaisse-Lagae F, Vanhoutte C, Rypens F et al. Anomalies of fetal development in GK rats. *Acta Diabetol* 1997; **34**:55–60.

102. Ishimura E, Nishizawa Y, Koyama H et al. Impaired vitamin D metabolism and response in spontaneously diabetic GK rats. *Miner Electrolyte Metab* 1995; **21**:205–10.

103. Ikeda Y, Olsen GS, Ziv E et al. Cellular mechanism of nutritionally induced insulin resistance in *Psammomys obesus.* Overexpression of protein kinase Cε in skeletal muscle precedes the onset of hyperinsulinemia and hyperglycemia. *Diabetes* 2001; **50**:584–92.

104. Schmitz-Pfeiffer C, Browne CL, Oakes ND et al. Alterations in the expression and cellular localization of protein kinase C isozymes ε and θ are associated with insulin resistance in skeletal muscle of the high-fat-fed rat. *Diabetes* 1997; **46**:169–78.

105. Yu HY, Inoguchi T, Kakimoto M et al. Saturated non-esterified fatty acids stimulate de novo diacyl-glycerol synthesis and protein kinase C activity in cultured aortic smooth muscle cells. *Diabetologia* 2001; **44**:614–20.

106. Griffin ME, Marcucci MJ, Cline GW et al. Free fatty-induced insulin resistance is associated with activation of protein kinase Cθ and alterations in the insulin signaling cascade. *Diabetes* 1999; **48**:1270–4.

107. Kautzky-Willer A, Krssak M, Winzer C et al. Increased intramyocellular lipid concentration identifies impaired glucose metabolism in women with previous gestational diabetes. *Diabetes* 2003; **52**:244–51.

108. Zierath JR, Houseknecht KL, Gnudi L, Kahn BB. High fat feeding impairs insulin stimulated GLUT4 recruitment via an early insulin-signaling defect. *Diabetes* 1997; **46**:215–23.

9

Immunology of gestational diabetes mellitus

Alberto de Leiva, Dídac Mauricio, Rosa Corcoy

Autoimmune gestational diabetes as a clinical entity

Pregnancy represents a distinct immunologic state: the fetus acts as an allograft to the mother, needing protection against potential rejection.[1,2] Humoral immunoreactivity does not change much during pregnancy, with the exception of a lowered immunoglobulin G concentration at a late phase, probably explained by placental transport.[3] Regarding cellular immunity, reduction,[4,5] elevation[6] and no variation[7] in the number of different lymphocytic populations have been reported. The final effect of pregnancy on previously active autoimmune processes is controversial[8,9] and multiple autoimmune disturbances may manifest during this period.[10] In diabetic pregnancy, immunological abnormalities occurring in diabetes are superimposed on immunological changes of pregnancy, eventually influencing maternal and fetal outcomes.

Type 1 diabetes mellitus (DM-1) is considered to be an autoimmune disorder progressing toward the selective destruction of the beta cells. Subjects with DM-1 frequently display evidence of autoimmune disorders specific to other organs, e.g. the thyroid and adrenal glands, the gastric mucosa, and antigliadin antibodies in childhood.

Gestational diabetes mellitus (GDM) is defined as an impairment of glucose tolerance first recognized at the index of pregnancy.[11] For this category of women, an increased risk of progression to Type 2 diabetes mellitus (DM-2) has been repeatedly reported.[12–15] Nevertheless, a subset of women with GDM depicts one or several autoantibodies (AA) against various pancreatic islet cell autoantigens, typically detected in DM-1,[16] as well as in high-risk subjects for the development of the disease, especially first-degree relatives (FDR) of patients with DM-1 (FDR-DM-1).[17] In DM-1A, selective destruction of the insulin-producing cells occurs mediated by T cells.

Autoimmune destruction of the beta cells is determined by multiple genetic susceptibilities and is modulated by undefined environmental factors. The autoimmune response may be detected for months or years before the clinical onset. Patients with DM-1 have an increased risk of other autoimmune disorders, including Graves' disease, thyroiditis, Addison's disease, celiac disease and pernicious anemia. A minority of patients with DM-1 have no known etiology and no evidence of autoimmunity (DM-1B; idiopathic DM-1) – most of these patients are of African or Asian origin. It is well known that autoimmunity against pancreatic islet cells may evolve in some instances as a highly aggressive process responsible for extreme insulinopenia, whereas in other cases it leads to a slow and non-aggressive process, practically asymptomatic, recognized by humoral auto-immunity markers. Over the past decade, islet AA have been demonstrated in the sera of a significant fraction (5–20%) of individuals with phenotypical characteristics of DM-2.[18–20] As a result, the term latent autoimmune diabetes of adulthood (LADA) has been incorporated to define this new clinical variant of diabetes.[18–20]

Therefore, autoimmune GDM is defined as occurring in a subgroup of women depicting humoral autoimmune markers against pancreatic islet cells in association with glucose intolerance at pregnancy. Due to its potential high risk for progression to clinically overt insulinopenia, women with autoimmune GDM may be considered as candidates for immune interventions.

Islet cell autoantibodies

Islet cell autoantibodies include AA to islet cell cytoplasm (ICA), to native insulin (IAA), to glutamic acid decarboxylase (GAD65A)[21–23] and to two tyrosinephosphatases (insulinoma-associated antigens IA-2A and IA-2betaA).[24–25] AA markers of immune destruction are present in 85–90% of new-onset DM-1 cases at the time that fasting hyperglycemia is first detected.[26]

The risk of developing DM-1 in FDR of patients with the disease is c. 5%, c. 15-fold higher than the risk in the general population (1:250–300 lifetime risk). Screening FDR can identify those at high risk for DM-1. Nevertheless, as many as 1–2% of healthy individuals display a single AA and they are at low risk of developing DM-1.[27] Due to the low prevalence of DM-1 in the general population (c. 0.3%), the positive predictive value (PPV) of a single AA is low.[28] The presence of combined islet cell AA is associated with a risk

of DM-1 of ≥ 90%.[27,29] Only c. 20% of subjects presenting with new-onset DM-1 express only a single AA. Children and young adults carrying certain human leucocyte antigen (HLA)-DR and/or DQB1 (D, R, Q and B refer to gene loci; see Genetic markers in auto-immune GDM) chains (*0602/*0603/*0301) are mostly protected from DM-1, but not from developing islet cell AA.[30] Screening of FDR of patients with DM-1, or of the general population, for islet cell AA is not recommended at present. Islet cell AA are usually measured in research protocols and clinical trials as surrogate end points. It is important that AA should be measured only in accredited laboratories with an established quality-control program and participation in a proficiency-testing protocol.

So far, no therapy has been recommended to prevent the clinical onset of DM-1 in islet-cell-AA-positive individuals.[31]

Cytoplasmic islet cell autoantibodies in gestational diabetes mellitus

ICA were first described in 1974:[32] the investigated serum was incubated with a slide of human pancreas and the antigen–antibody interaction was visualized by fluorescent microscopy. Only the cytoplasm of endocrine cells depicted fluorescence, showing the non-specific character of the antibodies for the beta cells.

Circulating antibodies against ICA have been demonstrated in the great majority of individuals with DM-1 both at the preclinical state and at the onset of clinically overt disease, and they persist in the circulation for various lengths of time. In pregnant women with DM-1, the reported frequencies of ICA are 11–62%.[33–35] ICA are transferred by the placenta,[33] but their passage has not been associated with fetal/neonatal morbidity. Nevertheless in a recent paper, Greeley et al report that elimination of transmission of autoantibodies prevents diabetes in nonobese mice.[36]

The present authors' group has investigated the frequency of ICA in the serum of pregnant women with DM-1 matched for age and disease duration and compared it with that of a population of non-pregnant women with DM-1. The aim was to assess the potential reactivation/suppression of the immune response during gestation. ICA were determined by indirect immunofluorescence on cryostat sections of human pancreas (blood type 0) with prolonged incubation with aprotinin,[37] validated by the International Immunology and Diabetes Workshops.[38] The results were reported in Juvenile Diabetes Foundation (JDF) units, with a cut-off titer of 5 JDF units. The observed frequency of ICA in the sera of women with DM-1 investigated in advanced pregnancy did not differ from that predicted by the known duration of the disease.[35]

Through the coordinated efforts of 22 hospital units throughout Spain, between 1987 and 1994, 2181 FDR were recruited by a procedure in concordance with the American Diabetes Association (ADA).[39] The investigation was also extended to 203 healthy control subjects without a family history of DM-1 and an additional subgroup of 33 HLA-identical siblings.[40,41] Also, all women presenting at the Obstetric Department of Hospital de la Santa Creu i Sant Pau, Barcelona, were screened for GDM following a standard protocol.[42] A sample of serum for ICA was obtained at the time of the first obstetric visit in 534 women with GDM compared with 65 control pregnant women with normal oral glucose tolerance test (OGTT) in all phases of pregnancy. ICA were present in the sera of 0.5% of the control group and 9.3% of FDR, and reached 21.2% in identical HLA siblings.

Prevalence of ICA in women with GDM was 13.3%, which was clearly higher than that of women with normal OGTT (3%; *P* < 0.03).

Serum ICA titers for a group of ICA-positive women with GDM (*n* = 38) were also compared with those of 66 DM-1 women screened as positive for ICA and investigated at clinical onset during the same period of sample collection as that of GDM group. Fig. 9.1 illustrates that ICA-positive women with GDM displayed a lower frequency of high titers (> 80 JDF units) and a higher frequency of low titers (< 20 JDF units) than the group of DM-1 subjects investigated at the time of diagnosis. Mean blood glucose values at the postpartum OGTT were higher in the subgroup of ICA-positive women with GDM than in the ICA-negative subgroup of women with GDM (Table 9.1). Frequency of impaired glucose tolerance (IGT)/DM was elevated in the ICA-positive group (18.9 versus 9.9%; *P* < 0.02), diabetes being demonstrated in 10.3% of ICA-positive women with previous GDM and only in 1.6% in those negative for ICA (*P* < 0.01).

Prevalence rates of 1.5–15% have been reported for ICA in GDM (Table 9.2).[15,43–58] These discordant results are probably explained

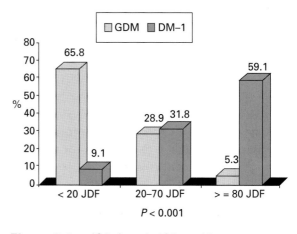

Figure 9.1. *ICA titers in ICA-positive women with GDM and Type 1 DM.*

GDM (n = 307)		ICA –	ICA +	P
Glycemia	0 min	5.35	5.62	0.015
Glycemia	30 min	8.92	9.57	0.004
Glycemia	60 min	8.79	9.62	0.03
Glycemia	120 min	6.20	7.29	0.002

Blood glucose in mM/l

Table 9.1. Blood glucose values at postpartum OGTT in ICA-negative and ICA-positive women with GDM.

Number of subjects	Prevalence %	Author
50	10	Steel, 1980
88	35	Ginsberg-Fellner, 1980
52	38	Rubinstein, 1981
39	5	Falluca, 1985
160	7.5	Freinkel, 1985
187	1.6	Catalano, 1990
181	2.8	Bell, 1990
307	12.4	Mauricio, 1992
55	11	Ziegler, 1993
241	2.9	Damm, 1994

Table 9.2. Prevalence of ICA in women with GDM.

by differences in investigated populations, methodology of assessing ICA, and dissimilar protocols of screening and diagnosing GDM.

The presence of ICA in GDM was first reported by Steel,[43] with a frequency of 10%. Freinkel showed a prevalence of 7.5%, being higher in those women showing more severe impairment of glucose tolerance.[15] Most recent publications have not offered different results.

Several studies have confirmed lower titers for ICA in women with autoimmune GDM than in relatives of newly diagnosed DM-1 subjects,[52,54,56,58–60] although ICA persistance in GDM appears higher in the long run.[61,62]

Insulin autoantibodies in gestational diabetes mellitus

For the measurement of IAA, a radioisotopic method that calculates the displaceable insulin radioligand binding after the addition of excess non-radiolabeled insulin is recommended. Results are reported as positive when the specific AA binding is > +2–3 standard deviations (SD) for healthy persons. Most laboratories use a cut-off value of 80–110 nIU/ml.

The recent introduction of a novel microassay for IAA, requiring only 20 µl of serum, has greatly facilitated IAA screening, particularly in children.[63] The presence of IAA in the sera of DM-1 subjects before initiating insulin therapy was first reported in 1982 by Palmer et al.[64] Since then, IAA have been detected in 18–50% of newly diagnosed DM-1 patients.[65,66] Overall, 4–6% of FDR are positive for IAA, a prevalence that is higher in young ICA-positive individuals. There are only a few reports on the prevalence of IAA in GDM, depicting rates of 0–3%. This group has measured IAA using the radiobinding assay described by Vardi et al. It was observed that pregnancy itself does not influence IAA levels and that only 0.98% (2 out of 203) of non-selected women at diagnosis of GDM depicted IAA in their sera before initiation of treatment – a frequency not significantly different to that of a control group (0%; 0 out of

106), and lower than that reported in FDR of subjects with DM-1 in the investigated population (4.7%) and in newly diagnosed DM-1 patients (16%).[67] Interestingly, the prevalence of IAA was higher in the group of ICA-positive women with GDM than in the ICA-negative group (11 versus 0.7%).

This group has recently shown that 44% of women receiving insulin therapy for GDM and 92% of insulin-treated DM-1 subjects developed insulin antibodies (IA) even after a short course of insulin administration.[69] Expressed as a percentage of insulin binding, the mean final binding was 9% in IA-positive women with GDM and 14% in DM-1 patients: these antibodies may persist up to 2 years after delivery. Concordance for IA status, and close relationships between IA titers in the maternal and cord blood samples, were also observed, supporting the IA transplacental passage from the mother to the fetus.[48] Materno-fetal morbidity was not different in those pregnancies exhibiting IA positivity compared to those that were not, with the exception of higher macrosomia rates in the small fraction of cases showing extreme IA titers (> 1000 nIU/ml).

Autoantibodies against glutamic acid decarboxylase (65 kDa isoform) and tyrosine phosphatase insulin antibodies in gestational diabetes mellitus

Baekkeskov et al[70] identified the pancreatic islet beta-cell autoantigen of relative molecular mass 64 kDa as glutamic acid decarboxylase (GAD), a major target of AA associated with the development of DM-1. GAD is the biosynthesizing enzyme of the inhibitory neurotransmitter gamma-aminobutyric acid (GABA). Pancreatic beta cells and a subpopulation of central nervous system neurons express high levels of this enzyme. Most patients with a rare neurologic disease called stiff-man syndrome have AA to GABA-secreting neurons. The 64 kDa antigen was found in beta cells as a hydrophilic-soluble 65 kDa form and a 64 kDa hydrophobic form.[71]

For the measurement of IA-2A and GAD65A, a dual micromethod and radioimmunoassay performed with ^{35}S-labeled recombinant human IA-2 and ^{3}H-labeled human recombinant GAD65 in a rabbit reticulocyte expression system is currently used by many laboratories.[72] Results are reported as positive when the signal is 99.7% (3 SD) of values in healthy controls.

In newly dignosed patients with DM-1, ICA positivity is depicted in 75–85% of cases, the presence of GAD65A in *c.* 60–70%, IA-2A in 40%, and IA-2betaA in 20%. IAA are positive in 90% of children who develop DM-1 before the age of 5, but in < 40% of cases developing the disease after the age of 12.

At present, a panel of IAA, GAD and IA-2A/IA-2betaA is now available for screening purposes of autoimmune diabetes, possibly with ICA used for confirmatory testing. It is likely that other islet cell antigens could lead to additional diagnostic and predictive tests for DM-1, e.g. GLIMA (glycosylated islet cell membrane-associated antigen)-38.[73] Antibody screening on finger-stick blood samples appears quite feasible in the future.

After the identification of IA-2 as a target beta-cell antigen, a few studies have shown a prevalence of IA-2 antibodies in GDM of 0–6.2%.[56–58,74,75]

At present, the best strategy for primary screening in order to detect FDR of DM-1 patients at high risk of developing the disease is the combined assessment of GADAb and IA2-Ab.[76] The first study, carried out in

Finland, identified 5% of women with GDM being positive for these antibodies. Another Scandinavian report showed a prevalence of 2.2% among women with diet-treated GDM.[77] Other investigations have displayed prevalence rates from 0% to > 10%.[52,55–58,60,74,75,78–82] Prevalence of GADAb and IA-2 Ab in DM-1 and GDM appears to be lower in African and Asian ethnic groups, as well as in southern compared to northern European countries.

The largest study on the prevalence of GAD65Ab in DM-2 is the United Kingdom Prospective Diabetes Study (UKPDS). Overall, 10% of patients tested positive for GAD65Ab and the prevalence was inversely proportional to age.[83] This investigation also depicted that 84% of GADAb-positive patients between the ages of 25 and 34 required insulin within 6 years, compared to 34% of those older than 55 years of age. No patient with DM-2 was positive for IA-2Ab alone. GAD65Ab-positive patients with DM-2 diabetes have lower fasting C-peptide levels and lower insulin responses to orally administered glucose than do GAD65Ab-negative patients, as well as fewer features of the metabolic syndrome, an indication of potential lower risk or cardiovascular events than average DM-2 subjects. An estimated 5–10% of patients with DM-2 have maturity-onset diabetes of youth, 10% may have LADA and another 5–10% may have diabetes due to rare genetic disorders. Most patients with GDM who are GAD65-positive require insulin during pregnancy and are at a high risk of developing DM-1 within 6 years.[84,85]

The present group investigated the relation between the presence of antibodies against ICA, GAD and residual beta-cell function during the first year after diagnosis at 3-month intervals. The presence of GADAb was associated with higher insulin requirements over this period.[86]

Grasso et al[87] found a prevalence rate of GADAb of 20% in a study of 101 classical DM-2 patients: only 4 of these 20 were positive for IA-2Ab. In comparison, 75% of patients with DM-1 were positive for GADAb, IA-2Ab, or both ($P < 0.0001$). The coincidence of IA-2Ab positivity in GADAb-positive patients with DM-2 was significantly lower than in patients with DM-1 (20 versus 73%; $P = 0.002$). In any case, measurement of IA-2Ab and GADAb was useful to identify those patients with DM-2 most likely to require insulin therapy.[88]

In a retrospective study, GADAb was measured in a group of 100 North American women with gestational diabetes and 100 matched non-diabetic control subjects. None (0%) of the 100 control specimens was positive; in contrast, 6% of women with GDM were AA positive. This result falls midway between the 0% reported from northern Italy and the 10% prevalence found in a German multicenter study.[57]

Genetic markers in autoimmune gestational diabetes mellitus

Although genetic markers hold promise for the future, they are currently only of limited clinical value in the evaluation and management of diabetic patients. To screen for the genetic susceptibility for autoimmune-mediated DM-1A, HLA typing is most useful. The HLA complex on chromosome 6p21.3 is a major susceptibility locus, IDDM1 (insulin-dependent diabetes mellitus). The HLA complex contains class I and II genes that code for several polypeptide chains. The class I genes are HLA-A, -B and -C. The loci of class II genes are designated by three letters: the first, (D) indicates the class, the second

(M, O, P, Q, R) the family and the third (A or B) the chain. Both classes of molecules are heterodimers: class I exhibits an alfa chain and beta2-microglobulin; class II exhibits alfa and beta chains. The function of the HLA molecules is to present short peptides to T cells to initiate the immune response. Multiple genetic reports have demonstrated an association between various HLA alleles and autoimmune disorders. In Caucasian DM-1 patients, HLA-D genes contribute as much as 50% of the genetic susceptibility.[89]

HLA-DQ genes appear to be critical to the HLA-associated risk of DM-1A. In any individual, four possible DQ dimers are encoded; positive risks for the disease are associated with alfa chains that have an arginine residue 52 and beta chains that lack an aspartic acid at residue 57. The highest genetic risk corresponds to those persons in whom all four HLA-DQ combinations meet this criterion (heterozygous for *HLA-DRB1*04-DQA1*0301-DQB1*0302* and *DRB1*03-DQA1*0501-DQB1*0201*), with an absolute lifetime risk for DM-1A in the general population of 1:12. On the contrary, people who are protected are those with *DRB1*15-DQA1*0201-DQB1*0602* (*Asp57*+) haplotypes.[90] People carrying the *B1*0401* and *BI*0405* subtypes of *DRB1*04* are susceptible, whereas the **0403* and **0406* subtypes are protective.

The insulin-gene locus (*IDDM2, MIM 125852*) has also been shown to contribute to disease susceptibility. The variable nucleotide tandem repeat upstream from the insulin gene on chromosome 11q is also useful for predicting the development of DM-1A.[91]

Recently, a genomewide linkage analysis for DM-1A susceptibility has been carried out in 408 multiplex families from Scandinavia.[92] The study verified the HLA and insulin gene region susceptibility loci, and, in addition, provided confirmation of locus *IDDM15* on chromosome 6q21. Suggestive evidence of additional susceptibility loci was depicted on chromosomes 2p, 5q and 16p.

The sequencing of the human genome and the formation of consortia should lead to advances in the identification of the genetic bases for both DM-1 and DM-2. So far, the genes of the HLA complex have been the most investigated genetic factors in autoimmune GDM. The information obtained from various reports shows discordant results.[15,45,48,49,52,55,93,94] In these protocols, the number of investigated subjects was small and the analyzed populations quite heterogeneous. Rubinstein et al[45] depicted a strong association between HLA DR3/DR4 and islet autoimmunity of women with GDM. A similar observation was provided by Freinkel et al,[15] showing a twofold increase in the frequency of DR3 and DR4 alleles in women with GDM. Ferber et al[94] investigated 184 German women with GDM; when compared with another group of 254 non-diabetic unrelated subjects, no elevation in the frequency of any HLA class allele was observed. Nevertheless, DR3 allele frequency was increased in GDM women with positivity to islet cell antibodies, particularly GAD (P = 0.002), as well as DR4 and *DQB1*0302* (P = 0.009). Sixty percent of islet antibody-positive women and 74% of women who developed DM-1 post-partum had a DR3/DR4-containing genotype. Combining the determination of susceptible HLA alleles (DR3 and DR4) with IAA measurements increased the sensitivity of identifying GDM women developing postpartum DM-1 to 92%. Several reports have not shown an association between increased prevalence of class II alleles and the presence of humoral islet cell autoimmune markers in women with GDM.[49,55,93] Finally, Damm et al[52] showed a trend towards an increased frequency of DR3/DR4 and a decreased frequency of DR2 in women with GDM developing DM-1.

Autoimmune gestational diabetes mellitus and the risk of developing postpartum DM-1A

A major issue regarding autoimmune GDM is that of the potential increased risk for the development of DM-1 either short term postpartum or at a longer follow-up. The present authors accept the proposal that the majority of women developing DM after GDM will develop DM-2;[12,15] nevertheless, a small but meaningful fraction will develop DM-1.

After delivery, the autoimmune process directed against beta cells may follow different pathways: (1) the restoration of normal glucose tolerance when pregnancy is over; (2) the appearance of DM-1 shortly after pregnancy; (3) slow deterioration of the insulin secretory capacity due to the continuous progression of autoimmune destruction of the residual population of beta cells, resulting in a long subclinical period (i.e. LADA).

Several studies have shown a higher prevalence of humoral autoimmune markers in those women with GDM presenting a higher degree of IGT.[15,57,58,78] For example, Freinkel et al[15] published a higher prevalence of ICA in those women with a more altered OGTT. Wittingham et al[58] showed higher prevalence of GADAb in women under insulin treatment during pregnancy. The derangement of the first phase of the insulin response to intravenous (IV) glucose in ICA-positive individuals was first recognized in FDR of patients with DM-1.[95] This group has demonstrated an impairment of the acute insulin response to glucose in ICA-positive women with previous GDM in the presence of normal OGTT, and the comparison between women with previous GDM associated with ICA positivity and ICA-positive FDR of subjects with DM-1 revealed

no difference in the results of the IV glucose tolerance test (Fig. 9.2).[54]

Clinical presentation of autoimmune diabetes varies, especially with age: classical rapid onset or slowly evolving (i.e. LADA). In the past the progression to DM-1 in women with GDM focused specifically on unequivocal clinical diagnosis with rapid onset; the first investigation on the prevalence of ICA in GDM provided the information that three out of five ICA-positive gestational diabetic women developed classical DM-1 shortly after pregnancy.[43] This group has reported a higher incidence of glucose tolerance impairment during the first year after delivery in ICA-positive women with

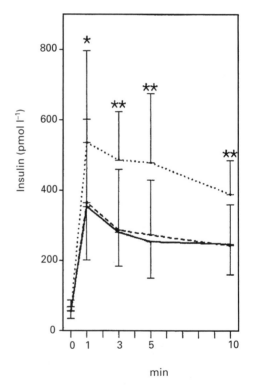

Figure 9.2. *Acute insulin response to intravenous glucose in islet cell antibody positive women with gestational DM(—), islet cell antibody positive first degree relatives of Type 1 diabetic subjects (---) and control women (....). From Mauricio et al.[54]*

GDM, as compared with ICA-negative individuals; moreover, diabetes mellitus, as diagnosed by OGTT, was present in 10.3% of ICA-positive women versus 1.6% in ICA-negative ones.[60] In a report by Catalano et al,[47] three ICA-positive women with previous GDM showed impaired tolerance after pregnancy, one of them clearly developing DM-1, and all three women depicted a diminished acute insulin response to IV glucose.

Some studies have investigated the long-term risk of DM-1 in women with autoimmune GDM. Ginsberg-Fellner et al[44] recorded that 73% of ICA-positive women with previous GDM were under insulin treatment after long-term follow-up. In a Danish study, low-titer ICA in GDM conferred a high risk of developing DM-1 2–11 years after the index of pregnancy, and all GAD-positive women later developed the disease.[52,80]

A large study with a follow-up period of up to 7 years revealed a higher risk of developing DM-1 in antibody-positive women with previous GDM than in antibody-negative ones (29 versus 2%),[57] and the risk increased with the number of antibodies present in the individuals' sera. In this investigation, the postulated prediction strategy for future DM-1 in women with GDM was similar to the one currently designed for studies among FDR of patients with DM-1, using the screening of combined AA with the assessment of the HLA risk markers.[76]

In this group's studies, a higher risk of developing IGT during the first year after pregnancy has been identified,[50,59,60] especially in those women carrying higher ICA titers (Fig. 9.3). It has also been established that ICA, GADAb and IA2-Ab positivity show PPV of 24, 25 and 43%, respectively, for the presence of abnormal glucose tolerance 1 year after delivery.[74]

A significant proportion of women with autoimmune GDM show only a minor impair-

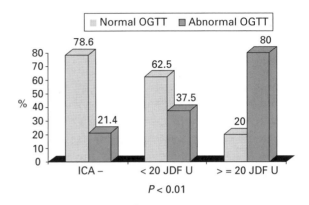

Figure 9.3. *Postpartum OGTT in women without islet cell antibodies and with low titer and high titer islet cell antibodies.*

ment of glucose tolerance, even several years after pregnancy, with a slow progression towards complete insulin deficiency. Interestingly, in a similar manner to that previously described in women with autoimmune GDM after the index of pregnancy, a recent Finnish investigation on FDR of LADA patients demonstrated that these subjects exhibit a decreased insulin secretory capacity in response to IV glucose, associated with risk-conferring genotypes in the population.[96]

Conclusions

Autoimmune GDM appears to be the result of the variable expression of autoimmunity against the beta cell, challenged by the higher functional demand associated with the insulin-resistant state of pregnancy. In this respect, autoimmune GDM can be considered as a distinct clinical entity. There are different time-course patterns in the progression of autoimmune GDM, from the restoration of normal glucose tolerance when pregnancy is over (even with eventual disappearance of autoimmune markers), to the appearance of DM-1 shortly after partum, to an established state of glucose intolerance which may eventually progress, slowly, to a non-insulin dependent state, manifested as LADA. Furthermore, the course of the autoimmune destruction of the residual beta-cell mass may be accelerated at any time-point, resulting in a rapid-onset form of DM-1.

Women with autoimmune GDM must be regarded as a high-risk group for the development of DM-1 in any of its clinical forms. These women are candidates for immuno-modulatory interventions to prevent diabetes after pregnancy.

References

1. Gleicher N. Pregnancy and autoimmunity. *Acta Haematol* 1986; **76**:68–77.
2. Lewis JE, Coulam CB, Moore S. Immunologic mechanisms in the maternal–fetal relationship. *Mayo Clin Proc* 1986; **61**:655–65.
3. Mauroluis GB, Buckley RH, Younger GB. Serum immunoglobulin levels during normal pregnancy. *Am J Obstet Gynecol* 1971; **109**:971–6.
4. Galluzzo A, Giordano C, Bompiani GF. Cell-mediated immunity in diabetic pregnancy. In: (Andreani D, Bompiani G, Di Mario U et al, eds) *Immunobiology of Normal and Diabetic Pregnancy*. (Wiley: Chichester 1990) 273–81.
5. Bulmer R, Hancock W. Depletion of circulating T lymphocytes in pregnancy. *Clin Exp Immunol* 1977; **29**:302–7.
6. Clements PJ, Yu DTY, Levy J, Pearson CM. Human lymphocytes subpopulation: effects on pregnancy. *Proc Soc Exp Biol Med* 1976; **152**:664–72.
7. Dodson MG, Kerman RH, Lange CF et al. T and B cells in pregnancy. *Obstet Gynecol* 1976; **49**:229–303.
8. Shonfeld Y, Schwarz RS. Immunologic and genetic factors in autoimmune diseases. *N Engl J Med* 1984; **311**:1019–29.
9. Giordano C. Immunobiology of normal and diabetic pregnancy. *Immunol Today* 1990; **11**:301–3.
10. Torry DS, McIntyre JA. The role of the antibody in pregnancy. In: (Andreani D, Bompiani G, Di Mario U et al, eds) Immunobiology of Normal and Diabetic Pregnancy. (Wiley: Chichester, 1990) 39–57.
11. Metzger BE, Coustan DM, and the Organizing Committee. Summary and recommendations of the Fourth International Workshop–Conference on Gestational Diabetes Mellitus. *Diabetes Care* 1998; **21**:B161–B167.
12. Kjos SL, Buchanan TA. Gestational diabetes mellitus. *N Engl J Med* 1999; **341**:1749–56.
13. Kjos SL, Peters RK, Xiang A et al. Predicting future diabetes in Latino women with gestational diabetes. Utility of postpartum glucose tolerance testing. *Diabetes* 1995; **44**:586–91.
14. Buchanan TA, Metzger BE, Freinkel N, Bergman RN. Insulin sensitivity and B-cell responsiveness to glucose during late pregnancy in lean and moderately obese women with normal glucose tolerance or mild gestational diabetes. *Am J Obstet Gynecol* 1990; **162**:1008–14.
15. Freinkel N, Metzger BE, Phelps RL et al. Gestational diabetes mellitus: heterogeneity of maternal age, weight, insulin secretion, HLA antigens, and islet cell antibodies and the impact of maternal metabolism on pancreatic B-cell and somatic development in the offspring. *Diabetes* 1985; **34**:1–7.
16. Schranz DB, Lernmark A. Immunology in diabetes: an update. *Diabetes Metab Rev* 1998; **14**:3–29.
17. Palmer JP. Predicting IDDM: use of humoral immune markers. *Diabetes Rev* 1992; **1**:104–15.
18. Tuomi T, Groop LC, Zimmet PZ et al. Antibodies to glutamic acid decarboxylase reveal latent autoimmune diabetes mellitus in adults with a non-insulin dependent onset of the disease. *Diabetes* 1993; **42**:359–62.
19. Turner R, Stratton I, Horton V et al, for the UK Prospective Diabetes Study (UKPDS) Group: UKPDS 25. Autoantibodies to islet cytoplasm and glutamic acid decarboxylase for prediction of insulin requirement in type 2 diabetes. *Lancet* 1997; **350**:1288–93.
20. Zimmet PZ, Tuomi T, Mackay JR et al. Latent autoimmune diabetes in adults (LADA): the role of antibodies to glutamic acid decarboxylase in diagnosis and prediction of insulin dependency. *Diabetic Med* 1994; **11**:299–303.
21. Baekkeskov S, Aanstoot HJ, Christgau S et al. Identification of the 64K autoantigen in insulin-dependent diabetes as the GABA-synthesizing enzyme glutamic acid decarboxylase. *Nature* 1990; **347**:151–6 [published erratum appears in *Nature* 1990; **347**:782.
22. Kaufman DL, Erlander MG, Clare-Salzler M et al. Autoimmunity to two forms of glutamate decarboxylase in insulin-dependent diabetes mellitus. *J Clin Invest* 1992; **89**:283–92.
23. Atkinson MA, Maclaren NK. Islet cell autoantigens in insulin dependent diabetes. *J Clin Invest* 1993; **92**:1608–16.
24. Lan MS, Wasserfall C, Maclaren NK, Notkins AL. IA-2, a transmembrane protein of the protein tyrosine phosphatase family, is a major autoantigen in insulin-dependent diabetes mellitus. *Proc Natl Acad Sci USA* 1996; **93**:6367–70.
25. Lu J, Li Q, Xie H et al. Identification of a second transmembrane protein tyrosine phosphtase, IA-2β, as an autoantigen in insulin-dependent diabetes mellitus: precursor of the 37-kDa tryptic fragment. *Proc Natl Acad Sci USA* 1996; **93**:2307–11.

26. American Diabetes Association. Report of the Expert Committee on the diagnosis and classification of diabetes mellitus. *Diabetes Care* 1997; **20**:1183–201.

27. Maclaren N, Lan M, Coutant R et al. Only multiple autoantibodies to islet cells (ICA), insulin, GAD65, IA–2 and IA–2β predict immune-mediated (type 1) diabetes in relatives. *J Autoimmun* 1999; **12**:279–87.

28. Harrison LC. Risk assessment, prediction and prevention of type 1 diabetes. *Pediatr Diabetes* 2001; **2**:71–82.

29. Verge CF, Gianani R, Kawasaki E et al. Prediction of type I diabetes in first-degree relatives using a combination of insulin, GAD, and ICA512bdc/IA–2 autoantibodies. *Diabetes* 1996; **45**:926–33.

30. Schott M, Schatz D, Atkinson M et al. GAD65 autoantibodies increase the predictability but not the sensitivity of islet cell and insulin autoantibodies for developing insulin dependent diabetes mellitus. *J Autoimmun* 1994; **7**:865–72.

31. Atkinson MA, Eisenbarth GS. Type 1 diabetes: new perspectives on disease pathogenesis and treatment. *Lancet* 2001; **358**:221–9.

32. Bottazo GF, Florin-Christensen A, Doniach D. Islet cell antibodies in diabetes mellitus with polyendocrine autoimmune deficiencies. *Lancet* 1974; **ii**:1279–82.

33. Tingle AJ, Lim G, Wright VJ et al. Transplacental passage of islet cell antibody in infants of diabetic mothers. *Pediatr Res* 1979; **13**:1323–5.

34. Falluca F, Di Mario U, Gargiulo P et al. Humoral immunity in diabetic pregnancy: interrelationships with maternal/neonatal complications and maternal metabolic control. *Diabetes Metab* 1985; **11**:387–95.

35. Mauricio D, Corcoy R, Codina M et al. Frequency of islet-cell antibodies is not different in pregnant versus non-pregnant type 1 diabetic women. *Diabetes* 1991; **40**:277A (abstract).

36. Greeley SA, Katsumata M, Yu L et al. Elimination of maternally transmitted autoantibodies prevents diabetes in nonobese diabetic mice. *Nat Med* 2002; **8**:399–402.

37. Pilcher CC, Elliot RB. A sensitive and reproducible method for the assay of human islet cell antibodies. *J Immunol Meth* 1990; **129**:111–17.

38. Bonifacio E, Boitard C, Gleichmann H et al. Assessment of precision, concordance, specificity, and sensitivity of islet cell antibody measurement in 41 assays. *Diabetologia* 1990; **33**:731–6.

39. ADA Ad Hoc Committee. Prevention of type 1 diabetes mellitus (Position Statement). *Diabetes Care* 1990; **31**:1026–7.

40. Grupo de Trabajo de la Sociedad Española de Diabetes. Proyecto multicéntrico sobre la prevención de diabetes mellitus insulinodependiente: informe I. *Anal Med Int* 1992; **9**:93–7.

41. Rodríguez M, García I, Marzo L et al. Estado actual de la Prediabetes en España. *Anal Esp Pediatr* 1994; **58**:32–9.

42. Corcoy R, Cerqueira MJ, Codina M et al. Diagnóstico de la diabetes gestacional: importancia del screening rutinario y utilidad relativa de los factores de riesgo. *Av Diabetol* 1988; **1**:90–4.

43. Steel JM, Irvine WJ, Clarke BF. The significance of pancreatic islet cell antibody an abnormal glucose tolerance during pregnancy. *J Clin Lab Immunol* 1980; **4**:83–5.

44. Ginsberg-Fellner F, Mark EM, Nechemias C et al. Islet cell antibodies in gestational diabetics. *Lancet* 1980; **2**:362–3.

45. Rubinstein P, Walker M, Krassner J et al. HLA antigens and islet cell antibodies in gestational diabetes. *Hum Immunol* 1981; **3**:271–5.

46. Falluca F, Di Mario, Gargiulo P et al. Humoral immunity in diabetic pregnancy: interrelationships with maternal/neonatal complications and maternal metabolic control. *Diabetes Metab* 1985; **11**:387–95.

47. Catalano PM, Tyzbir ED, Sims EAH. Incidence and significance of islet cell antibodies in women with previous gestational diabetes. *Diabetes Care* 1990; **13**:478–82.

48. Bell DSH, Barger BO, Go RCP et al. Risk factors for gestational diabetes in black population. *Diabetes Care* 1990; **13**:1196–201.

49. Stangenberg M, Agarwal N, Rahman F et al. Frequency of HLA genes and islet cell antibodies (ICA) and result of postpartum oral glucose tolerance tests (OGTT) in Saudi Arabian women with abnormal OGTT during pregnancy. *Diabetes Res* 1990; **14**:9–13.

50. Mauricio D, Corcoy R, Codina M et al. Islet cell antibodies identify a subset of gestational diabetic women with higher risk of developing diabetes mellitus shortly after pregnancy. *Diabetes Nutr Metab* 1992; **5**:237–41.

51. Ziegler AG, Hillebrand B, Rabl W et al. On the appearance of islet associated autoimmunity in offspring of diabetic mothers: a prospective study from birth. *Diabetologia* 1993; **36**:402–8.

52. Damm P, Kühl C, Buschard K et al. Prevalence and predictive value of islet cell antibodies and insulin antibodies in women with gestational diabetes. *Diabetic Med* 1994; **11**:558–63.

53. Kohnert K-D, Rjasasnowski I, Hehmke B et al. The detection of autoantibodies to pancreatic islet cells by immunoenzyme histochemistry. *Diabetes Res* 1994; **25**:1–12.

54. Mauricio D, Corcoy R, Codina M et al. Islet cell antibodies and beta cell function in gestational diabetic women: comparison to first-degree relatives of Type 1 (insulin-dependent) diabetic subjects. *Diabetic Med* 1995; **12**:1009–14.

55. Lapolla A, Betterle C, Sanzari M et al. An immunological and genetic study of patients with gestational diabetes mellitus. *Acta Diabetol* 1996; **33**:139–44.

56. Dozio N, Beretta A, Belloni C et al. Low prevalence of islet autoantibodies in patients with gestational diabetes mellitus. *Diabetes Care* 1997; **20**:81–3.

57. Füchtenbusch M, Ferber K, Standl E, Ziegler A-G, and participating centers. Prediction of type 1 diabetes postpartum in patients with gestational diabetes mellitus by combined islet cell autoantibody screening. A prospective multicenter study. *Diabetes* 1997; **46**:1459–67.

58. Wittingham S, Byron SL, Tuomilehto J et al. Autoantibodies associated with presymptomatic insulin-dependent diabetes mellitus in women. *Diabetic Med* 1997; **14**:678–85.

59. Mauricio D, Balsells M, Morales J et al. Islet cell autoimmunity in women with gestational diabetes and risk of progession to insulin-dependent diabetes mellitus. *Diabetes Metab Rev* 1996; **12**:275–85.

60. Mauricio D, Morales J, Corcoy R et al. Immunology of gestational diabetes: heterogeneity of islet cell antibodies. *Diabetes Rev* 1996; **4**:36–48.

61. Corcoy R, Albareda M, Ortiz A et al. In women with GDM, glutamic acid decarboxylase and tyrosine phosphatase antibodies increase after delivery. *Diabetologia* 2000; **43**:A19.

62. Panczel P, Kulley O, Luczay A et al. Detection of antibodies against pancreatic islet cells in clinical practice. *Orvosi Hetilap* 1999; **140**:2695–701.

63. Naserke HE, Dozio N, Ziegler AG, Bonifacio E. Comparison of a novel micro-assay for insulin autoantibodies with the conventional radiobinding assay. *Diabetologia* 1998; **41**:681–3.

64. Palmer JP, Asplin CH, Clemons P. Insulin antibodies in insulin dependent diabetics before insulin treatment. *Science* 1982; **222**:1337–9.

65. Karjalainen J, Salmena P, Ilonen J et al. A comparison of childhood and adult type I diabetes mellitus. *N Engl J Med* 1989; **320**:881–6.

66. Srikanta S, Richter AT, MacCulloch DK et al. Autoimmunity to insulin, beta-cell dysfunction and development of insulin-dependent diabetes mellitus. *Diabetes* 1986; **36**:139–42.

67. Vardi P, Dib SA, Tuttleman M et al. Competitive insulin antibody assay: prospective evaluation of subjects at high risk for development of type I diabetes mellitus. *Diabetes* 1987; **36**:1286–91.

68. Puig-Domingo M, Mauricio D, Morales J et al. Proyecto de la Sociedad Española de Diabetes sobre prediabetes tipo 1. *Av Diabetol* 1992; **5**:57–65.

69. Balsells M, Corcoy R, Mauricio D et al. Insulin antibody response to a short course of human insulin therapy in women with gestational diabetes. *Diabetes Care* 1997; **20**:1172–5.

70. Baekkeskov S, Aanstoot HJ, Christgau S et al. Identification of the 64K autoantigen in insulin dependent diabetes as the GABA-synthesizing enzyme glutamic acid decarboxylase. *Nature* 1990; **347**:151–6.

71. Tuomilehto J, Zimmet P, Mackay IR et al. Antibodies to glutamic acid decarboxylase as predictors of insulin-dependent diabetes mellitus before clinical onset. *Lancet* 1994; **343**:1383–5.

72. Maclaren N, Lan M, Coutant R et al. Only multiple autoantibodies to islet cells (ICA), insulin, GAD65, IA2 and IA2beta predict immune-mediated (type 1) diabetes in relatives. *J Autoimmun* 1999; **12**:279–87.

73. Aanstoot HJ, Kang SM, Kim J et al. Identification and characterization of glima 38, a glycosylated islet cell membrane antigen, which together with GAD65 and IA2 marks the early phases of autoimmune response in type 1 diabetes. *J Clin Invest* 1996; **97**:2772–83.

74. Albareda M, Corcoy R, Piquer S et al. Prevalence and predictive value of GAD and IA2 autoantibodies in a group of women with gestational diabetes related to ICA. *Diabetologia* 1998; **41**:A29.

75. Balaji V, Balaji M, Seshiah V et al. Autoimmune diabetes constitutes a sigificant proportion of patients diagnosed as gestational diabetes mellitus. *Diabetologia* 2000; **43**:A19.

76. Bingley PJ, Bonifacio E, Ziegler A-G et al on behalf of the Immunology of Diabetes Society. Proposed guidelines on screening for risk of type 1 diabetes. *Diabetes Care* 2001; **24**:398.

77. Damm P, Petersen J, Dyrberg T et al. Prevalence and predicitive value of GAD65 antibodies in women with gestational diabetes. *Diabetologia* 1995; **38**:A70.

78. Tuomilehto J, Zimmet P, Mackay IR et al. Antibodies to glutamic acid decarboxylase as predictors of insulin-dependent diabetes mellitus before clinical onset of disease. *Lancet* 1994; **343**:1383–5.

79. Beischer NA, Wein P, Sheedy MT et al. Prevalence of antibodies to glutamic acid decarboxylase in women who have had gestational diabetes. *Am J Obstet Gynecol* 1995; **173**:1563–9.

80. Petersen JS, Dyrberg T, Damm P et al. GAD65 autoantibodies in women with gestational or insulin dependent diabetes mellitus diagnosed during pregnancy. *Diabetologia* 1996; **39**:1329–33.

81. Fallucca F, Tiberti C, Torresi P et al. Autoimmune markers of diabetes in diabetic pregnancy. *Ann Ist Super Sanita* 1997; **33**:425–8.

82. Mitchell ML, Hermos RJ, Larson CA et al. Prevalence of GAD autoantibodies in women with gestational diabetes. A retrospective analysis. *Diabetes Care* 2000; **23**:1705–6.

83. Turner R, Stratton I, Horton V et al. UKPDS 25: autoantibodies to islet-cell cytoplasm and glutamic acid decarboxylase for prediction of insulin requirement in type 2 diabetes. *Lancet* 1997; **350**:1288–93.

84. Zimmet PZ. The pathogenesis and prevention of diabetes in adults: genes, autoimmunity, and demography. *Diabetes Care* 1995; **18**:1050–64.

85. Damm P, Kühl C, Buschard K et al. Prevalence and predictive value of islet cell antibodies and insulin autoantibodies in women with gestational diabetes. *Diabetic Med* 1994; **11**:558–63.

86. Mauricio D, Carreras G, Pérez A et al. Association of islet-cell and glutamic acid decarboxylase antibodies to beta cell function after the onset of type 1 diabetes in adult subjects. *Diabetic Nutr Metab* 1997; **10**:189–92.

87. Grasso YZ, Sethu S, Reddy K et al. Autoantibodies to IA-2 and GAD65 in patients with type 2 diabetes mellitus of varied duration: prevalence and correlation with clinical features. *Endocr Pract* 2001; **7**:339–45.

88. Mitchell M, Hermos RJ, Larson CA et al. Prevalence of GAD autoantibodies in women with gestational diabetes: a retrospective analysis. *Diabetes Care* 2000; **23**:1705–6 (letter to the editor).

89. Todd JA. Genetics of type 1 diabetes. *Pathol Biol (Paris)* 1997; **45**:219–27.

90. Redondo MJ, Kawasaki E, Mulgrew CL et al. DR- and DQ-associated protection from type 1A diabetes: comparison of DRB1*1401 and DQA1*0102–DQB1*0602*. *J Clin Endocrinol Metab* 2000; **85**:3793–7.

91. Bell GI, Horita H, Karam JH. A polymorphic locus near the insulin gene is associated with insulin-dependent diabetes mellitus. *Diabetes* 1984; **33**:176–83.

92. European Consortium for IDDM Gemome Studies. A genomewide scan for Type 1-diabetes susceptibility in Scandinavian families: identification of new loci with evidence of interactions. *Am J Hum Genet* 2001; **69**:1301–13.

93. Vambergue A, Fajardi I, Bianchi F et al. Gestational diabetes mellitus and HLA class II (-DQ, -DR) association: the DIAGEST Study. *Eur J Immunogenet* 1997; **24**:385–94.

94. Ferber K, Keller E, Albert ED, Ziegler A-G. Predictive value of human leucocyte antigen Class II typing for the development of islet autoantibodies and insulin-dependent diabetes postpartum in women with gestational diabetes. *J Clin Endocrinol Metab* 1999; **84**:2342–8.

95. Srikanta S, Ganda OP, Rabizadeh A et al. First degree relatives of patients with type 1 diabetes mellitus: islet cell antibodies and abnormal insulin secretion. *N Engl J Med* 1985; **313**:461–4

96. Vauhkonen I, Niskanen L, Knip M et al. Impaired insulin secretion in non-diabetic offspring of probands with latent autoimmune diabetes in adults. *Diabetologia* 2000; **43**:69–78.

10

The placenta in diabetic pregnancy

Gernot Desoye, Sylvie Hauguel-de Mouzon, Eleazar Shafrir

Introduction

The placenta is a complex organ of limited lifespan that is vital for fetal growth and successful gestation. It is a discriminatory interface that allows transport of oxygen and nutrients from the mother to the fetus whilst protecting the fetus from any harmful maternal environmental changes. In fulfilling its pleiotropic functions the placenta serves as a substitute for fetal organs until maturity, thereby sustaining and protecting fetal development. Owing to its position between the maternal and fetal circulation, the placenta is exposed to diabetes-associated endocrine and metabolic derangements of both mother and fetus. However, the tissue surfaces and molecular targets that may be affected are different, i.e. the trophoblast fronts to the maternal circulation whereas the feto-placental endothelium bathes in fetal blood.

Upon reviewing the literature no clear-cut picture of the effects of diabetes on the placenta emerges, most likely because of the variety of confounding factors that need to be controlled in comprehensive studies, such as the type of diabetes, the severity of disease, the modality of treatment and the quality of glycemic control. Critical for placental development and possible alterations by maternal diabetes is the time point of departures from excellent glycemic control. Given the complex processes that occur

in placental development in the first trimester (Fig. 10.1), any metabolic or endocrine insult will have long-ranging consequences for placental development and, hence, the fetus, as opposed to an insult late in gestation, a period which is characterized by an increase in placental mass without any major differentiation processes. The importance of glycemic control at the beginning of gestation for placental development is exemplified by morphometric data of placentae at term of gestation that correlate with the day-to-day variation in blood glucose levels only early in gestation.[1]

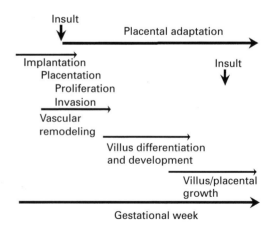

Figure 10.1. *Various stages of placental development may be differentially sensitive towards an endocrine or metabolic insult associated with a diabetic environment.*

There is also indirect evidence to suggest compromised placental development early in a diabetic pregnancy because maternal serum levels of human placental lactogen are lower in the first trimester, whereas those of placental protein 14, an endometrial hormone, are not.[2] Since placental lactogen is a trophoblast-specific hormone, and because its synthesis is mainly determined by trophoblast mass, by inference, trophoblast proliferation is impaired in such diabetic pregnancies in the first trimester. If this were true then it could explain the retarded growth of some fetuses early in these pregnancies.[3] What factors in the diabetic environment have a detrimental effect on placental, i.e. trophoblast, growth early in gestation is unclear, but hyperglycemia may be one of these.[4,5]

Pregnancy pathologies that are related to placental dysfunction, i.e. too shallow a trophoblast invasion into the maternal decidua in the first trimester, such as spontaneous abortions, pre-eclampsia and intrauterine growth restriction, occur more frequently when the mothers are diabetic. Insulin,[6] leptin[7] and isoprostanes,[8] but not glucose,[9] may be among the causative factors in the diabetic environment leading to such increases in invasion defects.

Placental morphology and composition

Improvements in glycemic control in recent years has led to less pronounced placental weight differences between normal and diabetic pregnancies,[10,11] although a tendency to heavier placentae in overt diabetes has remained, especially when neonates are heavier. The occurrence of placentomegaly as a result of an increase in parenchymal tissue cellularity, reflected by higher DNA contents,[12,13] in cases of increased weight of the neonate, confirms the close correlation of placental weight with that of the offspring. The placentae in diabetic pregnancies also contain more triglycerides and phospholipids than in normal pregnancies (Table 10.1).[12]

Essentially normal microscopical morphology is preserved in placentae from diabetic mothers with good glycemic control, regardless of the type of diabetes; however, some distinct alterations can be noted. A characteristic feature of placentae from diabetic pregnancies is the enlargement of the villous surface by 30–50% owing to the greater surface area in the periphery of the villous tree. Moreover, total length of villous capillaries (+30%), as

	Normal pregnancy	Gestational DM	Type 1 DM
DNA (grams)	1.40±0.07	1.71±0.12[†]	1.87±0.20[†]
Glycogen (grams)	4.67±0.29	6.57±0.60[†]	9.16±0.88[†]
Lipid			
TG (nmol)	1.38±0.10	2.20±0.25[†]	2.80±0.41[†]
PL (mgrams)	154±11	305±33[†]	338±37[†]
Cholesterol (grams)	2.20±0.17	2.26±0.21	2.71±0.32

* Data are mean ± SEM expressed per total placenta.
[†] $P < 0.05$ versus normal pregnancy.
DM, Diabetes mellitus; TG, triglyceride; PL, phospholipid, SEM, standard error of mean.

Table 10.1. Placental composition in normal and diabetic human pregnancies (from Diamant et al[12]).

well as the capillary surface area (+40%), are greater in diabetic placentae.[14] Together with changes on the endothelium (see below) and fetal erythrocytes that result in a shorter diffusion distance for oxygen,[15-17] this may be part of a mechanism to compensate for the impaired maternal–fetal transfer of diffusion-limited substances, predominantly of oxygen. Fetal hypoxia, which is the consequence of trophoblast basement-membrane thickening and intensified fetal metabolism, may stimulate placental synthesis of angiogenetic factors such as fetal growth factor (FGF)-2,[18] vascular endothelial growth factors (VEGF) and placental growth factor (PGF)-1. The resulting hypervascularization and the increase in the surface area of exchange facilitates oxygen diffusion across the placenta.

Trophoblastic basement membrane thickening may be attributed to increased amounts of collagen, predominantly of collagen type IV. Some collagens, e.g. types IV, V and VI, contain a higher proportion of carbohydrates and it may be conceived that this is due to non-enzymatic glycation. The villous stroma is slightly edematous and may impress by the over-representation of tissue macrophages (Hofbauer cells). Their ability to release interleukin (IL)-1, a hypoglycemic agent, may contribute to establishing a normoglycemic environment for the fetus. The total glycosaminoglycan content of the villous connective tissue is increased in diabetic pregnancies due to a higher proportion of hyaluronic acid subfractions and of heparan sulfate, whereas the proportion of dermatan sulfate is markedly decreased.

A hyperplasia of the endothelial cells may occur. The endothelial cells are in an active stage, as can be inferred from the arrangement of eu- and heterochromatin. The expression of adherens (vasculoendothelial cadherin, β-catenin) and tight (occludin, zonula occludens protein-1) junctional proteins is downregulated, which may alter placental barrier function.[19]

The continuous exposure to maternal hyperglycemia of the many proteins, such as enzymes, transporters and receptors, on the microvillous membrane of the syncytiotrophoblast may result in their non-enzymatic glycation. However, preliminary evidence demonstrates the formation of advanced glycation endproducts (AGE), predominantly around fetal vessels in stem villi.[20] Whether such non-enzymatic glycation accounts for some functional changes remains to be investigated.

Accumulating evidence points towards a participation of free oxygen radical overproduction in the induction of embryonic dysmorphogenesis in diabetic pregnancy. Hyperglycemia- stimulated activity of the mitochondrial electron transport chain is the intracellular process accounting for free radical generation.[21] In diabetic rat pregnancy, mitochondrial morphology is altered in ectodermal cells of day-9 embryos and in the neuroepithelium of day-10 embryos, but not in the brain, heart and liver of day-15 fetuses. Clear evidence shows that free oxygen radicals were involved in the mitochondrial large-amplitude swelling induced by hyperglycemia.[22,23] However, in human trophoblasts exposed to hyperglycemia this morphological alteration of the mitochondria was not observed, regardless of the time in gestation,[24] although trophoblast mitochondria can generate free oxygen radicals.[25] Also in diabetes, trophoblast mitochondria are morphologically normal, although the placenta shows signs of oxidative stress (Fig. 10.2).[26]

Collectively, these results suggest that the placenta in controlled diabetic pregnancy adapts to retain the essential anatomical structures for the efficient support of fetal growth. Consequently, any impaired placental function in maternal diabetes must be due to inadequate

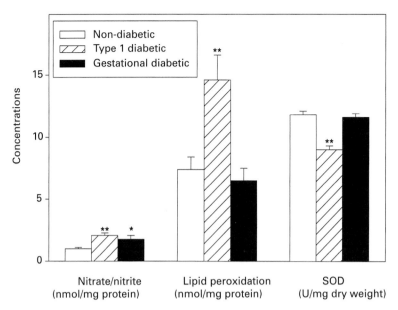

Figure 10.2. *Concentrations (mean ± SEM) of oxidative stress-related parameters in placental villi from healthy subjects, and patients with Type 1 and gestational diabetes mellitus. SOD, Superoxide dismutase, SEM, Standard error of mean. *P < 0.05; **P < 0.01 versus control. (Data taken from Pustovrh et al.[26])*

biochemical or physiological processes, such as metabolism and transport. The functional immaturity is locally restricted in structurally immature villi. In view of the large functional reserve of the placenta it must be presumed that the overall performance of the organ ultimately does not limit growth nor development of the human fetus.

Blood flow

Utero-placental and feto-placental blood flow determine materno–fetal exchange of substances whose transport is flow limited such as oxygen or glucose, although the latter is debated. In view of the above characterized diabetes-associated changes in placental structure, alterations in blood flow in both circulations in the placenta may be expected. In fact, blood flow may be reduced in both circula-

tions, resulting in increased resistance indices, but absence of changes has also been noted. These variations may reflect the different levels of glycemia achieved in the different studies and varying degrees of fetal oxygenation. There is no direct relationship between utero-placental blood flow and fetal birthweight in diabetes. Therefore, fetal macrosomia in diabetes should be explained on a metabolic basis rather than by flow-regulated increased placental transfer of nutrients, if it occurs at all.

Utero-placental blood flow may be compromised in diabetes by a number of contributing factors:

- inadequate opening of the spiral arteries by too shallow an invasion of the trophoblast – although there is no experimental evidence to support this hypothesis, the increased incidence in diabetes of pregnancy pathologies that are currently associated with impaired trophoblast invasion, such as pre-eclampsia, spontaneous abortions and growth restricted fetuses, suggests such a defect;

- narrowing of the lumen of placental bed arterioles because of fibrinoid necrosis and foam cell deposition (acute atherosis),[27,28] perhaps as a result of isoprostane action;[29]
- enlargement of placental villi in diabetes because of a greater mass of parenchymal tissue, resulting in a reduction of the inter-villous space volume;[1]
- imbalance in local prostacyclin/thromboxane production favoring the vaso-constrictive effect of thromboxane (Fig. 10.3);[30] this may be induced by maternal hyperglycemia;[31]
- hyperglycemia-induced reduction in trophoblast estradiol production,[32] which has a potent effect on uterine vasculature and, hence, intervillous perfusion.[33]

Because of the absence of innervation, feto-placental blood flow is autonomous and regulated by locally produced vasoactive substances such as eicosanoids, endothelins and nitric oxide. Neither the amounts nor the activities of nitric oxide synthase isoforms are altered in the placental endothelium in diabetes,[34–36] yet more nitrite is produced and placental nitrotyrosine residues are expressed at a higher level in diabetic than in control placentae.[35,37,38] Nitrotyrosines are formed either from nitrite by the activity of myeloperoxidase that is located on the endothelium of normal term placentae,[39] or by peroxynitrite action on amino acids. Peroxynitrite is the result of nitric oxide reacting with superoxide that is formed by hyperglycemia-associated increased substrate flow through the electron transport chain in mitochondria.

The expression of the manganese isoform of superoxide dismutase is higher in diabetic pregnancies,[35] but indirect evidence suggests that

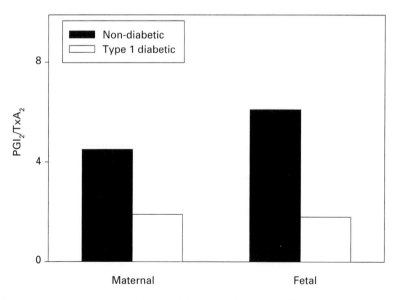

Figure 10.3. *Comparison of relative eicosanoid production (vasodilator/vasoconstrictor) in the maternal and fetal circulation of placentae from normal and Type 1 diabetic pregnancies. PGI_2, Prostacyclin I_2; TxA_2, thromboxane A_2. (Data taken from Kuhn et al.[30])*

catalase activity may be reduced in vessels of diabetic pregnancies perhaps as a result of inhibition by nitric oxide.[38] Therefore, H_2O_2 may accumulate in the feto-placental endothelium in diabetes producing a prostaglandin-mediated contraction that is even more pronounced in placental vessels from diabetic women as compared to control subjects.[40]

The feto-placental vasculature is quite tolerant towards hyperglycemia because only concentrations of circulating glucose > 160 mg/dl result in an increase in the resistance index.[41] This may be accounted for by attenuated responses to vasoconstrictors and vasodilators in diabetes compared to control placentae,[37,38] which may be caused in part by peroxynitrite interaction with placental vessels.[37] This is probably not the only mechanism altering placental vascular responses to vasoactive agents, because the vessels may become stiffened in diabetes as a result of progressive glycation and cross-linking of extracellular matrix proteins of the vessel walls.[42]

Whether expression levels of endothelins and their receptors are altered in diabetic placentae as compared to normal controls is unknown, but can be expected by inference from other tissues in diabetes.

Placental prostacyclin and thromboxane production are imbalanced in diabetes,[30,43] favoring the generation of vasoconstricting prostaglandins. However, the effect of this eicosanoid-induced contraction of vessels may be counterbalanced if the fetus is hypoxic, because hypoxia leads to a relaxation of fetal-placental vessels, which is even more pronounced in diabetes.[40]

Maternal–fetal transfer

Oxygen and iron

Umbilical cord erythroblast counts, erythropoietin and hemoglobin, as well as lactate levels, are elevated in diabetes, strongly suggesting that the fetuses are hypoxic. This is the result of an increased fetal oxygen consumption for glucose oxidation in the wake of fetal hyperglycemia, and of a reduced oxygen supply because of the structural and blood flow changes of the placenta discussed above. Although the significance of structural changes has been challenged recently,[46] the functional consequences can be seen clearly *in vitro* by a reduced transplacental transfer in diabetes of the highly diffusible antipyrine (Fig. 10.4)[47] and of L-glucose[48] that both cross the placenta by simple diffusion.

The human placenta is an extrarenal site of oxygen-sensitive erythropoietin production.[49] Elevated fetal levels of erythropoietin may originate from placental synthesis, but a definitive answer is pending. It is also unknown whether placental erythropoietin synthesis is altered in diabetes.

Augmented fetal hemoglobin synthesis for erythropoiesis during diabetic pregnancy increases fetal iron demand. The increase in placental syncytiotrophoblastic transferrin receptor expression associated with reduced cord serum ferritin concentration suggests that the fetus requires both increased placental iron transport and mobilization of fetal iron stores to support augmented erythropoiesis.[50] Despite this increase in transferrin receptor expression, binding of diferric transferrin is decreased proportionately to the severity of maternal disease. Increased glycosylation of the N-linked oligosaccharides of the receptor isolated from diabetic placentae may alter its three-dimensional structure or charge, thus reducing its binding affinity for transferrin.[51]

Whether iron regulatory protein (IRP)-1 and IRP-2 (which bind to iron-responsive elements on the mRNA of transferrin receptor and ferritin, thus coordinately stabilizing transferin receptor mRNA and inactivating

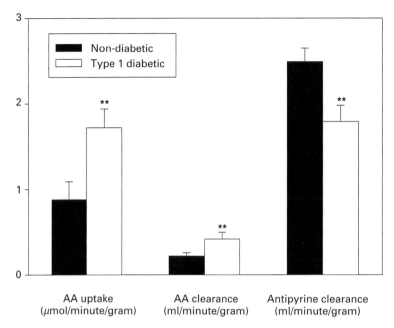

Figure 10.4. *Uptake and clearance [means ± standard deviation (SD)] into the fetal circulation of arachidonic acid (AA) in total placentae from normal and Type 1 diabetic pregnancies are increased, whereas clearance of the highly-diffusible antipyrine is reduced. **P < 0.01 versus normal. (Data taken from Kuhn et al.[47])*

translation of ferritin mRNA) are involved in these changes is unclear. Placental IRP-1 is more highly expressed in iron-deficient placentae, such as in diabetic pregnancies, suggesting a regulatory role in placental transferrin receptor expression.[52]

Glucose

The human fetus is almost totally dependent on maternal glucose passing through the placenta, since its own gluconeogenetic activity is minimal.[53] The key position of glucose for fetal maldevelopment in diabetes has prompted detailed studies into the molecular and regulatory mechanisms of maternal–fetal glucose transport and on their alterations in diabetes.

In most situations, transplacental glucose transport in the maternal-to-fetal direction follows a downhill gradient involving glucose

transporter (GLUT)-1 as the predominant GLUT isoform. The recently cloned GLUT8 is also ubiquitously expressed in the term placenta with lower expression levels in diabetes, but its role in placental glucose utilization is elusive.[54] The high-affinity isoform GLUT3[55] and the insulin-regulatable isoforms GLUT4[56] and GLUT12[57] have also been identified in the human placenta, but their location on endothelial cells and in the placental stroma, respectively, makes their direct contribution to maternal-to-fetal glucose transport unlikely. Rather, they are involved in glucose backtransfer from the fetus into the placenta and uptake into cells surrounding the placental endothelium.

Maternal-to-fetal glucose transport involves GLUT1 on the trophoblast, where it is located on the microvillous and on the basal membrane, facing the maternal and fetal circulation, respectively. The transport system has a high capacity with saturation reached at glucose levels > 20 mmol/l.[58] This system allows for a rapid transfer from the maternal to the fetal circulation.

Similar to other tissues, trophoblast GLUT1 is regulated by ambient glucose levels, i.e. it is upregulated under hypoglycemic and downregulated under hyperglycemic conditions, respectively. Loss of functional GLUT1 on the trophoblast surface is accounted for by lower GLUT1 transcript levels and, hence, translation,[59] as well as by a hyperglycemia-induced translocation of GLUT1 from the surface to intracellular sites.[60] Kinetic studies demonstrated that the loss of GLUT1 at the cell surface alters glucose uptake only at concentrations close to or > 15 mmol/l,[59] a concentration that is not reached in diabetic patients who are controlled. This GLUT1 response to hyperglycemia must be acquired during gestation, because it is absent in the first trimester trophoblast.[61] At this stage of gestation, ketone bodies[62] and insulin[61] appear to reduce or increase GLUT1 levels, respectively.

At term, Type 1 diabetes is associated with an increased expression of GLUT1 at the basement membrane, but not at the microvillous membrane, of the syncytiotrophoblast, whereas in gestational diabetes no such changes have been observed, regardless of offspring weight.[63–65] Total placental levels of GLUT1, GLUT3 and GLUT4 are unchanged in diabetes,[66] suggesting that the protein content of these transporters is not modified, although this awaits experimental confirmation.

Since transfer is determined by composite parameters such as the maternal–fetal concentration gradient, blood flow, surface area of exchange and diffusion distance, and placental metabolism, as well as the number and intrinsic activity of transporters, alterations in transporter levels alone will not predict *in vivo* changes. In gestational diabetes, maternal–fetal glucose transport as measured by placental perfusion was reduced when the mothers were treated with diet alone,[67] whereas when they received insulin, transport was higher as compared to the diet-treated group but not different from non-diabetic controls.[48] However, at a pathological glucose concentration of 8 mmol/l, no significant changes in maternal–fetal glucose transport were noted when the total placental weight was also taken into account (Fig. 10.5).[42,67] It appears as if the potential changes at the molecular level of transporters are counterbalanced by morphological changes such as increased area of exchange and basement membrane thickening resulting in increased diffusion distance. These data make it unlikely that the alterations in maternal–fetal glucose transport contribute to fetal macrosomia in diabetes, nor does it protect the fetus from glucose overload, at least not at the trophoblast level.

The high-affinity GLUT3 is located on the feto-placental vessels, and the insulin-regulatable

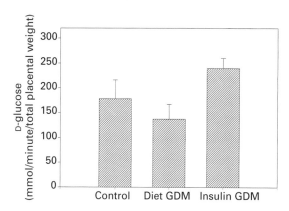

Figure 10.5. *Comparison of total maternal–fetal D-glucose transfer (mean ± SEM) across the placenta at 8 mmol/l external D-glucose in normal, diet-treated and insulin-treated gestational diabetic (GDM) pregnancies. (Data taken from Osmond et al.[48])*

GLUT4 and GLUT12 in the placental stroma, i.e. a portion of the placenta that is more exposed to fetal rather than maternal blood. The functional significance of these transporters is unclear, but the placenta may have developed mechanisms to take up glucose from the fetal circulation. In fact, glucose is also transported back from the fetus into the placenta[68] and the backflux is even increased in diabetes.[69] These transporters may extract glucose from the fetal circulation into the cells making up the endothelium, where glucose may then be stored as glycogen. The endothelium is also richly endowed with glycogenin, the protein precursor for glycogen synthesis, and glycogen is deposited predominantly around feto-placental vessels.[70] Therefore, the glycogen increments found in diabetes[11,12,70] may result from an increased glucose uptake from the feto-placental circulation. This would explain why the placenta in diabetes stores more glycogen than in non-diabetic pregnancies, although glycogen synthesis in the trophoblast is not stimulated by insulin or hyperglycemia. Whether or not fetal insulin by activating GLUT4 or GLUT12 stimulates glucose uptake into the endothelium – and subsequently glycogen synthesis is unknown – but a net effect of fetal insulin on glycogen levels in the placenta was found, with little increase in fetal liver glycogen.[71] The accumulated placental and fetal glycogen may then be broken down in case of fetal emergency demands such as prolonged labor. Because of the low levels of glucose-6-phosphatase,[72] lactate will then be the outflowing product. Collectively, these data suggest that the placenta may serve as a buffer for excess fetal glucose, at least at term of gestation, and it can be envisioned that an overflow of this buffer, i.e. when the storage capacity is exhausted, may result in permanent fetal hyperglycemia and hyperinsulinemia.[73]

Amino acids

Continuous growth of the fetus and the placenta depends on permanent net protein synthesis. Maternal amino acids provide by far the major source of nitrogen and, thus, are taken up by both the placenta and the fetus. Uptake of amino acids from the maternal and fetal circulation requires the presence of specific transport mechanisms on both surfaces of the placenta. The transport systems in the human term placenta resemble those described for various other tissues and cells.[74] Maternal and fetal-facing plasma membranes contain both common and distinct systems (systems ASC and t) for amino acid transport. The activity of transport systems may be coupled to an inward Na^+ gradient, but some are also Na^+ independent.

The efficient function of the Na^+-dependent transport systems requires low Na^+ concentrations in the syncytiotrophoblast, which in turn requires the presence of transport systems for pumping out the intracellular sodium. The most ubiquitous Na^+ transport system in animal cells is the Mg^{2+}-dependent Na^+/K^+-adenosine triphosphate (ATP)ase (enzyme catalogue number, EC 3.6.1.36), which is also present in human term placenta, where its activity in the basal trophoblast membrane is almost fourfold that of the microvillous membrane.[75] In placentae of Type 1 diabetic pregnancies, total activity of this enzyme is reduced, not because of a lower number of active molecules but due to an abnormal enzymatic function.[76]

For Na^+-independent transport systems one must assume passive diffusion of the amino acids along a concentration gradient. However, this is difficult to reconcile with the high placental concentrations of many amino acids as compared to the levels in the maternal or fetal circulation. A clear-cut explanation for this apparent discrepancy is still missing, but metabolism of amino acids by the placenta in general, or by the syncytiotrophoblast in particular, may influence transfer.

Some amino acids are taken up by the placenta from the fetal circulation. They are either metabolized and/or modified for release back into the fetal circulation. Such cycles have been demonstrated for glutamine–glutamate and asparagine–aspartate. The amide nitrogen of glutamine and asparagine may be required in the fetus for pyrimidine and purine synthesis, which in turn are building blocks for nucleic acids that are essential for rapid fetal growth.

Amino acid availability regulates placental transport systems. This 'adaptive control' can consistently be observed *in vitro* when placental tissue is cultured for several hours in the absence of amino acids.

In maternal diabetes, amino acid levels in maternal plasma, especially those of branched-chain amino acids, appear to be higher than in uncomplicated pregnancies, but this is not a consistent finding.[77] Conversely, infants of diabetic mothers generally have lower than normal plasma amino acid levels. As a result, the umbilical vein:maternal plasma level ratios are reduced in diabetic versus non-diabetic pregnancies.

Placental uptake and maternal–fetal transfer of amino acids in humans has not yet been studied *in vivo*, but in an *in vitro* system no significant difference was detected in the uptake of α-isobutyric acid by syncytiotrophoblast plasma membrane vesicles from normal and non-insulin-dependent gestational diabetic mothers of normal weight, i.e. non-macrosomic, offspring.[78] In similar experiments the Na^+-dependent uptake of methyl-α-isobutyric acid was measured, a non-metabolizable amino acid analogue, reflecting transporter system A. Detailed kinetic analyses revealed a lower initial rate of uptake, whereas equilibrium uptake was not different in vesicles of placentae from

diabetic mothers of macrosomic offspring, compared with normal pregnancies. System L appeared unaffected.[79] This strongly suggests that the activity of transporters may be altered, but total uptake is unchanged in the mother. However, when intact trophoblasts rather than isolated membrane vesicles were used for the uptake measurements, then α-isobutyric acid uptake was increased in women with impaired glucose tolerance as compared to non-diabetic controls.[80] Hence, different experimental models may lead to different results. Different diabetes-associated factors may also lead to opposing alterations and the net result is then determined by the prevalence of one of these. As an example, long-term hyperglycemia increases whereas hyperinsulinemia decreases L-arginine uptake into a trophoblast model;[81] however, the problem of model selection also becomes pertinent.

Maternal diabetes *per se* does not seem to impact on amino acid transporters located in the microvillous membrane per unit membrane protein. Despite an elevated total protein content of placentae from diabetic mothers, the increase in protein content is proportional to the increase in DNA, demonstrating that the amount of protein per cell has not increased.[13] Thus, one can infer an unaltered amino acid uptake per cell, but an increased uptake of the total placenta. However, one has to recall that the various transporter systems in the placenta can respond differently to maternal diabetes, requiring caution in generalizing inferences.

Lipids and fatty acids

At birth *c.* 8–12% of the fetal body mass is fat and about half of that fat is derived from maternal sources passing across the placenta over the whole period of gestation. The remainder may be due to the lipogenic activity of the fetal liver and other tissues. For most fatty acids a maternal–fetal concentration gradient exists and, hence, free fatty acids may traverse the placenta by simple diffusion, but an intermediate esterification of free fatty acids to triglycerides within the placenta may occur, followed by lipolysis and release into the fetal circulation.

Additional sources of fetal lipids are lipoprotein-borne triglycerides, phospholipids and cholesterol. Triglycerides cannot cross the placenta but will be hydrolyzed to free fatty acids and glycerol by lipoprotein lipase on the microvillous surface of the syncytiotrophoblast. There is about a fourfold difference in the maternal–fetal plasma concentration of lipoprotein-borne cholesterol, suggesting its transfer. This will be mediated by apolipoprotein B receptors on the microvillous membrane of the syncytiotrophoblast. The cholesterol taken up may then be stored, released on the fetal side or metabolized, in part serving as precursor for placental biosynthesis of steroid hormones. Similar to triglycerides, phospholipids are hydrolyzed into their constituents and can be stored within the placenta. Placental storage capacity, however, is limited and does not prevent excessive flow of lipids to the fetus in a condition of maternal lipid excess, such as occurs in diabetes.

Diabetes is associated with well-known alterations in the level and composition of maternal lipids. In particular, Type 1 diabetes in pregnancy is characterized by elevation of maternal plasma free fatty acids and triglycerides, as a result of loss of restraint on fatty acid mobilization from adipose tissue. The elevated lipid concentration promotes the transfer of free fatty acids and triglycerides across the placenta by increasing the maternal–fetal concentration gradient and by making other diabetes-related alterations that promote placental fat accumulation. Also, in non-diabetic women, concentrations of the free fatty acids myristate,

palmitate, stearate and linoleate in maternal venous blood and umbilical vein blood are correlated.[82]

The uptake of arachidonate into the perfused human term placenta in Type 1 diabetes is increased (Fig. 10.4). It is preferentially incorporated into triglycerides rather than into phospholipids of placental tissue and fetal effluent. Thus, transfer (Fig. 10.4) and distribution among lipid classes of arachidonic acid are altered in Type 1 diabetic pregnancies.[47] The linoleate content, among others, in placental tissues is higher, while 20:5 n-3/22:6 n-3 levels, and the ratios of 20:4 n-6/18:2 n-6 and 22:6 n-3/18:3 n-3, were reduced in diabetic pregnancies.[83] Therefore, a proportion of the arachidonic acid increments stored in the placenta in diabetes may also be derived by conversion of linoleate into arachidonic acid by elongation and desaturation reactions that occur in the human placenta.

Three to six times more arachidonate is converted to eicosanoids in a diabetic pregnancy than in normal placentae. In addition, the transfer of eicosanoids into the opposing circulation was doubled in placentae from Type 1 diabetics compared to normal placentae. The predominant direction of eicosanoid transfer in both groups of placentae was in the fetal-to-maternal direction. The relative amount of eicosanoids produced was also altered in placentae from Type 1 diabetic pregnancies, leading a lower ratio of prostacyclin I_2 to thromboxane A_2 (Fig. 10.3). This accounts for the imbalance in eicosanoid production, which is a strong contributing factor to placental vasoconstriction in diabetic pregnancies.[30]

Nucleotides

Nucleotides are transported from the mother to the fetus along a downhill concentration gradient by carrier-mediated transport mechanisms.

Transporters have been identified at the microvillous and basal membrane of the syncytiotrophoblast. Distinct from other tissues such as kidney and intestine, the transporter is Na[+] independent. Transporters for adenosine are also present on the endothelium of placental vessels and the umbilical cord. In diabetes the transporters on the endothelium of the umbilical cord are downregulated,[84] but not those on the trophoblast.[85] Because umbilical cord endothelial cells do not contribute to overall passage of nucleosides, it is expected that the fetus in a diabetic pregnancy is supplied with sufficient nucleosides to ensure adequate formation of nucleotides as building blocks for RNA and DNA.

Metabolism

The energy produced by the placenta from glucose is small. Most maternal glucose taken up by the placenta from non-diabetic pregnancies is passed as such to the fetus and only a small fraction undergoes glycolysis to lactate, which is also transferred to the fetus. There is only scant oxidation to CO_2.[58] The effect of diabetes on the activation of glucose-metabolizing pathways has not been studied in detail, but lactate release into the fetal and maternal circulation from *in vitro* perfused placentae is reduced in diet-treated gestational diabetes.[48,67] In addition, glycogen is accumulated in the placenta,[11,12] suggesting that placental glucose utilization is altered in maternal diabetes compared with the non-diabetic pregnancy. In addition, some increases in the activity of enzymes related to glucose catabolism, i.e. glycolysis, pentose phosphate and reduced nicotinamide adenine dinucleotide phosphate (NADPH)-generating pathways, are associated with diabetes, whereas those related to gluconeogenesis are unaffected.[86] Apart from these distinct changes, other pathways of placental metabolism appear not to be affected by changes in the maternal hormonal milieu different from liver and adipose tissue. This is because enzymes in the placenta are mainly constitutively expressed with little regulation by pathophysiological conditions, i.e. altered levels of hormones or increased effector concentration. Teleologically, this characteristic of the placenta confers metabolic stability to the fetus and protects it from the hormone-elicited metabolic changes in the maternal organism that are associated with diabetes.

There is only scant fatty acid oxidation in the placenta, but the capacity for fat uptake and transport is considerable. The extent of triglyceride transport varies with the species, it is limited in sheep, and moderate in human and rodent placenta. Most of the transport is indirect, involving the breakdown of the triglycerides to free fatty acids and glycerol, and re-esterification with intracellularly generated glycerol phosphate on the fetal side. Triglyceride transport across the placenta involves several lipase activities, active in the entry and release of triglycerides to and from the placenta.[87] Three triglyceride lipases have been identified in human placenta:[88] placental cytosol exhibits a pH 6 lipase activity which appears to be sensitive to hormonal activation; microvillous membranes contain a pH 8 enzyme with properties similar to lipoprotein lipase, a pH 5 lipase, presumably of lysosomal origin. With regard to the latter, a pH 4 lipase activity was found in human placenta, increasing in diabetic patients in correlation with birthweight[89] and decreasing with fetal growth retardation.[90]

Placental mitochondria

The placenta is rich in mitochondria. However, their capacity to generate oxidative energy is low in spite of considerable oxygen uptake, because of a potent ATPase bound to the mitochondria, which hydrolyzes a great portion of the newly elaborated ATP.[91,92] However, it is unclear in which placental cells the ATPase is located and, hence, whether low oxidative metabolism is a general characteristic of the human placenta or confined to distinct cell types. Mitochondria from cytotrophoblasts and the syncytiotrophoblast are different in architecture and function.[93] Cytotrophoblast mitochondria are larger than their syncytiotrophoblast counterpart, and they do not contain detectable cytochrome $P450_{scc}$. The respiratory chain of trophoblast mitochondria is a source of intracellular oxidants and endogenously produced nitric oxide modulates mitochondrion-dependent oxidative changes.[25] It is possible that diabetes-associated hyperglycemia results in an increased substrate flux through the Krebs cycle and the aldose reductase pathway, and, hence, may be associated with an increased generation of reactive oxygen species. To what extent this is increased in diabetes is unknown, but the level of oxidant stress response is below the threshold to produce morphological changes in the mitochondria that were seen in some gestational rat tissues.[24] The high cholesterol levels in placental mitochondria may confer some protection against changes in serum osmolarity that may be associated with diabetes.[94]

A tight coupling exists between the mitochondria and steroidogenesis in the placenta, by oxidation of a cholesterol side chain – the first step in the synthesis of estrogen and progesterone.[95,96] This occurs mainly in the heavy fraction of mitochondria and is mediated by the P450-'mixed-function oxidase', a cytochrome functioning as an alternative electron transfer system.[97] This cytochrome, often referred to as aromatase, affects sterol hydroxylation, which appears to be specific for the placenta.[98] Neither the aromatase reaction, catalyzing the conversion of C19 androgens to C18 estrogens, nor the NADPH-P450 reductase, are affected by diabetes.[99]

Placental leptin

Synthesis

Leptin, a 16 kDa protein which acts in the hypothalamus to regulate feeding and energy balance, was originally discovered as an adipocyte-derived hormone.[100] Leptin is also synthesized by several peripheral tissues including the placenta, which is quantitatively the second source of leptin production after adipose tissue. Besides its central anti-obesity effects, leptin serves a variety of roles in reproduction, early human development and pregnancy.[101,102] In early pregnancy, plasma leptin levels increase out of proportion with changes in adipose tissue mass of the mother, becoming maximal at the end of the first trimester[103] and returning to normal 24 hours after delivery.[104] These observations indicate that leptin production by the placenta contributes to an increase in maternal leptinemia. This is supported by data obtained with *in vitro* dually perfused human placenta showing that 95–98% of leptin synthesized within the placenta is delivered into the maternal circulation.[105,106] The similarity of placental and adipose leptins does not allow precise determination of their respective contributions to circulating levels. However, a similar production rate (0.03 ng/minute/gram) in both tissues suggests that the placenta makes a major contribution to maternal leptin levels.[106] Leptin is detected in fetal plasma as early as week 18 of gestation.[107] At term, 2–5% of placental leptin can be delivered to the umbilical circulation, and hence contribute to circulating plasma levels in the fetus.

Alternatively, fetal leptin may simply reflect fetal fat mass because leptin concentrations correlate with the adipose tissue mass over a wide range of fetal weights.[108,109] Indeed, leptin mRNA and protein are detected in human fetal fat from early stages of development until term.[106,110]

Regulation of production

Placental leptin production is increased in diabetic pregnancies requiring insulin therapy probably as a result of the fourfold augmentation in leptin mRNA expression (Fig. 10.6).[111] The stimuli responsible for augmented placental leptin gene expression are not yet identified, but insulin and hypoxia are two strong candidates for transcriptional regulation.[112,113] Hypoxia increases leptin production by trophoblast derived BeWo choriocarcinoma cells.[113,114] This is due to an upregulation of gene expression through a transcriptional mechanism that involves hypoxia-responsive *cis*-acting sequences.[114] 17-β-Oestradiol also stimulates leptin secretion by cultured human cytotrophoblast cells, suggesting that steroids synthesized locally participate in the regulation of placental leptin synthesis.[115] Regulation of leptin synthesis may also involve post-transcriptional mechanisms such as an activation of protein kinases A and C in choriocarcinoma cells.[116]

The fate of the high amounts of leptin synthesized in diabetic placentae is still debated. It is not known whether the leptin concentration

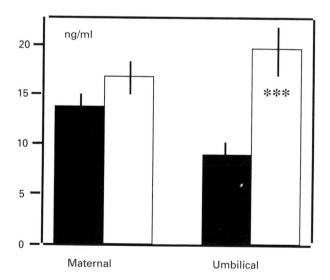

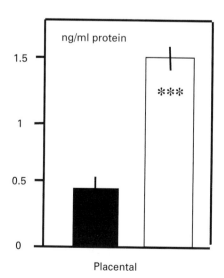

Figure 10.6. *Leptin concentrations (mean ± SEM) in plasma and placenta of Type 1 diabetic pregnancies. ***P < 0.001 versus control. Data taken from Lepercq et al.[111]*

ratio between maternal and fetal circulations is modified in diabetic pregnancies. For example, the increased placental production of leptin may contribute to fetal hyperleptinemia, a hallmark of diabetic pregnancies.[111,117,118] In the mother, conflicting data range from unchanged leptin levels in lean Type 1 and gestational diabetic women to increased levels in obese gestational diabetic women.[106,119] These findings suggest that leptin concentrations reflect maternal body mass index (BMI) or maternal weight gain rather than diabetes-induced metabolic defects. The effects of placental leptin in the fetus are even more speculative. It is unlikely that leptin directly controls fetal growth but an indirect regulation through stimulation of placental growth and/or metabolic pathways should be considered.[106]

Molecular pathways for leptin action

Similar to most cytokines, leptin transmits its biological action through binding to specific membrane receptors and activation of intracellular effectors. Five leptin receptor isoforms are generated by alternate splicing of a primary transcript.[120,121] They contain a common extracellular domain analogous to that of class I cytokine receptors and differ by the length of their intracellular region. None of these receptors have intrinsic kinase activity and they must activate Janus kinase proteins that initiate a phosphorylation cascade.[122] Short and long membrane receptors, as well as a soluble isoform, have been identified in the placenta and choriocarcinoma cells.[123–125] The activation of the endogenous receptors in trophoblast cells leads to the phosphorylation of p42–44 MAP (mitogen-activated protein) kinases and stimulation of DNA synthesis.[126] The same effects are induced by insulin, suggesting the existence of crosstalks between the insulin and leptin

signaling pathways in the placenta.[127,128] In Type 1 diabetes, the high placental leptin content in the face of an hyperinsulinemic milieu could contribute to stimulate MAP kinase pathways, ending up in increased mitotic activity and cell growth. Such functional interactions between leptin and insulin are potential mechanisms for diabetes-induced placental macrosomia. Besides its ability to activate the transmembrane receptors, placental leptin is able to bind to a soluble receptor which does not transduce a signal. In contrast with the amount of transmembrane receptors, which does not change, the concentration of soluble receptors is increased in Type 1 diabetes and may participate in the induction of leptin resistance in the mother or in blunting leptin action in the placenta.[125,126]

Insulin and insulin-like growth factor-1 in the regulation of placental growth

Mechanisms of action

The major effect of insulin in peripheral target tissues is the stimulation of glucose transport requiring the translocation of GLUT4 from an intracellular storage pool to the plasma membrane.[127] Except for one study showing that fetal insulin stimulates placental glucose uptake in the ewe,[128] the bulk of evidence indicates that glucose transport is not stimulated by insulin in the placenta.[129,130] This is in agreement with the findings that the insulin regulatable glucose transporter isoform GLUT4 is not translocated in response to insulin in placenta cells.[131,132] Hence, placental GLUT4 may differ structurally or functionally from 'classical' GLUT and may make only a minor contribution to overall placental glucose transport under insulin-stimulated states.

One possible approach to elucidate these issues is to characterize the intracellular pathways elicited by the activation of placental insulin and IGF-1 receptors. Classically, the autophosphorylation of insulin receptor (IR) triggers a cascade of reactions of phosphorylation inside the cell, allowing substrate molecules and protein adaptors to phosphorylate.[133] Despite a high insulin receptor density, which displays ample binding and effective tyrosine kinase (TK) activity,[134] limited biological effects mediated through insulin receptors have been described in the placenta.[135,136] The main pathway leading to the stimulation of DNA synthesis classically involves the MAP kinase cascade, whereas the metabolic effects are mostly mediated through the phosphatidylinositol-3 kinase (PI-3K) pathway.[133] In human choriocarcinoma JAr cells, MAP kinase is phosphorylated in response to insulin and this leads to the stimulation of DNA synthesis.[131] In the same trophoblast cell line, the PI-3K pathway is also stimulated in response to insulin, leading to the phosphorylation and activation of protein kinase B (PKB), a downstream target of PI-3K. However, in contrast to the pathways decribed in fat and muscle cells, PKB activation is neither associated with GLUT4 translocation nor with the stimulation of glycogen synthesis.[131] This indicates that the major effects of insulin in the placenta are directed towards the stimulation of mitogenic rather than metabolic signals.

Regulation of placental growth

The concept that insulin is a potent growth factor *in utero* was based on the increased size of rat, rabbit and monkey fetuses injected with insulin.[137–139] In humans, infants with excessive *in utero* insulin secretion, primary hepatic pathology and Beckwith–Wiedeman syndrome also exhibit increased birthweights. The feto-

placental overgrowth observed in pregnancies with Type 1 and gestational diabetes is associated with an hyperinsulinemic state in both the mother and fetus.[111,140] Hence, the insulin-mediated mechanisms which regulate placental growth are sufficient to explain the overgrowth of fetuses of diabetic mothers (see above). Besides insulin, the contribution of IGF and binding proteins has to be taken into account in order to understand increased somatic growth in hyperinsulinic states. The high structural homology shared by insulin and IGF-1 receptors supports the idea that common concurrent pathways lead to enhanced mitotic activity. Expression of IGF-1 receptors and their ability to autophosphorylate are increased in placenta from pregnancies complicated with Type 1 diabetes.[141,142] The contribution of IGF is also supported by the dramatic effects that gene disruption of IGF ligands and receptors elicit on feto-placental growth in mice.[143,144] The chief substrates for the IR and IGF-1 receptor TK include the IR substrates (IRS)-1–4), and the Src and collagen homologous protein Shc.[145] IRS-1 gene disruption leads to fetal growth restriction in mice, and decreases in insulin/IGF-1 stimulated glucose uptake and insulin resistance, suggesting that IRS-1- dependent signaling pathways regulate feto-placental growth. PI-3K knockout mice also display *in utero* growth restriction, strenghtening the essential role of the insulin signaling cascade for *in utero* growth.[146]

The close correlation between placenta and fetal size in normal and pathological pregnancies is a straighforward indication that placental growth is a major determinant of fetal growth. On the other hand, it is becoming evident that fetal genetics and endocrine milieu contribute to the regulation of placental growth and metabolism. The first demonstration that fetal genetic factors affect birthweight was obtained by screening the siblings of parents bearing a mutation in the glucokinase gene. The presence of the mutation in the fetus results in a reduced birthweight due to a decrease in fetal insulin secretion, indicating that genetic influences upon the fetal pancreas alter insulin-dependent fetal growth.[147] The contribution of genetic factors is further supported by the fact that despite similar maternal glycemic status, only half of the fetuses of Type 1 diabetic mothers become macrosomic,[148] whereas 50–80% of feto-placental macrosomia develops in fetuses of diabetic mothers.[149]

References

Because of space constraints only a small number of references could be cited. Priority was given to recent references. For a more comprehensive list of references the reader may wish to consult earlier reviews on this topic.[135,136,150]

1. Bjork O, Persson B. Placental changes in relation to the degree of metabolic control in diabetes mellitus. *Placenta* 1982; 3:367–78.

2. Pedersen JF, Sorensen S, Molsted-Pedersen L. Serum levels of human placental lactogen, pregnancy-associated plasma protein A and endometrial secretory protein PP14 in first trimester of diabetic pregnancy. *Acta Obstet Gynecol Scand* 1998; 77:155–8.

3. Brown ZA, Mills, JL, Metzger BE et al. Early sonographic evaluation for fetal growth delay and congenital malformations in pregnancies complicated by insulin-requiring diabetes. *Diabetes Care* 1992; 15:613–19.

4. Desoye G, Weiss U, Schmut O et al. Distinct effects of hyperglycemia in vitro on trophoblast proliferation and mitochondrial activity of placental trophoblasts at various stages of first trimester human pregnancy. *Diabetes* 2000; **49 (Suppl 1)**:A49.

5. Weiss U, Cervar M, Puerstner P et al. Hyperglycaemia in vitro alters the proliferation and mitochondrial activity of the choriocarcinoma cell lines BeWo, JAR and JEG-3 as models for human first-trimester trophoblast. *Diabetologia* 2001; **44**:209–19.

6. Shaw LM. Identification of insulin receptor substrate 1 (IRS-1) and IRS-2 as signaling intermediates in the alpha6beta4 integrin-dependent activation of phosphoinositide 3-OH kinase and promotion of invasion. *Mol Cell Biol* 2001; **21**:5082–93.

7. Castellucci M, De Matteis R, Meisser A et al. Leptin modulates extracellular matrix molecules and metallo-proteinases: possible implications for trophoblast invasion. *Mol Hum Reprod* 2000; 6:951–8.

8. Staff AC, Ranheim T, Henriksen T, Halvorsen B. 8-Iso-prostaglandin f(2alpha) reduces trophoblast invasion and matrix metalloproteinase activity. *Hypertension* 2000; 35:1307–13.

9. Weiss U, Arikan G, Haas J et al. Hyperglycemia in vitro alters the invasion of trophoblast from human first trimester placenta into extracellular matrix. *Diabetes* 2000; **49 (Suppl 1)**:A316.

10. Clarson C, Tevaarwerk GJ, Harding PG et al. Placental weight in diabetic pregnancies. *Placenta* 1989; 10:275–81.

11. Desoye G, Hofmann HH, Weiss PA. Insulin binding to trophoblast plasma membranes and placental glycogen content in well-controlled gestational diabetic women treated with diet or insulin, in well-controlled overt diabetic patients and in healthy control subjects. *Diabetologia* 1992; 35:45–55.

12. Diamant YZ, Metzger BE, Freinkel N, Shafrir E. Placental lipid and glycogen content in human and experimental diabetes mellitus. *Am J Obstet Gynecol* 1982; 144:5–11.

13. Winick M, Noble A. Cellular growth in human placenta. II. Diabetes mellitus. *J Pediatr* 1967; 71:216–19.

14. Mayhew TM, Sorensen FB, Klebe JG, Jackson MR. Growth and maturation of villi in placentae from well-controlled diabetic women. *Placenta* 1994; 15:57–65.

15. Mayhew TM, Sorensen FB, Klebe JG, Jackson MR. The effects of mode of delivery and sex of newborn on placental morphology in control and diabetic pregnancies. *J Anat* 1993; 183:545–52.

16. Mayhew TM, Sorensen FB, Klebe JG, Jackson MR. Oxygen diffusive conductance in placentae from control and diabetic women. *Diabetologia* 1993; 36:955–60.

17. Mayhew TM, Jackson MR, Boyd PA. Changes in oxygen diffusive conductances of human placentae during gestation (10–41 weeks) are commensurate with the gain in fetal weight. *Placenta* 1993; 14:51–61.

18. Arany E, Hill DJ. Fibroblast growth factor-2 and fibroblast growth factor receptor-1 mRNA expression and peptide localization in placentae from normal and diabetic pregnancies. *Placenta* 1998; 19:133–42.

19. Babawale MO, Lovat S, Mayhew TM et al. Effects of gestational diabetes on junctional adhesion molecules in human term placental vasculature. *Diabetologia* 2000; 43:1185–96.

20. Avila C, Tanji M, D'Agati V et al. Localization of advanced glycation end-products (AGEs) and its receptor (RAGE) in placenta of gestational and pre-gestational diabetes. *J Soc Gynecol Invest* 1999; 6(Suppl): 153A.

21. Nishikawa T, Edelstein D, Du XL et al. Normalizing mitochondrial superoxide production blocks three

pathways of hyperglycaemic damage. *Nature* 2000; **404**:787–90.

22. Yang X, Borg LAH, Siman CM, Eriksson UJ. Maternal antioxidant treatments prevent diabetes-induced alterations of mitochondrial morphology in rat embryos. *Anat Rec* 1998; **251**:303–15.

23. Yang X, Borg LAH, Eriksson UJ. Altered mitochondrial morphology of rat embryos in diabetic pregnancy. *Anat Rec* 1995; **241**:255–67.

24. Jones CJ, Weiss U, Siman CM, Desoye G. Mitochondria from human trophoblast and embryonic liver cells are resistant to hyperglycaemia-associated high-amplitude swelling. *Diabetologia* 2001; **44**: 389–91.

25. Goda N, Suematsu M, Mukai M et al. Modulation of mitochondrion-mediated oxidative stress by nitric oxide in human placental trophoblastic cells. *Am J Physiol* 1996; **217**:H1893–H1899.

26. Pustovrh C, Jawerbaum A, Sinner D et al. Membrane-type matrix metalloproteinase-9 activity in placental tissue from patients with pre-existing and gestational diabetes mellitus. *Reprod Fertil Develop* 2000; **12**:269–75.

27. Barth WH, Genest DR, Riley LE et al. Uterine arcuate artery Doppler and decidual microvascular pathology in pregnancies complicated by type I diabetes mellitus. *Ultrasound Obstet Gynecol* 1996; **8**:98–103.

28. Kitzmiller JL, Watt N, Driscoll SG. Decidual arteriopathy in hypertension and diabetes in pregnancy: immunofluorescence studies. *Am J Obstet Gynecol* 1981; **141**:773–9.

29. Halvorsen B, Staff AC, Henriksen T et al. 8-iso-prostaglandin F(2alpha) increases expression of LOX-1 in JAR cells. *Hypertension* 2001; **37**:1184–90.

30. Kuhn DC, Botti JJ, Cherouny PH, Demers LM. Eicosanoid production and transfer in the placenta of the diabetic pregnancy. *Prostaglandins* 1990; **40**:205–15.

31. Rakoczi I, Tihanyi K, Gero G et al. Release of prostacyclin (PGI2) from trophoblast in tissue culture: the effect of glucose concentration. *Acta Physiol Hung* 1988; **71**:545–9.

32. Hochberg Z, Perlman R, Benderli A, Brandes JR. The effect of glucose 2-deoxyglucose and insulin on estradiol secretion by cultured human trophoblast. *Biochem Biophys Res Commun* 1982; **108**:102–9.

33. Resnik R. Endocrine modulation of uterine blood flow in pregnancy. *Clin Perinatol* 1983; **10**:567–73.

34. Schoenfelder G, John M, Hopp H et al. Expression of inducible nitric oxide synthase in placenta of women with gestational diabetes. *FASEB J* 1996; **10**:777–84.

35. Lyall F, Gibson JL, Greer IA et al. Increased nitrotyrosine in the diabetic placenta: evidence for oxidative stress. *Diabetes Care* 1998; **21**:1753–8.

36. Di Iulio JL, Gude NM, King RG et al. Human placental nitric oxide synthase activity is not altered in diabetes. *Clin Sci (Lond)* 1999; **97**:123–8.

37. Kossenjans W, Eis A, Sahay R et al. Role of peroxynitrite in altered fetal-placental vascular reactivity in diabetes or preeclampsia. *Am J Physiol Heart Circ Physiol* 2000; **278**:H1311–H1319.

38. Figuroa R, Martinez E, Fayngersh RP et al. Alterations in relaxation to lactate and H_2O_2 in human placental vessels from gestational diabetic pregnancies. *Am J Physiol Heart Circ Physiol* 2000; **278**:H706–H713.

39. Hammer A, Desoye G, Dohr G et al. Myeloperoxidase-dependent generation of hypochlorite-modified proteins in human placental tissues during normal pregnancy. *Lab Invest* 2001; **81**:543–54.

40. Figueroa R, Omar HA, Tejani N, Wolin MS. Gestational diabetes alters human placental vascular responses to changes in oxygen tension. *Am J Obstet Gynecol* 1993; **168**:1616–22.

41. Roth JB, Thorp JA, Palmer SM et al. Response of placental vasculature to high glucose levels in the isolated human placental cotyledon. *Am J Obstet Gynecol* 1990; **163**:1828–30.

42. Bucala R, Tracey KJ, Cerami A. Advanced glycosylation products quench nitric oxide and mediate defective endothelium-dependent vasodilatation in experimental diabetes. *J Clin Invest* 1991; **87**:432–8.

43. Walsh SW, Parisi VM. The role of prostanoids and thromboxane in the regulation of placental blood flow. In: (Rosenfeld C, ed.) *The Uterine Circulation*. (Perinatology Press: Ithaca, NY, 1989) 273–98.

44. Widness JA, Teramo KA, Clemons GK et al. Direct relationship of antepartum glucose control and fetal erythropoietin in human type 1 (insulin-dependent) diabetic pregnancy. *Diabetologia* 1990; **33**:378–83.

45. Salvesen DR, Brudenell JM, Snijders RJ et al. Fetal plasma erythropoietin in pregnancies complicated by maternal diabetes mellitus. *Am J Obstet Gynecol* 1993; **168**:88–94.

46. Mayhew TM, Jairam IC. Stereological comparison of 3D spatial relationships involving villi and intervillous pores in human placentas from control and diabetic pregnancies. *J Anat* 2000; **197**:263–74.

47. Kuhn DC, Crawford MA, Stuart MJ et al. Alterations in transfer and lipid distribution of arachidonic acid in placentas of diabetic pregnancies. *Diabetes* 1990; **39**: 914–18.

48. Osmond DT, King RG, Brennecke SP, Gude NM. Placental glucose transport and utilisation is altered at term in insulin-treated, gestational-diabetic patients. *Diabetologia* 2001; **44**:1133–9.

49. Conrad KP, Benyo DF, Westerhausen-Larsen A, Miles TM. Expression of erythropoietin by the human placenta. *FASEB J* 1996; **10**:760–8.

50. Petry CD, Wobken JD, McKay H et al. Placental transferrin receptor in diabetic pregnancies with increased fetal iron demand. *Am J Physiol* 1994; **267**: E507–E514.

51. Georgieff MK, Petry CD, Mills MM et al. Increased N-glycosylation and reduced transferrin-binding capacity of transferrin receptor isolated from placentae of diabetic women. *Placenta* 1997; **18**:563–8.

52. Georgieff MK, Berry SA, Wobken JD, Leibold EA. Increased placental iron regulatory protein-1 expression in diabetic pregnancies complicated by fetal iron deficiency. *Placenta* 1999; **20**:87–93.

53. Kalhan S, Parimi P. Gluconeogenesis in the fetus and neonate. *Semin Perinatol* 2000; **24**:94–106.

54. Gorovitz N, Cui L, Busik JV, Ranalletta M, Haugel-de Mouzon S, Charron MJ. Regulation of hepatic GLUT8 expression in normal and diabetic models. *Endocrinology* 2003; in press.

55. Hauguel-de Mouzon S, Challier JC, Kacemi A et al. The GLUT3 glucose transporter isoform is differentially expressed within human placental cell types. *J Clin Endocrinol Metab* 1997; **82**:2689–94.

56. Xing AY, Challier JC, Lepercq J et al. Unexpected expression of glucose transporter 4 in villous stromal cells of human placenta. *J Clin Endocrinol Metab* 1998; **83**:4097–101.

57. Gude NM, Rogers S, Best JD et al. Reduced glucose uptake and expression of a novel glucose transporter in placentas from gestational diabetic pregnancies. *Placenta* 2001; **22**:A56. [In the abstract the transporter was designated GLUTx, but since then it has been termed GLUT12 (Rogers S, Macheda ML, Docherty SE et al. Identification of a novel glucose tranporter like protein GLUT12. *Am J Physiol Endocrinol Metab* 2002; **282**:E733–8.

58. Hauguel S, Desmaizieres V, Challier JC. Glucose uptake, utilization, and transfer by the human placenta as functions of maternal glucose concentration. *Pediatr Res* 1986; **20**:269–73.

59. Hahn T, Barth S, Weiss U et al. Sustained hyperglycemia in vitro down-regulates the GLUT1 glucose transport system of cultured human term placental trophoblast: a mechanism to protect fetal development? *FASEB J* 1998; **12**:1221–31.

60. Hahn T, Hahn D, Blaschitz A et al. Hyperglycaemia-induced subcellular redistribution of GLUT1 glucose transporters in cultured human term placental trophoblast cells. *Diabetologia* 2000; **43**:173–80.

61. Gordon MC, Zimmerman PD, Landon MB et al. Insulin and glucose modulate glucose transporter messenger ribonucleic acid expression and glucose uptake in trophoblasts isolated from first-trimester chorionic villi. *Am J Obstet Gynecol* 1995; **173**:1089–97.

62. Shubert PJ, Gordon MC, Landon MB et al. Ketoacids attenuate glucose uptake in human trophoblasts isolated from first-trimester chorionic villi. *Am J Obstet Gynecol* 1996; **175**:56–62.

63. Gaither K, Quraishi AN, Illsley NP. Diabetes alters the expression and activity of the human placental GLUT1 glucose transporter. *J Clin Endocrinol Metab* 1999; **84**: 695–701.

64. Jansson T, Wennergren M, Powell TL. Placental glucose transport and GLUT 1 expression in insulin-dependent diabetes. *Am J Obstet Gynecol* 1999; **180**:163–8.

65. Jansson T, Ekstrand Y, Wennergren M, Powell TL. Placental glucose transport in gestational diabetes mellitus. *Am J Obstet Gynecol* 2001; **184**:111–16.

66. Sciullo E, Cardellini G, Baroni MG et al. Glucose transporter (Glut1, Glut3) mRNA in human placenta of diabetic and non-diabetic pregnancies. *Early Preg* 1997; **3**:172–82.

67. Osmond DT, Nolan CJ, King RG et al. Effects of gestational diabetes on human placental glucose uptake, transfer, and utilisation. *Diabetologia* 2000; **43**: 576–82.

68. Reiber W, Malek A, Aegerter E et al. Bidirectional human placental glucose transfer in vitro prefers maternofetal direction. *Placenta* 1991; **12**:430A.

69. Thomas CR, Eriksson GL, Eriksson UJ. Effects of maternal diabetes on placental transfer of glucose in rats. *Diabetes* 1990; **32**:276–82.

70. Robb SA, Hytten FE. Placental glycogen. *Placenta* 1976; **83**:43–53.

71. Goltzsch W, Bittner R, Bohme HJ, Hofmann E. Effect of prenatal insulin and glucagon injection on the glycogen content of rat placenta and fetal liver. *Biomed Biochim Acta* 1987; **46**:619–22.

72. Barash V, Riskin A, Shafrir E et al. Kinetic and immunologic evidence for the absence of glucose-6-phosphatase in early human chorionic villi and term placenta. *Biochim Biophys Acta* 1991; **1073**:161–7.

73. Desoye G, Korgun ET, Ghaffari-Tabrizi N, Hahn T. Is fetal macrosomia in adequately controlled diabetic women the result of a placenta defect? – a hypothesis. *J Matern Fetal Neonat Med* 2003; in press.

74. Christensen HN. Role of amino acid transport and countertransport in nutrition and metabolism. *Physiol Rev* 1990; **70**:43–77.

75. Kelley LK, Smith CH, King BF. Isolation and partial characterization of the basal cell membrane of human placental trophoblast. *Biochim Biophys Acta* 1983; **734**:91–8.

76. Zolese G, Rabini RA, Fumelli P et al. Modifications induced by insulin-dependent diabetes mellitus on human placental Na+/K+-adenosine triphosphatase. *J Lab Clin Med* 1997; **130**:374–80.

77. Verhaeghe J, van Asche FA. Maternal amino acid metabolism during pregnancy. In: (Herrera E, Knopp RH, eds) *Perinatal Biochemistry*. (CRC Press: Boca Raton, 1992) 53–68.

78. Dicke JM, Henderson GI. Placental amino acid uptake in normal and complicated pregnancies. *Am J Med Sci* 1988; **295**:223–7.

79. Kuruvilla AG, D'Souza SW, Glazier JD et al. Altered activity of the system A amino acid transporter in microvillous membrane vesicles from placentas of macrosomic babies born to diabetic women. *J Clin Invest* 1994; **94**:689–95.

80. Foster MR, Birdsey TJ, Bruce C et al. Evaluation of amino acid transport in cytotrophoblast cells isolated from placentas of diabetic women. *Placenta* 2001; **22**:A57.

81. Eaton BM, Sooranna SR. In vitro modulation of L-arginine transport in trophoblast cells by glucose. *Eur J Clin Invest* 1998; **28**:1006–10.

82. Hendrickse W, Stammers JP, Hull D. The transfer of free fatty acids across the human placenta. *Br J Obstet Gynaecol* 1985; **92**:945–52.

83. Lakin V, Haggarty P, Abramovich DR et al. Dietary intake and tissue concentration of fatty acids in omnivore, vegetarian and diabetic pregnancy. *Prostaglandins Leukot Essent Fatty Acids* 1998; **59**:209–20.

84. Sobrevia L, Jarvis SM, Yudilevich DL. Adenosine transport in cultured human umbilical vein endothelial cells is reduced in diabetes. *Am J Physiol* 1994; **267**: C39–C47.

85. Osses N, Sobrevia L, Cordova C et al. Transport and metabolism of adenosine in diabetic human placenta. *Reprod Fertil Develop* 1995; **7**:1499–503.

86. Diamant YZ, Kissilevitz R, Shafrir E. Changes in the activity of enzymes related to glycolysis, gluconeogenesis and lipogenesis in placentae from diabetic women. *Placenta* 1984; **5**:55–60.

87. Shafrir E, Barash V. Placental function in maternal–fetal transport in diabetes. *Biol Neonate* 1987; **51**: 102–12.

88. Waterman IJ, Emmison N, Dutta-Roy AK. Characterisation of triacylglycerol hydrolase activities in human placenta. *Biochim Biophys Acta* 1997; **1394**:169–76.

89. Kaminsky S, Sibley P, Maresh M et al. The effects of diabetes on placental lipase activity in the rat and human. *Pediatr Res* 1992; **30**:541–3.

90. Kaminsky S, D'Souza SW, Massey RF et al. Effect of maternal undernutrition and uterine artery ligation on placental lipase activities in the rat. *Biol Neonate* 1991; **60**:201–6.

91. Martinez F, Meaney A, Espinosa-Garcia Ma T et al. Characterization of the F_1F_0-ATPase and the tightly-bound ATPase activities in submitochondrial particles from human term placenta. *Placenta* 1996; **17**:345–50.

92. Moriyama IS. Respiratory function of placentral mitochondria, especially oxidative phosphorylation and ATPase activity. *Acta Obstet Gynaecol Jap* 1976; **23**:10–13.

93. Martinez F, Kiriakidou M, Strauss III JF. Strunctural and functional changes in mitochondria associated with trophoblast differentiation: methods to isolate enriched preparations of syncytiotrophoblast mitochondria. *Endocrinology* 1997; **138**:2172–83.

94. Martinez F, Pardo JP, Flores-Herrera O, Espinosa-Garcia Ma T. The effect of osmolarity on human placental mitochondria function. *Int J Biochem Cell Biol* 1995; **27**:795–803.

95. Meigs RA, Shehan LA. Mitochondria from human term placenta. III. The role of respiration and energy generation in progesterone synthesis. *Biochim Biophys Acta* 1977; **489**:225–35.

96. Meigs RA, Moorthy KB. The support of steroid aromatization by mitochondrial metabolic activities of the human placenta. *J Steroid Chem* 1984; **20**:863–86.

97. Simpson ER, Mahendroo MS, Means GD et al. Aromatase cytochrome P450, the enzyme responsible for estrogen biosynthesis. *Endocrinol Rev* 1994; **15**: 342–55.

98. Yamada K, Ogawa H, Honda S et al. A GCM motif protein is involved in placenta-specific expression of human aromatase gene. *J Biol Chem* 1999; **274**:32, 279–86.

99. McRobie DJ, Korzekwa KR, Glover DD, Tracy TS. The effects of diabetes on placental aromatase activity. *J Steroid Biochem Mol Biol* 1997; **63**:147–53.

100. Zhang Y, Proenca R, Maffei M et al. Positional cloning of the mouse ob gene and its human homologue. *Nature* 1994; **372**:425–32.

101. Ahima R, Flier J. Leptin. *Annu Rev Physiol* 2000; **62**:413–37.

102. Henson M, Castracane V. Leptin in pregnancy. *Biol Reprod* 2000; **63**:1219–28.

103. Highman TJ, Friedman JE, Huston LP et al. Longitudinal changes in maternal serum leptin concentrations, body composition, and resting metabolic rate in pregnancy. *Am J Obstet Gynecol* 1998; **178**: 1010–15.

104. Masuzaki H, Ogawa Y, Sagawa N et al. Nonadipose tissue production of leptin: leptin as a novel placenta-derived hormone in humans. *Nature Med* 1997; **3**:1029–113.

105. Linnemann K, Malek A, Sager R et al. Leptin production and release in the dually in vitro perfused human placenta. *J Clin Endocrinol Metab* 2000; **85**:4298–301.

106. Lepercq J, Challier JC, Guerre-Millo M et al. Prenatal leptin production: evidence that human fetal adipose tissue produces leptin. *J Clin Endocrinol Metab* 2001; **86**:2409–13.

107. Schubring C, Kiess W, Englaro P et al. Levels of leptin in maternal serum, amniotic fluid, and arterial and venous cord blood: relation to neonatal and placental weight. *J Clin Endocrinol Metab* 1997; **82**:1480–3.

108. Clapp J, Kiess W. Cord blood leptin reflects fetal fat mass. *J Soc Gynecol Invest* 1998; **5**:300–3.

109. Jaquet D, Leger J, Levy-Marchal C et al. Ontogeny of leptin in human fetuses and newborns: effect of intrauterine growth retardation on serum leptin concentrations. *J Clin Endocrinol Metab* 1998; 83:1243–46.

110. Atanassova P, Popova L. Leptin expression during the differentiation of subcutaneous adipose cells of human embryos in situ. *Cells Tissues Organs* 2000; 166:15–19.

111. Lepercq J, Caüzac M, Lalhou N et al. Overexpression of placental leptin in diabetic pregnancies: a critical role for insulin. *Diabetes* 1998; 47:847–50.

112. Saladin R, De Vos P, Guerre-Millo M et al. Transient increase in obese gene expression after food intake or insulin administration. *Nature* 1995; 377:527–9.

113. Mise H, Sagawa N, Matsumoto T et al. Augmented placental production of leptin in preeclampsia: possible involvement of placental hypoxia. *J Clin Endocrinol Metab* 1998; 83:3225–9.

114. Grosfeld A, Andre J, Hauguel-de Mouzon S et al. Hypoxia-inducible factor 1 (HIF-1) transactivates the human leptin gene promoter. *J Biol Chem* 2002; 277:42953–7.

115. Chardonnens D, Cameo P, Aubert ML et al. Modulation of human cytotrophoblastic leptin secretion by interleukin-1alpha and 17beta-oestradiol and its effect on HCG secretion. *Mol Hum Reprod* 1999; 5:1077–82.

116. Yura S, Sagawa N, Ogawa Y et al. Augmentation of leptin synthesis and secretion through activation of protein kinases A and C in cultured human trophoblastic cells. *J Clin Endocrinol Metab* 1998; 83:3609–14.

117. Persson B, Westgreen M, Celsi G et al. Leptin concentrations in cord blood in normal newborn infants and offsprings of diabetic mothers. *Horm Metab Res* 1999; 31:467–71.

118. Oreke NC, Hutson-Presley L, Amini SB, Catalano PM. The effect of gender and gestational diabetes mellitus on cord leptin concentration. *Am J Obstet Gynecol* 2002; 187:798–803.

119. Kautzky-Willer A, Pacini G, Tura A et al. Increased plasma leptin in gestational diabetes. *Diabetologia* 2001; 44:164–72.

120. Tartaglia L, Dembski M, Weng X et al. Identification and expression cloning of a leptin receptor, OB-R. *Cell* 1995; 83:1263–71.

121. Cioffi AJ, Shafer AW, Zupancic TJ et al. Novel B219/OB receptor isoforms: possible role of leptin in hematopoiesis and reproduction. *Nature Med* 1996; 2:585–9.

122. Bjorbæk C, Uotani S, da Silva B, Flier JS. Divergent signaling capacities of the long and short isoforms of the leptin receptor. *J Biol Chem* 1997; 272:32,686–95.

123. Bodner J, Ebenbichler C, Wolf HJ et al. Leptin receptor in human term placenta: in situ hybridization and immunohistochemical localization. *Placenta* 1999; 20:677–82.

124. Lewandowski K, Horn R, O'Callaghan CJ et al. Free leptin, bound leptin, and soluble leptin receptor in normal and diabetic pregnancies. *J Clin Endocrinol Metab* 1999; 84:300–6.

125. Challier JC, Galtier, Bintein M et al. Placental leptin receptor isoforms in normal and pathological pregnancies. *Placenta* 2003; 56:92–9.

126. Cauzac M, Czuba D, Girard J et al. Transduction of leptin growth signals in placental cells is independent of JAK-STAT activation. *Placenta* 2003; 24:378–84.

127. Sheperd P, Kahn B. Glucose transporters and insulin action. *N Engl J Med* 1999; 341:248–57.

128. Simmons M, Jones M, Battaglia F, Meschia G. Insulin effect on fetal glucose utilization. *Pediatr Res* 1978; 12:90–2.

129. Challier JC, Hauguel-de Mouzon S, Desmaizières V. Effect of insulin on glucose transport and metabolism in the human placenta. *J Clin Endocrinol Metab* 1986; 62:803–7.

130. Schmon B, Hartmann M, Jones CJ, Desoye G. Insulin and glucose do not affect the glycogen content in isolated and cultured trophoblast cells of human term placenta. *J Clin Endocrinol Metab* 1991; 73: 888–93.

131. Boileau P, Cauzac M, Perreira MA et al. Dissociation between insulin-mediated signaling pathways and biological effects in placental cells: role of PKB and MAP kinase phosphorylation. *Endocrinology* 2001; 142: 3974–9.

132. Xing A, Caüzac M, Challier J et al. Unexpected expression of GLUT4 glucose transporter in villous stromal cells of human placenta. *J Clin Endocrinol Metab* 1999; 83:4097–101.

133. Saltiel AR, Kahn CR. Insulin signalling and the regulation of glucose and lipid metabolism. *Nature* 2001; 414:799–806.

134. Joost H, Steinfelder H, Schmitz-Salue C. Tyrosine kinase activity of insulin receptors from human placenta. *Biochem J* 1986; 233:677–81.

135. Desoye G, Shafrir E. Placental metabolism and its regulation in health and diabetes. *Mol Aspects Med* 1994; 15:505–682.

136. Hauguel-de Mouzon S, Shafrir E. Carbohydrate and fat metabolism and related hormonal regulation in normal and diabetic placenta. *Placenta* 2001; 22: 619–27.

137. Picon L. Effect of insulin on growth and biochemical composition of the rat fetus. *Endocrinology* 1967; 81:1419–21.

138. Susa J, McCormick K, Widess J et al. Chronic hyperinsulinemia in the fetal rhesus monkey. *Diabetes* 1979; 28:1058–63.

139. Fletcher J, Basset J. Increased placental growth and raised plasma glucocorticoid concentrations in fetal rabbits injected with insulin in utero. *Horm Metab Res* 1986; 18: 441–5.

140. Schwartz R, Gruppuso P, Petzold K et al. Hyperinsulinemia and macrosomia in the fetus of the diabetic mother. *Diabetes Care* 1994; **17**:640–8.

141. Bhaumick B, Danilkewich A, Bala R. Altered placental insulin and insulin-like growth factor-I receptors in diabetes. *Life Sci* 1988; **42**:1603–14.

142. Bhaumick B, Bala R. Increased autophosphorylation of insulin-like growth factor-I and insulin receptors in placentas of diabetic women. *Life Sci* 1989; **44**:1685–96.

143. Liu J, Baker J, Perkins A et al. Mice carrying null mutations of the genes encoding insulin-like growth factor I and type I IGF receptor. *Cell* 1993; **75**:59–72.

144. Eggenschwiler J, Ludwig T, Fisher P et al. Mouse mutant embryos overexpressing IGF-II exhibit phenotypic features of the Beckwith–Wiedemann and Simpson–Golabi–Behmel syndromes. *Genes Dev* 1997; **11**:3128–42.

145. White M. The IRS-signaling system: a network of docking proteins that mediate insulin and cytokine action. *Rec Prog Horm Res* 1998; **53**:119–38.

146. Bi L, Okabe I, Bernard DJ et al. Proliferative defect and embryonic lethalithy in mice homozygous for a deletion in the p110 alpha subunit of phosphoinositide 3-kinase. *J Biol Chem* 1999; **274**:10,963–8.

147. Hattersley A, Beards F, Ballantyne E et al. Mutations in the glucokinase gene of the fetus result in reduced birth weight. *Nature Genet* 1998; **19**:268–70.

148. Small M, Cameron A, Lunan C, MacCuish A. Macrosomia in pregnancy complicated by insulin-dependent diabetes mellitus. *Diabetes Care* 1987; **10**:594–9.

149. Shelley-Jones DC, Beischer N, Sheedy M, Walstab J. Excessive birth weight and maternal glucose tolerance – a 19 year review. *Aust NZ J Obstet Gynaecol* 1992; **32**: 318–24.

11

Amniotic fluid in non-diabetic and diabetic pregnancies
Marshall W Carpenter

Introduction

Biochemical, sonographic, immunologic and genetic analysis of amniotic fluid continues to offer significant insight into the environment and development of the human fetus that can inform clinical care decisions. Amniocentesis has been described as early as in 1880,[1] when Lambl first reported its use in managing hydramnios. Amniocentesis was employed to inject radiographic contrast material to document fetal anatomy by fluoroscopy in the early twentieth century.[2] By the 1950s the amniotic fluid itself was analyzed to ascertain fetal health: samples were obtained primarily for evidence of meconium passage. Several reports of successful fetal sex determination by identification of Barr bodies in amniocytes became a clinical tool in risk assessment for X-linked recessive traits.[3–6] By the mid-1960s estimation of severity of fetal hemolysis by spectrophotometric bilirubin analysis became common practice and fetal transfusion became a therapeutic option.

Prior to the 1960s, when the reported perinatal mortality in the third trimester of pregnancies complicated by chronic diabetes approached 25%, delivery was commonly induced by 36 weeks, after which time the highest risk of mortality was observed. Following general acceptance of amniotic fluid surfactant analysis in predicting risk of neonatal respiratory compromise in premature births,[7] clinical management of pregnancy in diabetic gravidas employed amniotic fluid studies to determine the risk of respiratory distress syndrome (RDS) in patients pre-emptively delivered pre-term.

Amniotic fluid insulin has been used in the third trimester to assay insulin treatment effect on fetal metabolism and to determine subsequent treatment to avoid diabetic fetopathy at birth. Amniotic fluid homeostasis may be affected by the maternal diabetic metabolic state to produce hydramnios. In contrast, utero-placental insufficiency secondary to hypertension, renal and vascular disease that may complicate maternal diabetes can produce oligohydramnios. Amniotic fluid volume estimation may potentially identify opportunities for fetal surveillance, treatment or delivery to improve perinatal outcome.

The following is a brief summary of factors thought to affect amniotic fluid homeostasis in non-diabetic and diabetic pregnancies. Additionally, this chapter will describe insulin and C-peptide amniotic fluid concentration changes in non-diabetic and diabetic pregnancies, and the association of increased amniotic fluid concentrations with pregnancy outcome.

Amniotic fluid volume homeostasis

Volume homeostasis in non-diabetic pregnancies

Volumetric and indicator dilution studies in human pregnancies have demonstrated a rise of volume from 30 ml at 10 weeks gestational age peaking at 780 ml at 32–35 weeks, with a fall to half those values at term.[8] However, marked individual variation exists in normal, uncomplicated pregnancies so that the 90% confidence limits of most studies are in the range of ±700 ml at 34 weeks and ±350 ml at term. The rate of decrease of amniotic fluid at term has been estimated as 150 ml/week.[9] These changes are also reflected in the clinical measurements of the amniotic fluid index, the sum of vertical dimensions of the amniotic fluid in each of the uterine four quadrants. In a series of 709 uncomplicated pregnancies, mean values of the index remained stable from 22 to 32 gestational weeks at 14 cm. However, the 95th centile values continued to rise from 21 cm at 22 weeks to 25 cm at 36 weeks.[10] Moreover, the 90% confidence limits increased from 12 cm at 22 weeks to 17.5 cm at 36 weeks.

Net volume change of amniotic fluid is predicated on the flux of solute, since no active transport of free water appears to occur. Net flux of water cannot be reliably studied, though daily turnover has been estimated as > 95%.[11] In the second half of pregnancy amniotic fluid is largely the product of fetal urine production, which has been observed to contribute to amniotic fluid as early as 8 weeks.[12] Fetal urine production increases from 110 ml/kg/24 hours at 25 weeks to 190 ml/kg/24 hours at 39 weeks.[13] Low urine volume is often associated with oligohydramnios in growth-restricted fetuses.[14] On the other hand, polyhydramnios is not reliably associated with increased urine production, even in fetuses without anatomic defects. In one study, only 10% of cases of polyhydramnios in normal fetuses demonstrate fetal urine production above the 95th centile.[15]

The interrelationship of the several forces that affect amniotic fluid volume is poorly understood, though individual maternal and fetal factors have been demonstrated. Several vasoactive hormones have been demonstrated in fetal tissues and their use in several experimental models produce expected effects on fetal renal hemodynamics. However, the regulatory role of hormones such as arginine vasopressin, epinephrine, atrial natriuretic peptide and others in maintaining basal fetal urinary production and amniotic fluid volume remains unknown.

Fetal lung fluid production is inhibited and absorbtion is increased by agents that increase intracellular cyclic adenosine monophosphate (AMP). Arginine vasopressin has a similar effect and has been shown to increase ovine amniotic fluid volume.[16] Prolactin functions as an osmoregulatory hormone in teleosts and amphibia. Prolactin receptors are found in fetal lung and decidua. These may play a role in production of pulmonary luminal fluid and, thus, amniotic fluid volume homeostasis.

The permeability of fetal membranes to water is positively associated with decidual prolactin.[17] Several aquaporins (mammalian water channel proteins 1, 3 and 8) found in a wide variety of tissues have also been found expressed in fetal membranes and placenta. Aquaporin-8 is the only type identified in amnion.[18] Factors modulating aquaporin expression in fetal tissues are not well described.

Reduced fetal swallowing activity has been observed in conditions thought to reduce fetal central nervous system (CNS) activity. However, factors that affect swallowing in the undisturbed fetus are unclear.

Disturbances in maternal homeostasis may also affect amniotic fluid volume. Acute maternal volume expansion[19] and/or decreased osmolarity have been shown to acutely increase amniotic fluid volume. However, these effects are apparently short-lived,[16] and are rapidly overcome by maternal and fetal compensatory mechanisms. Consequently, the interactions between maternal and fetal blood volume and osmolarity, and their potential chronic effects on amniotic fluid volume homeostasis, remain unknown.

Volume homeostasis in diabetic pregnancies

Manning[20] has observed the incidence of oligohydramnios (≤ 2 cm largest vertical pocket by sonography) to be related to the severity and duration of maternal diabetes, being found in 0.3% in those with gestational diabetes mellitus (GDM), in 1.3% of women with prepregnancy diabetes diagnosed < 10 years earlier and in 2.1% of pregnancies in women with longer duration diabetes. However, the association of oligohydramnios and placental insufficiency found in non-diabetic pregnancies may be masked by the metabolic rather than the ischemic compromise of the fetal state in diabetic gravidas, and by the predisposition of such pregnancies toward increased amniotic fluid volume.

The prevalence of hydramnios among human diabetic pregnancies is unclear. The several published case series differ in measurement methods, the gestational age and conditions of observation, and in the criteria used for both diabetes and hydramnios. Hydramnios in pregnancy in insulin-dependent diabetic mellitus (IDDM) patients has been reported to be as high as 26%,[21] 40 times that found in non-diabetic controls. Some GDM case series have described rates of 2%, about four times that in unaffected pregnacies.[22,23]

In explaining the association between maternal diabetes and hydramnios, one may be tempted to extrapolate from the osmotic diuresis of the hyperglycemic diabetic adult to the fetus of the hyperglycemic diabetic mother. Amniotic fluid and maternal glucose concentrations have a significant association, for example.[24] In one study, a cohort of 41 insulin-treated women hospitalized for glycemic control for c. 1 month, underwent amniocentesis prior to planned elective delivery at 38 weeks.[25] Compared to a non-diabetic cohort (n = 35) undergoing amniocentesis for planned repeat Cesarean section, those with diabetes demonstrated higher amniotic fluid glucose levels (39 ± 17 mg/dl in the diabetes group versus 24 ± 11 mg/dl in the control group) and amniotic fluid indices (16.6 ± 5.0 cm in the diabetes group versus 13.4 ± 3.5 cm in the control group). In the diabetic cohort, amniotic fluid glucose was found to be modestly associated with the amniotic fluid index ($r = 0.32$). However, this cohort of hospital-treated, largely obese, gravidas may not be representative of other groups of diabetic gravidae. Others have not found such an association.[26] Moreover, case series of diabetic gravidas with excellent metabolic control actually demonstrate an increased incidence compared to historical, less well-managed, controls.[27]

An interesting cohort study examined GDM patients' average glycemia and proportion of glucose values ≥ 120 mg/dl for 24 hours and for the 7 days prior to amniotic fluid volume determination (an amniotic fluid index measurement).[28] Only patients having two observations, one showing normal and one showing an elevated volume, were enrolled. Consequently, patients served as their own controls. A retrospective review of 399 patient records provided only 13 cases providing two amniotic fluid index measurements, one of which was > 20 cm. Higher mean glucose values were found for the day and week prior to the amniotic fluid assessment showing elevated volume compared to the lower volume measurement (115 versus 103 mg/dl and 111 versus 102 mg/dl, respectively). Additionally, the proportion of glucose measurements that were elevated was greater in the epochs before the elevated amniotic fluid volume was measured. Though the investigators found no association between the amniotic fluid index and gestational age among the 26 observations, they did not account for the probable confounding of their findings by the probable improvement in glycemic control found later rather than earlier in gestation among their subjects. Nevertheless, this study suggests that even mild shifts in average maternal glycemia may produce an increase in amniotic fluid volume.

That maternal diabetes may cause hydramnios is supported by one study which observed fetal urine flow in excess of the 95th centile in 32% of fetuses in diabetic pregnancies.[15] In contrast, VanOtterlo et al[29] found no increased urine flow in diabetic pregnancies affected with hydramnios. Studies in fetal lambs suggest that acute maternal hyperglycemia does produce increase fetal GFR and urine production.[30]

These observations suggest that the effect of maternal diabetes upon fetal urine production may require a chronic stimulus associated with maternal hyperglycemia and/or an induction of metabolic change in the kidney, neither of which may be identifiable in acute experimental models. Consequently, mediators of the chronic effect of maternal hyperglycemia, if any, on fetal renal function or, alternatively, upon other factors known to affect amniotic fluid volume homeostasis are unknown.

Amniotic fluid insulin and C-peptide

Early amniotic fluid insulin and C-peptide in non-diabetic and diabetic pregnancies

Reiher et al[31] have demonstrated positive immunohistologic staining for insulin in the embryonic fetal pancreas at 9 weeks in pregnancies complicated by diabetes. However, fetuses of non-diabetic gravidas do not appear to release insulin in response to acutely induced fetal hyperglycemia.[32] Subsequent studies have suggested that, prior to mid-pregnancy, the human fetus may produce more insulin in gravidas at high risk of subclinical glucose intolerance.[33] These observations suggest that in the fetus of the non-diabetic gravida, fetal insulin may not regulate fetal glycemia. However, maternal diabetic metabolic disturbances may impact on early fetal insulin production, and response, in the first half of human pregnancy.

There is little doubt that the greater part of insulin in amniotic fluid is of fetal origin. Amniotic fluid insulin is reduced in fetal growth retardation and fetal death. Its amniotic fluid concentration correlates with that in umbilical plasma.[34,35] Transport across the placenta or fetal membranes is minimal and is associated with the presence of maternal anti-insulin antibodies.[36]

Earlier studies of amniotic fluid insulin employed relatively insensitive insulin assays, such that only insulin values > 2 μIU/ml could be identified.[37,38] Even so, insulin could be identified as early as 13 gestational weeks. However, the limited sensitivity of these assays interfered with identifying developmental changes in human pregnancy. Weiss et al[34] demonstrated a developmental rise in amniotic fluid concentration in non-diabetic pregnancy from 1.3 to 5.1 µIU/ml (0.29 µIU/ml/week) between 13 and 25 weeks gestation. A cohort study of 77 non-diabetic and nine diabetic women found lower insulin concentrations from amniotic fluid samples from 15 to 18 weeks gestation compared to samples obtained at 19–22 weeks (42±2 versus 51±6 pmol/L), but no increase thereafter in non-diabetic gravidas.[39] Diabetic pregnancies actually demonstrated lower insulin values (32±3 pmol/l) than non-diabetic pregnancies. However, diabetic pregnancies went on to develop a twofold rise of insulin concentration from early to third trimester pregnancy.

Using a double antibody solid phase assay with a limit of test sensitivity of 0.03 µIU/ml, Carpenter et al[40] found a logarithmic association between gestational age and amniotic fluid insulin (log insulin = 0.104 weeks gestation – 1.665) that described a rise in concentration between 14 and 20 weeks of 0.6–2.6 µIU/ml, suggesting a maturational increase in fetal insulin production during early pregnancy.

Addressing the observation that fetal macrosomia was commonly observed in late pregnancy in diabetic pregnancy, Pedersen hypothesized that the chronic maternal hyperglycemia characterizing diabetes stimulates increased fetal insulin production that induces fetal macrosomia.[41,42] However, the developmental onset and character of this fetal response to increased transplacental fuel flux remains undefined. Amniotic fluid concentrations of insulin or C-peptide in early pregnancy may provide some insight into these questions.

A case–control study of women with and without GDM has documented an association with stored samples of amniotic fluid obtained in the early second trimester.[43] A weak association was also demonstrated in a cohort of older patients undergoing genetic amniocentesis.[44] However, both studies failed to measure insulin

in a number of stored samples, suggesting that the radioimmunoassay employed was insufficiently sensitive. Nevertheless, these studies suggest that subclinical maternal hyperglycemia may have an effect on fetal development prior to 20 weeks gestational age.

A subsequent prospective cohort study of non-diabetic subjects > 34 years of age used a high sensitivity immunometric insulin assay to identify a possible association between early fetal insulin production and subsequent maternal diabetes diagnoses and fetal growth. Amniotic fluid insulin concentration at 14–20 weeks, expressed as multiples of the gestational age-specified medians, was associated with an increase in the later diagnosis of GDM, independent of maternal weight and age, with an odds ratio (OR) adjusted for maternal age and mid-pregnancy weight of 1.9 [confidence interval (CI) = 1.3–2.4].[33]

The association of second trimester amniotic fluid insulin levels with subsequent fetal growth in women without diagnosed glucose intolerance is less clear. Hidvegi et al[45] were able to find an association, among women > 35 years of age, of 16–18 week amniotic insulin more than two standard deviations (2 SD) above the mean with subsequent increased birthweights, but only in female offspring. This finding is understandable, since the majority of women will not be hyperglycemic and will demonstrate fasting and postprandial glucose values within narrow confidence limits. Such a conservation of maternal plasma glucose concentration will obscure any true association of increased maternal glycemia and early amniotic fluid insulin concentrations on birthweight. However, examination of the association in women with glucose challenge test values > 130 mg/dl (presumably a group at risk for mild maternal hyperglycemia), demonstrated that 14–20 week amniotic fluid insulin concentrations appear to be associated with risk of birth macrosomia [adjusted OR = 3.1 (CI = 1.3–4.9)].[33] An amniotic fluid insulin value of 1.40 MoM achieves a screen sensitivity of 88% and specificity of 73% for fetal macrosomia.[46] These findings suggest that in older gravidas, some of whom may have chronic subclinical glucose intolerance, fetal environment in the second trimester may be sufficiently altered to stimulate acceleration of fetal insulin secretion and augment subsequent fetal growth.

Third trimester amniotic fluid insulin and C-peptide

Third trimester amniotic fluid insulin and C-peptide in non-diabetic pregnancies

Amniotic fluid insulin concentration has been found to be associated with birthweight in a case series of amniocentesis specimens from non-diabetic gravidas, 94% of which were collected after 28 weeks.[38] In women with historical risk factors for diabetes, Weiss et al[35] found that third trimester samples from 28 to 41 weeks correlated with birthweights independent of the degree of maternal glucose intolerance. Amniotic C-peptide has been shown to correlate with relative birthweight (age-specific centile) in non-diabetic pregnancy,[47] though others have not found C-peptide to be associated with absolute birthweight in non-diabetic pregnancy.[48] These data and those based on fetal plasma insulin suggest that fetal insulin production, release and/or renal clearance may be a marker for fetal size. The possibility that differences in the maternal glycemic profile among women with clinically normal glucose tolerances may affect late pregnancy growth remains unexplored.

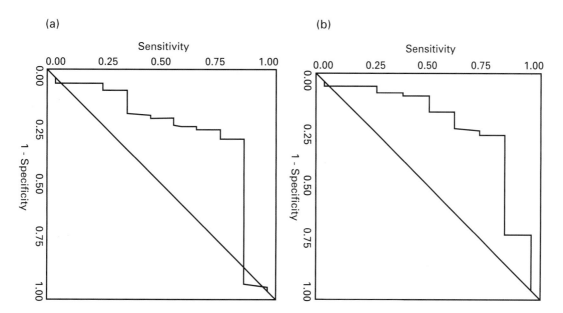

Figure 11.1. *(a) A receiver operator characteristic (ROC) curve illustrating sensitivity and specificity of a second trimester log amniotic fluid insulin MoM for subsequent development of gestational diabetes mellitus (GDM) among all 247 subjects. (b) A ROC curve demonstrating the same parameters of second trimester log amniotic fluid insulin MoM for subsequent fetal macrosomia (birthweight > 90th centile) among 60 subjects with 1 hour glucose challenge test values > 130 mg/dl.*

Third trimester amniotic fluid insulin and C-peptide in diabetic pregnancies

Studies of pregestational patients, those with GDM and non-diabetic controls have found higher amniotic fluid insulin concentrations in both diabetic groups compared to controls.[49] Weerasiri et al[49] also found that those with GDM who went on to develop postpartum diabetes had higher amniotic fluid insulin concentrations than those who reverted to a normal glucose tolerance after pregnancy. In a similarly designed study, Silverman et al[50] reported late gestation amniotic fluid insulin concentrations to be higher among 85 patients with pregestational diabetes (92±81 pM) and among 120 patients with GDM (74±76 pM) than among 37 control gravidas with a normal glucose tolerance (39±23 pM).

This effect appears to be mediated, in part, by the maternal glycemic profile. Kainer et al[51] examined the amniotic fluid insulin concentration in 25 IDDM gravidas at 32 and 34 weeks gestation. Twelve had amniotic fluid insulin concentrations > 8.2 µIU/ml, the 97th centile for 822

non-diabetic patients in their population. No measure of a glycemic profile at 14, 7 and 2 days prior to amniocentesis could be identified that demonstrated a statistically significant correlation with amniotic fluid insulin. Six subjects with elevated amniotic fluid insulin underwent a subsequent amniocentesis. Their amniotic fluid insulin and mean blood glucose values at each amniocentesis (18.5±6 µIU/ml and 112±13 mg/dl versus 7.7±0.4 µIU/ml and 94±13 mg/dl, respectively) were significantly correlated ($r = 0.7$).

Weiss et al[35] also found an association of amniotic fluid insulin not only with the diagnosis of GDM but also with neonatal characteristics that they labeled as diabetic fetopathy (macrosomia, hyperinsulinemia, hypoglycemia, polycythemia, hyperbilirubinemia, respiratory distress, etc.). They performed a weight-specified glucose tolerance test in 75 women with historic risk factors for GDM and found intolerance in 53. All 75 subject underwent subsequent glucose testing and amniocentesis for insulin assay. As Table 11.1 indicates,

	Diabetic fetopathy		Number	Sensitivity	Positive predictive value
	Present	Absent			
Postprandial GTT* glucose values (mg/dl)					
> 200	9	16	25	0.64	0.36
160–200	3	25	28	0.86	0.23
< 160	2	20	22	–	–
Amniotic fluid insulin					
> 97th centile	14[†]	0	14	1.0	1.0
≤ 97th centile	0	61[†]	61	–	–

† All 14 fetuses with diabetic fetopathy demonstrated elevated amniotic fluid and cord blood insulin concentrations (50±39 mIU/ml compared to 15.4±3.2 mIU/ml among pregnancies in the same cohort without evident diabetic fetopathy).
* Glucose tolerance test.

Table 11.1. Glucose intolerance and amniotic fluid insulin concentration association with diabetic fetopathy.

amniotic fluid insulin demonstrated a significantly greater test sensitivity and positive predictive accuracy for diabetic fetopathy than did the initial glucose tolerance test. These findings were consistent with those of Strangenberg et al,[52] who found an association of amniotic C-peptide levels in third trimester specimens with birthweight. The results suggest that fetal insulin production and/or renal clearance as manifest in amniotic fluid concentrations are biologically more proximate to the pathogenic processes producing diabetic fetopathy. These data should be viewed with some caution, however. The glucose tolerance test was performed between 20 and 28 weeks, and many amniocenteses were probably performed very late in pregnancy.

In a study wherein both fetal biometry and amniotic fluid insulin were measured at the same time, Schaefer-Graf et al[53] performed amniocentesis and measured abdominal circumference in 89 consecutive GDM and 32 consecutive Type 1 diabetic patients, all free of clinical vascular disease. They found a significant positive correlation between amniotic fluid insulin concentration and the relative abdominal circumference expressed as centiles ($r = 0.3$, $P = 0.0005$). They found that among fetuses with an abdominal circumference $\geq$ 80th centile the probability of elevated ($\geq$ 90th centile) amniotic fluid insulin was 0.48, in contrast to those having abdominal circumference < 80th centile where only 22% had an elevated amniotic fluid insulin concentration. These studies suggest that amniotic fluid measures of fetal insulin metabolism may offer more specific markers for diabetic fetopathy and may aid in guiding treatment.

C-peptide is released in equimolar amounts with insulin. Unlike insulin, which is cleared by the liver in widely varying proportions and by the kidney, C-peptide is cleared primarily by the kidney. Consequently, amniotic fluid C-peptide may correlate better with fetal insulin release. Amniotic C-peptide has been shown to correlate with the amniotic fluid insulin concentration in the third trimester in diabetic pregnancies.[54] The same study demonstrated that C-peptide amniotic fluid concentration among insulin-treated diabetic gravidas is similar to that of non-diabetic controls, though no pre- and post-treatment values were reported among the diabetic patients. C-peptide is also associated with fetal birthweight among diabetic gravidas.[54] However, others have not found the amniotic fluid C-peptide concentration to be associated with fetal growth in GDM and non-diabetic controls.[48] Arginine-stimulated amniotic fluid C-peptide and insulin have also been found associated with fetal macrosomia among insulin-treated diabetic pregnant women.[55] However, C-peptide assays may be potentially less stable in stored amniotic samples than insulin, thus limiting the utility of C-peptide assays as an investigative tool.

Conclusions

Amniotic fluid volume homeostasis and the impact of the maternal and fetal state upon it remain largely unexplored. Amniotic fluid volume peaks at nearly a liter in a human singleton pregnancy at 32–35 weeks, but with wide variation in normal pregnancies. By mid-pregnancy, fetal luminal pulmonary fluid, urine, fetal swallowing and transmembrane flux contribute to the amniotic fluid balance. Transmembrane water flux is wholly the result of osmotic and physical forces, since active transport of free water occurs. Vasoactive hormones may play a role in acute changes in amniotic fluid volume but their role in maintaining homeostasis in uncomplicated pregnancies is not clear. Prolactin functions in other species as an osmoregulatory hormone and may affect water transport across amnion. Maternal diabetes is associated with a higher prevalence of increased amniotic fluid volume. Though increased amniotic fluid glucose is associated with maternal hyperglycemia, it is unlikely that such exposed fetuses undergo an osmotically-driven diuresis.

Amniotic fluid insulin and C-peptide are primarily excreted from the fetus, thereby reflecting fetal pancreatic development and response to its intrauterine environment. Study of amniotic fluid insulin between 13 and 25 weeks demonstrates a rising amniotic fluid insulin concentration, probably from increased fetal renal excretion. As early as 14 weeks, the pancreatic production, and possibly renal clearance, of insulin is amplified in pregnancies complicated by maternal diabetes. Late pregnancy amniotic insulin values correlate with maternal diabetes status. Especially among less adequately controlled diabetic patients, the amniotic fluid insulin concentration correlates with maternal glycemic levels. Late pregnancy amniotic fluid insulin and C-peptide concentrations are associated with clinical signs of diabetic fetopathy demonstrated in the neonatal period.

References

1. Lambl D. Ein seltener Fall von Hydramnos. *Zentralbl Gynakol* 1881; 5:329.
2. Menees TO, Miller JD, Holly LE. Amniography: preliminary report. *Am J Roentgenol Radium Ther* 1930; 24:363–6.
3. Bevis DCA. The antenatal prediction of haemolytic disease of the newborn. *Lancet* 1952; 1:395–8.
4. Fuchs F, Riis P. Antenatal sex determination. *Nature* 1956; 177:330.
5. James F. Sexing foetuses by examination of amniotic fluid. *Lancet* 1956; 1:202.
6. Makowski EL, Prem K, Kaiser IH. Detection of sex of fetuses by the incidence of sex chromatin body in nuclei of cells in amniotic fluid. *Science* 1956; 123:542–3.
7. Gluck L, Kulovich MV, Borer RC et al. Diagnosis of the respiratory distress syndrome by amniocentesis. *Am J Obstet Gynecol* 1971; 109:440–5.
8. Brace RA, Wolf EJ. Normal amniotic fluid volume changes throughout pregnancy. *Am J Obstet Gynecol* 1989; 161:382–8.
9. Elliott PM, Inman WHW. Volume of liquor amnii in normal and abnormal pregnancy. *Lancet* 1961; 2:835–40.
10. Moore TK, Cayle JE. The amniotic fluid index in normal pregnancy. *Am J Obstet Gynecol* 1990; 162:1168–73.
11. Gitlin D, Dumate J, Morales C et al. The turnover of amniotic fluid protein in the human conceptus. *Am J Obstet Gynecol* 1972; 113:632–45.
12. Abrahamovich DR, Page KP. Pathways of water transfer between liquor amnii and the feto-placental unit at term. *Eur J Obstet Gynaecol* 1973; 3:155.
13. Lotgering FK, Wallenburg HCS. Mechanisms of production and clearance of amniotic fluid. *Semin Perinatol* 1986; 10:94–102.
14. Creasy RK. Biophysical aspects of management of the growth retarded fetus. *Semin Perinatol* 1984; 8:56–61.
15. Kurjak A, Kirkinen P, Latin V, Ivankovic D. Ultrasonic assessment of fetal kidney function in normal and complicated pregnancies. *Am J Obstet Gynecol* 1981; 141:266–70.
16. Nijland MJM, Ross MG, Kullama LK et al. DDAVP-induced maternal hypo-osmolality increased ovine fetal urine flow. *Am J Physiol* 1995; 268:R358–R365.
17. Josimovich JB, Merisko K, Boccella L. Amniotic prolactin control of amniotic and fetal extracellular fluid water and electrolytes in the rhesus monkey. *Endocrinology* 1977; 100:564–70.
18. Wang S, Kallichanda N, Song W et al. Expression of aquaporin-8 in human placenta and chorioamniotic membranes: evidence of molecular mechanism for intramembranous amniotic fluid resorption. *Am J Obstet Gynecol* 2001; 185:1226–31.
19. Goodlin RC, Anderson JC, Gallagher TF. Relationship between amniotic fluid volume and maternal plasma volume expansion. *Am J Obstet Gynecol* 1983; 146:505–11.
20. Manning F. Fetal biochemical and biophysical assessment. In: (Reece EA, Coustan DR, eds) *Diabetes Mellitus in Pregnancy*, 2nd edn. (Churchill Livingstone: New York, 1995) 251–60.
21. Rosenn B, Miodovnik M, Combs CA et al. Poor glycemic control and antepartum obstetric complications in women with insulin-dependent diabetes. *Int J Gynaecol Obstet* 1993; 43:21–8.
22. Jacobsen, JD, Cousins L. A population-based study of maternal and perinatal outcome in patients with gestational diabetes. *Am J Obstet Gynecol* 1989; 161:981–6.
23. Goldman M, Kitzmiller JL, Abrams B et al. Obstetrics complications with GDM. Effects of maternal weight. *Diabetes* 1991; 40(Suppl 2):79–82.
24. Weiss PAM, Hofmann H, Winter R et al. Amniotic fluid glucose values in normal and abnormal pregnancies. *Obstet Gynecol* 1985; 65:333–9.

25. Dashe J, Nathan L, McIntire DD, Leveno KJ. Correlation between amniotic fluid glucose concentration and amniotic fluid volume in pregnancy complicated by diabetes. *Am J Obstet Gynecol* 2000; **182**:901–4.

26. Cassady G. Amniocentesis. *Clin Perinatol* 1974; **1**:87–124.

27. Girz BA, Dovon MY, Papajohn M, Merkatz IR. Amniotic fluid volume in diabetic pregnancy. *J Matern Fetal Invest* 1992; **1**:237–40.

28. Bar-Hava I, Scarpelli S, Barnhard Y, Divon MY. Amniotic fluid volume reflects recent glycemic status in gestational diabetes. *Am J Obstet Gynecol* 1994; **171**:952–5.

29. VanOtterlo LC, Wladimiroff JW, Wallenburg HCS. Relationship between fetal urine production and amniotic fluid volume in normal pregnancy and pregnancy complicated by diabetes. *Br J Obstet Gynaecol* 1977; **84**:205–9.

30. Smith FG, Lumbers E. Effects of maternal hyperglycemia on fetal renal function in sheep. *Am J Physiol* 1988; **255**:F11–F14.

31. Reiher H, Fuhrmann K, Noack S et al. Age-dependent insulin secretion of the endocrine pancreas in vitro from fetuses of diabetic and nondiabetic patients. *Diabetes Care* 1983; **6**:446–51.

32. Adam P, Teramo K, Raiha N et al. Human fetal insulin metabolism early in gestation. Response to acute elevation of the fetal glucose concentration and placental transfer of human insulin-I-I31. *Diabetes* 1969; **18**:409–16.

33. Carpenter MW, Canick JA, Hogan JW et al. Amniotic fluid insulin at 14–20 weeks gestation: association with later maternal glucose intolerance and birth macrosomia. *Diabetes Care* 2001; **24**:1259–63.

34. Weiss P, Purstner P, Winter R, Lichtenegger W. Insulin levels in amniotic fluid of normal and abnormal pregnancies. *Obstet Gynecol* 1984; **63**:371–5.

35. Weiss PAM, Hofman H, Winter R et al. Gestational diabetes and screening during pregnancy. *Obstet Gynecol* 1984; **63**:776–80.

36. Menon R, Cohen R, Sperling M et al. Transplacental passage of insulin in pregnant women with insulin-dependent diabetes mellitus. Its role in fetal macrosomia. *N Engl J Med* 1990; **323**:309–15.

37. Casper D, Benjamin F. Immunoreactive insulin in amniotic fluid. *Obstet Gynecol* 1970; **35**:389–93.

38. Spellacy W, Buhi W, Bradley B, Holsinger K. Maternal, fetal and amniotic fluid levels of glucose, insulin, and growth hormone. *Obstet Gynecol* 1973; **41**:323–31.

39. Fallucca F, Sciullo E, Napoli A et al. Amniotic fluid insulin and C-peptide levels in diabetic and nondiabetic women during early pregnancy. *J Clin Endocrinol Metab* 1995; **80**:137–9.

40. Carpenter MW, Canick JA Star JA et al. A high-sensitivity assay for amniotic fluid insulin: characterization in 14–20 week specimens. *Obstet Gynecol* 1999; **94**:778–82.

41. Pedersen J. Weight and length at birth of infants of diabetic mothers. *Acta Endocrinol* 1954; **16**:330.

42. Pedersen J. *The Pregnant Diabetic and Her Newborn*, 2nd edn. (Williams & Wilkins: Baltimore, 1977).

43. Star JA, Canick J, Palomaki G et al. The relationship between second trimester amniotic fluid insulin and glucose levels and subsequent gestational diabetes. *Prenat Diag* 1997; **17**:149–54.

44. Carpenter MW, Canick JA, Star J et al. Fetal hyperinsulinism at 14–20 weeks and subsequent gestational diabetes. *Obstet Gynecol* 1996; **87**:89–93.

45. Hidvegi J, Paulin F, Megyeri J et al. Insulin concentration in amniotic fluid in mid-term pregnancy. *Orv Hetil* 1995; **136**:599–601.

46. Carpenter MW, Canick JA. Amniotic fluid insulin and C-peptide in normal and diabetic pregnancy. In: (Rao KA, Ross MG, eds) *Amniotic Fluid*. (Prism Books Pvt Ltd: Calcutta, 1999) 191–6.

47. Lin C, Moawad AH, River P et al. Amniotic fluid C-peptide as an index for intrauterine fetal growth. *Am J Obstet Gynecol* 1981; **139**:390–6.

48. Pschera H, Bersson B, Lunel N. Amniotic fluid C-peptide and cortisol in normal and diabetic pregnancies and pregnancies accompanied by fetal growth retardation. *Am J Perinatol* 1986; **3**:16–21.

49. Weerasiri T, Riley SF, Sheedy MT et al. Amniotic fluid insulin values in women with gestational diabetes as a predictor of emerging diabetes mellitus. *Aust NZ J Obstet Gynaecol* 1993; **33**:358–61.

50. Silverman BL, Rizzo TA, Cho NH, Betzger BE. Long-term effects of the intrauterine environment. *Diabetes Care* 1998; **21**:B142–B149.

51. Kainer F, Weiss PA, Huttner U et al. Levels of amniotic fluid insulin and profiles of maternal blood glucose in pregnant women with diabetes type-I. *Early Hum Develop* 1997; **49**:97–105.

52. Strangenberg M, Persson B, Vaclavinkova V. Amniotic fluid volumes and concentrations of C-peptide in diabetic pregnancies. *Br J Obstet Gynaecol* 1982; **89**:536–42.

53. Schaefer-Graf UM, Engel A, Henrich W et al. Relationship between amniotic fluid insulin levels and fetal abdominal circumference at time of amniocentesis in pregnancies with diabetes. *Am J Obstet Gynecol* 2000; **182**:S78.

54. Lin C, River P, Moawad A et al. Prenatal assessment of fetal outcome by amniotic fluid C-peptide levels in pregnant diabetic women. *Am J Obstet Gynecol* 1981; **141**:671–6.

55. Fallucca F, Gargiulo P, Troili F et al. Amniotic fluid insulin, C-peptide concentrations, and fetal morbidity in infants of diabetic mothers. *Am J Obstet Gynecol* 1985; **153**:534–40.

12

Classification of diabetic pregnancy
Yasue Omori

Introduction

The objective of every pregnant mother is to have a healthy baby. After many years of research and clinical applications, the normalization of blood glucose has been set as a goal of diabetes control before, during and after pregnancy. In order to determine the appropriate treatment and attain euglycemia, an appropriate classification of diabetic pregnancy that enables specific treatment strategies is paramount.

Thus far, several classifications of diabetic pregnancy have been made and each classification has unique features, and some have been more widely used than others. However, advances in the understanding of the pathophysiology of different forms of diabetes mellitus (DM) over the years has in one way or another necessitated some changes in even the most widely used classification of pregnancy complicated by diabetes. A review of the classifications of diabetic pregnancy from the past to the present will be discussed in this chapter.

The White Classification

Priscilla White, who worked at Joslin Clinic, Boston, was one of the most important pioneers in the field of diabetes and pregnancy. (see also Chapter 2.) In 1949, she developed a classification of diabetes in pregnancy that incorporated fetal risks based on the duration of maternal diabetes, the age of onset of diabetes and the presence or absence of maternal

Class A	It consists of subclinical diabetics. The diagnosis of diabetes is made upon the basis of a glucose tolerance test (GTT). These patients do not require insulin and can be controlled by dietary regulation (chemical diabetes).
Class B	The onset of diabetes has occurred in adult life, age over 20. Duration is under 10 years, no vascular lesions.
Class C	The onset of diabetes is from age 10 to 19. Duration is between 10 and 19 years. There are no vascular lesions.
Class D	The onset of diabetes is under age 10. Duration is over 20 years or they have calcification of vessels of legs or retinopathy.
Class E	Calcification of pelvic arteries.
Class F	Nephropathy excluding pyelitis or acute nephritis.

Table 12.1. *White's classification of diabetes in pregnant women (from White).[1]*

vascular complications (Table 12.1).[1] The validity of this classification is demonstrated in Table 12.2, in which the percentage of fetal survival of 278 pregnant diabetic women under her treatment is shown.[2] This classification was accepted worldwide because White demonstrated the relationship between the conditions of diabetic mothers and perinatal fetal or newborn morbidity. In 1965, White[3] added Class R for those patients with proliferative retinopathy. Moreover, in 1971, she added two more classes: FR, those with the characteristics of Class F and Class R, and Class G, which included those women who have had multiple failures in pregnancy.[4] Finally, in 1980, Hare and White[5] revised the White Classification, as shown in Table 12.3. The characteristics of this revised classification were: (1) the separation of gestational diabetes mellitus (GDM) and Class

A; (2) the omission of Classes E and G; and (3) the addition of Classes H and T (Class T was applied based on the work of Tagatz et al[6]). Although the White Classification had initially been used worldwide for three decades, except for Class T, its application became obsolete after the United States came up with a new classification of DM: Type 1 DM, Type 2 DM, GDM and other causes.[7] During White's era there was no awareness of the differences between Type 1 and Type 2 diabetes. Buchanan[8] pointed out that the White Classification could be simplified because of the current understanding of the pathogenesis of diabetes, the impact of pregnancy on maternal diabetes and the effect on the fetus. From the standpoint of the metabolic impact of pregnancy on maternal diabetes, the most important distinctions to be made are: (1) the differentiation between pregestational diabetes and GDM; (2) the differentiation between pregestational Type 1 [previously called insulin-dependent diabetes mellitus (IDDM)] and pregestational Type 2 [previously called non-insulin dependent diabetes mellitus (NIDDM)].

The application of the White Classification in Japan was very difficult, because in Japan the prevalence of Type 2 DM outnumbers that of Type 1, even in juvenile diabetic patients whose diabetes onset or duration is unclear. In 1983, Omori et al[9,10] reported their application of the White Classification of 100 diabetic women who had 127 deliveries; GDM women with transient abnormal glucose intolerance were excluded. Upon application of the White Classification to these 127 cases, Class B was found in 52 cases (40.9%), Class C in only two cases and Class D in only one case. In addition, 66 cases (52.0%) were unclassified. At the same time, it was attempted to classify pregnant diabetic women using the C-peptide response (CPR) after the meal tolerance test: it was concluded that the classification of

Class of diabetes	Fetal survival (%)
Class A: Chemical diabetes	100
Class B: Maturity onset (age over 20 years), duration under 10 years, no vascular lesions	67
Class C: Age 10 to 19 years at onset or 10 to 19 years' duration, no vascular lesions	48
Class D: Under age 10 at onset or over 20 years' duration or calcification of vessels of legs or hypertension or benign retinopathy	32
Class E: Calcification of pelvic arteries	13
Class F: Nephropathy	3

Table 12.2. Classification of diabetes in pregnant women (from White).[2]

Gestational diabetes	Abnormal GTT, but euglycemia maintained by diet alone
	Diet alone insufficient, insulin required
Class A	Diet alone, any duration or onset age
Class B	Onset age 20 years or older and duration less than 10 years
Class C	Onset age 10–19 years or duration 10–19 years
Class D	Onset age under 10 years, duration over 20 years, background retinopathy, or hypertension (not pre-eclampsia)
Class R	Proliferative retinopathy or vitreous hemorrhage
Class F	Nephropathy with over 500 mg/day proteinuria
Class RF	Criteria for both classes R and F coexist
Class H	Arteriosclerotic heart disease clinically evident
Class T	Prior renal transplantation

All classes below A require insulin therapy. Classes R, F, RF, H, and T have no onset/duration criteria but usually occur in long-term diabetes. The development of a complication moves the patient to the lower class.

Table 12.3. *The White Classification (revised by Hare and White).[5]*

pregnancy complicated by Type 1 and Type 2 DM is more useful than the White Classification in Japan.

Classification of pregnant diabetic women using the Pedersen Classification

Jørgen Pedersen revised the White Classification in 1965, as shown in Table 12.4. He omitted Class E and incorporated Class R (proliferative retinopathy) into Class F (Table 12.4). (see also Chapter 3.)

This revised classification was not generally used, but Pedersen often used it in his papers and books.[11] Pedersen and Pedersen[12] also made their own classification of pregnant diabetic women using factors that resulted in a poor prognosis during the current pregnancy. This classification has been named the prognostically bad signs in pregnancy (PBSP) classification. These factors are: clinical pyelonephritis, precoma or severe acidosis,

toxemia or those who could be designated neglectors. A neglector was defined as a woman who failed to follow the recommended regimen, irrespective of the cause, e.g. psychopathy, low intelligence, first attendance late in pregnancy (< 60 days before the calculated term), poor social circumstances and lack of proper information.[11]

Pedersen's classifications made a great contribution to the improvement of the condition

A	Chemical diabetes (diet ± oral drugs)		
	Age of onset (years)	*Duration (years)*	*Retinopathy benign*
B	≥ 20 and	< 10	Absent
C	10–19 or	10–19	Absent
D	< 10 or	≥ 20	Present
F	Nephropathy and/or proliferative retinopathy		

Table 12.4. *White's Classification as applied in the Rigshospital.[11]*

of pregnant diabetic mothers and fetal prognosis at that time. However, this classification was not universally adopted.

Hare[13] stated in his book his opinion with regard to the classification of diabetes in pregnancy:

It would seem that any new system of classification would have to have several features. First, it needs to be relatively simple so that it has utility not only for specialized workers in the field, but also for obstetricians and internists in general. Second, it must address both the maternal and fetal side of the equation. Thus, it has to have clinical utility and correlation with fetal outcome. Moreover, it will have to take into consideration the type of maternal diabetes, the presence or emergence of maternal complications, the severity of the metabolic derangement, and any subsequent effect on maternal health.

Two simple classifications

As mentioned above, Hare[13] pointed out that the classification of diabetes in pregnancy needs to be simple. At King's College Hospital, London, classification of diabetes in pregnancy was the epitome of simplicity.[14,15] It consisted of only three groups:

(1) diabetes diagnosed during pregnancy, whether it remits thereafter (GDM) or not;
(2) established diabetes with few or no signs of complications;
(3) established diabetes with major complications.

Essex and co-workers[14,15] wrote that if glucose tolerance reverts to normal after delivery, then it is defined as GDM. Moreover, with regard to point (3), it was reported that the number of patients with severe background or proliferative retinopathy and/or nephropathy was

c. 10% of their practice.[14] Essex et al[15] tried to solve the problem by advising women with major complications to avoid pregnancy.

Gabbe[16] also divided pregnancies complicated by DM into three groups: (1) patients with recent onset of pregestational diabetes (White Classes B and C); (2) patients with pregestational diabetes who have vascular complications (White Classes D, F, R and H); and (3) women with GDM. These classifications were not used worldwide.

World Health Organization classification

There is no formal classification of diabetic pregnancy by the WHO; however, GDM is included under its classification of diabetes. Considering the importance of these developments, the present author would like to introduce the WHO classification of diabetes. The WHO developed the classification of diabetes in cooperation with the National Diabetes Data Group (NDDG) and the American Diabetes Association (ADA).[17] Thereafter, the WHO reported its classification in 1985,[18] 1994[19] and 1999.[20]

In 1980, the WHO presented its classification of DM (Table 12.5). This technical report did not include any special definition or diagnostic procedure for pregnant women. The WHO's classification of diabetes in 1985 was almost the same as that in 1980, except for the addition of malnutrition-related DM.[18] The report said, 'The category of gestational diabetes should be applied only to women in whom glucose intolerance is first detected during pregnancy. Reclassification is necessary post partum.' However, their diagnostic criteria for pregnant women were the same as all adults. There were no major changes in the WHO's classification of diabetes in 1994. A new terminology, gestational impaired glucose tolerance (GIGT) was

A. Clinical classes
Diabetes mellitus
Insulin-dependent type – Type 1
Non-insulin-dependent type – Type 2
(*a*) non-obese
(*b*) obese
Other types including diabetes mellitus associated with certain conditions and syndromes:
(1) pancreatic disease, (2) disease of hormonal etiology, (3) drug- or chemical-induced
condition, (4) insulin receptor abnormalities, (5) certain genetic syndromes, (6) miscellaneous.
Impaired glucose tolerance
(*a*) Non-obese
(*b*) Obese
(*c*) Impaired glucose tolerance associated with certain conditions and syndromes
Gestational diabetes
B. Statistical risk classes (subjects with normal glucose tolerance but substantially increased
risk of developing diabetes)
Previous abnormality of glucose tolerance
Potential abnormality of glucose tolerance

Table 12.5. *Classification of diabetes mellitus and other categories of glucose intolerance (from National Diabetes Data Group[17]).*

introduced in this report. GIGT is ideally the proper term for GDM, although the criteria of GIGT was irrational because the fasting blood glucose level was too high.

The WHO revised their classification of diabetes in 1999 following the revision of diabetes classification by the ADA.[20] In the report of a WHO consultation in 1999, under the topics of gestational hyperglycemia and diabetes, they described that diabetic women who become pregnant do not have GDM but have 'diabetes mellitus and pregnancy' and should be treated accordingly, before, during and after pregnancy.

American Diabetes Association classification of diabetic pregnancy

In 1979, the NDDG of NIH in the United States made the classification and diagnosis of DM,

and other categories of glucose intolerance, based on their vast knowledge and data in order to set a standard universal criteria.[7] No other classification and diagnosis of diabetes has ever been discussed in such detail. The NDDG classified diabetes into clinical classes and statistical risk classes. The clinical classes include: Type 1 (IDDM), Type 2 (NIDDM), other types including DM associated with certain conditions and syndromes, impaired glucose tolerance (IGT) and GDM (Table 12.5).

Each class was explicitly explained under former terminology, associated factors, clinical characteristics and diagnostic criteria. The only classification with regard to pregnancy was GDM. GDM was defined as a class restricted only to pregnant women in whom the onset or recognition of diabetes, or IGT, occurs during pregnancy. Thus, diabetic women who become pregnant are not included in this class. In addition, after pregnancy terminates, the women must be reclassified, either into DM or IGT, if her postpartum plasma glucose levels meet the criteria for those classes, or into previous abnormality of glucose tolerance (PreAGT). In the majority of gestational diabetics, glucose tolerance returns to normal postpartum, and the subject can be reclassified as PreAGT. GDM is recommended as a separate class because of the special clinical features of the diabetes developing in pregnancy. Patients with asymptomatic, newly diagnosed diabetes in pregnancy, in whom there is no prior adverse obstetric history and in whom good control can be maintained with diet alone, are still at increased risk for perinatal morbidity and mortality. There is also an increased frequency of viable fetal loss. Clinical recognition of GDM is important because: (1) in a setting where high-risk pregnancies can be managed effectively, therapy can prevent much of the associated perinatal morbidity and mortality; and (2) these women are at higher risk of developing diabetes 5–10 years after parturition. In c. 1–2% of all pregnancies, GDM will develop. Indications for giving an oral glucose tolerance test (OGTT) include glycosuria, a family history of diabetes in a first-degree relative, a history of stillbirth or spontaneous abortion, the presence of a fetal malformation in a previous pregnancy, a previous large-for-gestational-age (LGA) baby, obesity in the mother, a high maternal age, and a parity of five or more. The presence of more than one of these factors is especially indicative of increased risk.[18]

Apparently, because it was believed that the explanations of GDM were thoroughly expounded on in the summary of the GDM workshops, classification of diabetic pregnancy gradually disappeared to be replaced by discussions of GDM.

The concept of GDM in the ADA has been changed by the influences of the second[21] and third[22] international workshop–conferences on GDM. In 1997, the expert committee on the diagnosis and classification of DM of the ADA changed the diagnostic criteria of DM from a fasting glucose level of 140 mg/dl (7.8 mmol/l) to 126 mg/dl (7.0 mmol/l); at the same time they modified the definition of GDM.[23] No section about the classification of diabetic pregnancy could be found in this report, which was entirely focused on GDM.

The expert committee defined GDM as 'any degree of glucose intolerance with onset or first recognition during pregnancy'. This definition applies regardless of whether insulin or only diet modification is used for treatment, or of whether the condition persists after pregnancy. In addition, this definition does not exclude the possibility that unrecognized glucose intolerance may have antedated or begun concomitantly with the pregnancy. It is also suggested that: 'Six weeks or more after pregnancy ends, the woman should be reclassified into one of the following categories; (1) diabetes, (2) IGF, (3) IGT, (4) normoglycemia. In the majority of cases of GDM, glucose regulation will return to normal after delivery.'

There are two problems with regard to GDM as diagnosed by the ADA. First, a 100 gram OGTT is still being used for the diagnosis of GDM in the United States, while other countries are using a 75 gram OGTT. Second, slight IGT induced by pregnancy and diabetes first diagnosed during pregnancy are combined into one category by the ADA.

Definition and diagnostic criteria of gestational diabetes mellitus of the Japan Diabetes Society

The Committee for the Classification and Diagnosis of Diabetes Mellitus in Japan's Diabetes Society adopted the ADA's

Time in pregnancy	Normal (%)		GDM (%)		Diabetes mellitus (%)	
1st trimester	202/250	(80.8)	33/250	(13.2)	15/250	(6.0)
2nd trimester	374/417	(89.7)	32/417	(7.7)	11/417	(2.6)
3rd trimester	702/749	(93.7)	37/749	(4.9)	10/749	(1.3)
Total	1278/1416	(90.3)	102/1416	(7.2)	36/1416	(2.5)

Using Diagnostic Criteria of Japan Society of Obstetrics and Gynecology. 75 gram OGTT: Fasting 100, 1 hour 180 2 hour 150 mg/dl, two values met or exceeded.

Table 12.6. *Frequency of GDM by 75 gram OGTT in 1416 women. January 1980 – March 1998: Diabetes Center Tokyo Women's Medical University.*

classification and diagnosis of diabetes in 1999.[24,25] Like the ADA's classification, this report also did not include the classification of pregnant diabetics, it was solely about GDM. With regard to GDM, they stated that 'GDM is a state of glucose intolerance occurring or detected for the first time during pregnancy' and 'glucose intolerance milder than diabetic type may affect the infant and mother adversely'.[25]

Japan's Diabetes Society persisted that the patients diagnosed as diabetics by a 75 gram OGTT have to be treated as pregnant diabetics not GDM patients. Moreover, 'the deterioration of glucose tolerance usually develops after the second trimester of pregnancy'; therefore, patients who show diabetic type or diabetic retinopathy during the first trimester are likely to have had diabetes since before pregnancy. It is more appropriate to regard them as 'pregnant women with diabetes' rather than as 'GDM'. By using a 75 gram OGTT, GDM is diagnosed when either 2 points among fasting plasma glucose, 1 hour plasma glucose or 2 hour plasma glucose exceeded 100, 180 or 150 mg/dl, respectively. This diagnostic criteria for GDM was made by Sugawa and Takagi[26] in their report for the Committee for Nutrition and Metabolism of Japan's Society of Gynecology and Obstetrics in

1984. The Committee of Japan's Diabetes Society on the Diagnostic Criteria of Diabetes Mellitus decided to adopt this criteria for the diagnosis of GDM in Japan in 1999.

It has been reported that juvenile-onset diabetics diagnosed under the age of 30 in Europe and the USA have Type 1 DM.[27] Ninety-five percent of diabetic patients in Japan have Type 2 DM, and even juvenile-onset diabetic patients have Type 2 diabetes. Figure 12.1 shows the age at onset and type of diabetes of 3025 Japanese diabetic patients diagnosed under the age of 30 who were registered at the Diabetes Center, Tokyo Women's Medical University (TWMU) School of Medicine.[28] The number of Type 1 diabetic patients tends to decrease from the age of 15 and the number of Type 2 diabetic patients increases from 10 years of age. One of the characteristics of Type 2 DM is that there are no symptoms for a long time from the onset of the disease; sometimes, Type 2 DM is first detected during pregnancy.

Table 12.6 shows the frequency of GDM diagnosed by a 75 gram OGTT in 1416 Japanese pregnant women. These patients were referred to the Diabetes Center, TWMU School of Medicine, by obstetricians because of glycosuria, family history or previous delivery of macrosomia, etc., from 1980 to March 1998. The OGTT results

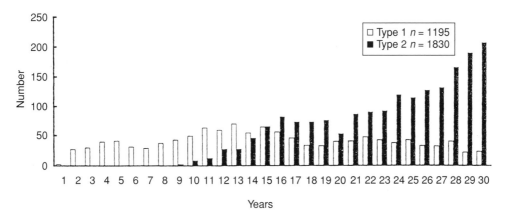

Figure 12.1. *Age of onset and type of diabetes in Japanese diabetic patients diagnosed under the age of 30. (Diabetes Center, Tokyo Women's Medical University School of Medicine n = 3025, 1960–1998, Uchigata[28]).*

demonstrate that the frequency of GDM is highest (13.2%) in the first trimester. The frequency of pregnant women diagnosed as Type 2 diabetic also shows the same tendency as GDM: this frequency is highest during the first trimester. It is suggested that the patients' slightly abnormal glucose tolerance or Type 2 DM existed before pregnancy but was undiagnosed.

Table 12.7 shows the frequency of congenital malformations and diabetic retinopathy among GDM patients and pregnant diabetic women diagnosed during pregnancy based on the present author's experiences at the Diabetes Center, TWMU School of Medicine, from 1985.1–1997.12. Universally, the general frequency of congenital malformations among newborns born to diabetic mothers is c. 4–10%.[29–31] However, the frequency of congenital malformations of newborns of pregnant diabetic mothers diagnosed as such during pregnancy is 12.7%, as compared to 1.9% of babies of mothers with GDM.

Moreover, 4.2% of pregnant diabetic women diagnosed during pregnancy had proliferative retinopathy and 12.7% had simple retinopathy. The simple or proliferative retinopathy affected

	Cases	Congenital malformations	Simple retinopathy	Proliferative retinopathy
GDM	104/1571 (6.6%)	*(104 deliveries, 105 babies)* 2/105 (1.9%)	0	0
Pregnant diabetic women diagnosed during pregnancy	71/1571 (4.5%)	*(71 deliveries, 71 babies)* 9/71 (12.7%)	9/71 (12.7%)	3/71 (4.2%)

Table 12.7. *Congenital malformations and diabetic retinopathy among GDM patients and pregnant diabetics diagnosed during pregnancy. (Diabetes Center, TWMU, 1985.1–1997.12).*

by hyperglycemia would take > 10 years to develop. GDM is usually known as a pre-stage of diabetes, especially for Type 2 DM, and should not include Type 2 diabetics first diagnosed during pregnancy. If Type 2 diabetes is first detected during pregnancy, then it should be called Type 2 diabetes diagnosed during pregnancy.

O'Sullivan and Mahan,[32] who developed the diagnostic criteria for GDM by using a 100 gram OGTT in 1964, defined GDM as 'a transient abnormality of glucose tolerance during pregnancy'.[33] This would be a more appropriate definition for GDM.

References

1. White P. Pregnancy complicating diabetes. *Am J Med* 1949; 7:609–16.
2. White P. Classification of obstetric diabetes. *Am J Obstet Gynecol* 1978; **130**:228–30.
3. White P. Pregnancy and diabetes, medical aspect. *Med Clin N Am* 1965; **49**:1015–24.
4. White P. Pregnancy and diabetes. In: (Marble A, White P, Bradley RF, Krall LP, eds) *Joslin's Diabetes Mellitus*, 11th edn. (Lea and Febiger: Philadelphia, 1971) 581–98.
5. Hare JW, White P. Gestational diabetes and the White Classification. *Diabetes Care* 1980; 3:394–6.
6. Tagatz GE, Arnold NI, Goetz FC et al. Pregnancy in a juvenile diabetic after renal transplantation. *Diabetes* 1975; 24:497–501.
7. National Diabetes Data Group. Classification and diagnosis of diabetes and other categories of intolerance. *Diabetes* 1979; 12:1039–63.
8. Buchanan TA. Diabetic pregnancy – classification. In: (Reece EA, Coustan DR, eds) *Diabetes Mellitus in Pregnancy*, 2nd edn. (Churchill Livingstone: 1995) 67.
9. Omori Y, Minei S, Akihisa R et al. Classification of diabetes in pregnant diabetics using CPR response in Japan. *Proceedings of the 16th Annual Meeting of DPSG in EASD*, Leuven, 11–13, 1983.
10. Omori Y, Mimei S, Akihisa R et al. Classification of diabetes in pregnant diabetics using CPR response in Japan. *J Japan Diabetes Soc* 1983; **26**: 239 [in Japanese].
11. Pedersen J. *The Pregnant Diabetic and her Newborn*, 2nd edn. (Munksgaard: Copenhagen, 1977) 202.
12. Pedersen J, Pedersen LM. Prognosis of the outcome of pregnancies in diabetics. A new classification. *Acta Endocrinol (Kbh)* 1965; **50**:70–8.
13. Hare WJ. Classification of diabetes in pregnancy. In: (Hare JW, ed.) *Diabetes Complicating Pregnancy – The Joslin Clinic Method*. (Alan RL: New York, 1989) 36–9.
14. Essex NL, Pyke DA, Watkins PJ et al. Diabetic pregnancy. *Br Med J* 1973; 4:89–93.
15. Essex NL, Pyke DA. Management of maternal diabetes in pregnancy. In: (Sutherland HW, Stowers JM, eds) *Carbohydrate Metabolism in Pregnancy and the Newborn*. (Springer-Verlag: Berlin, 1978) 357.
16. Gabbe SG. Management of diabetes mellitus in pregnancy. *Am J Obstet Gynecol* 1985; **153**:824–8.
17. WHO. *WHO Expert Committee on diabetes mellitus*, second report. WHO Technical Report Series 646, Geneva, 1980.
18. WHO. *Report of a WHO study group on diabetes mellitus*. WHO Technical Report Series 727, Geneva, 1985.
19. WHO. *Report of a WHO study group; prevention of diabetes mellitus*. WHO Technical Report Series 844, Geneva, 1994.
20. WHO. *Report of a WHO consultation; definition, diagnosis and classification of diabetes and its complications*. WHO, Geneva, 1999.
21. Freinkel N (ed.). Proceedings of the second international workshop – conference on gestational diabetes mellitus. Summary and recommendations. *Diabetes* 1985; **34 (Suppl 2)**:123–6.
22. Metzger B and the Organizing Committee. Summary and recommendations of the third international workshop – conference on gestational diabetes mellitus. *Diabetes* 1991; **40 (Suppl 2)**:197–201.
23. The Expert Committee on the diagnosis and classification of diabetes mellitus. Report of the Expert Committee on the diagnosis and classification of diabetes mellitus. *Diabetes Care* 1997; **20**:1183–97.
24. The committee of Japan Diabetes Society on the diagnostic criteria of diabetes mellitus. Report of the committee on the classification and diagnostic criteria of diabetes mellitus. *J Japan Diabetes Soc* 1999; **42**:385–404. [in Japanese].
25. The committee of the Japan Diabetes Society on the diagnostic criteria of diabetes mellitus, Kuzuya T, Nakagawa S, Satoh J et al. Report of the committee on the classification and diagnostic criteria of diabetes mellitus. *Diabetes Res Clin Pract* 2002; **55**:65–85.
26. Sugawa T, Takagi S. Report of the Committee for Nutrition and Metabolism, the Japan Society of Gynecology and Obstetrics. A proposal of a guideline for the diagnosis of glucose intolerance particularly of gestational diabetes mellitus. *J Japan Soc Gynecol Obstet* 1984; **36**:2055–8.
27. Laasko M, Pyorala K. Age of onset and type of diabetes. *Diabetes Care* 1985; 8:114–17.
28. Uchigata Y. Long-term outcomes of type 2 diabetes in adolescence. In: (Silink M, Kida K, Rosenbloom J, eds.) *Type 2 Diabetes in Children and Adolescence* (Martin-Dunitz: London) in press.

29. Reece EA, Eriksson JU. Congenital malformations: epidemiology, pathogenesis, and experimental methods of induction and prevention. In: (Reece EA, Coustan DR, eds) *Diabetes Mellitus in Pregnancy*, 2nd edn. (Churchill Livingstone: 1995) 119–54.

30. The Diabetes Control and Complications Trial Research Group. Pregnancy outcomes in the Diabetes Control and Complications Trial. *Am J Obstet Gynecol* 1996; **174**:1343–53.

31. Omori Y, Mimei S, Testuo T et al. Current status of pregnancy in diabetic women. A comparison of pregnancy in IDDM and NIDDM. *Diabetes Res Clin Pract* 1994; **24 (Suppl)**:S273–S278.

32. O'Sullivan JB, Mahan CM. Criteria for the oral glucose tolerance test in pregnancy. *Diabetes* 1964; **13**:278–85.

33. O'Sullivan JB. Gestational diabetes and its significance. In: (Camerini–Davalos R, Cole HS, eds) *Early Diabetes* (Academic Press: New York, 1970) 339–44.

13

Detection and diagnostic strategies for gestational diabetes mellitus

Boyd E Metzger, Yoo Lee Kim

Introduction

Gestational diabetes mellitus (GDM) is recognized as one of the most common medical complications of pregnancy. The most widely used definition of GDM ('carbohydrate intolerance of varying degrees of severity with onset or first recognition during pregnancy') has been accepted for more than two decades.[1,2] Nevertheless, for many years, there has been much debate and controversy concerning optimal strategies for detection and diagnosis of GDM. Some of the debate derives from differences of opinion about what degree of glucose intolerance should be labeled as GDM. Therefore, it is to be expected that there are different viewpoints on how to detect GDM. The participants of the second and third workshop–conferences on GDM,[3,4] and the American Diabetes Association (ADA), recommended that all pregnant women undergo blood glucose testing to classify glucose tolerance. Although a large majority of practicing obstetricians indicated that they follow this policy,[5] the American College of Obstetricians and Gynecologists has not formally endorsed the practice of universal blood glucose testing.[6–9] The fourth international workshop–conference on GDM conducted a detailed review and discussion of the issues related to detection and diagnosis of GDM. More 'flexible' positions were taken concerning screening and diagnostic criteria for GDM[1] than had been recommended by the contributors to the previous workshop–conferences.[3,4] With respect to screening, a strategy for potential 'exclusion from blood glucose testing' on the basis of below-average risk for GDM, rather than performing blood glucose testing of all pregnant women, was offered.[1] On the issue of diagnostic criteria, the Summary and Recommendations[1] state that 'data presented at the workshop–conference indicated that the infants of women who meet these lower (Carpenter–Coustan)[10] criteria are at similar risk for perinatal morbidity, including macrosomia, as those patients identified using the NDDG [National Diabetes Data Group] criteria'.[2] Thus, Carpenter–Coustan criteria were recommended for interpretation of the 100 gram oral glucose tolerance test (OGTT). In addition, criteria for interpretation of a 75 gram 2 hour OGTT were proposed, but not endorsed.[1] It was also acknowledged that the recommendation by the World Health Organization (WHO) that levels of glycemia during pregnancy should be interpreted according to the criteria used outside of pregnancy[11] has gained acceptance in some centers. This practice was likewise not endorsed.[1] The recommendations of the ADA's Position Statement on Gestational Diabetes Mellitus[12] closely paralleled those of the fourth international workshop–conference.[1]

The objectives in presenting this chapter are to assess key information that has become available since the fourth international workshop–conference, and to evaluate new approaches to detection and diagnosis of GDM that have been recommended in the interim. These reports indicate that the polarization of opinion about the detection and diagnosis of GDM may actually have intensified, rather than abated, since the Summary and Recommendations of the fourth international Workshop–Conference on GDM were published.[1] In addition, the Hyperglycemia and Adverse Pregnancy Outcome (HAPO) study was initiated in 1999 and is still continuing.[13] The objective of the HAPO study is to determine what degree of glucose intolerance short of diabetes conveys a clinically important risk for adverse perinatal outcome. The data that are being collected in the HAPO study should permit the selection of outcome-based criteria for the diagnosis of GDM. Therefore, for the interim, the primary focus has been on recent studies that having bearing on the problems of detection and diagnosis of GDM in conjunction with a less comprehensive review of historically important earlier reports.

Screening strategies

There is no debate about the fact that when overt diabetes mellitus (DM) occurs during pregnancy it is associated with adverse maternal and fetal outcomes. Since early diabetes, especially Type 2 DM, is usually asymptomatic, virtually all caregivers are alert to the need to detect and treat this condition. Therefore, they all engage in some form of a screening process.

Indeed, it has been acknowledged that systematically taking a personal and family medical history represents a form of screening or, at least, an assessment of risk. Furthermore, though the presence of glucosuria is neither very sensitive, nor specific, for the identification of diabetes during pregnancy, it remains a common practice in many clinics and offices to test urine for glucose and protein at each prenatal visit. The differences then are not whether to screen for glucose intolerance during pregnancy, but rather revolve about the following four questions: (1) what level or severity of glucose intolerance should be identified and treated; (2) how prevalent is the condition; (3) which patients require blood glucose testing in order to identify the individuals that need to be detected; and (4) are the sensitivity, specificity and reproducibility of the screening procedure that is recommended adequate to serve the intended purpose? Some of these questions have remained controversial for nearly three decades. In the meantime, the need to resolve the issues has become acute because the prevalences of GDM, Type 2 DM in children, and Type 2 DM in younger and older adults have all increased substantially over the past 10–20 years. In the sections that follow, it has been attempted to provide an overview of the contemporary issues that relate to detection of GDM.

Use of high-risk characteristics as a screening tool

Historically, investigators and clinicians were well aware of the serious adverse outcomes associated with maternal diabetes, and instances of DM being present during pregnancy with its disappearance postpartum were documented many years before GDM became designated as a distinct entity.[14] These factors prompted some clinicians to begin testing for diabetes during pregnancy among women with a history of previous 'bad obstetric outcomes', those with severe obesity or with a strong family history of diabetes. When definitions of abnormal glucose tolerance in pregnancy were proposed, many continued to apply the strategy of limiting testing to such high-risk subjects. On the other hand, in the 1950s, it was a was a common practice to use the measurement of blood glucose concentration 1 hour after ingesting a 50 gram glucose load as a screening test for glucose intolerance or DM. It was in this context that O'Sullivan and coworkers developed the 50 gram glucose challenge test (GCT)[15,16] in concert with the criteria that they proposed for interpretation of a 100 gram OGTT during pregnancy.[15] In the original study, a sensitivity of *c.* 80% was achieved with the proposed cut-off value of 130 mg/dl (venous whole blood). O'Sullivan's group,[16] and others in years following,[17–20] demonstrated much higher yields of GDM by performing the GCT on all pregnant women rather than doing blood glucose testing only on those with high-risk characteristics. Furthermore, it was more cost-effective, since fewer diagnostic OGTT were performed on the basis of a GCT than when high-risk characteristics were used to select women for a full diagnostic test. Nevertheless, selecting subjects for diagnostic tests on the basis of high-risk characteristics remains popular, in part because it does not require blood glucose testing on two separate occasions.

Screening based on risk stratification

For many years, some experts have advised that risk assessment for GDM should be conducted as part of the initial prenatal evaluation and that those considered high risk on the basis of historical factors should undergo initial blood glucose testing early in pregnancy.[21] This strategy has also been suggested in the Summary and Recommendations report of each of the four international workshop–conferences on GDM.[1,3,4,22] However, in practice, this point is commonly overlooked, resulting in a delay in the detection of GDM until after the 24–28 week window is reached, i.e. the standard or routine time for testing. Published reports based on careful analyses of data from the Toronto Tri-Hospital Study,[23,24] and other data confirming low prevalences of GDM among younger women,[25] prompted the participants of the fourth international workshop–conference[1] and the ADA Expert Committee[12] to recommend a strategy for potential 'exclusion from blood glucose testing' on the basis of below-average risk for GDM (Table 13.1) rather than relying on the former strategy of testing only on the basis of perceived 'high risk'. It is important to emphasize that this approach requires that all of the low-risk characteristics are present in an individual to qualify for exclusion from blood glucose testing. As indicated in the Summary and Recommendations of the fourth international workshop–conference,[1] when blood glucose testing is required, either a one-step procedure (diagnostic test performed on all subjects) or a two-step procedure (initial screening test in all cases, with the diagnostic test reserved for those above a defined threshold value) is acceptable.

A number of groups have reported results of their efforts to apply the fourth international workshop–conference and ADA-endorsed guidelines for the identification of subjects to be excluded from blood glucose testing based on their low-risk characteristics.[1,12] Williams et al[26] analyzed their screened population and those with a diagnosis of GDM using the NDDG criteria[2] that were also used in the Toronto Tri-Hospital study.[23,24] They found that if the recommendations of the fourth

GDM risk	Strategy
Low risk	**Blood glucose testing not routinely required if all of the following characteristics are present:** Member of an ethnic group with a low prevalence of GDM No known diabetes in first-degree relatives Age < 25 years Weight normal before pregnancy No history of abnormal glucose metabolism No history of poor obstetric outcome
Average risk	**Perform blood glucose testing at 24–28 weeks in the following:*** All subjects not classified as low risk or high risk Subjects initially designated high risk that did not have GDM at early testing
High risk	**Perform blood glucose testing as soon as feasible after booking if one or more of the following characteristics are present:** Severe obesity according to local standards Strong family history of Type 2 diabetes mellitus Previous history of GDM or glucose intolerance outside of pregnancy Glucosuria If GDM is not diagnosed, blood glucose testing should be repeated at 24–28 weeks, or at any time a patient has symptoms or signs that are suggestive of hyperglycemia.

* Blood glucose testing by: (1) the two-step procedure: 50 gram glucose challenge test (GCT) followed by a diagnostic oral glucose tolerance test (OGTT) in those meeting the threshold value in the GCT; or (2) a one-step procedure: diagnostic OGTT performed on all subjects.

Table 13.1.   Screening strategy for detecting gestational diabetes mellitus (GDM).[1] GDM risk assessment should be ascertained at the first prenatal visit.

international workshop–conference and the ADA[1,12] had been applied, few cases with GDM would have been missed (4%); however, most (c. 90%) would still have required blood glucose testing. Danilenko-Dixon et al[27] did a retrospective analysis of 18,504 women who were universally screened for GDM with the 50 gram GCT over an 11 year interval at the Mayo Clinic, Rochester, MN. They also found that use of the guidelines[1,12] would have failed to subject only a small proportion (3%) of the women with GDM to screening but would have required that 90.4% of the population receive the GCT. Moses et al[28] reported that lean Caucasian women, < 25 years of age, had a prevalence of GDM that was 2.8%, compared to 6.3% overall, and suggested that the published guidelines for identifying pregnancies that could be excluded from blood glucose testing[1,12] required further study. It should be noted, however, that Moses et al[28] used criteria for the diagnosis of GDM that yield a much higher prevalence of GDM than is the case when the NDDG[2] or Carpenter-Coustan[10] criteria are applied. The strategy for identifying cases to be excluded from blood glucose testing has been formally tested only for the application of the NDGG criteria.[2]

Some novel approaches to identification of subjects at low risk have been reported. Southwick and Wigton[29] found a prevalence of GDM of 1.5% (only 9.2% with a positive GCT) among young (< 20 years of age) Hispanic women and they suggested that blood glucose testing of this subgroup of young pregnant women might not be warranted. Young et al[30] looked at the prevalence of a positive GCT and of GDM in a group of 352 women that were seen for prenatal care with a second pregnancy after an interval of ≤ 4 years. All had a negative GCT (< 7.8 mmol/l) during the index pregnancy, but < 10% would have qualified for exclusion from blood glucose testing on the basis of low-risk characteristics. In the second pregnancy, 12 had a positive GCT but none met the NDDG diagnostic criteria for GDM[2] on the diagnostic OGTT. They concluded that women with a normal GCT in one pregnancy have a minimal risk of GDM in the near future and could be excluded from blood glucose testing in a pregnancy occurring within the next 4 years.

Blood glucose screening tests (two-step procedure)

GCT

The GCT that was described briefly in the previous section is the screening test most commonly used by those who employ a two-step procedure for GDM detection and diagnosis. It is important to consider several factors in reaching a decision about how to use the GCT. These include: (1) the proportion of screened subjects that one is willing to subject to the diagnostic test; (2) what are the diagnostic criteria that will be used in the interpretation of the OGTT? and (3) what are the desired levels of sensitivity and specificity? Although use of the GCT has been implemented successfully in many clinical settings, the test has limitations

and many critics. It is relatively complex and involves administration of a specific glucose load. At threshold values that achieve the desired degree of sensitivity, it has relatively low specificity. Furthermore, results are not highly reproducible. As a result, many variations of the 1 hour GCT have been explored.

Doing the GCT in the fasting state and postprandially has been compared in two studies, with opposing conclusions being reached and no reasons for the difference being apparent.[31,32] Thus, there does not appear to be a clear advantage of doing the GCT after an overnight fast. Many investigators have proposed using cut-off values for a positive GCT other than the ≥ 7.8 mmol/l plasma glucose concentration that was extrapolated by the NDDG[2] from the original whole-blood glucose cut-off value of > 7.2 mmol/l originally used by O'Sullivan et al[16] with different levels of sensitivity and specificity reported. For example, there is evidence that the cut-off values needed to obtain similar levels of sensitivity and specificity may be different for making a diagnosis of GDM with the NDDG criteria than with the Carpenter–Coustan criteria.[33,34] Others have proposed that higher specificity can be achieved without loss of sensitivity by varying the value for a positive test according to the interval between the last intake of food and the time of the GCT.[23,24,35,36] Use of 50 grams of glucose polymer[37] or a quantity of jelly beans equivalent to 50 grams of glucose[38] as test doses have been advocated as ways to improve palatability of the test dose (less nausea or vomiting that require the test be redone) while maintaining performance similar to that seen with the usual GCT procedure. Although some of these proposed alternatives are appealing, just now, none of these modified GCT procedures has been used widely and none has consistently been found to be superior to the standard way of doing the GCT.

Analysis of samples collected at random times

Collecting blood samples for the measurement of glucose concentrations without regard to time of day or interval since the last food intake (random sampling) has also been advocated as a simpler and adequate method for blood glucose screening.[39] However, others have found this approach to be very insensitive for the detection of subjects with degrees of glucose intolerance short of overt DM.[40,41]

Fasting plasma glucose as a screening test

Many investigators have found a relatively strong correlation between the concentrations of fasting plasma glucose (FPG) and postprandial plasma glucose (PPG) in non-pregnant subjects with normal and abnormal glucose metabolism [impaired glucose tolerance (IGT) or early Type 2 DM]. For example, the association between FPG and PPG was used to identify individuals at high risk for IGT as candidates for enrollment in the Diabetes Prevention Program (DPP). The DPP recently demonstrated that progression from IGT to DM could be prevented or delayed by lifestyle changes or the use of metformin.[42]

The concentration of FPG has also been examined as a means of detecting subjects at risk for GDM (Table 13.2).[43–47] Some investigators have reported an upper level for FPG that has high specificity for the diagnosis of GDM (≥ 90%);[43,44,46,47] however, such levels are insufficient as the sole marker for GDM since most cases have FPG values below the putative threshold. Other investigators have attempted to identify a level of FPG that can specifically exclude individuals with GDM. In individual studies, various cut-off values have been recommended because certain blood glucose levels could exclude approximately one third to one half of the population from further testing with this 'simple test'.[43,46]

There are significant limitations in most of these studies that reduce the ability to extrapolate the findings to the obstetric population at large. First, measurements of FPG and the diagnostic OGTT were performed on an entire unselected population of pregnant subjects in only two of the studies.[45,46] Population-based measurements are important in order to verify that an upper level of FPG truly has acceptably high specificity for the presence of GDM. For example, it has recently been shown that women with normal carbohydrate metabolism who are severely obese failed to show a fall in FPG during pregnancy and actually tended to have a small increase.[48] The report does not contain the FPG values from the obese subjects; however, the inter-quartile ranges given for the values in early pregnancy and the subsequent upward trend in values that was observed indicate that in the third trimester, values > 5.8 mmol/l were present in some of the obese pregnant subjects with a normal glucose tolerance. It is also important to establish that putative lower cut-off levels truly have sufficient specificity to be used to exclude GDM in normal weight and lean women, subgroups that, for example, represent a relatively high proportion of cases in many Asian populations. In addition, the utility of FPG as a screening tool is linked to the criteria used for a diagnosis of GDM. This is clearly illustrated in the report by Reichelt et al,[46] (Table 13.2). The optimal sensitivity-specificity relationship for the detections of DM during pregnancy (WHO criteria)[11] was found for an FPG ≥ 4.9 mmol/l; whereas, sensitivity for the detection of gestational IGT (WHO criteria)[12] was much lower at this level of FPG. Instead, a value of 4.5 mmol/l was chosen as the lower limit cut-off for excluding GDM or gestational IGT. This value had a sensitivity of 82% and a negative predictive value (NPV) of 97%, and could be used to eliminate about half the

Authors	Population studied	Diagnostic criteria	Assay method	Screening/ diagnostic algorithm	Results FPG (mmol/l)	Sensitivity (%)	Specificity (%)	PPV (%)	NPV (%)
Agarwal et al[43]	United Arab Emirates Selected by positive GCT Mean age: 30.2±5.62 years n = 368	Carpenter–Coustan	Glucose oxidase	Prospective 50 gram GCT: if ≥7.8, 100 gram 3 hour OGTT†	4.4* 5.3†	97 79	28 91	38 80	95 90
Atilano et al[44]	USA Selected by positive GCT 54% White; 19% Hispanic; 11% Asian; 8% Black; 8% other n = 512	NDDG	Not reported	Retrospective 50 gram GCT: if ≥7.8, 100 gram 3 hour OGTT	FPG (mmol/l) 5.8	Sensitivity (%) 20.2	Specificaty (%) 99.7	PPV (%) 95.8	NPV (%) 81.4
Perucchini et al[45]	Switzerland Unselected 63% White; 19% Asian; 6% African; 12% other Mean age: 28.4±0.2 years BMI: 23.8±0.2 n = 520	Carpenter–Coustan	Hexokinase	Prospective all subjects had: 50 gram GCT and 100 gram 3 hour OGTT	Threshold (mml/l) GCT: 7.8 – FPG: 4.8	Sensitivity (%) 59 81	Specificity (%) 91 76		
Reichelt et al[46]	Brazil Consecutive ≥ 20 years 45% White; 14% Black; 41% mixed Mean age: 27.9±5.5 years BMI: 26.1±4.1 n = 5010	WHO DM 2 hour PG ≥ 11.1 Gestational IGT ≥ 7.8, < 11.1	Glucose oxidase	Prospective All subjects had 75 gram 2 hour OGTT	**Diabetes mellitus** FPG (mmol/l) 4.9 **Gestational IGT** FPG 4.5*	Sensitivity (%) 88 81	Specificity (%) 78 54	PPV (%) 1.3 12	NPV (%) 100 97
Sacks et al[47]	USA Selected by positive GCT n = 968	NDDG	Glucose oxidase	Retrospective 50 gram GCT: if ≥7.8, 100 gram 3 hour OGTT	FPG (mmol/l) 4.9 4.7 4.5	Sensitivity (%) 80 90 95	Specificity (%) 40 21 11		

BMI, Body mass index; DM, diabetes mellitus; GCT, glucose challenge test; IGT, impaired glucose tolerance; NDDG, National Diabetes Data Group; NPV, negative, predictive value OGTT, oral glucose tolerance test, PG, plasma glucose; PPV, positive predictive value; WHO, World Health Organization.
* Value suggested as cut-off below which the prevalence rate of GDM is so low that the full diagnostic OGTT need not be done.
† Value suggested as cut-off with a sufficiently high specificity for the diagnosis of GDM so that the full diagnostic OGTT need not be done.

Table 13.2. *Fasting plasma glucose (FPG) as a screening tool for the detection of gestational diabetes mellitus (GDM).*

population from the need for the diagnostic OGTT.

In the aggregate, the studies that are summarized in Table 13.2 do not make a convincing case that a single measurement of FPG can be cost-effectively substituted for the 1 hour GCT as a screening test. In the largest, most complete, study from Brazil,[46] the cut-off would have to be set at 4.5 m/mol/l and 49% of the subjects would have to undergo an OGTT to ensure the detection of *c.* 81% of GDM cases. Finally, in the studies summarized in Table 13.2, the specific levels of FPG that have been suggested as high or low cut-off values vary. This may result from true differences among populations. Alternatively, variation may result from different analytical methods or specific analytical instruments that were employed for the studies. Either option means that use of FPG to screen for subjects at increased or low risk for GDM would have to be validated for each center and population before implementation.

Methodological and instrumentation issues

The comments about methodology and instruments above serve as an introduction to a further discussion of the potential utility of measuring the capillary blood glucose concentration with strip and meter technology to identify subjects who should have a diagnostic OGTT. During fasting, concentrations of glucose in capillary and venous blood are similar, but concentrations differ postprandially, being higher in capillary than in venous blood. Though whole blood is sampled for most analyses by stripmeter techniques, glucose is actually measured in a plasma ultrafiltrate with many of the techniques that are currently in use. However, the validity of a given method is ultimately established by the precision and accuracy of the measurements. Careful review of published data that analyzed

these technologies[49,50] indicated that a lack of precision would be an important issue for most systems. Thus, to maintain the desired sensitivity, thresholds for positive tests would have to be lowered to values that would reduce specificity and greatly increase the number of cases referred for OGTT. In addition, when precision and accuracy are deemed to be adequate, it remains essential to establish stability over time and to participate in a standardized external quality assurance scheme. Such schemes are not typically available for office-based procedures. Dillon et al[51] have proposed a scheme that combines meter-based and laboratory testing at the time of the GCT. They found that meter values of 6.1 and 8.6 mmol/l predicted plasma glucose values in the laboratory of < 7.5 or > 7.5 mmol/l (threshold for positive GCT) with 95% confidence. Thus, they could confidently discharge those with meter values < 6.1 mmol/l without further testing or waiting for laboratory analyses to be completed, and could immediately schedule the diagnostic OGTT without confirming a result in the laboratory in those with meter values ≥ 8.6 mmol/l. For those with a meter value between 6.1 and 8.6 mmol/l the decision regarding further testing was deferred until the plasma glucose concentration was determined in the laboratory. Although this appears to be a workable approach, only clinical laboratory-based and certified methods should be used for the analysis of diagnostics tests.

Blood glucose tests (one-step procedure)

Some investigators and clinicians favor using the one-step process (the diagnostic test) in all subjects that require blood glucose testing (as defined by the risk-assessment scheme outlined above). This approach may be cost-effective under two circumstances. First, if the diagnostic test that is used is not complicated to administer, e.g. a single sample drawn 2 hours after a 75 gram glucose load,[52] then it approaches the standard GCT in simplicity. Secondly, in populations that have a very high prevalence of GDM, as is the situation among Pima women and a number of other Native American tribes, a high proportion will have a positive GCT and require the diagnostic OGTT. In this circumstance, it is cost-effective to administer the full diagnostic test to all subjects.

Diagnostic oral glucose tolerance test

There has been a longstanding lack of consensus about the optimal diagnostic test and criteria for interpretation of glucose tolerance in pregnancy. As indicated in the Introduction, criteria that are based on the original epidemiological study of OGTT in pregnancy by O'Sullivan and Mahan[15] have been widely used in North America and in numerous centers in other countries. In that study, O'Sullivan's group's objective was to devise a scheme that identified women at risk for DM outside of pregnancy sometime in the future. That objective was fulfilled in O'Sullivan's group's landmark long-term follow-up of the original cohort of women[15,53] and has been validated extensively in other populations.[54–59] Evidence that GDM may be associated with adverse perinatal events was found later.[16,60,61] O'Sullivan and Mahan's criteria for the interpretation of OGTT in pregnancy were based on measurements in whole blood.[15] The NDDG provided the first guidelines for the extrapolation from whole blood to plasma glucose equivalents.[2] Because most laboratories now use an enzymatic method for measurement of glucose concentrations, rather than using the AutoAnalyzer technology that prevailed when the NDGG criteria were derived, other formulae for extrapolating values from the original whole-blood values found in the O'Sullivan and Mahan study[15] have been proposed.[10,62]

In addition, a large number of individuals from a broad spectrum of clinical and research backgrounds have advocated many other procedures and criteria for the diagnosis of GDM over the past three decades. Investigators have offered criteria derived from OGTT that were performed in certain specific groups of subjects. In some instances these were populations of pregnant women, in other cases they were derived from studies in a general population of non-pregnant subjects. No large studies have been completed in which the primary objective was to establish diagnostic criteria by determining the level of hyperglycemia that is specifically and independently associated with a clinically significant increase in the risk of adverse pregnancy outcome. Gilmer et al[63] reported values for an area under the curve for a 2 hour OGTT that could predict risk of neonatal hypoglycemia. These issues will be considered in detail in a later section.

Many groups have reported evidence that the 'usual' criteria for the diagnosis of GDM fail to capture a significant proportion of the cases at risk for adverse outcomes. In fact, evidence has been reported that suggests that the relationship between maternal glycemia and macrosomia is a continuum.[64–66] The participants in the fourth international workshop–conference on GDM[1] concluded that data presented at the conference indicated that the infants of women who meet these lower (Carpenter–Coustan)[10] criteria are at similar risk for perinatal morbidity, including macrosomia, as those patients identified using the NDDG criteria.[2] Others have reported higher than expected rates of complications and morbidity in cases with one-abnormal value on the diagnostic OGTT.[67,68] Still others have reported an increase in adverse outcomes, in particular macrosomia, among GCT-positive cases with non-diabetic or normal OGTT values by NDDG criteria[24,65,69,70] and among cases meeting the WHO criteria for IGT, or similar levels of glycemia.[71–73] Other investigators have failed to confirm the above findings, or emphasize the potential role of confounding factors such as obesity, and continue to counsel against adopting more inclusive criteria for the diagnosis of GDM.[74–76] In concluding this part of the discussion, it is important to indicate that two issues commonly overlooked in reports that compare morbidities among cases with GDM with those having lesser degrees of glucose intolerance and or normal glucose metabolism. These are the confounding effects of treatment of GDM and the potential impact of knowledge of glucose levels or classification of glucose tolerance status on medical decision-making.

Conclusions

Recommendations of the fourth international workshop–conference on GDM

As indicated previously, participants in the fourth international workshop–conference on GDM concluded that 'data presented at the workshop–conference indicated that the infants of women who meet these lower (Carpenter– Coustan)[10] criteria are at similar risk for perinatal morbidity, including macrosomia, as those patients identified by using the NDDG criteria'.[2] Thresholds for interpretation of both 100 gram and 75 gram OGTT were recommended,[1] and are presented in Tables 13.3 and 13.4, respectively; these recommendations have received both support and criticism (see above). At the time of the report, information on outcomes in pregnancies with GDM diagnosed with the criteria recommended for the 75 gram OGTT were lacking and the use of these criteria and the WHO IGT criteria were not endorsed for clinical use

Specimen	mg/dl[†]	mmol/l[†]
Fasting	95	5.3
1 hour	180	10.0
2 hour	155	8.6
3 hour	140	7.8

* The test should be performed in the morning after an overnight fast of at least 8 hours but not > 14 hours and after at least 3 days of unrestricted diet (≥ 150 gram carbohydrate/day) and physical activity. The subject should remain seated and should not smoke throughout the test.
† The cut-off values are those proposed by Carpenter and Coustan[10] for extrapolation of the whole-blood glucose values found by O'Sullivan and Mahan[15] to plasma or serum glucose concentrations. Two or more of the venous plasma concentrations must be met or exceeded for a positive diagnosis.

Table 13.3. *Diagnosis of gestational diabetes mellitus (GDM) 100 gram oral glucose tolerance test[†] (OGTT).* *

Specimen	mg/dl[†]	mmol/l[†]
Fasting	95	5.3
1 hour	180	10.0
2 hour	155	8.6

* The test should be performed in the morning after an overnight fast of at least 8 hours but not > 14 hours and after at least 3 days of unrestricted diet (≥ 150 gram carbohydrate/day) and physical activity. The subject should remain seated and should not smoke throughout the test.
[†] Cut-off values for the 75 gram, 2 hour OGTT in pregnancy are, of necessity, arbitrary. The lack of definitive data relating such test results to perinatal outcome made it difficult for the panel and the organizing committee of the fourth international workshop–conference on GDM to arrive at a consensus.[1,12]

Table 13.4. *Diagnosis of gestational diabetes mellitus (GDM): 75 gram oral glucose tolerance test (OGTT)*.*

until such data became available from studies of large numbers of subjects. Some additional information is now available for consideration. In the Brazil GDM project, *c.* 5000 pregnant women underwent a 75 gram OGTT.[73] In that cohort, 2.4% met the ADA 75 gram OGTT criteria for GDM.[1,12] However, a recent preliminary report suggests that more women meet the diagnostic threshold for GDM when challenged with 100 gram of glucose than when they receive a 75 gram test dose.[77]

Recommendations of the present authors

One consequence of applying lower glycemic thresholds in the interpretation of the OGTT was entirely predictable; namely, that the prevalence of GDM varies with the criteria that are applied to the population in question. In published studies, the magnitude of the difference is not constant from one population to another, but the relative change is substantial. Data from several studies that have been reported over the past few years are summarized in Table 13.5.[71,73–75] The choice of criteria has major implications for both the cost and complexity

of prenatal care. The controversial issues that have been summarized in this report will continue until data such as those from the ongoing HAPO study[13] help to define criteria for the diagnosis of GDM that are based on the specific relationships between maternal glycemia and perinatal outcome. After weighing all of these outstanding issues, the present authors advise established programs to continue using one of the recommended screening/diagnostic strategies[1,12] for routine clinical care, and encourage more population-based data be collected. It is hoped that this overview of the issues will be of assistance in making a choice for those establishing new programs, clinics or practices.

References

1. Metzger, BE, Coustan DR, The Organizing Committee. Summary and recommendations of the fourth international Workshop–Conference on Gestational Diabetes Mellitus. *Diabetes Care* 1998; **21 (Suppl 2)**:161–7.
2. National Diabetes Data Group (Metzger BE, member). Classification and diagnosis of diabetes mellitus and other categories of glucose intolerance. *Diabetes* 1979; 28:1039–57.
3. Freinkel N. Summary and recommendations of the second International Workshop–Conference on Gestational Diabetes Mellitus. *Diabetes* 1985; **34(Suppl 2)**:123–6.

Authors	Population studied	Diagnostic criteria	Assay method	Screening/ diagnostic algorithm	Prevalence	
Deerochanawong et al[71]	Thailand Randomly selected n = 709	WHO IGT: 2 hour PG ≥ 7.8 NDDG GDM	Glucose oxidase	Prospective All subjects had: 50 gram GCT; if ≥ 7.8, 100 gram OGTT	WHO GCT (+) NDDG	15.7% 11.7% 1.4%
Rust et al[74]	USA Selected: positive GCT n = 434	NDDG Carpenter–Coustan (C–C) Sacks	Not reported	Retrospective 50 gram GCT; if ≥ 7.8, 100 gram 3 hour OGTT	R Risk NDDG C/C Sacks	1 1.5 1.7
Schmidt et al[73]	Brazil Consecutive ≥ 20 years n = 4977	WHO[11] ADA 75 gram[12]	Glucose oxidase	Prospective All subjects had 75 gram OGTT	WHO ADA	7.2% 2.4%
Schwartz et al[75]	USA Unselected n = 8857	NDDG Carpenter–Coustan (C–C)	Glucose oxidase	Retrospective 50 gram GCT; if ≥ 7.8, 100 gram 3 hour OGTT	GCT (+) NDDG C–C	18.7% 3.2% 5.0%

ADA, American Diabetes Association; GCT, glucose challenge test; IGT, impaired glucose tolerance; NDDG, National Diabetes Data Group; OGTT, oral glucose tolerance test; PG, plasma glucose; R Risk, relative risk; WHO, World Health Organization.

Table 13.5. *Impact of diagnostic criteria on the prevalence of gestational diabetes mellitus (GDM).*

4. Metzger BE, Organizing Committee. Summary and recommendations of the third International Workshop–Conference on Gestational Diabetes Mellitus. *Diabetes* 1991; **40(Suppl 2)**:197–201.

5. Wilkins-Haug L, Horton JA, Cruess DF, Frigoletto FD. Antepartum screening in the office-based practice: findings from the collaborative Ambulatory Research Network. *Obstet Gynecol* 1996; **88**:483–9.

6. ACOG Technical Bulletin. *Management of diabetes mellitus in pregnancy*. Number 48, April 1978.

7. ACOG Technical Bulletin. *Management of diabetes mellitus in pregnancy*. Number 92, May 1986.

8. ACOG Technical Bulletin. *Diabetes and pregnancy*. Number 200, December 1994.

9. ACOG Practice Bulletin. *Gestational diabetes*. Number 30, September 2001.

10. Carpenter MW, Coustan DR. Criteria for screening tests for gestational diabetes. *Am J Obstet Gynecol* 1982; **144**:763–73.

11. Alberti KGMM, Zimmet PZ (for the WHO Consultation). Definition, diagnosis and classification of diabetes mellitus and it complications. Part 1: Diagnosis and classification of diabetes mellitus. Provisional report of a WHO consultation. *Diabet Med* 1998; **15**:539–53.

12. The Expert Committee on the diagnosis and classification of diabetes mellitus. Report of the Expert Committee on the diagnosis and classification of diabetes mellitus. *Diabetes Care* 1997; **28**:1083–97.

13. HAPO Study Cooperative Research Group. The Hyperglycemia and Adverse Pregnancy Outcome (HAPO) Study. *Int J Gynecol Obstet* 2002; **78**:69–77.

14. Hadden D. A historical perspective on gestational diabetes. *Diabetes Care* 1998; **21 (Suppl 2)**:B3–B4.

15. O'Sullivan JB, Mahan CM. Criteria for the oral glucose tolerance test in pregnancy. *Diabetes* 1964; **13**:278–85.

16. O'Sullivan JB, Mahan CM, Charles D, Dandrow RV. Screening criteria for high-risk gestational diabetic patients. *Am J Obstet Gynecol* 1973; **116**:895–900.

17. Lavin JP. Screening of high-risk and general populations of gestational diabetes: clinical application and cost analysis. *Diabetes* 1985; **34 (Suppl 2)**:24–7.

18. Marquette GP, Klein VR, Niebyl JR. Efficacy of screening for gestational diabetes. *Am J Perinatol* 1985; **2**:7–9.

19. Coustan DR, Nelson C, Carpenter MW et al. Maternal age and screening for gestational diabetes: a population based study. *Obstet Gynecol* 1989; **73**:557–61.

20. Griffin ME, Coffey M, Johnson H et al. Universal vs. risk factor-based screening for gestational diabetes mellitus: detection rates, gestation at diagnosis and outcome. *Diabet Med* 2000; **17**:26–32.

21. Mestman JH, Anderson GV, Barton P. Carbohydrate metabolism in pregnancy. *Am J Obstet Gynecol* 1971; **109**:41–5.

22. Freinkel N, Josimovich J, Conference Planning Committee. American Diabetes Association Workshop–Conference on Gestational Diabetes. Summary and recommendations. *Diabetes Care* 1980; **3**:499–501.

23. Naylor CD, Sermer M, Chen E, Farine D. Selective screening for gestational diabetes mellitus. *N Engl J Med* 1997; **337**:1591–6.

24. Sermer M, Naylor CD, Farine D et al, for the Toronto Tri-Hospital Gestational Diabetes Investigators. The Toronto Tri-Hospital Gestational Diabetes Project. *Diabetes Care* 1998; **21 (Suppl 2)**:B33–B42.

25. Sacks DA, Abu-Fadil S, Karten GJ et al. Screening for gestational diabetes with the one-hour 50-g glucose test. *Obstet Gynecol* 1987; **70**:89–93.

26. Williams CB, Iqbal S, Zawacki CM et al. Effect of selective screening for gestational diabetes. *Diabetes Care* 1999; **22**:418–21.

27. Danilenko-Dixon DR, Winter JTV, Nelson RL, Ogburn PL. Universal versus selective gestational diabetes screening: application of 1997 American Diabetes Association recommendations. *Am J Obstet Gynecol* 1999; **181**:798–802.

28. Moses RG, Moses J, Davis WS. Gestational diabetes: do lean young Caucasian women need to be tested? *Diabetes Care* 1998; **21**:1803–6.

29. Southwick RD, Wigton TR. Screening for gestational diabetes mellitus in adolescent Hispanic Americans. *J Reprod Med* 2000; **45**:31–4.

30. Young C, Kuehl TJ, Sulak PJ, Allen SR. Gestational diabetes screening in subsequent pregnancies of previously healthy patients. *Am J Obstet Gynecol* 2000; **182**:1024–6.

31. Coustan DR, Widness JA, Carpenter MW et al. Should the fifty-gram, one-hour plasma glucose screening test for gestational diabetes be administered in the fasting or fed state? *Am J Obstet Gynecol* 1986; **154**:1031–5.

32. Lewis GF, McNally C, Blackman JD et al. Prior feeding alters the response to the 50-g glucose challenge test in pregnancy. *Diabetes Care* 1993; **16**:1551–6.

33. Bonomo M, Gandini ML, Mastropasqua A et al, for the Definition of Screening Methods for Gestational Diabetes Study Group of the Lombardy Section of the Italian Society of Diabetology. Which cutoff level should be used in screening for glucose intolerance in pregnancy? *Am J Obstet Gynecol* 1998; **179**:179–85.

34. Monteros AE, Parra A, Hidalgo R, Zambrana M. The after breakfast 50-g, 1-hour glucose challenge test in urban Mexican pregnant women: its sensitivity and specificity evaluated by three diagnostic criteria for gestational diabetes mellitus. *Acta Obstet Gynecol Scand* 1999; **78**:294–8.

35. Sermer M, Naylor CD, Gare DJ et al. Impact of time since last meal on the gestational glucose challenge test. *Am J Obstet Gynecol* 1994; **171**:607–16.

36. Cetin M, Cetin A. Time-dependent gestational diabetes screening values. *Int J Gynecol Obstet* 1997; **56**:257–61.

37. Reece EA, Gabrielli S, Abdalla M et al. Diagnosis of gestational diabetes by use of a glucose polymer. *Am J Obstet Gynecol* 1989; **160**:383–4.

38. Lamar ME, Kuehl TJ, Cooney AT et al. Jelly bean as an alternative to a fifty-gram glucose beverage for gestational diabetes screening. *Am J Obstet Gynecol* 1999; **181**:1154–7.

39. Stangenberg M, Persson B, Nordlander E. Random capillary blood glucose and conventional selection criteria for glucose tolerance testing during pregnancy. *Diabetes Res* 1985; **2**:29–33.

40. Nasarat AA, Johnstone FD, Hasan SAM. Is random plasma glucose an efficient screening test of abnormal glucose tolerance in pregnancy? *Br J Obstet Gynaecol* 1988; **95**:855–60.

41. McElduff A, Goldring J, Gordon P, Wyndham L. A direct comparison of the measurement of a random plasma glucose and a post-50 g glucose load glucose, in the detection of gestational diabetes. *Aust NZ J Obstet Gynecol* 1994; **34**:28–30.

42. Diabetes Prevention Research Group. Reduction in the incidence of type 2 diabetes with lifestyle intervention or metformin. *N Engl J Med* 2002; **346**:393–403.

43. Agarwal MM, Hughest PF Punnose J, Ezimokhai M. Fasting plasma glucose as screening test for gestational diabetes in a multi-ethnic, high-risk population. *Diabet Med* 2000; **17**:720–6.

44. Atilano LC, Parritz AL, Lieberman E et al. Alternative methods of diagnosing gestational diabetes mellitus. *Am J Obstet Gynecol* 1999; **181**:1158–61.

45. Perucchini D, Fischer U, Spinas GA et al. Using fasting plasma glucose concentrations to screen for gestational diabetes mellitus. *Br Med J* 1999; **319**:812–15.

46. Reichelt AJ, Franco LJ, Spichler ER et al. Fasting plasma glucose is a useful test for the detection of gestational diabetes. *Diabetes Care* 1998; **21**:1246–9.

47. Sacks DA, Greenspoon JS, Fotherington N. Could the fasting plasma glucose assay be used to screen for gestational diabetes? *J Reprod Med* 1992; **37**:907–9.

48. Mills JL, Jovanovic L, Knopp R et al. Physiological reduction in fasting plasma glucose concentration in the first trimester of normal pregnancy: the diabetes in early pregnancy study. *Metabolism* 1998; **47**:1140–4.

49. Carr SR, Slocum J, Tefft L et al. Precision of office-based blood glucose meters in screening for gestational diabetes. *Am J Obstet Gynecol* 1995; **173**:1267–72.

50. Carr SR. Screening for gestational diabetes mellitus. A perspective in 1988. *Diabetes Care* 1998; **21 (Suppl 2)**: B14–B18.

51. Dillon AE, Menard MK, Rust P et al. Glucometer analysis of one-hour glucose challenge samples. *Am J Obstet Gynecol* 1997; **177**:1120–3.

52. Pettitt DJ, Knowler WC, Baird R, Bennett PH. Gestational diabetes: infant and maternal complications of pregnancy in relation to third-trimester glucose tolerance in the Pima Indians. *Diabetes Care* 1980; **3**:458–64.

53. O'Sullivan JB. The interaction between pregnancy, diabetes, and long-term maternal outcome. In: (Reece EA, Coustan DR, eds) *Diabetes Mellitus in Pregnancy:*

Principles and Practice. (Churchill Livingstone: New York, 1988) 575–85.

54. Mestman JH, Anderson GV, Guadalupe V. Follow-up study of 360 subjects with abnormal carbohydrate metabolism during pregnancy. *Obstet Gynecol* 1972; **39**:421–5.

55. Grant PT, Oats JN, Beischer NA. The long-term follow-up of women with gestational diabetes. *Aust NZ J Obstet Gynaecol* 1986; **26**:17–22.

56. Dornhorst A, Bailey PC, Anyaoku V et al. Abnormalities of glucose tolerance following gestational diabetes. *Q J Med* 1990; **77**:1219–28.

57. Damm P, Kühl C, Bertelsen A, Molsted-Pedersen L. Predictive factors for the development of diabetes in women with previous gestational diabetes mellitus. *Am J Obstet Gynecol* 1992; **167**:607–16.

58. Metzger BE, Cho NH, Roston SM et al. Prepregnancy weight and antepartum insulin secretion predict glucose tolerance five years after gestational diabetes mellitus. *Diabetes Care* 1993; **16**:1598–605.

59. Kjos SL, Peters RK, Xiang A et al. Predicting future diabetes in Latino women with gestational diabetes: utility of early postpartum glucose tolerance testing. *Diabetes* 1995; **44**:586–91.

60. O'Sullivan JB, Charles D, Mahan CM, Dandrow RV. Gestational diabetes and perinatal mortality rate. *Am J Obstet Gynecol* 1973; **116**:901–4.

61. Gabbe SG, Mestman JH, Freeman RK et al. Management and outcome of class A diabetes mellitus. *Am J Obstet Gynecol* 1977; **127**:465–9.

62. Sacks DA, Abu-Fadil S, Greenspoon JS, Fotheringham N. Do the current standards for glucose tolerance testing in pregnancy represent a valid conversion of O'Sullivan's original criteria? *Am J Obstet Gynecol* 1989; **161**: 638–41.

63. Gilmer MD, Beard RW, Brooke FM, Oakley NW. Carbohydrate metabolism in pregnancy. Part II. Relation between maternal glucose tolerance and glucose metabolism in the newborn. *Br Med J* 1975; **3**:402–4.

64. Sacks, DA, Greenspoon JS, Abu-Fadil S et al. Toward universal criteria for gestational diabetes: the 75-gram glucose tolerance test in pregnancy. *Am J Obstet Gynecol* 1995; **172**:607–14.

65. Sermer M, Naylor CD, Gare DJ et al, for the Toronto-Tri Hospital Gestational Diabetes Investigators. Impact of increasing glucose intolerance on maternal-fetal outcomes in 3637 women without gestational diabetes. *Am J Obstet Gynecol* 1995; **173**:146–56.

66. Jensen DM, Damm P, Sorensen B et al. Clinical impact of mild carbohydrate intolerance in pregnancy: a study of 2904 nondiabetic Danish women with risk factors for gestational diabetes. *Am J Obstet Gynecol* 2001; **185**:413–19.

67. Berkus M, Langer O. Glucose tolerance test: degree of glucose abnormality correlates with neonatal outcome. *Obstet Gynecol* 1993; **81**:344–8.

68. Lindsay MK, Graves W, Klein L. The relationship of one abnormal glucose tolerance test value and pregnancy complications. *Obstet Gynecol* 1989; **73**:103–6.

69. Leikin EL, Jenkins JH, Pomerantz GA, Klein L. Abnormal glucose screening tests in pregnancy a risk factor for fetal macrosomia. *Obstet Gynecol* 1987; **69**:570–3.

70. Bevier WC, Fischer R, Jovanovic L. Treatment of women with an abnormal glucose challenge test (but a normal oral glucose tolerance test) decreases the prevalence of macrosomia. *Am J Perinatol* 1999; **16**:269–75.

71. Deerochanawong C, Putiyanum C, Wongsuryrat M et al. Comparison of National Diabetes Data Group and World Health Organization criteria for detecting gestational diabetes mellitus. *Diabetologia* 1996; **39**:1070–3.

72. Moses RG, Moses M, Russell KG, Schier GM. The 75-g glucose tolerance test in pregnancy. *Diabetes Care* 1998; **21**:1807–11.

73. Schmidt MI, Duncan BB, Reichelt AJ et al. Gestational diabetes mellitus diagnosed with a 2-h 75-g OGTT and adverse pregnancy outcomes. *Diabetes Care* 2001; **24**:1151–5.

74. Rust OA, Bofill JA, Andrew ME et al. Lowering the threshold for the diagnosis of gestational diabetes. *Am J Obstet Gynecol* 1996; **175**:961–5.

75. Schwartz ML, Ray WN, Lubarsky SL. The diagnosis and classification of gestational diabetes mellitus: is it time to change our tune? *Am J Obstet Gynecol* 1999; **180**:1560–71.

76. Penninson EH, Egerman RS. Perinatal outcomes in gestational diabetes: a comparison of criteria for diagnosis. *Am J Obstet Gynecol* 2001; **184**:1118–21.

77. Mello G, Cioni R, Martini E et al. Lack of concordance between 75-G and 100-G glucose loads for the diagnosis of gestational diabetes mellitus. *Program and Abstract Book of the Diabetic Pregnancy Study Group of the EASD, 34th Annual Meeting*, 2002, 45.

14

Gestational diabetes in developing countries

Liliana S Voto, Matías Uranga Imaz, Miguel Margulies

Introduction

The Argentine Republic, included among the developing countries, has severe deficiencies regarding the socio-economical situation, medical care, women's status, prenatal care, and maternal and perinatal morbidity and mortality. According to the Latin-American & Caribbean Regional Office of UNICEF,[1] the risk of maternal mortality in the developed compared with the developing world in 1990 was 1:1800 versus 1:48, with an incidence of 1:140 for South America. In Argentina, the estimated number of maternal deaths in 1990 was 690 (maternal mortality rate per 100,000 liveborns = 100), while in 1997 this figure was reduced to 605 (maternal mortality rate for 1980–1997 = 85).[2]

The Argentine Ministry of Health[3] reports that in 2000 the total number of maternal deaths was 245, with a maternal mortality rate of 3.5. These figures refer to the whole country; however, different Argentine provinces show wide variations, ranging from six (rate = 1.4) in Buenos Aires to 23 (rate = 17.7) in the province of Formosa.

The main cause of maternal death in Argentina is hemorrhage, mostly associated with complications of illegal abortion, followed by hypertension.[4]

Definition and classification

Gestational diabetes mellitus (GDM) is defined as carbohydrate intolerance diagnosed for the first time during pregnancy. Although no significant difference is observed in the incidence of fetal malformations between GDM patients and the general population, the former show elevated rates of perinatal morbidity and mortality due to macrosomia, intrauterine sudden death, acute fetal distress and cesarean section.[5–8]

Hare and White[9] agree in the definition that GDM comprises those cases detected during pregnancy. Glycemia may or may not be controlled with diet only, requiring insulin administration in refractory patients. The White Classification identifies several types of GDM:

Class A: Cases detected and evolving at any time before pregnancy and controlled with diet only

Class B: Cases appearing after the age of 20 and with < 10 years of evolution

Class C: Cases appearing between the ages of 10 and 19 or with 10–19 years of evolution

Class D: Cases appearing before the age of 10 and with > 20 years of evolution, presenting with retinopathy

Class R: Proliferative retinopathy or vitreous hemorrhage

Class F: Nephropathy with > 500 mg/day proteinuria

Class RF: Criteria for Classes R and F coexist

Class H: Clinically apparent atherosclerotic cardiac disease

Class T: Previous renal transplant.

Frequency

Most authors mention a frequency of GDM of 2–12% depending on the population studied and the geographical location. In Argentina, the frequency observed varies for each center. For instance, the Argerich Hospital[10] had an incidence of 6.5% between 1991 and 1995, while in the Sardá Maternity Hospital the frequency in 1989 was 3.7–5%.[11] In the Juan A Fernández Hospital the incidence for the period of 1994–2001 was 0.44% (total number of deliveries = 16,287; total number of diabetic patients = 72). All these centers are situated in the capital city. Votta et al[10] mention that, in 1998, Alvariños found an incidence of GDM for Buenos Aires of 2.3%.

Argentina, as most underdeveloped countries, lacks year-by-year statistical records, but during 1999, 2000 and 2001 a total of 200 cases of demises in women due to GDM were recorded, without any specification regarding pregnant status or the woman's age.[12]

Pathophysiology

Numerous hormonal changes occur during gestation that increase insulin requirements. The appearance of human placental lactogen (hPL)[13] and the increase in prolactin concentrations enhance free fatty acids (FFA) through the mobilization of lipid reserves; this, in turn, causes a certain degree of resistance to insulin in peripheral tissues.[14] Also, the increase in estrogen concentration reduces glucose tolerance.[15] Moreover, the placental insulin receptors present during pregnancy have proteolytic enzymes with the ability to degrade insulin molecules and therefore consume insulin.[16]

The consequent maternal hyperglycemia produces fetal hyperglycemia because glucose crosses the placenta by facilitated diffusion,[17] positioning fetal glycemia 20–30% below maternal levels.[18] This fetal hyperglycemic state stimulates the fetal pancreas, therefore increasing insulin levels and leading to:

- macrosomy due to adipose tissue accumulation allowed for by the insulin antilipolytic effect;
- lung immaturity due to insulin–cortisol competition in the formation of surfactant at the pneumonocytes level;[19]
- polyhydramnios due to osmotic diuresis in a hyperglycemic fetus;[20]
- and intrauterine sudden death, or increased incidence of acute fetal distress in metabolically decompensated patients due to increased ketonic bodies and fetal metabolic acidosis with intolerance to uterine contractions.

Fetal–neonatal hypoglycemia secondary to pancreatic hypertrophy causes severe neonatal disturbances and even cerebral palsy.

Risk factors

Pedro B Landabure was a direct disciple of Bernardo Houssay. On 28 December 1954 he founded the Argentine Society of Diabetes, and presided over it during the period from 1955 to 1956. He pioneered investigations on diabetes mellitus (DM) in Argentina and Latin America and described the Landabure Syndrome as consisting of:

- history of macrosomic neonates (newborns weighing > 4000 grams);
- maternal obesity (> 10% maternal weight increase with respect to height and age);
- family history of DM;
- intrauterine fetal death;
- history of fetal congenital malformations;
- habitual abortion;
- prematurity;
- low birthweight;
- polihydramnios;
- glycosuria in pregnancy;
- perinatal mortality;
- multiparity and maternal age > 35 years.

In 1981 Pedersen[21] developed the prognostically bad signs of diabetic pregnancy, which disagree with the White Classification in one category. Pedersen's ill prognosis signs are:

- moderate to severe ketoacidosis;
- gestational hypertension;
- chronic pyelonephritis;
- maternal negligence.

Overweight and obesity play an important role not only because of their high frequency, but also because of their contribution to the development of GDM.[22] Universal GDM screening is more effective than that based on risk factors, detecting more cases, allowing for an earlier diagnosis and showing better perinatal results.[23]

Diagnosis and follow-up

The Argentine approach to diagnosis and follow-up this pathology is similar to that recommended by international guidelines. The difference, as in all developing countries, lies in the reticence of low-income pregnant women to attend health care centers, the lack of home and telephonic follow-up, non-compliance with treatment, and elevated numbers of undetected high-risk pregnant women.

Any patient presenting with risk factors (obesity, weight > 10% for height and age, history of DM, macrosomia, etc.) should be intensively investigated because these variables strongly influence DM epidemiology. Some of the risk factors mentioned previously, such as habitual abortion, polihydramnios and preterm labor, hold less importance but should also be taken into account.

According to the American College of Obstetrics and Gynecology (ACOG) guidelines,[24] a 50 gram, 1 hour glucose challenge test should be performed on these patients at 24–28 weeks gestation without any previous diet. This screening test renders positive results at a threshold of 130–140 mg/dl. After that, an oral glucose tolerance test (OGTT) should be performed with a previous 72 hour, 30 cal/kg hypercarbohydrate diet. Two or more measurements over normal values in the curve (exclus-ive of fasting value) diagnose GDM. A unique increased measurement is defined as a non-pathologic abnormal curve, requiring a strict follow-up of the patient.

On diagnosing GDM, a dietary plan should be instituted as the patient's initial treatment. The number of calories in the diet is calculated based on the patient's ideal body weight. The calories required for 1 kg of weight (30–35 cal/kg ideal body weight) is multiplied by the ideal body weight (in kg), resulting in the total calories the patient should eat daily. To avoid glycemic variations, the total caloric intake should be evenly distributed among three meals and a snack before bedtime. The intake generally consists of 30 cal/kg actual weight. In cases when the actual weight exceeds estimations, in > 10%, a theoretical overweight should be calculated with 40–50% of carbohydrates.

After determining the diet, ambulatory fasting and 1 hour postprandial glycemic profiles should be performed in the hospital to keep glycemic levels at 80 mg% fasting and 120 mg% postprandial.

According to the ACOG guidelines,[24,25] NPH insulin use should be considered at an initial fasting dose of 4 units (U) whenever nutritional therapy fails, defining failure as fasting glucose levels > 95 mg/dl, 1 hour postprandial values > 130–140 mg/dl, or 2 hour postprandial valules > 120 mg/dl. Glucose corrections consist of 1 U of crystalline Neutral Protamine Hagedorn NPH insulin per 10 mg/dl of fasting glycemia > 150 mg/dl, and 1 U/10 mg/dl of postprandial glycemia > 200 mg/dl. The total daily crystalline insulin dose should be calculated and the following day two thirds of that dose should be administered before breakfast and one third in the evening.[25]

These glycemic profiles should be continued once a week at the hospital on an ambulatory basis until delivery. If the patient requires insulin admi-nistration, she should be hospitalized until her glycemia normalizes, and until she learns how to self-administrate insulin and correct her glucose levels by ambulatory hospital follow-up.

On the day of delivery, half the required insulin dose should be administered and hourly glycemic measurements should be performed, correcting them when values > 200 mg/dl are detected. Ambulatory follow-up is as effective as hospitalization both in previously diabetic and in gestational diabetic women, to maintain an adequate glucose level, and to reduce perinatal morbidity and mortality. Additionally, the former is

Year	1994	1995	1996	1997	1998	1999	2000	2001	Total
Maternal age (years)									
19–34	7	7	2	5	5	3	2	9	40 (55.5%)
> 34	3	4	2	4	3	2	6	8	32 (44.4%)
History of infant mortality									
No	8	6	3	9	6	5	7	16	60 (83.3%)
Yes	2	5	1	0	2	0	1	1	12 (16.7%)
Prenatal care									
With	8	9	4	9	8	5	8	14	65 (90.0%)
Without	2	2	0	0	0	0	0	3	7 (9.7%)
Gestational age at first visit (weeks)									
20–30	4	4	2	2	2	1	3	3	21 (29.2%)
< 20	4	5	2	5	3	2	5	9	35 (48.6%)
> 30	2	2	0	2	3	2	0	5	16 (22.2%)
Total numbers of diabetic patients	10	11	4	9	8	5	8	17	72

Data from the Maternal–Infant Department, Juan A Fernández Hospital, from 1994 to 2001: total number of deliveries, 16,287; total number of diabetic patients, 72.

Table 14.1. *Characteristics of the diabetic pregnant population.*

significantly more cost-effective. However, in Argentina, as in most of the region, the low socio-economical status prompts physicians to hospitalize patients to monitor them adequately.

When the estimated fetal weight is > 4500 grams then a Cesarean section may reduce the probability of neonatal brachial plexus injury.[24]

Personal experience at the Juan A Fernández Hospital

The Juan A Fernández Hospital is a tertiary level, high-risk pregnancy referral center.

Between 1994 and 2001, the Maternal–Infant Department assisted 72 pregnant women with a diagnosis of DM; in 55% of the cases the women were between the ages of 19 and 34, and in 45% of the cases the women were > 34 years of age (Table 14.1). Seventeen percent of the patients had a history of perinatal mortality. Seven women (9.7%) lacked prenatal care. Gestational age at the first prenatal visit was > 30 weeks in 22.2% of the cases.

The most frequently associated maternal pathologies (Table 14.2) were urinary infection and hypertension. Hospitalization during gestation was required for 48.6% of the patients.

Year	1994	1995	1996	1997	1998	1999	2000	2001	Total
Secondary maternal pathology									
Hemorrhage*	0	1	0	0	0	0	0	1	2 (2.8%)
Urinary infection	2	2	1	0	0	0	0	0	5 (6.9%)
PROM	1	0	0	1	0	1	0	0	3 (4.2%)
Rhesus factor	0	0	0	1	0	0	0	0	1 (1.4%)
Hypertension	0	0	0	0	1	0	1	3	5 (6.9%)
Anemia	0	0	0	0	1	0	0	0	1 (1.4%)
Cardiopathies	0	0	0	0	0	1	0	0	1 (1.4%)
No secondary pathology	7	8	3	7	6	3	7	13	54 (75.0%)
Hospitalization during pregnancy									
No	4	4	1	6	3	3	5	11	37 (51.4%)
Yes	6	7	3	3	5	2	3	6	35 (48.6%)
Gestational age at delivery (weeks)	0	0	0	1	0	1	0	0	2 (2.8%)
20–28	4	4	1	1	2	1	3	1	17 (23.6%)
29–36	6	7	3	7	6	3	5	16	53 (73.6%)
37–42									
Total number of diabetic patients	10	11	4	9	8	5	8	17	72

Data from the Maternal–Infant Department, Juan A Fernández Hospital, from 1994 to 2001: total number of deliveries 16,287; total number of diabetic patients, 72.
*Second half of pregnancy; PROM, premature rupture of membranes.

Table 14.2. *Pregnancy evolution in 72 diabetic pregnant women.*

Gestational age at delivery was > 37 weeks in 74% of the population.

Cesarean sections were performed in 51.3% of the cases (Table 14.3). There were four intrauterine death. Neonates were vigorous at 1 and 5 minutes after birth in 88 and 93% of the cases, respectively. High and low birthweights were observed in 18.16 versus 15% of the newborns, respectively. Neonatal assess-ment detected an 18% incidence of preterm babies.

Six neonates (Table 14.4) required hospital-ization in Neonatal Intensive Care Unit (NICU). Five newborns presented with respira-tory distress syndrome, mechanical ventilation was required in two cases. There was one neonatal death, giving an overall perinatal sur-vival rate of 93%.

Year	1994	1995	1996	1997	1998	1999	2000	2001	Total
Mode of delivery									
Spontaneous	3	5	3	2	6	1	6	9	35 (48.6%)
Cesarean section	7	6	1	7	2	4	2	8	37 (51.4%)
Fetal status									
Alive	10	11	4	9	7	4	7	16	68 (94.4%)
Dead	0	0	0	0	1	1	1	1	4 (5.6%)
Apgar score at 1 minute									
Severely depressed	0	1	0	0	0	0	1	0	2 (2.9%)
Moderately depressed	1	2	0	1	2	0	0	0	6 (8.8%)
Vigorous	9	8	4	8	5	4	6	16	60 (88.3%)
Apgar score at 5 minutes									
Severely depressed	0	0	0	0	0	0	0	0	0
Moderately depressed	1	3	0	0	0	0	1	0	5 (7.4%)
Vigorous	9	8	4	9	7	4	6	16	63 (92.6%)
Birthweight									
Low	1	2	0	1	1	1	2	2	10 (14.7%)
High	2	2	1	3	1	1	0	2	12 (17.6%)
Adequate	7	7	3	5	5	2	5	12	46 (67.6%)
Gestational age at delivery (excludes fetal deaths) (weeks)									
20–32	0	0	0	1	0	0	0	1	2 (3.0%)
33–36	3	3	1	0	1	2	2	0	12 (17.6%)
> 36	7	8	3	8	6	2	5	15	54 (79.4%)
Total number of diabetic patients	10	11	4	9	8	5	8	17	72

Data from the Maternal–Infant Department, Juan A Fernández Hospital, from 1994 to 2001: total number of deliveries, 16,287; total number of diabetic patients, 72; total number of neonates, 68.

Table 14.3. *Mode of delivery and fetal outcome.*

Year	1994	1995	1996	1997	1998	1999	2000	2001	Total
Stay in Neonatal Intensive Care Unit									
No	10	10	4	8	7	3	6	14	62 (91.2%)
Yes	0	1	0	1	0	1	1	2	6 (8.8%)
Neonatal pathology									
Prematurity	1	1	0	1	0	1	1	1	6 (8.8%)
Severe RDS	1	1	0	0	0	1	1	1	5 (7.4%)
Non-rhesus jaundice	0	1	0	0	0	0	0	2	3 (4.4%)
Malformations	0	0	0	1	0	0	0	1	2 (2.9%)
Assisted ventilation									
Yes	0	0	0	0	0	1	1	0	2 (2.9%)
No	10	11	4	9	7	3	6	16	66 (97.1%)
Perinatal mortality									
Alive	10	11	4	8	7	4	7	16	67 (93.1%)
Dead	0	0	0	1	1	1	1	1	5 (6.9%)

Data from the Maternal–Infant Department, Juan A Fernández Hospital, from 1994 to 2001: total number of deliveries, 16,287; total number of diabetic patients, 72; total number of neonates, 68.
RDS, respiratory distress syndrome.

Table 14.4. Neonatal evolution.

Conclusions

From this group's personal experience, it can be concluded that, despite late first prenatal visits, when pregnant women receive prenatal care before birth, perinatal results are acceptable. However, the question remains as to how many diabetic patients never reach prenatal care, are never detected, or approach the hospital to deliver a dead or macrosomic fetus without a final diagnosis of the pathology that has led to this end.

These are the deficiencies of a developing country which lacks a continuous, efficient maternal–infant policy, in contrast to highly trained medical staff, who cannot achieve the desired reduction in maternal, fetal and neonatal morbidity and mortality. This not only affects the care of patients with DM; unknown numbers of young women die of hemorrhage and infections. This is a consequence of the absence of prenatal care, with patients reaching health centers at the last minute, some of which lack the facilities to make a fast diagnosis and provide timely treatment.

Argentine physicians are aware of risk factors and prevention of fetal malformations by achieving periconceptional glycemic control through preconception care.[26] However, at present this can only be applied to a minority of fertile age women from higher socioeconomic backgrounds who can comply with prenatal care guidelines The aim is to make this case standard, fighting against hundreds of obstacles that hinder the way towards the preventive care of women's health.

References

1. UNICEF. *Oficina Regional para América Latina y el Caribe: Mortalidad materna. Estrategia para su reducción en América Latina y el Caribe. Análisis y recomendaciones para la región,* 1999.

2. Jurgens, Esther (TACRO). Estado Mundial de la Infancia 1999. In: (UNICEF, ed) *Oficina Regional para América Latina y el Caribe: Mortalidad materna. Estrategia para su reducción en América Latina y el Caribe. Análisis y recomendaciones para la región,* 1999.

3. Ministerio de Salud de la República Argentina, www.msal.gov.ar.

4. Lomuto, Celia, Ministerio de Salud. *Programa Nacional de Estadísticas de Salud, Estadísticas Vitales: Información Básica 2000* 2001, 5 (44).

5. Gabbe SG, Mestman JG, Freeman RK et al. Management and outcome of class A diabetes mellitus. *Am J Obstet Gynecol* 1977; **127**:465–9.

6. Widness JA, Cowett RM, Coustan DR et al. Neonatal morbidities in infants of mothers with glucose intolerance in pregnancy. *Diabetes* 1985; **34 (Suppl 2)**:61–5.

7. Freinkel N, Metzger BE, Phelps RL et al. Gestational diabetes mellitus. Heterogeneity of maternal age, weight, insulin secretion, HLA antigens and islet cell antibodies and the impact of maternal metabolism on pancreatic B-cell and somatic development in offspring. *Diabetes* 1985; **34 (Suppl 2)**:1–7.

8. O'Sullivan JB, Charles D, Mahan CM et al. Gestational diabetes and perinatal mortality rate. *Am J Obstet Gynecol* 1973; **116**:901–4.

9. Hare JW, White P. Gestational diabetes and the White classification. *Diabetes Care* 1980; **3**:394.

10. Votta RM, Parada NM. Endocrinopatías y embarazo. In: *Compendio de Obstetricia.* (López Libreros Editores SRL: Buenos Aires, 1998) 206–11.

11. *Estadísticas del Hospital Materno–Infantil Ramón Sardá 1989–1991.* División Estadística. Sistema Informático Perinatal.

12. Ministerio de Salud de la República Argentina, Dirección de Estadística e Información de Salud, www.msal.gov.ar.

13. Spellacy WN. Human placental lactogen (HPL): the review of protein hormone important to obstetrics and gynecology. *South Med J* 1969; **62**:1054–7.

14. Van Assche FA, Hoet JJ, Lock PMB. The endocrine pancreas of the pregnant mother, fetus and newborn. In: (Beard R, Nathanielzs P, eds) *Fetal Physiology and Medicine.* (WB Saunders: London, 1976) 121.

15. Malkhoff RK, Costrini NV, Matute ML, Kim HJ. Metabolic modifications by the hormones in pregnancy. In: (Carmeni-Dávalos RA, Cole HJ, eds) *Early Diabetes in Early Life.* (Academic Press, New York, 1975).

16. Freinkel N, Goodner CJ. Carbohydrate metabolism in pregnancy. 1. The metabolism of insulin by human placental tissue. *J Clin Invest* 1960; **9**:116.

17. Adam PA, Teramo K, Raiha N et al. Human fetal insulin metabolism early in pregnancy. Response to acute elevation of the the fetal glucose concentration and placental transfer of human insulin I-131. *Diabetes* 1969; **18**:409–16.

18. Obenshain SS, Adam PA, King KC et al. Human fetal insulin response to sustained maternal hyperglycemia. *N Engl J Med* 1970; **283**:566–70.

19. Smith BT, Giroud C, Robert M, Avery M. Insulin antagonism of cortisol action on lecithin synthesis by cultured fetal lung cells. *J Pediatr* 1975; **87**:953–5.

20. Pell JH. Progress in the knowledge and management of the pregnant diabetic patient. *Am J Obstet Gynecol* 1962; **83**:47.

21. Pedersen J. *La diabética gestante y su recién nacido.* (Editorial Salvat: Buenos Aires, 1981).

22. Etchegoyen GS, de Martini ER. Gestational diabetes. Determination of relative importance of risk factors. *Medicina (Buenos Aires)* 2001; **61**:235–8.

23. Griffin ME, Coffey M, Johnson H et al. Universal vs. risk factor-based screening for gestational diabetes mellitus: detection rates, gestational diagnosis and outcome. *Diabet Med* 2000; **17**:26–32.

24. ACOG. ACOG issues new guidelines for management of gestational diabetes. *Obstet Gynecol* 2001; **98**:525–38.

25. Koremblit E, Uranga Imaz F, López R et al. Diabetes y embarazo. I. Terapia insulínica precoz en la diabetes clase A. *Revista de la Sociedad de Obstetricia y Ginecología de Bs As* 1986; **65**:69.

26. Ray JG, O'Brien TE, Chan WS. Preconception care and the risk of congenital anomalies in the offspring of women with diabetes mellitus: a meta-analysis. *Q J Med* 2001; **94**:435–44.

15

Diabetes following gestational diabetes mellitus

Peter Damm, Jeannet Lauenborg, Lars Mølsted-Pedersen

Diabetes mellitus and impaired glucose tolerance in women with previous gestational diabetes mellitus

Although glucose tolerance returns to normal in the majority of women with gestational diabetes mellitus (GDM) shortly after delivery, there is substantial evidence that these women have an increased risk of developing overt diabetes later in life (Table 15.1). In his classical studies, O'Sullivan[1–3] found a 36% incidence of diabetes in women with previous GDM 22–28 years after pregnancy, and an even higher incidence of diabetes in former GDM women was reported in a Hispanic American population from Los Angeles.[4,5] Two newer, carefully performed North American follow-up studies of former GDM women reported very different results, i.e. a relatively low incidence of abnormal glucose tolerance (11%) with a mean follow-up of 3 years[6] versus a 41% incidence of diabetes with a mean follow-up of 5 years.[7]

Thus, it is difficult to obtain a consistent message from the published studies (Table 15.1). This is probably due to heterogeneity of both the patient populations studied and of how GDM was diagnosed in the previous pregnancy.

Methodological considerations

It is a major problem that different diagnostic tests and criteria for GDM have been used. It seems logical that the higher blood glucose level needed to fulfil the criteria for the diagnosis of GDM would increase the risk of subsequent development of diabetes. In the majority of studies, GDM was diagnosed during pregnancy as it should be. In the study from Aberdeen,[8,9] GDM was assumed to have occurred based on the findings of an abnormal intravenous glucose tolerance test (IVGTT) in the postpartum period. This tends to select GDM women with relatively more profound metabolical aberrations since glucose tolerance normally improves shortly after pregnancy.[10] In contrast to most other studies, O'Sullivan[1] only included GDM subjects with a normal glucose tolerance after pregnancy, in accordance with the GDM definition used at that time.

At follow-up, the majority of the studies applied a 75 gram oral glucose tolerance test (OGTT) evaluated by the World Health Organization (WHO-1985)[11] or the National Diabetes Data Group (NDDG)[12] criteria. These two sets of criteria are very similar, but the NDDG criteria will probably give a slightly lower incidence rate of IGT.[13] Both sets of criteria have also been applied to a 100 gram OGTT,[2,7] a procedure that tends to

City, Country (Reference)	n*	Diagnostic test in pregnancy	Length of follow-up (years)	Diagnostic test at follow-up (diagnostic criteria)	Abnormal glucose tolerance (DM + IGT)	Control group (DM + IGT)
Arizona, USA (65)	233	75 gram OGTT	4–8	75 gram OGTT (WHO)	10% DM	(+)
Aberdeen, Scotland (8,9)	112	IVGTT	up to 22	IVGTT	35% (6% DM, 29% IGT)	
Uppsala, Sweden (66)	80	IVGTT	1–8	IVGTT	33% (16% DM, 17% IGT)	
Los Angeles, USA (4,5)	89	100 gram OGTT	12–18	Interview	65% DM	
Boston, USA (3)	615	100 gram OGTT	22–28	100 gram OGTT (WHO)	36% DM	+(5.5% DM)
Port-of-Spain, Trinidad (67)	60	75 gram OGTT	3–7	75 gram OGTT (WHO)	79% (62% DM, 17% IGT)	
London, England (68)	56	50 gram OGTT	6–12	75 gram OGTT (WHO)	64% (39% DM, 25% IGT)	
Los Angeles, USA (59)	246	100 gram OGTT	5–8 weeks	75 gram OGTT (NDDG)	19% (10% DM, 9% IGT)	
Vermont, USA (19)	103	100 gram OGTT	7 weeks	75 gram OGTT (NDDG)	22% (3% DM, 4% IGT)†	
Melbourne, Australia (23)	881	50 gram OGTT	up to 17	75 gram OGTT (WHO)	28% (12% DM, 16% IGT)	+(1% DM)
Stockholm, Sweden (25)	145	50 gram OGTT	3–4	75 gram OGTT (WHO)	25% (3.4% DM, 22% IGT)	+(4% IGT)
Copenhagen, Denmark (26)	241‡	50 gram OGTT	2–11	75 gram OGTT (WHO)	34% (3.7% Type 1 DM, 13.7% Type 2 DM, 17% IGT)	+(5.3% IGT)
Providence, USA (6)	350	100 gram OGTT	up to 10	75 gram OGTT (NDDG)	11% (7% DM, 4% IGT)	
Chicago, USA (7)	274	100 gram OGTT	up to 5	100 gram OGTT (NDDG)	57% (41% DM, 16% IGT)	
San Diego, USA (38)	94	100 gram OGTT	6 weeks	75 gram OGTT (NDDG)	34% (16% DM, 18% IGT)	
Los Angeles, USA (23)	671	100 gram OGTT	up to 7	75 gram OGTT (NDDG)	22% DM	
London, England (18)	192	75 gram OGTT	up to 7	75 gram OGTT (WHO)	49% (22% DM, 27% IGT)	
Madrid, Spain (17)	788	75 gram OGTT	3–6 months	75 gram OGTT (WHO)	20% (15% DM, 5% IGT)	
Barcelona, Spain (16)	120	75 gram OGTT	up to 1	75 gram OGTT (WHO)	14% (2% DM, 12% IGT)	
Lund, Sweden (27)	229	75 gram OGTT	1	75 gram OGTT (WHO)	31% (9%, 22%)	+(1.7% IGT)

DM, Diabetes mellitus; IGT, impaired glucose tolerance; IVGTT, intravenous glucose tolerance test; NDDG, National Diabetes Data Group; OGTT, oral glucose tolerance test; WHO, World Health Organization.
* Number of women with GDM.
† Fifteen per cent non-diagnostic.
‡ Diet-treated GDM women only.

Table 15.1.   Follow-up studies of women with previous gestational diabetes (GDM).

slightly overestimate the incidence of diabetes if corrections for the increased glucose load are not made. Recently, American Diabetes Association (ADA)[14] and WHO-1998[15] recommendations have also been used.[16–18]

Not all women with GDM during a specific period are available for participation in a follow-up examination several years later. It is, however, important that the women who are investigated at follow-up constitute a representative and large subset of the initial GDM population to ensure that the study material is not skewed in any way that can affect the results. Nevertheless, only a few studies give information regarding the participation rate and the representativity of the study participants. If, for example, women who required insulin treatment during pregnancy are overrepresented at follow-up compared with women who could be managed on diet alone, as in the studies by Catalano et al[19] and Metzger et al,[20] too high an incidence of abnormal glucose tolerance at follow-up can be expected. This kind of bias is likely to occur since women with a more severe disease generally are more compliant with respect to medical follow-up examinations. It has been documented[7,20] that GDM women with significantly increased fasting plasma glucose (FPG) at diagnosis, and who therefore were treated with insulin, have a significantly higher risk of developing overt diabetes later in life than GDM women who were treated with diet alone. However, it should be considered that the plasma glucose level at which insulin therapy is initiated varies between different studies. According to the definition of GDM, a subset of the insulin-treated GDM women would have Type 1 diabetes with accidental onset during pregnancy. In a Danish population, the majority of these women could be discharged from hospital after delivery without insulin treatment, but a nearly 100% incidence of subsequent development of diabetes was reported.[21] When comparing follow-up studies it is therefore important to know what the treatment/metabolic status during the index of pregnancy was. The current GDM definition also allows women with undiagnosed Type 2 diabetes antedating pregnancy to be categorized as having GDM. Thus, in populations with a high incidence of these women a relatively high rate of abnormal glucose tolerance in the post-partum period might consequently be found.

The incidence of overt diabetes in the general population is increasing with age. Hence, the time span between the index of pregnancy and the follow-up examination should be considered when comparing studies. Accordingly, some studies[7,22,23] performing life-table analyses found much higher estimates of the cumulative incidence rate of diabetes than the crude incidence rates.

It has generally been assumed that GDM is associated with an increased risk for later development of Type 2 diabetes and not for Type 1 diabetes, but very few studies have addressed this question.

Another very important factor when comparing different studies is the heterogeneous ethnic mixture of the populations. The background incidence of both Type 1 and Type 2 diabetes varies considerably among different populations.

These methodological problems underline the significance of an appropriate control group of women. Such control groups have only been included in relatively few of the follow-up studies of women with previous GDM; a net excess of diabetes on 30,[3] 11,[24] 3,[25] 17[26] and 9%[27] was found in women with previous GDM compared to controls.

Copenhagen series

The participation rate in present authors' study[26] was high (81%), and the participants representative for the total GDM population. All women with GDM were treated by diet only during pregnancy and they were diagnosed by uniform criteria in the same laboratory. Ethnically, the material was homogeneous with 90% Scandinavian Caucasians. At follow-up, glucose tolerance was evaluated according to the WHO-1985 criteria,[11] and a clear distinction between Type 1 and Type 2 diabetes[28,29] was made. With a 6 year median observation time since the index of pregnancy, 34.4% of the 241 women with previous GDM had developed an abnormal glucose tolerance; 3.7% had Type 1 diabetes, 13.7% had Type 2 diabetes and 17.0% had IGT. The routine was to perform an OGTT *c.* 2 months postpartum in women with GDM and diabetes was diagnosed in four women (three Type 1 and one Type 2) at this examination. Some women had well-known diabetes at follow-up but more than half of the women with Type 2 diabetes were diagnosed for the first time at the follow-up study.[26,30,31] Among the controls, none had diabetes but IGT was found in 5.3%. Women who developed Type 1 diabetes were younger and leaner than the GDM women who did not, with a high prevalence of the Type-1-diabetes-typical human leucocyte antigen (HLA) DR types DR3 and DR4, and of the autoimmune markers islet cell antoantibodies[30] and glutamic acid decarboxylase.[32] Thus, it is very likely that women who develop Type 1 diabetes after pregnancy already had an ongoing beta-cell destruction during pregnancy which was unmasked by the pregnancy-induced insulin resistance, as is also indicated by other workers (for a review see Mauricio and de Leiva[33]). In this study Type 1 diabetes tended to be diagnosed earlier after pregnancy than Type 2 diabetes; it is likely that some of the GDM women developing diabetes have maturity onset diabetes of the young (MODY). This is supported by the fact that MODY-typical gene mutations have been found in *c.* 5% of women with GDM.[34,35]

In conclusion, women with GDM have a considerably increased risk of developing DM (both Type 1 and Type 2) or IGT in the years following pregnancy. The incidence of abnormal glucose tolerance seems to increase with increasing follow-up time since pregnancy.[1,23,24,36] Up to 20% of the women with previous GDM who develop overt diabetes will, at least in some populations, develop Type 1 diabetes, a fact that may have been underestimated in some studies.

Predictive factors for development of overt diabetes in women with previous gestational diabetes mellitus

Having confirmed that women with GDM are at risk for subsequent development of overt diabetes, it is important to be able to predict which women among those with previous GDM are at highest risk. Many potential predictive factors, e.g. plasma glucose, plasma insulin, weight and age, are associated; hence, it is necessary to control for covariance and confounding factors in the analysis of predictive factors for diabetes development, a fact not always taken into account.

Tables 15.2 and 15.3 summarize the predictive factors for future diabetes identified by multivariate analysis. Predictor variables differ naturally among the different populations studied; however, some common features are present.

The majority of GDM women who in the postpartum period still have an abnormal OGTT (although are not overtly diabetic) will normalize their glucose tolerance within 1

Risk factor	References
Maternal overweight	17
Low gestational age at diagnosis of GDM	19*
High fasting glucose at GDM diagnosis	19*
High post-stimulatory glucose in pregnancy	7,17,38
Low fasting insulin at diagnosis	7
Low C-peptide/glucose score during OGTT at diagnosis	17
Previous history of GDM	38

OGTT, Oral glucose tolerance test.
* Impaired glucose tolerance or diabetes.

Table 15.2. *Risk factors for development of diabetes or abnormal glucose tolerance within 6 months after pregnancy in women with gestational diabetes mellitus (GDM) (identified with multivariant analysis).*

Risk factor	References
Increasing maternal age	22
Maternal overweight	6,* 7, 22
High fasting glucose at the diagnostic OGTT	6,* 23, 26, 37*
High glucose during the diagnostic OGTT	6,* 22, 23, 26, 27, 37,* 39
High fasting glucose postpartum	37*
High glucose during postpartum OGTT	23, 26, 37*
Abnormal OGTT postpartum	23, 26
Insulin treatment during pregnancy	27, 37*
Low insulin secretion during the diagnostic OGTT	7, 26
Poor beta-cell compensation for insulin resistance during pregnancy	39
Increased basal glucose production during pregnancy	39
Preterm delivery	26
Low gestational age at diagnosis of GDM	23

OGTT, Oral glucose tolerance test.
* Impaired glucose tolerance or diabetes.

Table 15.3. *Risk factors for development of diabetes or abnormal glucose tolerance after the postpartum period in women with gestational diabetes mellitus (GDM) (identified with multivariant analysis).*

year.[37] However, these women do *a priori* have a more disturbed glucose metabolism compared with women with a normal glucose tolerance postpartum, and are therefore expected to have an increased risk of diabetes development later in life. In agreement with this, the best predictor for later development of diabetes is elevated glucose levels during an OGTT in the postpartum period. The significance of this finding is underlined by the fact that it was found in two very different popula-tions, Hispanic Americans[23] and Danish Caucasians,[26] with relative risks as high as 11 and 5, respectively. Several studies have shown that the more glucose tolerance is affected during pregnancy, then the higher the risk for future development of abnormal glucose tolerance.[6,7,19,22,23,26,37,38] Maternal overweight, a well-known risk factor for development of Type 2 diabetes, was also a risk factor in some studies.[6,7,17,22]

Interestingly, a low and relatively insufficient insulin secretion during pregnancy pre-dicted development of diabetes in several studies,[7,17,26,39] in accordance with studies in non-GDM populations where a low insulin response to intravenous (IV) and oral glucose has been found to predict development of Type 2 diabetes.[40–42] From Los Angeles it was reported that an additional pregnancy or weight gain after the GDM pregnancy increased the risk of subsequent overt diabetes.[43]

Although women with GDM as a group have a low prevalence of autoimmune markers of Type 1 diabetes (ICA, GAD), it has been shown that the presence of one or more of these is highly predictive for the later develop-ment of Type 1 diabetes.[30,44–46]

Pre-Type 2 diabetes characteristics in glucose tolerant women with previous gestational diabetes mellitus

Type 2 diabetes is characterized by insulin resistance/decreased insulin sensitivity, pri-marily in skeletal muscle, and decreased insulin secretion,[47,48] and it is still unknown which is the primary defect in the patho-genesis of Type 2 diabetes. In normoglycaemic individuals insulin sensitivity as well as insulin secretion have been found to predict develop-ment of diabetes.[49]

Several studies have documented decreased insulin sensitivity in lean as well as obese glucose-tolerant women with previous GDM.[50–55] The decreased insulin sensitivity is mainly caused by a reduced non-oxidative glucose metabolism in skeletal muscle tissue, the cellular background for which is not known.[51] A relatively decreased insulin secretion in lean and obese glucose-tolerant women with previous GDM has also been found.[16,50,52,53,55,56] Thus, women with pre-vious GDM exhibit the metabolic profile of Type 2 diabetes despite a normal glucose tolerance several years after the GDM pregnancy.

Conclusions

The prevalence of Type 1 and Type 2 diabetes is increasing worldwide.[57] Thus, prevention and early diagnosis of diabetes will be of major clinical significance in the future. It is known that Type 2 diabetes is often asymptomatic during the early years after onset – it has been estimated that the onset of the disease occurs at least 4–7 years before the clinical diagnosis, since > 20% of newly diagnosed Type 2 dia-betic patients have micro- or macrovascular diabetic complications.[48,58] Although not all women who have had GDM will develop dia-betes their risk as a group is markedly increased, making a regular assessment of their glucose tolerance mandatory in the years following pregnancy. Substantial evidence indicates that an OGTT should be performed c. 2 months postpartum in all women with GDM because: (1) a high frequency of ab-normal glucose tolerance is found at this time,[7,19,23,26,37,59] (2) the result of the OGTT is highly predictive for the development of later overt diabetes.[23,26] Plasma insulin during OGTT is also a very good predictor of later diabetes,[7,26,31] but measurement of plasma insulin during the diagnostic OGTT will in many centres be impractical for other than scientific purposes.

It is now been well described in very different populations that the risk for development of Type 2 diabetes can be reduced significantly in subjects with IGT by lifestyle changes with increased physical activity, weight loss and a healthy diet.[60–63] Also, intervention with metformin has been found to reduce the progression to diabetes.[63] A common characteristic for these studies was that the subjects were seen repeatedly over a long period of time. In prior GDM women with IGT, Buchanan et al[64] found an improvement in insulin sensitivity by prophylactic treatment with an insulin-sensitizing drug. During the 3 month period of their study no significant effect on glucose tolerance could be demonstrated; however, it is possible that a prolonged treatment would be more efficient.

The prevalence of ICA and GAD autoantibodies in GDM pregnancy is low, but the predictive value for later Type 1 diabetes is high. Thus, ICA and GAD autoantibody-positive GDM women could in the future be candidates for intervention trials with the aim to prevent or postpone the development of Type 1 diabetes. However, routine screening of women with GDM for ICA and/or GAD does not seem to be indicated before a safe intervention therapy of antibody-positive women is available.

Women with GDM should be advised to lose weight after pregnancy if they are obese, to eat a low-fat diet and to have an active lifestyle, including physical activity. These measures will all theoretically improve insulin sensitivity and thereby prevent or delay development of overt diabetes. Concerning pharmacological intervention to prevent diabetes, the results are promising but further documentation is needed before final conclusions can be drawn. Furthermore, women with previous GDM should be instructed to have a regular check of their glucose tolerance, e.g. by an OGTT with 1 or 2 year intervals, to secure early diagnosis of overt diabetes. To implement all or some of these measures it is necessary to offer a long-term, continuous programme to women with previous GDM, including education, stimulation and testing. At present only very few clinics are able to offer these facilities. However, based on the available evidence, a major aim during the next decade will be to implement such programmes in the daily clinical life for the benefit of women with previous GDM.

References

1. O'Sullivan JB. Diabetes mellitus after GDM. *Diabetes* 1991; **29 (Suppl 2)**:131–5.
2. O'Sullivan JB. Subsequent morbidity among gestational diabetic women. In: (Sutherland HW, Stowers JM, eds) *Carbohydrate Metabolism in Pregnancy and the Newborn*. (Churchill Livingstone: Edinburgh, 1984) 174–180.
3. O'Sullivan JB. The Boston gestational diabetes studies: review and prospectives. In: (Sutherland HW, Stowers JM, Pearson DWM, eds) *Carbohydrate Metabolism in Pregnancy and the Newborn*. (Springer-Verlag: Berlin, 1989); 287–94.
4. Mestman JH, Anderson GV, Guadalupe V. Follow-up study of 360 subjects with abnormal carbohydrate metabolism during pregnancy. *Obstet Gynecol* 1972; **39**: 421–5.
5. Mestman JH. Follow-up studies in women with gestational diabetes mellitus. The experience at Los Angeles Country/University of Southern California Medical Center. In: (Weiss PAM, Coustan DR, eds) *Gestational Diabetes*. (Springer-Verlag: Vienna, 1988) 191–8.
6. Coustan DR, Carpenter MW, O'Sullivan PS, Carr SR. Gestational diabetes: predictors of subsequent disordered glucose metabolism. *Am J Obstet Gynecol* 1993; **168**: 1139–45.
7. Metzger BE, Cho NH, Roston SM, Radvany R. Prepregnancy weight and antepartum insulin secretion

predict glucose tolerance five years after gestational diabetes mellitus. *Diabetes Care* 1993; **16**:1598–605.

8. Stowers JM. Follow-up of gestational diabetic mothers treated thereafter. In: (Sutherland HW, Stowers JM, eds) *Carbohydrate Metabolism in Pregnancy and the Newborn*. (Churchill Livingstone: Edinburgh, 1984) 181–3.

9. Stowers JM, Sutherland HW, Kerridge DF. Long-range implications for the mother. The Aberdeen experience. *Diabetes* 1985; **34 (Suppl 2)**:106–10.

10. Kühl C. Glucose metabolism during and after pregnancy in normal and gestational diabetic women. 1. Influence of normal pregnancy on serum glucose and insulin concentration during basal fasting conditions and after a challenge with glucose. *Acta Endocrinol* 1975; **79**:709–19.

11. World Heath Organization. *Diabetes mellitus: report of a WHO study group*. World Health Organization, Geneva, 1985.

12. National Diabetes Data Group. Classification and diagnosis of diabetes mellitus and other categories of glucose intolerance. *Diabetes* 1979; **28**:1039–57.

13. Motala AA, Omar MAK. Evaluation of WHO and NDDG criteria for impaired glucose tolerance. *Diabetes Res Clin Pract* 1994; **23**:103–9.

14. The Expert Committee on the diagnosis and classification of diabetes mellitus. Report of the Expert Committee on the diagnosis and classification of diabetes mellitus. *Diabetes Care* 1997; **20**:1183–97.

15. World Health Organization. *Report of the World Health Organization: Definition, diagnosis and classification of diabetes mellitus and its complications*. (WHO: Geneva, Switzerland, 1999).

16. Costa A, Carmona F, Martinez-Roman et al. Postpartum reclassification of glucose tolerance in women previously diagnosed with gestational diabetes mellitus. *Diabet Med* 2000; **17**:595–8.

17. Pallardo F, Herranz L, Garcia-Ingelmo T et al. Early postpartum metabolic assessment in women with prior gestational diabetes. *Diabetes Care* 1999; **22**:1053–8.

18. Kousta E, Lawrence NJ, Penny A et al. Implications of the new diagnostic criteria for abnormal glucose homeostasis in women with previous gestational diabetes. *Diabetes Care* 1999; **22**: 933–7.

19. Catalano PM, Vargo KM, Bernstein IM, Amini SB. Incidence and risk factors associated with abnormal postpartum glucose tolerance in women with gestational diabetes. *Am J Obstet Gynecol* 1991; **165**:914–19.

20. Metzger BE, Bybee DE, Freinkel N et al. Gestational diabetes mellitus. Correlations between the phenotypic and genotypic characteristics of the mother and abnormal glucose tolerance during the first year postpartum. *Diabetes* 1985; **34 (Suppl 2)**:111–15.

21. Buschard K, Hougaard P, Mølsted-Pedersen L, Kühl C. Type 1 (insulin-dependent) diabetes mellitus diagnosed during pregnancy: a clinical and prognostic study. *Diabetologia* 1991; **33**:31–5.

22. O'Sullivan JB. Gestational diabetes: factors influencing the rates of subsequent diabetes. In: (Sutherland HW, Stowers JM, eds.) *Carbohydrate Metabolism in Pregnancy and the Newborn*. (Springer-Verlag: Berlin, 1979) 425–35.

23. Kjos SL, Peters RK, Xiang A et al. Predicting future diabetes in Latino women with gestational diabetes. Utility of early postpartum glucose tolerance testing. *Diabetes* 1995; **44**:586–91.

24. Henry OA, Beischer NA. Long-term implications of gestational diabetes for the mother. In: (Oats JN, ed.) *Baillière's Clinical Obstetrics and Gynaecology*. (Baillière Tindall: London, 1991) 461–83.

25. Persson B, Hanson U, Hartling SG, Binder C. Follow-up of women with previous GDM. Insulin, C-peptide, and proinsulin responses to oral glucose load. *Diabetes* 1991; **40 (Suppl 2)**:136–41.

26. Damm P, Kühl P, Bertelsen A, Molsted-Pedersen L. Predictive factors for the development of diabetes in women with previous gestational diabetes mellitus. *Am J Obstet Gynecol* 1992; **167**:607–16.

27. Aberg AEB, Jönsson EK, Eskilsson I et al. Predictive factors of developing diabetes mellitus in women with gestational diabetes. *Acta Obstet Gynecol Scand* 2002; **81**:11–16.

28. Faber OK, Binder C. C-peptide response to glucagon. A test for residual beta-cell function in diabetes mellitus. *Diabetes* 1977; **26**:605–10.

29. Madsbad S, Krarup T, McNair T et al. Practical clinical value of C-peptide response to glucagon stimulation in the choice of treatment in diabetes mellitus. *Acta Med Scand* 1981; **210**:153–6.

30. Damm P, Kühl C, Buschard K et al. Prevalence and predictive value of islet cell antibodies and insulin autoantibodies in women with gestational diabetes. *Diabet Med* 1994; **11**:558–63.

31. Damm P, Kühl C, Hornnes PJ, Molsted-Pedersen L. A longitudinal study of plasma insulin and glucagon in women with previous gestational diabetes. *Diabetes Care* 1995; **18**:654–65.

32. Petersen JS, Dyrberg T, Damm P et al. GAD65 autoantibodies in women with gestational or insulin dependent diabetes mellitus during pregnancy. *Diabetologia* 1996; **39**:1329–33.

33. Mauricio D, de Leiva A. Autoimmune gestational diabetes mellitus: a distinct clinical entity? *Diabetes Metab Res Rev* 2001; **17**:422–8.

34. Weng J, Ekelund M, Lehto J et al. Screening for MODY mutations, GAD antibodies, and type 1 diabeets-associated HLA genotypes in women with gestational diabetes mellitus. *Diabetes Care* 2002; **25**:68–71.

35. McLellan JA, Barrow BA, Levy JC et al. Prevalence of diabetes mellitus and impaired glucose tolerance in parents of women with gestational diabetes. *Diabetologia* 1995; **38**:693–8.

36. Hanson U, Persson B, Hartling SG, Binder C. Increased molar proinsulin-to-insulin ratio in women with previous

gestational diabetes does not predict later impairment of glucose tolerance. *Diabetes Care* 1996; **19**:17–20.

37. Lam KSL, Li DF, Lauder IJ et al. Prediction of persistent carbohydrate intolerance in patients with gestational diabetes. *Diabetes Res Clin Pract* 1991; **12**:181–6.

38. Greenberg LR, Moore TR, Murphy H. Gestational diabetes mellitus: antenatal variables as predictors of postpartum glucose intolerance. *Obstet Gynecol* 1995; **86**:97–101.

39. Buchanan TA, Xiang AH, Kjos S et al. Antepartum predictors of the development of type 2 diabetes in Latino women 11–26 months after pregnancies complicated by gestational diabetes. *Diabetes* 1999; **48**:2430–6.

40. Skarfos ET, Selinus KI, Lithell HO. Risk factors for developing non-insulin dependent diabetes: a 10 year follow up of men in Uppsala. *Br Med J* 1991; **303**:755–60.

41. Charles MA, Fontbonne A, Thibult N et al. Risk factors for NIDDM in white population. Paris prospective study. *Diabetes* 1991; **40**:796–9.

42. Saad MF, Knowler WC, Pettitt DJ et al. A two-step model for development of non-insulin-dependent diabetes. *Am J Med* 1991; **90**:229–35.

43. Peters RK, Kjos SL, Xiang A, Buchanan TA. Long-term diabetogenic effect of single pregnancy in women with previous gestational diabetes mellitus. *Lancet* 1996; **27**:227–30.

44. Catalano, PM, Tyzbir ED, Sims EAH. Incidence and significance of islet cell antibodies in women with previous gestational diabetes. *Diabetes Care* 1991; **13**:478–82.

45. Steel JM, Irvine WJ, Clarke BF. The significance of pancreatic islet cell antibody and abnormal glucose tolerance during pregnancy. *J Clin Lab Immunol* 1980; **4**:83–5.

46. Mauricio D, Corcoy RM, Codina M et al. Islet cell antibodies identify a subset of gestational diabetic women with higher risk of developing diabetes mellitus shortly after pregnancy. *Diabetic Nutr Metab* 1992; **5**:237–41.

47. DeFronzo RA, Bonadonna RC, Ferrannini E. Pathogenesis of NIDDM. A balanced overview. *Diabetes Care* 1992; **15**:318–68.

48. Beck-Nielsen H, Groop LC. Metabolic and genetic characterization of prediabetic states. Sequence of events leading to non-insulin-dependent diabetes mellitus. *J Clin Invest* 1994; **94**:1714–21.

49. Lillioja S, Mott DM, Spraul M et al. Insulin resistance and insulin secretory dysfunction as precursors of non-insulin-dependent diabetes mellitus. Prospective studies of Pima Indians. *N Engl J Med* 1993; **329**:1988–92.

50. Ryan EA, Imes S, Liu D et al. Defects in insulin secretion and action in women with a history of gestational diabetes. *Diabetes* 1995; **44**:506–12.

51. Damm P, Vestergaard H, Kühl C, Pedersen O. Impaired insulin-stimulated nonoxidative glucose metabolism in glucose-tolerant women with previous gestational diabetes. *Am J Obstet Gynecol* 1996; **174**:722–9.

52. Kautzky-Willer A, Prager R, Waldhausl W et al. Pronounced insulin resistance and inadequate beta-cell

secretion characterize lean gestational diabetes during and after pregnancy. *Diabetes Care* 1997; **20**:1717–23.

53. Ward WK, Johnston CLW, Beard JC et al. Abnormalities of islet B-cell function, insulin action, and fat distribution in women with histories of gestational diabetes: relationship to obesity. *J Clin Endocrinol Metab* 1985; **61**:1039–45.

54. Catalano PM, Tyzbir ED, Wolfe RR et al. Carbohydrate metabolism during pregnancy in control subjects and women with gestational diabetes. *Am J Physiol* 1993; **264**:E60–E67.

55. Damm P. Gestational diabetes mellitus and subsequent development of overt diabetes mellitus – a clinical, metabolic and epidemiological study. *Danish Med Bull* 1998; **45**:495–509.

56. Byrne MM, Sturis J, O'Meara NM, Polonsky KS. Insulin secretion in insulin-resistant women with a history of gestational diabetes. *Metabolism* 1995; **44**:1067–73.

57. Amos AF, McCarty DJ, Zimmet P. The rising global burden of diabetes and its complications: estimates and projections to the year 2010. *Diabet Med* 1997; **14 (Suppl 5)**:S1–S85.

58. Harris, MI, Klein R, Welborn TA, Knuiman MW. Onset of NIDDM occurs at least 4–7 yr before clinical diagnosis. *Diabetes Care* 1992; **15**:815–19.

59. Kjos SL, Buchanan TA, Greenspoon JS et al. Gestational diabetes mellitus: the prevalence of glucose intolerance and diabetes mellitus in the first two months post partum. *Am J Obstet Gynecol* 1990; **163**:93–8.

60. Eriksson, KF, Lindgärde F. Prevention of Type 2 (non-insulin-dependent) diabetes mellitus by diet and physical exercise. *Diabetologia* 1991; **34**:891–8.

61. Pan XR, Li GW, Hu YH et al. Effects of diet and exercise in preventing NIDDM in people with impaired glucose tolerance. *Diabetes Care* 1997; **20**:537–44.

62. Tuomilehto J, Lindstrom J, Eriksson JG et al. Prevention of type 2 diabetes mellitus by changes in lifestyle among subjects with impaired glucose tolerance. *N Engl J Med* 2001; **344**:1390–2.

63. Knowler WC, Barrett-Connor E, Fowler SE et al. Reduction in the incidence of type 2 diabetes with lifestyle intervention or metformin. *N Engl J Med* 2002; **346**:393–403.

64. Buchanan TA, Xiang AH, Peters RK et al. Response of pancreatic β-cells to improved insulin sensitivity in women at high risk for type 2 diabetes. *Diabetes* 2000; **49**:782–8.

65. Pettitt DJ, Knowler WC, Baird HR, Bennett PH. Gestational diabetes: infant and maternal complications of pregnancy in relation to third-trimester glucose tolerance in the Pima Indians. *Diabetes Care* 1980; **3**:458–64.

66. Berne C, Dimeny E. A follow-up study of women with gestational diabetes mellitus. In: (Weiss PAM, ed.) *Kohlenhydratstoffwechslungen und schwangerschaft.* (Verlag Wilhelm Maudrich: Wien, 1987) 282–7.

67. Ali Z, Alexis SD. Occurence of diabetes mellitus after gestational diabetes in Trinidad. *Diabetes Care* 1990; **13:** 527–9.

68. Dornhorst A, Bailey PC, Anyaoku V et al. Abnormalities of glucose tolerance following gestational diabetes. *Q J Med* 1990; **284:**1219–28.

16

Nutrient delivery and metabolism in the fetus
William W Hay

Introduction

Fetuses of diabetic mothers have markedly different growth rates and develop considerably different body compositions. Fetuses of poorly controlled diabetics who have wide swings in meal-associated plasma concentrations of glucose and fatty acids tend to be macrosomic, with large amounts of subcutaneous adipose tissue. In contrast, severely diabetic pregnant women, particularly those with vascular disorders and hypertension, frequently produce smaller placentae that transfer fewer nutrients to the fetus; their fetuses tend to be growth restricted and relatively devoid of body fat. To appreciate how such disparate patterns of growth can occur, it is important to understand the basic aspects of nutrient transport to the fetus. In the following discussion, data from a variety of animal models, principally sheep, are used to augment and support the more limited information from humans.

Nutrients for the fetus

The principal metabolic nutrients in the fetus are glucose and amino acids. Glucose (including its metabolic product lactate) serves as the principal substrate in the fetus for maintenance energy production and expenditure, energy storage in glycogen and adipose tissue, and the energy requirements of protein synthesis and growth. Amino acids, while primarily providing the structural basis for protein synthesis and growth, also serve as oxidative substrates for energy production. Fatty acids are also taken up by the fetus, where they are primarily used for structural components of membranes and for growth of adipose tissue. In humans, fatty acid oxidation occurs readily after birth, even in preterm infants, indicating that the lack of marked fatty acid oxidation in the fetus is primarily due to the ready supply and oxidation of glucose, lactate, and amino acids. Hormonal regulation of metabolic substrate utilization and growth in the fetus, including the effects of insulin and the insulin-like growth factors (IGF), is important but secondary to the supply of nutrient substrates.[1–5]

Role of the placenta in nutrient transfer to the fetus

The placenta plays a key role in nutrient transfer to the fetus. The placenta contains membrane transporter proteins for glucose, lactate and fatty acids that facilitate their transport to the fetus by concentration gradients. The placenta also actively concentrates and then transfers amino acids to the fetal plasma, processes aided by the unique positioning of specific amino acid transporter proteins and systems on the maternal-facing and fetal-facing trophoblast membranes. The placenta also consumes nutrient substrates at a very high metabolic rate, producing part of the transplacental nutrient substrate gradient for glucose and fatty acids, as well as specific metabolic products of glucose, lipid and amino acid metabolism that then provide a unique fetal plasma nutrient milieu. Placental–fetal metabolic interaction, in which certain substrates transported directly to the fetus by the placenta are then metabolized into products for both fetal and, in turn, placental metabolism, also provides a unique fetal nutrient metabolic milieu and tissue/organ-specific metabolic pathways.[1–5]

Nutrient supply and fetal metabolic rate

Estimates of carbon supply to the fetus are compared with requirements for energy production and storage in Table 16.1.[5–7] The fetal glucose/oxygen metabolic quotient, an index of that fraction of fetal oxygen consumption that could be accounted for by complete oxidation of glucose uptake and utilization, is < 1.0.[5] Furthermore, the fraction of fetal glucose utilization that actually produces CO_2 is only c. 0.5–0.6[8] (Table 16.2).[8] Thus, carbon substrates other than glucose are required to meet the oxidative requirements imposed by the rate of fetal oxygen consumption; these include lactate and amino acids principally, as there is little evidence for fatty acid oxidation in the fetus.

	Carbon (gram/kg/day)	Calories (kcal/kg/day)
Requirement		
Accretion in carcass: non-fat (human)	3.2	32
Accretion in carcass: fat (human)	3.5	33
Excretion as CO_2	4.4	0
Excretion as urea	0.2	2
Excretion as glutamate	0.3	2
Heat (measured as O_2 consumption)	0.0	50
Total	**11.6**	**119**
Uptake		
Amino acids	3.9	45
Glucose	3.7	26
Lactate	1.7	21
Fatty acids	1.1–2.2	17–34
Total	**10.4–11.5**	**109–126**

Table 16.1. Estimated human fetal nutrient substrate balance in late gestation (adapted from Battaglia and Meschia,[5] Hay[6] and Sparks et al[7]).

Substrate	Oxidation fraction	Carbon for oxidation (mmol/minute/kg)	Fraction of fetal VO_2
Glucose	0.55	0.09	0.29
Lactate	0.72	0.14	0.50
Amino acids	0.30	0.03	0.09
Total	–	–	0.88

* Estimates derived from data in fetal sheep in late gestation.

Table 16.2. *Fetal carbon substrate oxidation in relation to fetal oxygen consumption (VO_2) (from Battaglia and Meschia,[5] Hay et al,[8,12] Sparks et al[10] and Meznarich et al[11])**

At markedly reduced rates of glucose supply to the fetus, fetal glucose utilization rates decrease proportionally.[8,9] Under such short-term conditions (hours to days), fetal oxygen consumption remains near normal, indicating active reciprocal oxidation of other substrates, such as glucose released from glycogen, lactate, amino acids, fatty acids and ketoacids.[10–12] Over longer periods of reduced glucose supply (> 2 weeks), fetal oxygen consumption tends to decrease by up to 25–30%. Because the rate of fetal growth decreases at the same time and to the same extent, the reduction in fetal oxygen consumption with prolonged nutrient deficiency and decreased fetal growth probably represents the oxidative requirements of the decreased protein synthetic rate.

Similar to nutrient deprivation, excess delivery of nutrients to the fetus, such as with experimental glucose infusion into the fetus or mother, decreases amino acid oxidation, but has little effect on fetal metabolic rate. A maximal increase of *c.* 15% has been observed in fetal sheep infused directly with glucose. The balance of excess glucose consumption under these conditions maximizes glycogen stores and, in those fetuses that can produce abundant fat such as the human, augments the growth of adipose tissue. There is little evidence that excess amino acids enhance the growth of lean body mass or linear growth. Thus, fetuses of diabetic mothers tend primarily to be macrosomic (i.e. obese).

Fetal carbohydrate supply and metabolism

The rate of glucose transfer from maternal to fetal plasma and the net rate of fetal glucose uptake are directly related to the maternal glucose concentration (Fig. 16.1a).[13] Fetal growth rate, glycogen deposition, and fat production and storage in adipose tissue also are directly related to fetal glucose supply and uptake. Thus, it is not surprising that fetuses of hyperglycemic, diabetic mothers tend to contain more hepatic and muscle glycogen and body fat than do fetuses of more normally glycemic mothers, whether they are diabetic or not. In contrast to the direct relationship between maternal glucose concentration and uterine and fetal glucose uptake rates, the partition of uterine glucose uptake into fetal and utero-placental glucose uptakes is separately regulated by fetal glucose concentration (Fig. 16.1a).[13,14] A relatively higher fetal glucose concentration will diminish placental-to-fetal glucose transfer in favor of placental glucose consumption, while a relatively lower fetal glucose concentration will

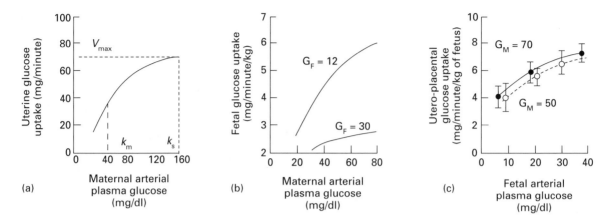

Figure 16.1. *(a) Schematic representation of effect of maternal glucose concentration on uterine glucose uptake, based on experiments in which glucose was infused into pregnant sheep after an overnight fast to produce a large variety of maternal arterial blood glucose concentrations. Fick's principle measurements were then made of net uterine glucose uptake rates versus the maternal arterial blood glucose concentration, which shows saturation kinetics with an approximate k_m value in the physiological range of maternal glucose concentration (c. 50–60 mg/dl) (adapted from Hay et al[13]). (b) Fetal glucose uptake (net transfer of glucose from placenta to fetal circulation) plotted against maternal arterial glucose concentration showing a saturable dependence of fetal glucose uptake on maternal glucose concentration. In addition, this relationship is left-shifted as the fetal glucose concentration is decreased, showing that as the fetal glucose concentration decreases relative to that of the mother, which increases the maternal–fetal glucose concentration gradient, placental-to-fetal glucose transfer increases, (adapted from Hay et al[14]). (c) Net rate of utero-placental glucose consumption in sheep, expressed per kilogram of fetus, plotted against fetal arterial plasma glucose. Solid line, values measured while maternal arterial plasma glucose was clamped at c. 70 mg/dl; dashed line, values measured while maternal arterial plasma glucose was clamped at c. 50 mg/dl. These data show that although the maternal glucose concentration determines glucose entry into the utero-placenta and fetus, actual utero-placental glucose consumption is regulated largely by the fetal glucose concentration (adapted from Hay et al[14]). (Reproduced with permission from Hay.[35])*

limit placental glucose consumption and enhance transfer of glucose into the fetal plasma. The concentration of glucose in the fetal plasma declines relative to that in the maternal plasma over the second half of gestation. This increases the transplacental glucose concentration gradient in later gestation, providing a greater driving force to supply glucose for the increasing glucose requirements of the growing fetus.[15] The decrease in fetal glucose concentration over the second half of gestation represents an absolute increase in glucose clearance. At least three principal mechanisms are responsible for this increase in glucose clearance: the size, cellularity

and glucose metabolic rate of the brain increases relative to other fetal tissues and organs; there is progressive development of fetal insulin secretion by the expanding mass of pancreatic islets and beta cells; finally, there is increased growth of insulin-sensitive tissues, primarily skeletal muscle, but also the heart and adipose tissue.

Placental glucose transport

Glucose transporters

Placental glucose uptake and transfer are mediated by Na^+-dependent transport systems on both the maternal-facing microvillous and fetal-facing basal plasma membranes of the syncytiotrophoblast.[16–18] The predominant molecular isoforms of glucose transporters (GLUT) in the placenta are GLUT1 and GLUT3. GLUT1 is localized in both microvillous and basal plasma membranes of the syncytiotrophoblast, as well as endothelial cells[19–23] and the amnion.[24] Expression of the higher affinity GLUT3 isoform in the human placenta is controversial; its mRNA has been demonstrated in high levels, but GLUT3 protein has been found in variable abundance among studies.[25] Participation of GLUT3 in glucose uptake and transport has not been confirmed, although in sheep placenta, cytochalasian binding assays indicate that GLUT3 might account for as much as 40% of glucose uptake by the end of gestation.[26] Despite considerable study, the regulation of placental glucose transporter expression and activity remain poorly defined.[27–32] Placental GLUT1 is acutely upregulated by hypoxia and hyperglycemia, while hypoglycemia leads to downregulation. Chronic changes in glycemia generally are associated with diminished expression. *In vitro* studies indicate that changes in GLUT concentrations are related to transport capacity, but this has not been demonstrated *in vivo*, except in experiments in which the transporters were competitively blocked by pharmacologic inhibitors.

Kinetics of glucose uptake and transport by the placenta

Although the effect of the maternal glucose concentration on net placental-to-fetal glucose transfer demonstrates saturation kinetics,[13] this relationship does not necessarily define the quantitative characteristics of placental-to-fetal glucose transport capacity, because as maternal glucose concentration and placental glucose transport are increased, both fetal glucose concentration and the utilization rate

increase. Other studies in which glucose was infused directly into the fetus have shown degrees of increase (slope) and saturation of fetal glucose utilization rates occurring at about the same fetal glucose concentrations as determined by maternal glucose infusions.[33] Thus, the maternal glucose infusion approach reflects fetal glucose consumption kinetics as well as those of placental-to-fetal glucose transfer. To address this experimental problem, different studies have used glucose clamp procedures to regulate the maternal-to-fetal glucose concentration gradient at different maternal and fetal glucose concentrations.[34] As shown in Fig. 16.1b, placental-to-fetal glucose transfer is sensitive to a change in fetal glucose concentration, regardless of the maternal glucose level.[35]

Thus, at almost any maternal glucose concentration utero-placental glucose consumption is directly related to the fetal glucose concentration (Fig. 16.1c). In fact, when the transplacental glucose concentration is abolished, *c.* 75% of the glucose consumed by the utero-placenta is supplied by the fetal circulation.[5] These observations imply that the fetal side of the utero-placenta is markedly more permeable to glucose than the maternal side. They also indicate that changes in the fetal glucose concentration have a strong influence on placental glucose flux and metabolism. The importance of this regulation of placental-to-fetal glucose transfer and net utero-placental glucose consumption by fetal glucose concentration is highlighted by observations in chronically hypoglycemic pregnant sheep in which fetal glucogenesis developed.[15,36] This rate of fetal glucose production contributes glucose molecules to the fetal glucose pool and sustains fetal glucose utilization at near-normal rates. As a result, the placental-to-fetal glucose concentration gradient and the placental-to-fetal glucose transfer rate are relatively reduced; under these circumstances, utero-placental glucose consumption is maintained at near-normal rates for the level of maternal glycemia. Fetal glucose production can compensate for a reduced maternal glucose supply and sustain placental as well as fetal glucose utilization requirements.

Several other placental factors may affect placental glucose transport, including placental surface area, thickness of the various cell and tissue layers between the maternal and fetal plasma, rates of uterine and umbilical blood flow, and the placental glucose consumption rate. The effect of changes of placental thickness on glucose transport has not been studied, but there appears to be a direct relation between the maternal-to-fetal arterial glucose gradient and the amount of intervening placental and vascular tissue layers.[37] Whether such tissue layers increase the gradient by glucose consumption or by imposing a barrier to transport, or both, is not known.

Gestational changes in placental glucose transfer

Placental glucose transport increases markedly over gestation. In sheep, the increase in transport capacity accounts for c. 60% of the increase in placental glucose transport, with an increase in the transplacental glucose concentration gradient accounting for the remaining 40%.[38] This increased transport capacity most likely reflects the growth of the surface area of the trophoblast and increased numbers of glucose transporters.[26–28] It has not been determined if an increase in trophoblast membrane glucose transporter concentrations occurs as well. The regulation of this developmental increase in glucose transporter abundance, other than by remodeling of the trophoblast membrane surface area, is not known.

Fetal glucose uptake and utilization

Glucose utilization rate in near-term fetal sheep is c. 5–7 mg/minute/kg.[39] This value is similar to those measured in term human newborn infants using stable isotope tracer methodology,[40] and is about half the value that occurs at mid-gestation in fetal sheep[9] when fetal growth, protein turnover and fractional synthetic rates also are about twice those closer to term. The high correlation between fetal glucose utilization and growth rates indicates that glucose probably serves a major role as the energy supply for the protein synthesis required for growth. Indeed, fetal growth restriction is directly related to glucose deprivation.[41] Table 16.3 presents estimated utilization rates of glucose in several fetal organs and the remaining carcass of fetal sheep in late gestation. All organs are dependent on the plasma glucose concentration for their specific rate of glucose uptake, while skeletal muscle, heart and liver develop insulin sensitivity in later gestation. It still is not known to what extent basal insulin concentration affects glucose uptake by specific organs and tissues in the fetus. However, an acute decrease in the fetal plasma insulin concentration (studies in fetal sheep), such as by somatostatin infusion, does not affect measurements of the fetal glucose utilization rate. These procedures do, however, lead to an increase in the fetal glucose concentration. Thus, the basal plasma insulin concentration in the fetus appears to regulate glucose production but not utilization, the latter is more under the control of the plasma glucose concentration.

Fetal glucose transporters

GLUT1 is found throughout the fetal tissues and on all endothelial cells, and probably accounts for the majority of basal tissue

	Glucose utilization rate (mg/minute/kg fetus)	Percentage of total
Whole fetus (sheep, measured)	5.0	100
Whole fetus (human, estimated)	6.0–8.0	100
Brain (sheep, measured)	0.8	16
Brain (human, estimated)	4.0	50–67
Heart (sheep, measured)	0.65	13
Lungs (sheep, estimated)	0.1	2
Liver (sheep, measured)	0.1	2
Red blood cells (human, estimated)	0.1	2
Gut (sheep, estimated)	?	?
Carcass/skeletal muscle (estimated, sheep)	3.25	65
Total of organs accounted for		
Sheep	5.0	100
Human	8.2	103–137

* Based on data in fetal sheep and estimates for human fetuses for brain.

Table 16.3. Metabolic rates in the fetus that account for glucose utilization (adapted from Battaglia and Meschia,[5] Hay[6] and Sparks et al[7]).

glucose uptake from the fetal plasma. GLUT4 is found in the heart, adipose tissue and skeletal muscle. In the fetal sheep, the GLUT1 protein concentration is upregulated by hypoglycemia and hypoinsulinemia in skeletal muscle and adipose tissue, while there is no change in the brain.[42] In contrast, hyperglycemia appears to downregulate GLUT1 protein concentrations in most tissues.[43–46] Insulin-responsive GLUT4 protein is upregulated by hypoglycemia,[42] but in response to hyperglycemia it is initially upregulated and then downregulated towards normal, or to less than normal, levels in skeletal muscle and adipose tissue.[47,48] Acute hyperinsulinemia decreases the fetal glucose concentration and increases the whole fetal glucose utilization rate,[8] but it has been difficult to demonstrate in which organs this increased glucose utilization rate takes place. Hyperinsulinemia also appears to have acute effects on increasing protein

concentrations for both GLUT1 and GLUT4.[47,48] In humans, there is considerable evidence for insulin lowering the plasma glucose concentration in the preterm and term newborn. The principal action of insulin in the human fetus, however, is to promote lipid formation and deposition in adipose tissue. In this situation, substrate supply (glucose, fatty acids and triglycerides, and glycerol) probably is as, or is more than, important as insulin itself. Different studies among species, tissues studied, gestational ages, and conditions of glycemia and insulinemia show considerable variability and complexity of changes in glucose transporter concentrations during fetal life.[49]

Kinetics of the glucose utilization rate in the fetus

The capacity for glucose utilization in the human fetus can only be estimated from measurements in prematurely born infants or in animal models such as the sheep. In preterm humans, doubling or even tripling of glucose utilization rate (GUR) from basal is possible.[50] GUR in fetal sheep follows Michaelis–Menten kinetics,[8] and is relatively limited to a doubling of basal GUR. This capacity is variable, however, as increased entry of glucose into the fetal plasma from the placenta increases fetal glucose concentration and insulin secretion, which, in turn, augments fetal glucose utilization, thus limiting further increases in the fetal glucose concentration.[51,52] Glucose and insulin clamp experiments in fetal sheep, in which glucose or insulin or both are infused until GUR reaches maximal rates, have shown that plasma glucose and insulin concentrations act independently (i.e. additively) to increase glucose utilization and oxidation.[8] Furthermore, while both glucose and insulin enhance fetal GUR according to saturation kinetics, it is not known how this effect is partitioned among different fetal organs. Despite wide changes in glucose utilization, the relative proportion of glucose oxidized during short-term 3–4-hour studies – c. 55% – does not change significantly over the entire range of glucose utilized. Furthermore, because oxygen consumption, and thus the fetal metabolic rate, do not vary significantly, if at all, under these circumstances, oxidation of other carbon substrates, such as amino acids and lactate, must increase in compensation. Indeed, acute hypoglycemia in fetal sheep leads to a near doubling of the rate of leucine oxidation relative to the rate of leucine disposal from the plasma.[53] In the human fetus, glucose and/or insulin may promote lipogenesis more than oxidation. This may occur because the human fetus naturally produces adipose tissue in late gestation, similar to adult humans in whom higher rates of glucose utilization are partitioned more into glucose storage in adipose tissue fat than into oxidation. Glucose carbon also contributes significantly to the formation of glycogen, which is stored primarily in skeletal muscle, but also in the heart,

liver and lung, and to the carbon contained in amino acids and synthesized proteins.

In contrast to the acute effect of increased fetal plasma insulin concentrations to increase fetal glucose utilization and decrease fetal plasma glucose concentrations, an acute decrease of fetal plasma insulin concentration, for example, with somatostatin infusion, does not appear to affect the fetal glucose concentration or glucose utilization.[54] It is possible that the decrease in insulin concentration allows fetal glucose production to develop under these conditions, which would limit glucose transfer to the fetus from the placenta, preventing a measurable increase in fetal glucose concentration. A chronic decrease of fetal plasma insulin concentration, however, either by pancreatectomy or streptozotocin injection (a drug that leads to destruction of the pancreatic beta cells) into the fetus,[55–57] results in an increased fetal plasma glucose concentration. As discussed above, fetal hyperglycemia decreases placental to fetal glucose transfer. Chronic hyperglycemia in fetal sheep is also associated with decreased peripheral tissue insulin sensitivity and glucose utilization capacity,[58] as well as the potential release of insulin's normal inhibition of hepatic glucose production.

As a result of chronic fetal glucose deprivation, from whatever cause, fetal growth rate diminishes; the insulin concentration is reduced in hypoglycemic, glucose-deprivation conditions, and placental-to-fetal glucose transfer is reduced as a result of fetal hyperglycemia. These results indicate that the predominant growth-regulating effect of insulin in the fetus is its capacity to enhance glucose utilization, not just to independently and directly affect protein synthesis, breakdown and net balance, even though such processes clearly are positively regulated with acute increases in the fetal plasma insulin concentration. Examples of

Acute: mild–moderate
  Hyperglycemia
  Increased insulin production, secretion and hyperinsulinemia
  Increased glucose utilization and oxygen consumption
  Mild arterial hypoxemia
  Increased placental lactate production, and fetal lactate uptake and utilization

Acute: severe
  Increased fetal oxygen consumption
  Arterial hypoxemia and metabolic acidosis
  Decreased placental perfusion leading to fetal demise

Chronic
  Decreased insulin secretion and/or synthesis if hyperglycemia is marked and constant
  Increased insulin secretion and/or synthesis if hyperglycemia is variable
  Increased ratio of placental glucose consumption to placental glucose transfer
  Increased erythropoietin production

Box 16.1. Fetal responses to increased glucose supply (adapted from Hay[1]).

metabolic effects of increased glucose supply to the fetus are shown in Box 16.1.[1]

Fetal insulin secretion

Glucose-stimulated fetal insulin secretion (measured as an acute increase in fetal plasma insulin concentration) increases more than fivefold during the second half of gestation in fetal sheep.[59,60] Similar results appear to occur in human fetuses, derived from studies of human fetal islets *in vitro* and insulin secretion in preterm infants.[61] Fetal insulin secretion can also be modified by the degree, duration and pattern of changes in the fetal plasma glucose concentration. Experiments in fetal sheep,[62] for example, have shown that sustained, marked, relatively constant hyperglycemia actually decreases fetal insulin secretion. Similar results have been obtained in studies in rats.[63,64] Such observations contrast with the fetuses of gestational diabetic women in whom hyperglycemia stimulates fetal insulin secretion.[65] Insulin secretion is augmented in gestational diabetic women in whom there is a strong tendency to develop increasingly

exaggerated, meal-associated hyperglycemia in late gestation,[66] and in fetal sheep whose mothers received intermittent, pulsatile boluses of glucose intravenously.[67] Thus, a principal cause of enhanced fetal insulin secretion is variability in the magnitude and the intermittent nature of fetal glucose concentration. Fatty acids also stimulate fetal insulin secretion; their concentrations are increased in pregnant diabetics and in their fetuses in late gestation, perhaps contributing to augmented insulin secretion.[66] Acute and chronic hypoglycemia, and probably hypoaminocidemia as well, diminish fetal insulin secretion.[54] Responsible mechanisms are not known, although presumably glucose activates insulin gene response elements, and both glucose and amino acids are necessary to develop mechanisms that regulate insulin secretion from the beta cell. Recent studies in rats and sheep indicate that low protein diets in the mother, fetal amino acid deficiency, chronic fetal hypoglycemia and intrauterine fetal growth restriction might decrease fetal insulin secretion by decreased growth of the endocrine pancreas.[68,69]

Effect of other hormones on fetal glucose metabolism

Fetal thyroid hormone indirectly enhances fetal glucose utilization by increasing the fetal metabolic rate (oxygen consumption).[70] Changes in fetal plasma cortisol concentrations during late gestation have little effect on fetal glucose concentrations or on the rates of glucose utilization.[71] However, fetal plasma cortisol concentrations do increase in very late gestation, at which time cortisol-dependent increases in fetal hepatic glycogenolytic and gluconeogenic enzyme activities develop. These may enhance the glucogenic capacity of the fetus, thereby contributing to the endogenous glucose production observed in normal fetuses just before term and at the time of delivery.[72] Glucagon and circulating catecholamines (adrenal epinephrine and spillover norepinephrine from peripheral nerve endings) are normally present in modest concentrations in the fetal plasma, but they do stimulate fetal glucogenesis when infused into the fetus. Catecholamines promote glucose production at physiological levels,[73] but glucagon must reach relatively high concentrations in the fetal plasma to do this.[74]

Insulin, IGF and other growth factors

Acute changes in fetal plasma IGF-I concentrations appears to have little or no acute effect on fetal glucose kinetics.[75] Glucose does, however, act at the transcriptional level to regulate the production and plasma concentrations of both IGF-I and -II.[76] Plasma insulin also independently promotes IGF-I synthesis.[76,77] These observations indicate that the intracellular supply and/or concentration of glucose, which is controlled by both plasma glucose and insulin concentrations, can regulate fetal IGF-I production. In turn, increased plasma IGF-I concentrations can inhibit protein breakdown,[77] as does insulin,[78]

although this effect of IGF-I occurs primarily at higher glucose concentrations. Thus, both insulin and IGF-I indirectly enhance the capacity for glucose to promote the fetal nitrogen balance and growth. In fetal sheep, an acute increase in the fetal insulin concentration activates proteins in the mitogen activated protein (MAP) kinase cascade but glucose does not, indicating that insulin might have independent and direct effects on stimulating protein synthesis, cell growth and cell replication.[79] Similarly, acutely increased insulin concentrations in fetal sheep promote amino acid utilization and net nitrogen balance.[80] Such effects are probably short-lived, in that chronic infusions of insulin do not increase growth of lean tissues very much; instead, they contribute more to enhancing lipid production and storage in adipose tissue. In humans, as in experimental animal models, there is considerable evidence of insulin lowering plasma glucose concentrations: in humans, this occurs in the preterm as well as the term newborn. The principal action of insulin in the human fetus, however, is to promote lipid formation and deposition in adipose tissue. In this situation, substrate supplies (glucose, fatty acids and triglycerides, and glycerol) probably are as or more important than insulin itself.

Fetal glucose carbon contribution to glycogen formation

Many fetal tissues, including the placenta, as well as the brain, liver, lung, heart and skeletal muscle, produce glycogen over the second half of gestation.[81] Liver glycogen content increases with gestational age (Fig. 16.2) and is the most important store of glycogen for systemic glucose needs, because only the liver contains sufficient glucose-6-phosphatase for release of glucose into the circulation.[82] Skeletal muscle glycogen content increases during late gestation, whereas lung glycogen content decreases with loss of glycogen-

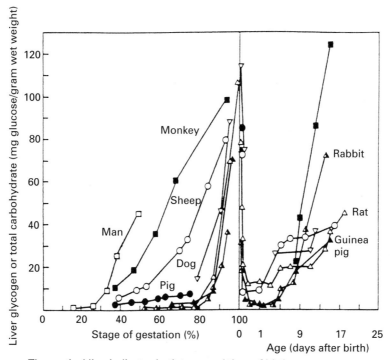

The vertical line indicates both term and time of birth.
□ Man (Szendi, 1936; Villee, 1954)
■ Rhesus monkey (Shelley, 1960; and unpublished data)
○ Sheep (Shelley, 1960)
● Pig (Mendel & Leavenworth, 1907; McCance & Widdowson, 1959)
▽ Dog (Demant, 1887; Schlossmann, 1938)
△ Rat (Stuart & Higgins, 1935; Martinek & Mikulas, 1954; Jacquot, 1955; Stafford & Weatherall, 1960)
▲ Rabbit (Szendi, 1936; Jost & Jacquot, 1955; Shelley, unpublished)
▲ Guinea-pig (Aron, 1922; Shelley, unpublished)

Figure 16.2. *Liver glycogen in various species before and after birth. Hepatic glycogen content in several species is shown to increase again with gestational age, decrease precipitously during the immediate postnatal period and increase again with a normal neonatal diet (from Shelly[81]).*

containing alveolar epithelium, development of type II pneumocytes and onset of surfactant production.[83] Cardiac glycogen concentrations decrease with gestation as cellular hypertrophy develops. Despite this decrease, the cardiac glycogen content is essential for postnatal cardiac energy supply and cellular function; in fact, deficits of cardiac glycogen are associated with shortened survival time during periods of anoxia.[84] Fetal glycogen synthetic rates vary from low, steady rates of accumulation in species with relatively long gestations, such as the human and sheep, to exceptionally high rates in species such as the rat that have relatively short gestations. In larger, more slow-growing fetuses (e.g. sheep, monkey, human), glycogen synthesis by the liver accounts for only a small (< 10%) portion of fetal glucose utilization.[85]

Fetal glucogenesis
Tracer studies in humans[86] and sheep[13] have shown the same specific activity or enrichment

ratio of tracer glucose to non-labeled glucose in fetal as in maternal plasma. This demonstrates that the only source of glucose in the fetus is from the maternal plasma, otherwise, new glucose production into the fetal plasma from either the fetus itself or from the placenta would dilute the tracer glucose coming from the mother along with unlabeled glucose, thus lowering the fetal enrichment ratio. Furthermore, studies in fetal sheep have shown that the net uptake of glucose by the fetus from the placenta invariably is equal to the fetal glucose utilization rate, independently measured with glucose tracers.[39,87,88] Thus, there is no evidence for fetal glucose production under normal conditions. Also, there is little if any fetal glucogenesis under the conditions of short-term (1–4 hour) changes in maternal and fetal glucose concentrations, the placental-to-fetal glucose transfer, and fetal glucose utilization rates. Measurable rates of fetal glucose production only develop significantly after prolonged periods (several days) of decreased fetal glucose supply, and sustained fetal hypoglycemia and hypoinsulinemia.[54–56,89] The capacity of the fetus to make new glucose molecules from non-glucose substrates (e.g. lactate, amino acids and glycerol) varies considerably among species. In nearly all cases this appears to be a late gestational development, augmented by cortisol activation of phosphoenolpyruvate carboxykinase, the rate-limiting step for gluconeogenesis, and glucose-6-phosphatase, the enzyme necessary for release of glucose from the liver into the circulation.[57]

Fetal lipid metabolism

Placental lipid metabolism and fetal lipid supply

The amount and type of fatty acid or complex lipid transported by the placenta varies among species. Lipid transport varies according to the transport capacity of the placenta; it is greatest in the hemochorial placenta of the human, guinea pig and rabbit, and least in the epithelio-chorial placenta of the ruminant and the endotheliochorial placenta of the carnivores.[90] There are many lipid substances in the plasma that are transported across the placenta that are essential for placental and fetal development, even if they do not contribute to nutritional or energy metabolism. Also, brown fat is common to all fetuses; it is essential for postnatal thermogenesis, even if the neonate is not 'fat' with white adipose tissue. Furthermore, many lipid substances entering the fetus are qualitatively different from those taken up by the uterus and utero-placenta, implying active placental metabolism of individual lipid substances. More complex pathways include lipoprotein dissociation by placental lipoprotein lipase activity, triglyceride uptake and metabolism (including metabolic pathways of oxidation, and chain-lengthening, synthesis and interconversion pathways), and release into the fetal plasma as free fatty acids (FFA) or lipoproteins.[91] A schema of placental lipid uptake, metabolism, transport and metabolic interaction with the fetus is shown in Fig. 16.3.[4,91]

The fetal impact of maternal plasma FFA and lipid concentrations is reflected in the fetal lipid content and adipose tissue development. Fatter human fetuses develop in pregnant women who have higher plasma concentrations of fatty acids and other lipids, particularly among women with diabetes during pregnancy. Experimentally, diabetic rats have increased FFA, and their fetuses have carcass and hepatic lipid contents that are twofold increased above normal.[92] Similarly, rabbits fed oil-rich diets show increased neonatal adipose stores.[93] In humans, umbilical venous–arterial fatty acid concentration differences in cord blood samples show that the net flux of non-esterified

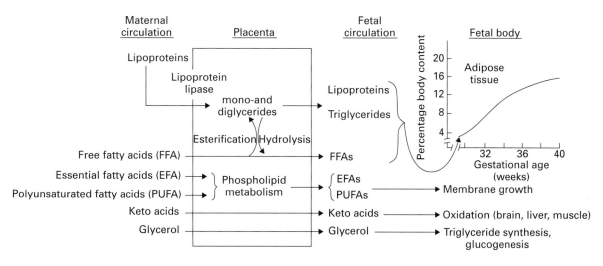

Figure 16.3. *Schematic of placental–fetal interrelationships in humans for various aspects of placental lipid metabolism, fetal lipid uptake and metabolism, and fetal lipogenesis into adipose tissue (adapted from Hay[1,4]).*

fatty acids into the fetus from the maternal circulation can account for the fetal requirement of fatty acids during the end of pregnancy.[94] Other estimates that are based on fetal lipid accumulation, as well as *in vitro* transfer experiments, estimate that as much as 50% of fetal fatty acid requirements are transferred across the human placenta.[95] Similar estimates have been made in the rat using the incorporation of ^3H from ^3H_2O into fatty acids, indicating that fatty acids are derived about equally from maternal and fetal fatty acid synthesis sources.[96] Estimates in the rabbit[97] and the monkey[98] indicate that in these species, placental fatty acid transfer across the placenta could account for all fetal fat deposition in late gestation. Overall, therefore, it appears that there is a relatively direct relationship between the permeability of the placenta to lipids, especially fatty acids, and the adiposity of the fetus at term. Human fetuses develop the most fat (15–18% of body weight at term), guinea pigs are second at *c.* 12%, rabbits third at *c.* 7%, and the sheep, because there appears to practi-

cally no fatty acid transfer except for essential fatty acids across the ovine placenta, only *c.* 3% (Fig. 16.4).

Fetal lipid metabolism

Physiological changes that develop in the fetus in late gestation and increase nutrient utilization, such as the increase in plasma insulin concentration, act to enhance net maternal-to-fetal fatty acid and lipid transport by increasing fatty acid utilization in the fetus (largely to develop adipose tissue).[7] Increased utilization of fatty acids by fetal tissues lowers fetal plasma fatty acid concentrations relative to those in the maternal plasma and increases the maternal-to-fetal fatty acid concentration gradients. For example, human maternal venous blood concentrations of fatty acids are directly related to the umbilical artery FFA concentrations and the umbilical vein-artery concentration differences of FFA.[99] Similar observations have been made in the rabbit[97] and the guinea pig.[100] In guinea pig placentae perfused

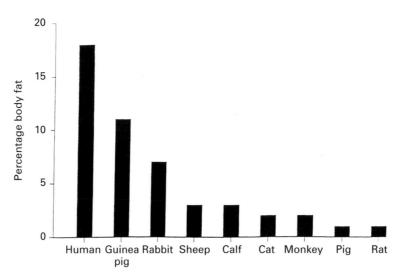

Figure 16.4. *Fetal fat content at term as a percentage of fetal body weight among species (adapted from Hay,[1,2] Battaglia and Meschia,[5] and Sparks et al.[7]*

in vitro, lowering the fatty acid concentrations in the fetal side perfusate relative to that in the maternal side perfusate independently increases fatty acid transfer across the placenta.

Placental amino acid uptake and transport to the fetus

Growth of placental amino acid transport capacity

As pregnancy advances, the increasing protein synthetic and nitrogen balance demands of the growing fetus are met by an appropriate increase in placental amino acid transport. This enhanced transport is facilitated by increases in placental perfusion, trophoblast membrane exchange area, transporter concentrations in the trophoblast membranes and alterations in trophoblast membrane potential differences. Some amino acid transport systems also increase their transport activity over gestation.[101–105] Vectoral transport of amino acids from maternal to fetal plasma is further aided by adding transporter activity at the microvillous maternal-facing membrane that increases placental amino acid uptake, and by adding transporter activity at the basal fetal-facing membrane that facilitates transport of amino acids into the fetal plasma.

Fetal amino acid uptake

Amino acids are actively concentrated in the trophoblast intracellular matrix by Na^+/K^+-adenosine triphosphate-(ATP)ase-F and H^+-dependent transporter proteins at the maternal-facing microvillous membrane of the trophoblast and then transported into the fetal plasma producing fetal–maternal plasma concentration ratios ranging from 1.0 to > 5.0.[106] This active transport process is decreased by hypoxia and inhibitors of protein synthesis,[107,108] while hypoaminoacidemia increases transport, indicating that synthesis of the transporters is in part responsible for their functional state.[109] Peptide uptake has also been observed. For example, protein molecules as small as albumin and as large as gamma-globulin pass from maternal to fetal plasma by pinocytosis with increasing efficiency as gestational age progresses.[110] This additional amount of protein probably provides little nutritional value, as shown by studies in the fetal lamb in which total amino nitrogen uptake is not different from the total amino nitrogen uptake in the form of amino acids.

Additional studies in sheep show that net total fetal amino acid uptake can account for up to 30–40% of the combined carbon requirements for oxidative metabolism and deposition in fetal protein, glycogen and fat, as well as providing 100% of the fetal nitrogen requirements.[111,112] The placenta and fetus also interact in a variety of ways to ensure amino acid supply to a large and complex set of vital developmental, metabolic and signaling processes that are unique to fetal growth and development (Fig. 16.5).[6]

Fetal amino acid metabolism

Fetal amino acid oxidation

Evidence for a relatively high rate of fetal oxidation of amino acids comes from three

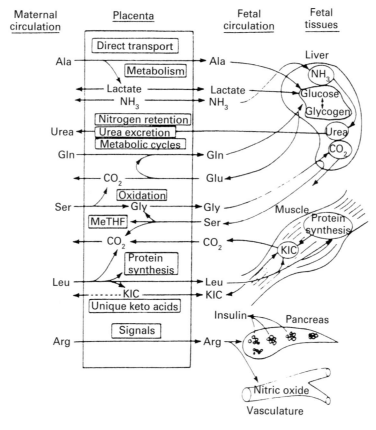

Figure 16.5. *Schematic representation of a variety of placental–fetal metabolic interactions with respect to amino acid uptake by the placenta, metabolism in the trophoblast cells, direct transfer to the fetus, signaling of fetal vascular and metabolic processes, and utilization in fetal tissues. Ala, alanine; Gln, glutamine; Glu, glutamate; Ser, serine; Gly, glycine; Leu, leucine; KIC, α-ketoisocaproic acid; Arg, arginine; MeTHF, methyltetrahydrofolate; NH₃, ammonia, (Adapted from Hay.[4,6])*

observations: amino acids are taken up by the fetus in excess of their rate of deposition in fetal protein;[111] fetal urea production rates are quite high;[113] fetal infusions of carbon-labeled amino acids have produced fetal production and excretion of labeled carbon dioxide.[114] The urea production rate in fetal sheep can account for c. 0.46 gram/day/kg of nitrogen excretion, which is c. 25% of fetal nitrogen uptake in amino acids. This magnitude of urea production also can account for up to c. 0.2 gram/day/kg of carbon, equal to c. 2% of total fetal carbon uptake and representing c. 6% of fetal carbon uptake in amino acids.[115] Such fetal urea production rates are large, exceeding neonatal and adult weight-specific rates, indicating relatively rapid protein turnover and oxidation in the fetus. Direct measurement of fetal amino acid oxidation has been made using carbon-labeled isotopic tracers of selected amino acids, including leucine, lysine, alanine, tyrosine, glycine, and serine.[115] Oxidation rates have been calculated for leucine (c. 25% of utilization), lysine (c. 10% of utilization) and glycine (c. 13% of utilization). The studies also demonstrate that the fetal oxidation–disposal rate ratio is directly related to the excess umbilical uptake of these amino acids above that required for protein accretion and to the plasma concentration of the amino acid.[111,116]

Fetal protein synthesis and turnover

The net umbilical uptakes of several non-essential amino acids are less than their total rate of utilization, emphasizing the need for a relatively high rate of fetal amino acid production.[113] Protein synthetic rates also are quite high. Fractional protein synthetic rate (k_S) and fractional growth rate (k_G) in fetal sheep have been compared using two tracers, ^{14}C-leucine

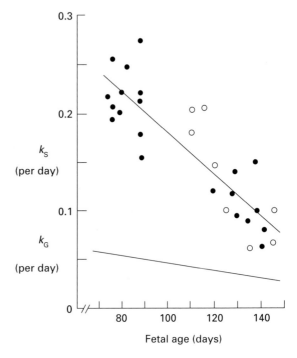

Figure 16.6.   *Fractional rate of protein synthesis (k_S) over gestation in fetal sheep studied with leucine (●) and lysine (○) radioactive tracers compared with the fractional rate of growth (k_G) in the lower portion of the figure (——) (adapted from Battaglia and Meschia,[5] Meier et al[116] and Kennaugh et al[117])*

and ^{14}C-lysine, at different gestational ages (Fig. 16.6).[116,117] The higher protein synthetic rate in the mid-gestation fetus is proportional to the higher metabolic rate and glucose utilization rate at that stage of gestation. Thus, protein synthesis per millimole of oxygen consumed is quite constant from mid-gestation until term.[118] The same appears to be true for the relationship between protein synthesis and glucose consumption.[119] The reduction in the protein synthetic rate over gestation is also related to the changing proportion of body mass contributed by the major organs. For example, the body-weight-specific mass of skeletal muscle, which has a relatively lower k_S increases more than other organs in late gestation, which would contribute to a decrease in the whole-body k_G.[120] Many anabolic endocrine–paracrine factors, such as insulin, pituitary and placental growth hormone, placental lactogen, IGF (somatomedins), and epidermal growth factors increase in late gestation. A direct relationship with such growth factors cannot be made, however, since most studies suggest an increasing concentration or secretion of these substances over gestation.[121] Simultaneous increases in binding proteins and changes in receptor density and binding capacity also develop that interact with and regulate the action of the various growth factors, thereby modulating their direct effects on promoting protein synthesis and cell growth.

Fetal skeletal muscle amino acid metabolism

Skeletal muscle in the fetal sheep takes up both essential and non-essential amino acids from the circulation,[122] reflecting the relatively high rate of protein synthesis and nitrogen accretion of the fetus. Under hyperinsulinemic conditions, in which glucose and amino acids are also infused to maintain normal concentrations, net uptake of most amino acids by skeletal muscle increases, reflecting reduced rates of proteolysis more than increased rates of protein synthesis. Protein synthesis is more strongly regulated by the plasma concentration of amino acids than by insulin alone. IGF-I acts similarly to insulin. Glucose utilization also increases the net protein balance, perhaps simply by substituting its carbon for that of amino acids in the tricarboxylic acid cycle, indicating that a positive energy balance and the provision of amino acids allow insulin to promote nitrogen accretion most effectively.[123,124]

Acknowledgements

Preparation of this manuscript was supported in part by research grants HD20761, HD28794 and DK52138 (WW Hay, PI) from the National Institutes of Health.

References

1. Hay Jr WW. Nutrition and development of the fetus: carbohydrates and lipid metabolism. In: (Walker WA, Watkins JB, eds) *Nutrition in Pediatrics (Basic Science and Clinical Applications)*, 2nd edn. (Decker Europe Inc.: Neuilly-sur-Seine, France, 1996) 364–78.
2. Hay Jr WW. Energy and substrate requirements of the placenta and fetus. *Proc Nutr Soc* 1991; 50:321–36.
3. Hay Jr WW, Wilkening RB. Metabolic activity of the placenta. In: (Thorburn GD, Harding R, eds) *Textbook of Fetal Physiology*. (Oxford Medical Publications: Oxford, 1994) 30–47.
4. Hay Jr WW. Metabolic interrelationships of placenta and fetus. *Placenta* 1995; 16:19–30.
5. Battaglia FC, Meschia G. *An Introduction to Fetal Physiology*. (Academic Press: Orlando, 1986).
6. Hay Jr WW. Fetal requirements and placental transfer of nitrogenous compounds. In: (Polin RA, Fox WW, eds) *Fetal and Neonatal Physiology*. (WB Saunders Co.: Philadelphia, 1991) 431–4.
7. Sparks JW, Girard J, Battaglia FC. An estimate of the caloric requirements of the human fetus. *Biol Neonate* 1980; 38:113–19.
8. Hay Jr WW, DiGiacomo JE, Meznarich HK et al. Effects of glucose and insulin on fetal glucose oxidation and oxygen consumption. *Am J Physiol* 1989; 256:E704–E713.
9. DiGiacomo JE, Hay Jr WW. Fetal glucose metabolism and oxygen consumption during sustained maternal and fetal hypoglycemia. *Metabolism* 1990; 39:193–202.
10. Sparks JW, Hay Jr WW, Bonds D et al. Simultaneous measurements of lactate turnover rate and umbilical lactate uptake in the fetal lamb. *J Clin Invest* 1982; 70:179–92.
11. Meznarich HK, Hay Jr WW, Sparks JW et al. Fructose disposal and oxidation rates in the ovine fetus. *Q J Exp Physiol* 1987; 72:617–25.
12. Hay Jr WW, Meyers SA, Sparks JW et al. Glucose and lactate oxidation rates in the fetal lamb. *Proc Soc Exp Biol Med* 1983; 73:553–63.
13. Hay Jr WW, Meznarich HK. Effect of maternal glucose concentration on uteroplacental glucose consumption

and transfer in pregnant sheep. *Proc Soc Exp Biol Med* 1988; 190:63–9.

14. Hay Jr WW, Molina RD, DiGiacomo JE et al. Model of placental glucose consumption and transfer. *Am J Physiol* 1990; 258:R569–R577.

15. Molina RD, Meschia G, Battaglia FC et al. Maturation of placental glucose transfer capacity in the ovine pregnancy. *Am J Physiol* 1991; 261:R697–R704.

16. Ingermann RL, Bissonette JM, Koch PL. Glucose-sensitive and -insensitive cytochalasin-B binding proteins from microvillous plasma membranes of human placenta: identification of the D-glucose transporter. *Biochim Biophys Acta* 1983; 730:57–63.

17. Johnson JW, Smith CH. Glucose transport across the basal plasma membrane of human placental synctiotrophoblast. *Biochim Biophys Acta* 1985; 815:44–50.

18. Stacy TE, Weedon P, Haworth C et al. Fetomaternal transfer of glucose analogues by sheep placenta. *Am J Physiol* 1978; 234:E32–E37.

19. Johnson LW, Smith CH. Monosaccharide transport across microvillous membrane of human placenta. *Am J Physiol* 1980; 238:C160–C168.

20. Eaton BM, Mann GE, Yudilevich DL. Kinetics and specificity of glucose transport on the fetal side of the guinea-pig placenta. *J Physiol (Lond)* 1979; 301:87–88.

21. Jansson T, Wennergren M, Illsley MP. Glucose transporter protein expression in human placenta throughout gestation and in intrauterine growth retardation. *J Clin Endocrinol Metab* 1993; 77:1554–62.

22. Takata K, Kasahara T, Kasahara M et al. Localization of erythrocyte/HepG2-type glucose transporter (GLUT1) in human placental villi. *Cell Tiss Res* 1992; 267:407–12.

23. Hahn T, Hartmann M, Blaschitz A et al. Localisation of the high affinity glucose transporter protein GLUT1 in the placenta of human, marmoset monkey (*Callithrix jacchus*) and rat at different developmental stages. *Cell Tiss Res* 1995; 280:49–57.

24. Wolf HG, Desoye G. Immunohistochemical localization of glucose transporters and insulin receptors in human fetal membranes at term. *Histochemistry* 1993; 100:379–85.

25. Hahn T, Desoye G. Ontogeny of glucose transport systems in the placenta and its progenitor tissues. *Early Preg Biol Med* 1966; 2:168–82.

26. Ehrhardt RA, Bell AW. Developmental increases in glucose transporter concentration in the sheep placenta. *Am J Physiol* 1997; 273:R1132–R1141.

27. Das UG, Hay Jr WW, Devaskar SU. Placental glucose transporter (GLUT–1) in fetal sheep is regulated by time-dependent changes in glucose and insulin concentrations. *Pediatr Res* 1996; 39:1828, 307A.

28. Sadiq HF, Morgenthaler TA, Schroeder RE et al. Effects of hypoxia and glucose on placental glucose transporters. *Pediatr Res* 1994; 35:1224, 206A.

29. Reid GJ, Flozak AS, Simmons RA. Increased expression of glucose transporter protein-1 (GLUT-1) in the growth retarded placenta. *J Soc Gynecol Invest* 1995; 2:193.

30. Bassett NS, Currie MJ, Woodall SM et al. The effect of maternal IGF-I treatment on placental GLUT gene expression. *Proceedings of the Thorburn Symposium*, Hamilton Island, Queensland, Australia, 1994.

31. Barth S, Hahn T, Zechner R et al. Prolonged hyperglycemia in vitro affects glucose transporter protein GLUT1 and glucose uptake in cultured term trophoblast cells. *Placenta* 1994; 15:A4.

32. Hay Jr WW, Carver TD, Aldoretta PW. Effect of acute and chronic hypo- and hyperglycemia on placental glucose transport capacity in pregnant sheep. *Proceedings of the First International Meeting of World Placental Associations*, Sydney, Australia, 1994.

33. Hay Jr WW, Meznarich HK, DiGiacomo JE et al. Effects of insulin and glucose concentrations on glucose utilization in fetal sheep. *Pediatr Res* 1988; 23:281–7.

34. Hay Jr WW, Molina RD, DiGiacomo JE et al. Model of placental glucose consumption and glucose transfer. *Am J Physiol* 1990; 258:R569–R577.

35. Hay Jr WW. Placental function. In: (Gluckman PD, Heymann MA, eds) *Scientific Basis of Pediatric and Perinatal Medicine*, 2nd edn. (Edward Arnold: London, 1996) 213–27.

36. DiGiacomo JE, Hay Jr WW. Fetal glucose metabolism and oxygen consumption during sustained maternal and fetal hypoglycemia. *Metabolism* 1980; 39:193–202.

37. Kulhanek JF, Meschia G, Makowski EL et al. Changes in DNA content and urea permeability of the sheep placenta. *Am J Physiol* 1974; 226:1257–63.

38. Molina RD, Meschia G, Battaglia FC et al. Gestational maturation of placental glucose transfer capacity in sheep. *Am J Physiol* 1991; 261:R697–R704.

39. Hay Jr WW, Sparks JW, Wilkening RB et al. Fetal glucose uptake and utilization as functions of maternal glucose concentration. *Am J Physiol* 1984; 246:E237–E242.

40. Kalhan SC, Savin SM, Adam PAJ. Measurement of glucose turnover in the human newborn with glucose-1-^{13}C. *J Clin Endocrinol Metab* 1976; 43:704–7.

41. Carver TD, Quick Jr AN, Teng, CC et al. Leucine metabolism in chronically hypoglycemic, hypoinsulinemic growth restricted fetal sheep. *Am J Physiol* 1997; 272:E107–E117.

42. Das UG, Schroeder RE, Hay Jr WW et al. Chronic hypoglycemia causes time-dependent changes in ovine fetal GLUT 1 & GLUT 4 protein expression. *Pediatr Res* 1995; 37:60A.

43. Schroeder RE, Doria-Medina CL, Das UG et al. Effect of maternal diabetes upon fetal rat myocardial and skeletal muscle glucose transporters. *Pediatr Res* 1997; 41:11–19.

44. Schroeder RE, Devaskar UP, Trail SE et al. Effect of maternal diabetes on the expression of genes regulating fetal brain glucose uptake. *Diabetes* 1993; **42**:1487–96.

45. Das UG, Schroeder RE, Hay Jr WW et al. Chronic hyperglycemia causes time-dependent changes in ovine fetal GLUT 1 & GLUT 4 protein expression. *Pediatr Res* 1995; **37**:305A.

46. Das UG, Schroeder RE, Hay Jr WW, Devaskar SU. Time-dependent and tissue-specific effects of circulating glucose on fetal ovine glucose transporters. *Am J Physiol* 1999; **276**: R809–817.

47. Anderson MS, He J, Flowers-Ziegler J et al. Effects of selective hyperglycemia and hyperinsulinemia on glucose transporters in fetal ovine skeletal muscle. *Am J Physiol* 2001; **50**:R1256–R1263.

48. Anderson MS, Ziegler JA, Das UG et al. Glucose transporter protein responses to selective hyperglycemia or hyperinsulinemia in fetal sheep. *Am J Physiol* 2001; **281**:R1545–R1552.

49. Klip A, Tsakiridis T, Marette A et al. Regulation of expression of glucose transporters by glucose: a review of studies in vivo and in cell cultures. *FASEB J* 1994; **8**:43–53.

50. Zarlengo KM, Battaglia FC, Fennessey P, Hay Jr WW. Relationship between glucose utilization rate and glucose concentration in preterm infants. *Biol Neonate* 1986; **49**:181–9.

51. Philipps AF, Carson BS, Meschia G et al. Insulin secretion in fetal and newborn sheep. *Am J Physiol* 1978; **235**:E467–E474.

52. Carson BS, Philipps AF, Simmons MA et al. Effects of a sustained fetal insulin infusion upon glucose uptake and oxygenation. *Pediatr Res* 1980; **14**:147–52.

53. van Veen LCP, Teng C, Hay Jr WW et al. Leucine disposal and oxidation rates in the fetal lamb. *Metabolism* 1987; **36**:48–53.

54. DiGiacomo JE, Hay Jr WW. Effect of hypoinsulinemia and hyperglycemia on fetal glucose utilization and oxidation. *Am J Physiol* 1990; **259**:E506–E512.

55. Hay Jr WW, Meznarich HK, Fowden AL. Effect of streptozotocin of rates of ovine fetal glucose utilization, oxidation and production in the sheep fetus. *Metabolism* 1988; **38**:30–7.

56. Fowden AL, Hay Jr WW. The effects of pancreatectomy on the rates of glucose utilization, oxidation and production in the sheep fetus. *Q J Exp Physiol* 1988; **73**:973–84.

57. Fowden AL. The endocrine regulation of fetal metabolism and growth. In: (Gluckman PD, Johnston BM, Nathanielsz PW, eds) *Advances in Fetal Physiology: Reviews in Honor of GC Liggins*. (Perinatology Press: Ithaca, 1989) 229–43.

58. Aldoretta PW, Hay Jr WW. Chronic hyperglycemia induces insulin resistance and glucose intolerance in fetal sheep. *Pediatr Res* 2001; **49**:307A.

59. Aldoretta PW, Gresores A, Carver TD, Hay Jr WW. Maturation of glucose-stimulated insulin secretion. *Biol Neonate* 1998; **73**:375–86.

60. Philipps AF, Carson BS, Meschia G et al. Insulin secretion in fetal and newborn sheep. *Am J Physiol* 1978; **235**:E467–E474.

61. Van Assche FA, Hoet JJ, Jack PMB. Endocrine pancreas of the pregnant mother, fetus, and newborn. In: (Beard RW, Nathanielsz PW, eds) *Fetal Physiology and Medicine*, 2nd edn. (Dekker: New York, 1984) 127–52.

62. Carver TD, Anderson SM, Aldoretta PW et al. Glucose suppression of insulin secretion in chronically hyperglycemic fetal sheep. *Pediatr Res* 1995; **38**:754–62.

63. Kervran A, Randon J. Development of insulin release by fetal rat pancreas *in vitro*. *Diabetes* 1980; **29**:673–78.

64. Kervran A, Guillaume M, Jost A. The endocrine pancreas of the fetus of diabetic pregnant rat. *Diabetologia* 1978; **15**:387–93.

65. Cowett RM. Hypoglycemia and hyperglycemia in the newborn. In: (Polin RA, Fox WW, eds) *Fetal and Neonatal Physiology*. (WB Saunders: Philadelphia, 1992) 406–18.

66. Freinkel N, Phelps NL, Metzger BE. Intermediary metabolism during normal pregnancy. In: (Sutherland HW, Stowers JM, eds) *Carbohydrate Metabolism in Pregnancy and the Newborn*. (Springer-Verlag: New York, 1979) 1–31.

67. Carver TD, Anderson SM, Aldoretta PW et al. Effect of low-level plus marked 'pulsatile' hyperglycemia on insulin secretion in fetal sheep. *Am J Physiol* 1996; **271**:E865–E871.

68. Fowden AL, Hill DJ. Intrauterine programming of the endocrine pancreas. *Br Med Bull* 2001; **60**:123–42.

69. Dahri S, Reusen B, Remacle C, Hoet JJ. Nutritional influences on pancreatic development – potential links with non-insulin-dependent diabetes. *Proc Nutr Soc* 1995; **54**:345–56.

70. Fowden AL, Silver MA. The effects of thyroid hormones on oxygen and glucose metabolism in the sheep fetus during late gestation. *J Physiol* 1995; **482**:203–13.

71. Barnes RJ, Comline RS, Silver M. Effect of cortisol on liver glycogen concentrations in hypophysectomized, adrenalectomized and normal foetal lambs during late or prolonged gestation. *J Physiol* 1978; **275**:567–79.

72. Fowden AL, Comline RS, Silver M. The effects of cortisol on the concentration of glycogen in different tissues in the chronically catheterized fetal pig. *Q J Exp Physiol* 1985; **70**:23–32.

73. Padbury JF, Ludlow JK, Ervin MG et al. Thresholds for physiological effects of plasma catecholamines in fetal sheep. *Am J Physiol* 1992; **252**:E530–E537.

74. Devaskar SU, Ganguli S, Styer D et al. Glucagon and glucose dynamics in sheep: evidence for glucagon resistance in fetus. *Am J Physiol* 1984; **246**:E256–E265.

75. Liechty EA, Boyle DW, Moorehead H et al. Effects of circulating IGF-I on glucose and amino acid kinetics in the ovine fetus. *Am J Physiol* 1996; **271**:E177–E185.

76. Oliver MH, Harding JE, Breier BH et al. Glucose but not mixed amino acid infusion regulates plasma insulin-like growth factor-I concentrations in fetal sheep. *Pediatr Res* 1993; **34**:62–5.

77. Han VKM, Fowden Al. Paracrine regulation of fetal growth. In: (Ward RHT, Smith SK, Donnai D, eds) *Early Fetal Growth and Development.* (RCOG Press: London, 1994) 275–91.

78. Liechty EA, Boyle DA, Moorehead H et al. Effect of hyperinsulinemia on ovine fetal leucine kinetics during prolonged maternal fasting. *Am J Physiol* 1992; **263**:E696–E702.

79. Stephens E, Thureen PJ, Goalstone ML et al. Fetal hyperinsulinemia increases farnesylation of p21 Ras in fetal tissues. *Am J Physiol* 2001; **281**:E217–E223.

80. Thureen PJ, Scheer B, Anderson SM, Hay Jr WW. Effect of hyperinsulinemia on amino acid utilization in the ovine fetus. *Am J Physiol* 2000; **279**:E1294–E1304.

81. Shelley HJ. Glycogen reserves and their changes at birth and in anoxia. *Br Med Bull* 1961; **17**:137–43.

82. Dawkins MJR. Biochemical aspects of developing function in newborn mammalian liver. *Br Med Bull* 1961; **22**:28–33.

83. Shellhase E, Kuroki Y, Emrie PA et al. Expression of pulmonary surfactant apoproteins in the developing rat lung. *Clin Res* 1989; **37**:208A.

84. Mott JC. The ability of young mammals to withstand total oxygen lack. *Br Med Bull* 1961; **17**:144–8.

85. Sparks JW. Augmentation of glucose supply. *Semin Perinatol* 1979; **3**:141–55.

86. Marconi A, Cetin E, Davoli A et al. An evaluation of fetal glucogenesis in intrauterine growth retarded pregnancies: steady state fetal and maternal enrichments of plasma glucose at cordocentesis. *Metabolism* 1993; **42**:860–4.

87. Hay Jr WW, Sparks JW, Quissel BJ et al. Simultaneous measurements of umbilical glucose uptake, fetal utilization rate, and fetal turnover rate of glucose. *Am J Physiol* 1981; **240**:E662–E668.

88. Gleason CA, Rudolph AM. Gluconeogenesis by the fetal sheep liver in vivo. *J Dev Physiol* 1985; **7**:185–194.

89. DiGiacomo JE, Hay Jr WW. Regulation of placental glucose transfer and consumption by fetal glucose production. *Pediatr Res* 1989; **25**:429–34.

90. Widdowson EM. Growth and composition of the human fetus and newborn. In: (Assali NS, ed.) *Biology of Gestation, Volume 2.* (Academic Press: New York, 1968) 1–48.

91. Coleman RA. Placental metabolism and transport of lipid. *Fed Proc* 1986; **45**:2519–23.

92. Goldstein R, Levy E, Shafrir E. Increased maternal–fetal transport of fat in diabetes assessed by polyunsaturated fatty acid content in fetal lipids. *Biol Neonate* 1985; **47**:343–49.

93. Stammers JP, Elphic MC, Hull D. Effect of maternal diet during late pregnancy on fetal lipid stores in rabbits. *J Dev Physiol* 1983; **5**:395–404.

94. Elphick MC, Hull D, Sanders RR. Concentrations of free fatty acids in maternal and umbilical cord blood during elective cesarean section. *Br J Obstet Gynaecol* 1976; **83**:539–44.

95. Dancis J, Jansen V, Kayden JH et al. Transfer across perfused human placenta. III. Effect of chain length on transfer of free fatty acids. *Pediatr Res* 1974; **8**:796–9.

96. Hummel L, Simmermann T, Wagner H. Quantitative evaluation of the fetal fatty acid synthesis in the rat. *Acta Biol Med Germ* 1978; **37**:229–32.

97. Elphick MC, Hull D. The transfer of free fatty acids across the rabbit placenta. *J Physiol (Lond)* 1977; **264**:751–66.

98. Portman OW, Behrman RE, Soltys P. Transfer of free fatty acids across the primate placenta. *Am J Physiol* 1969; **216**:143–7.

99. Hendrickse W, Stammers JP, Hull D. The transfer of free fatty acids across the human placenta. *Br J Obstet Gynaecol* 1985; **92**:945–53.

100. Thomas CR, Lowy C. Placental transfer of free fatty acids: factors affecting transfer across the guinea pig placenta. *J Dev Physiol* 1983; **5**:323–32.

101. Ayuk PT, Sibley C, Donnai P et al. Development and polarization of cationic amino acid transporters and regulators in the human placenta. *Am J Physiol* 2000; **278**:c1162–c1171.

102. Mahendran D, Donnai P, Glazier JD et al. Amino acid (system A) transporter activity in microvillous membrane vesicles from the placentas of appropriate and small for gestational age babies. *Pediatr Res* 1993; **34**:661–5.

103. Mahendran D, Byrne S, Donnai P et al. Na+ Transport, H+ concentration gradient dissipation, and system A amino acid transporter activity in purified microvillous plasma membrane isolated from first-trimester human placenta: comparison with the term microvillous membrane. *Am J Obstet Gynecol* 1994; **171**:1534–40.

104. Novak DA, Beveridge MJ, Malandro M, Seo J. Ontogeny of amino acid transport system A in rat placenta. *Placenta* 1996; **17**:643–51.

105. Malandro MS, Beveridge MJ, Kilberg MS, Novak DA. Ontogeny of cationic amino acid transport systems in rat placenta. *Am J Physiol* 1994; **267**:C804–C811.

106. Smith CH, Moe AJ, Ganapathy V et al. Nutrient transport pathways across the epithelium of the placenta. *Annu Rev Nutr* 1992; **12**:183–206.

107. Milley JR. Protein synthesis during hypoxia in fetal lambs. *Am J Physiol* 1987; **252**:E519–E524.

108. Milley JR. Uptake of exogenous substrates during hypoxia in fetal lambs. *Am J Physiol* 1988; **254**: E572–E524.

109. Smith CH. Incubation techniques and investigation of placental transport mechanisms in vitro. *Placenta* 1981; **2**:163–8.

110. Dancis J, Lind J, Oratz M et al. Placental transfer of proteins in human gestation. *Am J Obstet Gynecol* 1961; **82**:167–71.

111. Lemons JA, Adcock 3rd EW, Jones Jr MD et al. Umbilical uptake of amino acids in the unstressed fetal lamb. *J Clin Invest* 1976; **58**:1428–34.

112. Marconi AM, Battaglia FC, Meschia G et al. A comparison of amino acid arteriovenous differences across the liver, hindlimb and placenta in the fetal lamb. *Am J Physiol* 1989; **257**:E909–E915.

113. Gresham EL, James EJ, Raye JR et al. Production and excretion of urea by the fetal lamb. *Pediatrics* 1972; **50**:372–9.

114. van Veen LCP, Teng C, Hay Jr WW et al. Leucine disposal and oxidation rates in the fetal lamb. *Metabolism* 1987; **36**:48–53.

115. Battaglia FC, Meschia G. Fetal nutrition. *Annu Rev Nutr* 1988; **8**:43–61.

116. Meier PR, Peterson RG, Bonds DR et al. Rates of protein synthesis and turnover in fetal life. *Am J Physiol* 1981; **240**:E320–E324.

117. Kennaugh JM, Bell AW, Teng C et al. Ontogenetic changes in the rates of protein synthesis and leucine oxidation during fetal life. *Pediatr Res* 1987; **22**:688–92.

118. Bell AW, Kennaugh JM, Battaglia FC et al. Uptake of amino acids and ammonia at mid-gestation by the fetal lamb. *Q J Exp Physiol* 1989; **74**:635–43.

119. Sparks JW. Human intrauterine growth and nutrient accretion. *Semin Perinatol* 1984; **8**:74–93.

120. Waterlow JL, Garlick PJ, Millward DJ. *Protein Turnover in Mammalian Tissues and in the Whole Body*. (Elsevier/North-Holland Biomedical Press: Amsterdam, 1978).

121. Milner RDG, Hill DJ. Interaction between endocrine and paracrine peptides in prenatal growth control. *Eur J Pediatr* 1987; **146**:113.

122. Wilkening RB, Boyle DW, Teng C et al. Amino acid uptake by fetal ovine hindlimb under normal and euglycemic hyperinsulinemic states. *Am J Physiol* 1994; **266**:E72–E78.

123. Liechty EA, Boyle DW, Moorehead H et al. Increased fetal glucose concentration decreases ovine fetal leucine oxidation independent of insulin. *Am J Physiol* 1993; **265**:E617–E623.

124. Liechty EA, Lemons JA. Changes in ovine fetal hindlimb amino acid metabolism during maternal fasting. *Am J Physiol* 1984; **246**:E430.

17

Regulation of fetal growth
David J Hill

Introduction

Human fetal growth potential is influenced by multiple factors including the parental genome, placental sufficiency, and environmental factors such as maternal nutrition and lifestyle.[1] However, many pathological variations in term infant size can be associated with changes in the fetal production or action of insulin. The increased somatic tissue mass of the infant of the poorly controlled diabetic mother is thought to result primarily from fetal hyperinsulinemia as a result of maternal hyperglycemia. Such infants have hyperplasia of the beta cells. However, the pattern of overgrowth is complicated, consisting of visceromegaly of the liver, heart, adrenal and lungs, and subcutaneous adiposity, in addition to a modest increase in skeletal length.[2] Insulin is an important factor in fetal growth and infants born with nesidioblastosis or the Beckwith– Wiedemann syndrome, conditions associated with hypersecretion of insulin, exhibit enhanced fetal somatic growth. On the other hand, transient neonatal diabetes or pancreatic agenesis result in growth retardation. Both fetal over- and undergrowth are associated with altered expression of peptide growth factors, especially the insulin-like growth factors (IGF), which are widely expressed, and control organ cell mass and differentiation. One of many tissues shown to depend greatly on IGF availability and action for ordered development is the endocrine pancreas. This chapter will examine the relationship between the IGF axis and the development of appropriate pancreatic islet cell mass, thus providing for adequate insulin availability. It will also consider the long-term consequences of an inappropriate islet cell mass for adult Type 2 diabetes.

Trophic actions of insulin and insulin-like growth factors

It has been difficult to reproduce the organomegaly and limited skeletal overgrowth seen in the hyperinsulinemic human fetus by animal experimentation. The best-documented model of fetal hyperinsulinemia has been in the rhesus monkey. After 3 weeks of pharmacological insulin infusion the fetus had an elevated body weight consisting of an enlarged liver, heart and spleen, but with no changes in the weights of other organs or in the skeletal length.[3] The trophic effects of insulin during fetal growth may result from several separate, but interactive, mechanisms. Firstly, insulin supports the uptake and utilization of nutrients by insulin-sensitive fetal tissues leading to cellular hypertrophy.

Secondly, insulin may have direct mitogenic actions. Thirdly, the growth-promoting effects of insulin may involve the release of secondary hormones, such as IGF or IGF binding proteins (IGFBP).

Insulin receptors are found in all fetal tissues, and in human fetal liver the population is maximal between 19 and 25 weeks.[4] Insulin is metabolically active *in utero*. When fetal lambs in the third trimester were placed on a glucose clamp and infused with insulin, a rise in oxygen consumption, glucose uptake and glucose utilization resulted.[5] Insulin acts directly as a mitogen on isolated embryonic and fetal tissues, and on mammalian embryonic stem cells.[6,7] Disruption of the two insulin genes in the mouse by homologous recombination resulted in no embryonic lethality, but severe intrauterine growth retardation affected most tissues, with the exception of the brain.[8] These animals developed severe diabetes immediately after suckling and died within 48 hours of birth with ketoacidosis.[8] A pancreas was present with exocrine tissue and islets, the latter containing all endocrine cell types including beta cells, which were detected by using a β-galactosidase marker derived from a *LacZ* gene inserted at the *Ins2* locus. Inactivation of either the *Ins1* or the *Ins2* locus individually resulted in a compensatory increase in beta-cell mass compared to wild-type animals at 2–4 months of age.[9] This provides direct evidence for insulin being a major trophic hormone prior to birth.

Insulin and IGF are structurally related molecules, both of which are essential for optimal embryonic and fetal development. Two species of IGF exist, IGF-I and IGF-II, with an approximate molecular size of 7.6 kDa. The liver is a major site of expression both in fetal and postnatal life, although almost all tissues have been shown to express these peptides in the human and animal fetus,[10] suggesting a predominantly

autocrine or paracrine role. In the fetus the most abundant species is IGF-II. A high-affinity type-1 IGF receptor is ubiquitous in developing tissues and recognizes IGF-I with an order of magnitude greater binding affinity than for IGF-II. The mitogenic, anti-apoptotic and other effects on cell differentiation of IGF are primarily mediated by the type-1 receptor, and its intracellular activation of insulin receptor substrates (IRS)-1 and -2. The IGF are seldom found in free form but are complexed to one of six distinct classes of specific IGFBP.[10] These serve not only as carrier proteins to extend the biological half-life of the ligands, but also modulate their biological actions by either interacting or competing with the type-1 IGF receptors. A large proportion of the IGF/IGFBP complexes in extracellular fluids, stored within the extracellular matrix, are probably inaccessible to the cell-surface receptors. Their availability depends on modification of the IGFBP by specific proteases resulting in a reduced binding affinity for IGF. Such proteases have been identified for IGFBP-2–5.[10] Thus, while IGF-I and IGF-II are present in the circulation, this may serve predominantly as an extracellular store. Controlled proteolysis of IGFBP and extracellular matrix molecules is likely to be the key regulatory step in the bioavailability and subsequent actions of IGF-I and IGF-II.

Targeted gene deletions of IGF and their receptors have demonstrated the profound importance of the IGF axis to normal fetal growth (Table 17.1). By interbreeding, combination gene 'knockouts' have been obtained. Deletion of the *IGF-I* gene yielded homozygotes that had birthweights *c.* 60% of those of normal zygotes, some of which died within 6 hours of birth.[11] However, some of the mutant mice survived to adulthood, but females were infertile due to a failure of ovarian follicular development. Using a similar strategy to delete IGF-II, it was found that the *IGF-II* gene is

Receptor	Size reduction (%)
IGF-I, IGF-II, insulin	40 at birth
IGF type-1 receptor, IR	50–60
IRS-1 or IRS-2	60
IRS-1 + IRS-2	Lethal
IGF-II + IGF type-1 receptor	70
IGF-II + IRS-2	70

IR, Insulin receptor; IRS, insulin receptor substrate.

Table 17.1. Effects of insulin-like growth factor (IGF)/insulin axis gene knockout on size at birth in the mouse.

parentally imprinted and is only transmitted from the male allele in the majority of tissues, exceptions being the choroid plexus and meninges where the gene is active on both alleles.[12] IGF-II-deficient homozygotes had a similar growth deficiency at birth to animals lacking IGF-I, demonstrating that both species have a role in prenatal growth. However, IGF-II-deficient mice were fertile. Deletion of the type-1 IGF receptor, which is primarily responsible for the signaling of both mitogenesis and differentiation by both IGF-I and IGF-II, yielded homozygous animals which were only 45% of normal weight at delivery, and died within minutes of birth.[13] This was due to a failure to breathe and probably resulted from a widespread muscle hypoplasia, including that of the respiratory muscles. Double gene knock-out involving both the IGF-I and type-1 receptor genes resulted in a similar phenotype to that found after deletion of the receptor alone, however co-deletion of IGF-II and the type-1 receptor yielded a subgroup of animals with only 30% of normal birthweight at term and grossly retarded skeletal development. This suggests that an additional receptor to the type-1 form may also contribute to IGF-II signaling. IGF-II also binds to the IGF type-II/mannose-6-phosphate receptor that is believed to act as a degradation pathway for IGF-II.[14] Deletion of this receptor leads to increased birth size, presumably because of a prolonged presence of IGF-II. However, there is also evidence that the effects of IGF-II may be mediated by the insulin receptor (IR).[15] In *IgfIr* –/– mouse fibroblasts transfected with human IR, IGF-II stimulates cell proliferation through the IR.[16] Additionally, there are two isoforms of the insulin receptor (IR-A and IR-B) in humans and rodents, resulting from a different splicing of exon 11.[17–19] IR-A, but not IR-B, was found to bind IGF-II with an affinity close to that of insulin.[17] These data suggest that IGF-II could, perhaps partly compensate for the absence of insulin in the insulin knockout mice by binding and activation of the IR or IGF type-1 receptor.

The above series of studies demonstrates that neither IGF-I nor IGF-II are crucial for key morphological events in early development, but that they act as 'true' growth factors, contributing to the expansion of stem cell populations and the progression of cell differentiation. While both IGF-I and IGF-II contribute to fetal growth, the size of the placenta was normal following deletion of the IGF-I and type-1 receptor genes, while reduced after deletion of IGF-II.[13] This suggests that a high local expression of IGF-II in placenta may contribute to its development. Recently, it was demonstrated that the radiation-induced mouse mutation minute (Mnt)[20] has lost expression of *Igf2* in meso-dermal tissues and in the placenta, thus leading to intrauterine growth restriction (IUGR) with subsequent catch-up growth postnatally.

In the human infant with IUGR, IGF-I concentrations in blood are lower than in age-matched control infants, while levels of IGF-II are unaltered.[21] Conversely, in macrosomic infants of diabetic mothers, circulating levels of IGF-I and IGF-II are elevated.[22,23] While this suggests that fetal IGF-I expression may be closely related to growth rate in the last trimester of pregnancy, this association may not be the determining biological parameter since circulating levels of IGFBP-1 are substantially elevated in the growth-retarded infant.[24] This may limit IGF availability to its high-affinity IGF receptors.

Animal models of fetal growth manipulation

When fetal growth in the rat is restricted, either by uterine vessel ligation or by maternal fasting, there is a reproducible reduction in IGF-I mRNA levels in fetal tissues and of circulating IGF-I, and an increase in the hepatic expression and circulating levels of IGFBP-1 and IGFBP-2.[25,26] Fetal pancreatectomy in sheep caused a significant decrease in circulating levels of IGF-I and a relative fetal growth retardation. This occurred despite the maintenance of euglycemia. Replacement of insulin in the pancreatectomized sheep fetus significantly increased the growth rate compared to saline-treated controls.[27] These studies show that even when nutritional availability is optimal, insulin is obligatory for the maintenance of IGF synthesis and growth rate in the third trimester sheep fetus. Moreover, insulin was also able to

decrease the expression of IGFBP-1 mRNA within ovine or rat fetal hepatocytes, while increased circulating IGFBP-1 accompanied the relative hypoinsulinemia seen when experimental fetal growth retardation was induced in the fetal rat or rabbit by maternal fasting or by ligation of the uterine vessels. Thus, in addition to direct metabolic and mitogenic actions of insulin on fetal tissues, insulin can regulate the IGF and IGFBP presence. IUGR in rats and humans results in a reduced population of pancreatic beta cells at birth.[28,29] Maternal calorie restriction by 50% in rat from day 15 of gestation until term showed that the beta-cell mass was reduced in the newborn due to a reduction in the number of islets.[30] If a normal diet was restored at birth, then the beta-cell mass returned to that of controls by weaning. However, continuation of energy restriction during neonatal life led to irreversible changes in the beta-cell mass. A more severe 65% restriction of *ad libitum* food intake to the pregnant rat was applied for differing times during gestation: 1–7, 7–14 or 14–21 days.[31] All regimes gave rise to newborns with reduced body weights, but the pancreatic weight was only reduced after 14–21 days malnutrition. Protein restriction in an otherwise isocalorific diet provides a useful model, given the major role of amino acids as insulin secretogogues for the fetal islets, glucose responsiveness developing only 2 days before birth.[32] A reduction of dietary protein to 8% throughout gestation resulted in a reduced pancreatic weight at birth with a reduced beta-cell mass, islet cell size and pancreatic vascularity.[33–35] Pancreatic blood flow was also impaired.

IUGR is a risk factor for both perinatal disease and diseases of later life. Barker[36] showed that a strong inverse correlation exists between mortality from cardiovascular disease below 65 years of age and birthweight. Similarly, the relative risk for prevalence of syndrome X, consisting of Type 2 diabetes, hypertension and hyperlipidemia, is 18-fold higher in men born at < 2.5 kg compared to those > 4 kg.[36,37] The at-risk individuals were thin at birth with a low ponderal index. Impaired glucose tolerance can be detected as early as 7 years of age in children who had low birthweights and were thin.[38] This implies that programming of the metabolic axis can occur in early life that is modulated by the intrauterine environment. For Type 2 diabetes this may result from an altered development and insulin-secreting capacity of the endocrine pancreas, or by altered insulin sensitivity of target tissues. Each has been associated with a different phenotype of newborn, the development of insulin resistance correlating with thinness at birth and in childhood, and with a low maternal body mass index (BMI), but Type 2 diabetes with insulin deficiency being associated with a high BMI in childhood and a high maternal BMI.[39] The latter would represent many infants of poorly controlled diabetic mothers. It is possible that perturbations of prenatal growth may lead to inappropriate beta-cell ontogeny and result in a population of beta cells qualitatively ill-suited to subsequently manage metabolic stress. As mentioned previously, a reduced availability of insulin prenatally is a major contributor to IUGR, as demonstrated using insulin gene knockout mice[9] whose birthweights were 25% less than heterozygote littermates at birth, and the severe growth retardation of human infants with pancreatic agenesis.[40]

Development of the endocrine pancreas

Insulin release can be altered rapidly by a change in the secretion rate of individual beta cells but prolonged physiological challenge may result in an increased total beta-cell mass. In the rat fetus, the cellular area immunostained for insulin increases twofold over 2 days just prior to term, due to both beta-cell replication and recruitment, and maturation of undifferentiated beta-cell precursors.[41] In mouse embryos, dorsal and ventral pancreatic buds appear at day E (embryonic) 9.5 from mid-gut endoderm, and fuse by E16–17.[42] Each bud forms highly branched structures, and the acini and ducts are distinguishable at E14.5, with amylase being detectable in acinar tissue. Endocrine cells appear early in bud development and represent 10% of the pancreas by E15.5. Initially they exist as individual cells or small clusters close to the pancreatic ducts and only form mature islets, with outer alpha cells and an inner mass of beta and D cells, a few days before birth. This is seen by the early third trimester in humans. The growth and cytodifferentiation of the pancreas depends on mesenchymal–epithelial interactions. Pancreatic mesenchyme accumulates around the dorsal gut epithelium, inducing pancreatic bud formation and branching. Endocrine cells develop from the pancreatic duct epithelial cells and undergo a lineage progression and replication that has been modeled by Teitelman.[43,44] Within this model the appearance of alpha cells would constitute a default pathway and subsequent epigenetic effects would generate other endocrine cell types. These epigenetic signals are likely to include the expression of lineage-specific transcription factors and the effects of peptide growth factors within the total environment of the pancreatic rudiment.

Neogenesis of islets is rapid in the fetus and continues throughout neonatal life in the rat, but ceases shortly after weaning.[45] This derives not only from beta-cell replication but also from the recruitment and maturation of undifferentiated beta-cell precursors.[46] Conversely, the rate of mitosis in adult pancreatic beta cells is normally low, c. 3% replication rate of beta cells day.[47] What then precipitates a change to an adult phenotype of non-proliferative beta cells? A transient wave of apoptosis occurs in neonatal rat islets between 1 and 2 weeks of age.[48–50] The number of apoptotic cells within rat islets increases threefold at 14 days after birth, compared to either 4 or 21 days.[50] At this time, islet beta cells also contain an increased presence of immunoreactive inducible nitric oxide synthase (iNOS), suggesting that endogenous levels of NO within islets may be functionally linked to developmental beta-cell apoptosis. This is unlikely to be an exclusive pathway since beta-cell apoptosis has also been linked to the actions of peroxynitrite and to Fas activation.[51,52] Fas is a transmembrane cell-surface receptor protein related to the tumor necrosis factor (TNF)-α receptor family. Activation by the Fas ligand results in an intracellular signaling cascade terminating in apoptosis. However, the beta-cell mass is not altered appreciably at the time of neonatal apoptosis, suggesting that a new population of beta cells compensates for the loss by apoptosis. Increased numbers of insulin-positive cells are seen near to the ductal epithelia after 12 days, suggesting the generation of new islets to maintain the beta-cell mass. Recently, it has been reported that a similar wave of beta-cell apoptosis occurs in the human fetus during the third trimester.[53] It is hypothesized by the present author that partial replacement of beta cells neonatally provides a cell population suited to metabolic control in later adult life. Any aberrant apoptotic deletion of fetal-type cells, or the parallel neogenesis of adult-type islets, is likely to alter the ability of the animal to deal with metabolic or autoimmune stress in later life.

Transcription factors and islet development

The development of cells within the ductal epithelium into an endocrine lineage is controlled in part by a specific expression sequence of transcription factors (Fig. 17.1).[54] One of the most important is Pdx1,[55] which is expressed early in endocrine lineage commitment for cells within or adjacent to the ducts, is then silenced, but is re-expressed late in the separation of the beta cell lineage. In the mature beta-cell, Pdx1 transactivates the insulin and glucose transporter (GLUT2)-2 gene promoters. Pdx1 expression precedes insulin and glucagon expression in the mouse embryo, is localized to proliferating ductal epithelial cells, becomes further restricted to differentiating beta, D and PP cells, is lost from presumptive alpha cells, and finally becomes restricted to mature beta cells.[56,57] Pdx1 knockout mice form pancreatic ducts but little further endocrine differentiation or morphogenesis occurs.[58] Pdx1 appears to have a dual role; as an inducer of an early endocrine cell lineage, and in the maturation of beta cells and the control of insulin gene expression. Mutations in Pdx1 in humans results in mature onset diabetes of the young (MODY).[59] Cells within the ducts with the potential to commit to an endocrine lineage express Pdx1, Hnf6, Hnf3β and Hlxb9, the latter controlling migration away from the ducts. Hnf3β is a transcriptional regulator of Pdx1, and is itself regulated by Hnf6. Hnf6 also controls expression of neurogenin 3 (Ngn3), which continues to be expressed throughout islet formation until the point of final commitment of the endocrine lineages. Thus, the pre-endocrine cell type derived from ducts during early development has a transcription factor signature of Pdx1, Ngn3, Isl1, Nkx2.2, Beta2 and Pax6. Subsequent differentiation of beta cells requires the additional expression Nkx6.1 and Pax4, and a reduction in the expression of Ngn3 and Beta2. Deletion of Pax4 by homologous recombination in mice caused a complete loss of pancreatic beta and D cells, but an increased number of alpha

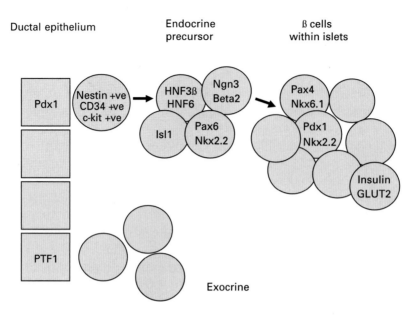

Figure 17.1. *Pattern of transcription factor expression associated with the neogenesis of pancreatic beta (β) cells from ductal epithelium to mature islet. Pdx1 expression within the ductal cells is a marker of focal production of an endocrine stem lineage, which expresses the stem cell markers nestin, c-kit and CD34. Pdx1 expression is then silenced as precursor endocrine cells express neurogenin 3 (Ngn3), Nkx2.2, Pax6, Isl1 and hepatocyte nuclear factors (HNF)-3β and -6. As beta cells become functionally active they re-express Pdx1, and express Pax4 and the glucose transporter GLUT2.*

cells.[60] Conversely, knockout of the *Pax6* gene decreased the presence of all endocrine cell types in the pancreas, but the presence of alpha cells was totally abolished.[61,62] Mice lacking *Pax4* and *Pax6* fail to develop any mature endocrine cells in the pancreas.[61] Both of these *Pax* genes are normally expressed during developmental islet cell neogenesis and may distinguish the alpha and beta cell lineages.

Growth factors and islet development

The ordered development of the endocrine pancreas is also dependent on the availability and actions of peptide growth factors originating from the ductal epithelium, the juxtaposing mesenchyme and the developing acinar.

Fibroblast growth factors (FGF) are involved in early pancreatic induction from gut endoderm,[63] and in the expansion of islet cell precursors and their commitment to beta cells. In the developing rat pancreas,[64] FGF receptors are normally absent from isolated adult islets;[65] however, in both the rat and mid-trimester human fetus FGF-2 and its high-affinity receptor, FGFR1, have been localized to the ductal epithelial cells, and to small developing islets.[66,67] FGFR4 was highly expressed in a model of fetal rat islet development *in vitro*.[68] Major ligands for FGFR4 include FGF-1 and FGF-7;[69] and FGF-7 is a potent contributor to beta-cell neogenesis. Systemic injection of FGF-7 into adult rats for up to 2 weeks caused a rapid increase in DNA synthesis within the ductal epithelium of intercalating, intra- and interlobular ducts[70] within 24 hours. Pancreatic duct hyperplasia followed, especially in the intralobular ducts adjacent to islets, but a progression to endocrine cells was not seen. When FGF-7 was expressed within the embryonic liver of transgenic mice, driven by an ApoE (Apolipoprotein E) promoter, pancreatic duct hyperplasia was seen, with increased numbers of ductal cells containing immunoreactive insulin.[71] During development of the endocrine pancreas, FGF-7 is expressed within the mesenchyme adjacent to the pancreatic ducts.[64] Recently, FGF-10 has been also been shown to be expressed within pancreatic mesenchyme in the mouse embryo, and its absence causes a failure of ductal branching and an absence of Pdx1-expressing endocrine progenitor cells.[72]

Vascular endothelial growth factor (VEGF) is a potent mitogen for endothelial cells both *in vitro* and *in vivo*, and also increases vascular permeability.[73] Two of its high-affinity, tyrosine kinase (TK)-type receptors are Flt-1 and Flk-1. Flk-1 mRNA is expressed within RINm2F islet cells, as well as in fetal rat islets where VEGF is able to increase the insulin content.[74] In intact fetal rat pancreas, immunoreactive Flk-1 was localized to pancreatic ductal cells and vascular endothelium, suggesting that ductal cells may also be a target for VEGF action. Using porcine fetal and adult rat ducts, VEGF was found to enhance cell replication and insulin content, implying that beta-cell neogenesis was also occurring.[75] Recently, Lammert et al[76] demonstrated, by targeted overexpression, that VEGF acts as a morphogen to induce endocrine cell commitment within the pancreatic ducts, leading to islet cell hyperplasia. While VEGF therefore induces an angiogenic response in support of an increasing islet cell mass, it also acts directly as a mitogen and morphogen for ductal epithelium. Hepatocyte growth factor (HGF) is expressed within tissue mesenchyme in the embryo and fetus, and during postnatal tissue regeneration.[77] Its receptor, the TK *met*,

is expressed within adjacent epithelial tissues, which are target sites for mitogenic and morphogenic actions of HGF. In the human fetus *met* is found on cells within the pancreatic ducts, while in adults *met* mRNA and peptide are localized to islet beta cells.[78] Conversely, HGF mRNA is abundant in pancreatic stroma. Recently, a transgenic overexpression of HGF to beta cells was shown to increase insulin release and islet cell replication once islets were transplanted to donor animals.[79]

The IGF potentiate beta-cell growth, maturation and function, and are expressed by beta cells in early life.[80] They appear to act via the type-1 IGF receptor and its activation of IRS-2 within the beta cells (Fig. 17.2). Complete disruption of IRS-2 in mice carrying a heterozygous mutation for the IGF-IR (*Irs2–/–*, *Igf1r+/–* mice) resulted in a severe absence of beta cells in 4-week-old animals.[81] This phenotype was more pronounced than the 50–60% reduction in beta cells observed in islets of *Irs2–/–* mice.[81] The analysis of *Igf1r+/–* and *Igf1r+/–*, and

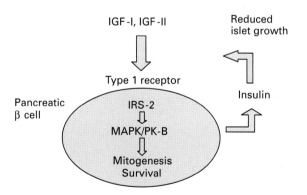

Figure 17.2. *Pathways whereby insulin-like growth factor (IGF)-I or -II act via the IGF type-1 receptor to activate mitogenesis and prevent apoptosis within pancreatic beta (β) cells. Mitogenesis is mediated via the ras-mitogen-activated protein kinase (MAPK) pathway, while cell survival is mediated via protein kinase B (PKB). Insulin acts locally to limit beta cell mass in a short loop negative feedback.*

Irs2+/– mice also revealed a reduction of 30–50% in the islet area of insulin-positive cells, which was less severe than that in *Igf1r+/–* and *Irs2–/–* animals. These observations suggest that the IGF-IR and IRS-2 signaling pathway is critical for beta-cell development. Interestingly, mice carrying a null mutation of IRS-1 and heterozygous mutation for IRS-2 (*Irs1–/–* and *Irs2+/–*) displayed insulin resistance associated with normal islet morphology but a twofold increase of the beta-cell area at 4 weeks or 4 months of age.[81] These data suggest that IRS-1 is not necessary for the maintenance of the beta-cell mass but that IRS-2 is crucial for a compensatory effect of the insulin resistance, causing islet hyperplasia.

IGF-II mRNA is greatest in the fetal pancreas, being expressed within islet cells and focal clusters of ductal epithelial cells, but declines during the neonatal period.[82,83] Conversely, IGF-I mRNA is low but detectable in fetal life, rises to adult levels within 2 weeks of birth, but is expressed mainly in the exocrine pancreas. Using transgenic mice, Petrik et al[84] showed that overexpression of IGF-II caused a four- to fivefold increase in the mean islet size at birth, affecting all endocrine cell types, but that the total number of mature islets was not altered (Table 17.2). This implies that *in vivo* IGF-II functions as a growth factor for existing islet cells but does not promote islet neogenesis. Between postnatal days 7 and 21 of normal development a transient wave of apoptosis destroys a proportion of beta cells in both the rat and the mouse,[85,86] to be replaced both from ductal neogenesis and from proliferation of remaining islet cells. This normal islet remodeling is thought to change the overall phenotype of the beta-cell mass from a fetal pattern of poor glucose responsiveness to a postnatal phenotype of rapid glucose responsiveness.[87] This developmental islet cell apoptosis coincides temporally with a diminished pancreatic expression of islet IGF-II.[86] IGF can prevent apoptosis in many cell types, and Petrik et al[86] have shown that endogenous IGF-II within isolated neonatal rat islets could protect them from cytokine-induced apoptosis. This protection was lost by weaning, when islets no longer expressed IGF-II but could be replaced with exogenous IGF-II. Functional proof that changes in IGF-II availability provoke developmental beta-cell apoptosis was obtained from transgenic mice overexpressing IGF-II in skin, leading to increased circulating levels which did not fall postnatally.[88] Here, the neonatal wave of beta-cell apoptosis was suppressed. In studies by others, using transgenic mice expressing IGF-II within beta cells, the disruption in developmental apoptosis within

Gene modification	Phenotype
IGF-II transgenic	Increased islet size, altered remodeling
IGF-II–/–	Reduced islet size
IRS-2–/–	Severe reduction in islet cell presence
IRS-1–/–	Increased islet cell mass due to peripheral insulin resistance
Insulin–/–	Increased islet size

IRS, Insulin receptor substrate; –/– homozygotic gene deletion.

Table 17.2. Effects of insulin-like growth factor (IGF)/insulin gene manipulation in mice on islet size.

the islets resulted in glucose intolerance in older animals.[89] The IGFs are usually associated with high-affinity IGFBP in biological fluids that are widely expressed in human and rat fetal tissues. In addition to extending the biological half-life of IGF, the IGFBP also modulate IGF action on tissues, including islets. Overexpression of IGFBP-5 in mice in multiple tissues resulted in reduced mean islet size at birth with a particular deficiency in beta cells.[90] It is likely that the excess IGFBP sequestrated endogenous IGF leading to reduced beta-cell proliferation and/or an increased developmental apoptosis.

Stem cells within the developing pancreas

Previously, it has been difficult to identify endocrine progenitor cells from other epithelial cells in the ductal epithelium, or to decide if a distinct subpopulation of precursor cells exists. Recently, specific progenitor markers have been identified in other cell lineages that may assist in recognizing islet precursor cells. Nestin is an intermediate filament protein that is abundantly expressed in neuroepithelial stem cells in embryogenesis, but is absent from nearly all mature central nervous system (CNS) cells.[91] Immature pancreatic endocrine cells share characteristics with developing neuronal cells, since transcription factors such as Ngn3 are implicated in the development, phenotype determination and maintenance of function in both. Recent studies indicate that there is a subpopulation of nestin-positive cells dispersed within adult islets that can differentiate into pancreatic endocrine, exocrine and hepatic phenotypes *in vitro*.[92,93] This group and others have also reported the presence of nestin-immunoreactive cells within and adjacent to the pancreatic ducts in the late gestation fetal and postnatal rat, which have a high incidence of proliferation, as determined by the presence of proliferating cell nuclear antigen (Fig. 17.3).[93,94] The abundance of nestin-immunoreactive cells within both ducts and islets was decreased following induced fetal growth restriction produced by feeding a low-protein diet to the mother. A subpopulation of

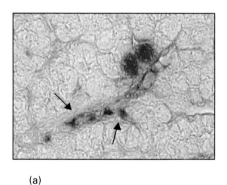

(a)

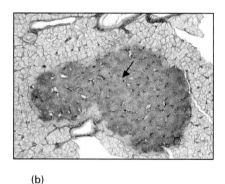

(b)

Figure 17.3. *Immunocytochemical localization of nestin as a marker of pre-endocrine stem cells within the juvenile rat pancreas (black arrows). Nestin-positive cells appear both in the pancreatic ducts (**a**) and within the mature islets (**b**). Mature beta cells are co-stained for insulin (red).*

pancreatic ductal cells also contained immuno-reactive c-*kit* and CD-34;[94] c-*kit* is a transmembrane protein whose ligand is a stem cell factor (SCF), which is of critical importance for early epithelial stem cell differentiation in hematopoiesis or gametogenesis. Recent studies suggest that SCF and c-*kit* have been involved in the growth and development of hepatic and islet progenitor cells.[95,96]

A regeneration of islet mass can occur following a pathological beta-cell loss. Histological evidence of islet cell neogenesis and regeneration have been found in recent-onset human Type 1 diabetes, particularly in children. Neogenesis was found in association with centroacinar and ductular cells leading to the formation of large, beta-cell-rich islets.[97–99] A 90% pancreatectomy in the young rat induces regeneration of both exocrine and endocrine tissue.[100] New beta cells are derived by both neogenesis and cell replication within the remaining islets.[101] Enhanced IGF-I mRNA expression was reported in duct cells, capillary endothelium and new endocrine cells,[102] while VEGF mRNA was rapidly upregulated. Partial pancreatectomy in the juvenile rat leads to a reduction in the expression of Pdx1, GLUT2 and insulin mRNAs,[103] most likely due to the associated hyperglycemia. Islet cell neogenesis can be induced in the adult hamster by obstruction of the pancreatic duct.[104] Ductal cell proliferation occurs within 14 days, leading to a cell outgrowth after 21 days forming new, small islets containing either glucagon, insulin or both. A second wave of proliferation occurs in islet cells after 8 weeks, leading to a total twofold increase in islet cell mass.[105] IGF-II mRNA is increased 10 days after pancreatic duct obstruction and is coincident with the commencement of ductal cell proliferation.[106] IGF-II released from ducts was capable of suppressing beta-cell apoptosis during co-culture with islets.[107] These findings support the notion

that an increase in beta-cell number can occur in early postnatal life, and that this involves changes in local growth factor and transcription factor expression.

The present author's group have utilized a model in which the young rat is rendered diabetic with a moderate dose of streptozotocin (STZ) 4 days after birth. This results in destruction of c. 60–70% of the beta cells within 72 hours and causes a transient hyperglycemia that is returned to the normal physiological range within 16 days post-STZ.[108,109] These changes are superimposed upon the normal islet remodeling seen in rodents between postnatal days 7 and 21. The beta-cell destruction caused by STZ is rapidly reversed, with the beta-cell mass having returned to some 70% of controls by weaning. This is due both to a repopulation from within islets and from neogenesis at the pancreatic ducts. The ratio of small to large islets is significantly increased within 8 days and is maximal at 12 days, as new islets are formed. Increased mitotic activity is apparent in the pancreatic ductal epithelium as early as 48 hours after STZ treatment, accompanied by an increased presence of FGF-7 within the adjacent mesenchyme. By 4 days post-STZ small clusters of cells immunopositive for Pdx1 and Ngn3 have budded from the ducts. Cells immunopositive for nestin and/or c-*kit* are observed in controls throughout the study period adjacent to the ducts, while nestin-positive cells are also dispersed throughout the islets. Their abundance increases in the ductal compartment within 4 days of STZ treatment, and this is maximal by 8 days. However, the nestin-positive cells within the islets do not demonstrate an increased number until 16 days after STZ, accompanied by an intense immunocytochemical presence of HGF and IGF-II within the islets, and an increased number of islet cells immunopositive for Nkx6.1 and NKx2.2.

Co-staining within cells of nestin with Pdx1, Nkx2.2, Nkx6.1 or with insulin is never seen.

This suggests that during islet regeneration two distinct processes are occurring. Firstly, islet cell neogenesis is induced at the pancreatic duct, possibly initiated by growth factors such as FGF-7, and involves nestin-immunopositive possible precursors that subsequently express Pdx1 and Ngn3. However, nestin-positive precursors within existing, mature islets may mount a secondary regenerative response in which new beta cells are formed without an apparent expression of Ngn3, but resulting in increased numbers of islet cells expressing Nkx2.2 and Nkx6.1, and the presence of HGF and IGF-II. This model is consistent with the findings of others. Waguri et al[110] induced diabetes with alloxan in the mouse, and demonstrated an islet regeneration involving both ductal neogenesis and the replication of cells within the islets. Following a total elimination of beta cells within the islets of adult mice with STZ two new populations appeared, some cells co-expressing somatostatin, insulin and Pdx1, and others expressing only GLUT2,[111,112] and these were potentiated by insulin treatment. Clearly, there is substantial plasticity in the endocrine pancreas of the juvenile rodent deriving from resident stem cell populations. In humans this period of islet remodeling occurs in the third trimester, and suggests that considerable capacity for recovery of islet cell mass may occur following discrete fetal insults. The exact mechanisms responsible for fetal environmental programming of islet phenotype, insulin availability and risk of later diabetes are now being revealed.

Programming of the fetal pancreas

A reduced dietary protein provided to rats throughout gestation caused a profound reduction in pancreatic weight at birth with a reduced beta-cell mass, islet cell size and pancreatic vascularity.[33–35] The offspring of the low-protein (LP) fed animals have been shown to exhibit abnormal circulating amino acid profiles, with a particular deficiency in taurine.[113] If nutritional restriction is lifted at birth the islet morphology will partly recover, but if extended until weaning or beyond the changes are irreversible and lead to glucose intolerance in later life. Islets isolated in late fetal life following LP administration during pregnancy showed a lower basal insulin release and a blunted insulin release in response to glucose, arginine or leucine.[114] These models show a strong effect of nutritional sufficiency on fetal islet development, but that the neonatal period is also a time of islet plasticity that will have lifelong consequences for glucose homeostasis. The mechanisms by which a LP diet alters islet development involves changes to local peptide growth factor presence and action. A LP diet causes a decreased rate of beta-cell replication, an increase in apoptosis, and a lower pancreatic expression of IGF-II and VEGF.[115] Analysis of beta-cell cycle kinetics *in situ* by detection of cell-cycle-specific proteins suggested that cycle length was increased by a LP diet, with an extended G1 phase. This may reflect a cell cycle block in which cells are not progressing to DNA synthesis due to the deficiency of a trophic progression factor, such as IGF-II, or result from a permanent reprogramming of cell cycle kinetics which may be imprinted on a precursor cell population prior to beta-cell differentiation. Analysis of pre-endocrine stem cell number, assessed by the presence of immunoreactive nestin or *c-kit*, showed a significant reduction in the offspring of animals receiving a LP diet in both the pancreatic ducts and within islets (Fig. 17.4).[116] This correlated with the deficiency of beta cells within individual islets,

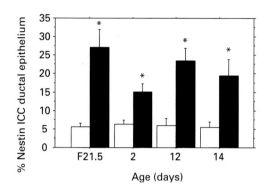

Figure 17.4. *Percentage of nestin-positive cells determined by immunocytochemistry (ICC) within the pancreatic ductal epithelium of rats between 21.5 days gestation (F21.5) and 14 days postnatally following feeding of the mother with a control diet (20% protein, ■) or a low-protein diet (LP; 8% protein, □) since conception. Figures represent mean values ± standard deviation for six to 10 animals; *P < 0.05 or better versus LP diet.*

suggesting that the nutritional deficiency had reduced stem cell plasticity through a change in resident stem cell populations. Such a restriction of cell plasticity may account for the risk of glucose intolerance in later life. In the Goto-Kahizaki (GK) rat model of Type 2 diabetes fetal IGF-II production is defective,[117] and these animals have impaired regeneration of beta cells following partial pancreatectomy.[118] Both observations indicate a possible deficiency of pre-endocrine stem cells that may be associated with an inappropriately low availability of IGF-II. A similar mechanism may explain why induced IUGR in the rat fetus using uterine vessel ligation yields offspring that are prone to Type 2 diabetes in later life.[119]

Strategies for the reprogramming of a developmentally induced risk of diabetes have centered on selective food supplementation at an epidemiological level[120] and the identification of key micronutrients at an experimental level. Taurine is normally an abundant sulphur-containing amino acid in most tissues, including

the pancreas,[121] and is synthesized from methionine and cysteine. It has a variety of functions related to glucose metabolism including liver glycogenesis, glycolysis and glucose oxidation.[122] Taurine levels were shown to be reduced in maternal blood and seriously depleted in fetal blood of rats given a LP diet during pregnancy.[113] The fetal deficit may be related to a reduced activity of placental taurine transporters seen in IUGR. Taurine supplementation of pregnant rats given a LP diet was able to restore pancreatic vascularity and glucose- and amino acid-dependent insulin release from islets isolated in late gestation,[114] while exogenous taurine was able to enhance secretogogue-induced insulin release from isolated fetal islets from LP fed animals.[123] Taurine supplementation alone was also able to reverse the deficits seen in fetal and neonatal beta-cell proliferation in response to a LP diet, and decrease islet cell apoptosis.[124] The proportion of islet cells demonstrating immuno-reactive IGF-II in early life was decreased following exposure to a LP diet, but this was restored by taurine, which appeared to delay the age-related loss of IGF-II in neonatal islets. There is considerable evidence from other tissues for an anti-apoptotic action of taurine[125,126] through mechanisms including an inhibition of the Fas pathway.[127] A LP diet caused an increase in the presence of immunoreactive Fas and the Fas ligand within islets, being greatest at the time of neonatal developmental apoptosis at day 14. Both Fas and Fas ligand presence were reduced by taurine supplementation. Also, taurine addition to culture medium or to the maternal diet prevented interleukin (II)-1- and TNFα-induced apoptosis in isolated islets,[128] and restored insulin secretion.[129] Thus, it appears that selective nutritional components can have a profound effect on endocrine pancreatic development and have the potential to offset environmentally induced damage in early life, and possibly the risk of transmission of Type 2 diabetes.

Conclusions

Insulin is a major drive to embryonic and fetal growth, acting in concert with the IGF axis. Overgrowth or undergrowth of the human infant is associated with an altered beta-cell mass, and altered insulin and IGF production. The IGF are mitogens and survival factors for pancreatic beta cells, while insulin acts to limit the beta-cell mass. The development of pancreatic beta cells occurs by a process of neogenesis from the pancreatic duct, and involves the activation and development of pre-endocrine stem cells. This process is controlled by the sequential expression of transcription factors, and is, in part, driven by locally expressed growth factors. IUGR can alter IGF expression in tissues, limit pre-endocrine stem cell number, and result in a compromised beta-cell mass and phenotype, and abnormal insulin secretion. This is associated with Type 2 diabetes in later life. Such fetal programming of metabolism might be reversible with targeted nutritional supplementation of the mother.

Acknowledgements

For those studies performed by the author gratitude is expressed to the Canadian Institute for Health Research, the Canadian Diabetes Association and the Juvenile Diabetes Research Foundation for financial support.

References

1. Fowden AL. Growth and metabolism. In: (Harding R, Bocking AD, eds.) *Fetal Growth and Metabolism*. (Cambridge University Press: Cambridge, 2001) 44–69.

2. Naeye RL. Infants of diabetic mothers: a quantitative morphological study. *Pediatrics* 1965; 35:980–8.

3. Susa JB, Neave C, Sehgal P et al. Chronic hyperinsulinaemia in the fetal rhesus monkey: effects of physiological hyperinsulinaemia on fetal growth and composition. *Diabetes* 1984; 33:656–60.

4. Newfeld ND, Scott M, Kaplan SA. Ontogeny of the mammalian insulin receptor. *Dev Biol* 1980; 78:151–60.

5. Carson BS, Phillips AF, Simmons MA et al. Effects of a sustained insulin infusion upon glucose uptake and oxygenation in the ovine fetus. *Pediatr Res* 1980; 14:147–52.

6. Girbau M, Gomez JA, Lesniak MA, De Pablo F. Insulin and insulin-like growth factor I both stimulate metabolism, growth and differentiation in the post-neurula chick embryo. *Endocrinology* 1987; 121:1477–82.

7. Raynor MJ, Graham CF. Clonal analysis of the change in growth phenotype during embryonal carcinoma differentiation. *J Cell Sci* 1982; 58:331–4.

8. Duvillié B, Cordonnier N, Deltour L et al. Phenotypic alterations in insulin-deficient mutant mice. *Proc Natl Acad Sci USA* 1997; 94:5137–40.

9. Duvillie B, Currie C, Chrones T et al. Increased islet cell proliferation, decreased apoptosis and greater vascularization leading to beta-cell hyperplasia in mutant mice lacking insulin. *Endocrinology* 2002; 143:1530–7.

10. Hill DJ. Insulin-like growth factors and receptors. In: (Crighton J, ed.) *Encyclopedia of Molecular Medicine*. (John Wiley and Son: New York, 2001) 1768–71.

11. Liu J-P, Baker J, Perkins AS et al. Mice carrying null mutations of the genes encoding insulin-like growth factor I (*Igf*1) and type 1 IGF receptor (*Igf*1r). *Cell* 1993; 75:59–72.

12. De Chiara TM, Efstratiadis A, Robertson EJ. A growth-deficiency phenotype in heterozygous mice carrying an insulin-like growth factor II gene disrupted by targeting. *Nature* 1990; 345:78–80.

13. Baker J, Liu J-P, Robertson EJ, Efstratiadis A. Role of insulin-like growth factors in embryonic and postnatal growth. *Cell* 1993; 75:73–82.

14. Butler AA, LeRoith D. Minireview: tissue-specific versus generalized gene targeting of the *igf*1 and *igf*1r genes and their roles in insulin-like growth factor physiology. *Endocrinology* 2001; 142:1685–88.

15. Werner H, LeRoith D. The role of the insulin-like growth factor system in human cancer. *Adv Cancer Res* 1996; 68:183–223.

16. Morrione A, Valentinis B, Xu S et al. Insulin-like growth factor II stimulates cell proliferation through the insulin receptor. *Proc Natl Acad Sci USA* 1997; 94:3777–82.

17. Frasca F, Pandini G, Scalia P et al. Insulin receptor isoform A, a newly recognized, high affinity insulin-like growth factor II in fetal and cancer cells. *Mol Cell Biol* 1999; 19:3278–88.

18. Vidal H, Auboeuf D, Beylot M, Riou JP. Regulation of insulin receptor mRNA splicing in rat tissues. Effect of fasting, aging and diabetes. *Diabetes* 1995; 44:1196–201.

19. Sbraccia P, Giaccari A, DíAdamo M et al. Expression of the two insulin isoforms is not altered in the skeletal muscle and liver of diabetic rats. *Metabolism* 1998; 47:129–32.

20. Cattanach BM, Peters J, Ball S, Rasberry C. Two imprinted gene mutations: three phenotypes. *Hum Mol Genet* 2000; 9: 2263–73.

21. Lassarre C, Hardouin S, Daffos F et al. Serum insulin-like growth factor binding proteins in the human fetus. Relationships with growth in normal subjects and in subjects with intrauterine growth retardation. *Pediatr Res* 1991; 9:219–21.

22. Delmis J, Drazancic A, Ivanisevic M, Suchanek E. Glucose, insulin, HGH and IGF-I levels in maternal serum, amniotic fluid and umbilical venous serum: a comparison between late normal pregnancy and pregnancies complicated with diabetes and fetal growth retardation. *J Perinatol Med* 1992; 20:47–56.

23. Yan-Jun L, Tsushima T, Minei S et al. Insulin-like growth factors (IGFs) and IGF-binding proteins (IGFBP-1, -2 and -3) in diabetic pregnancy: relationship to macrosomia. *Endocr J* 1996; 43:221–31.

24. Wang HS, Lim J, English J et al. The concentration of insulin-like growth factor-I and insulin-like growth factor binding protein-1 in human umbilical cord serum at delivery: relationship to birth weight. *J Endocrinol* 1991; 129:459–64.

25. Price WA, Rong L, Stiles AD, D'Ercole AJ. Changes in IGF-I and -II, IGF binding protein, and IGF receptor transcript abundance after uterine artery ligation. *Pediatr Res* 1992; 32:291–5.

26. Straus DS, Ooi GT, Orlowski CC, Rechler MM. Expression of the genes for insulin-like growth factor-I (IGF-I), IGF-II, and IGF-binding proteins-1 and -2 in fetal rat under conditions of intrauterine growth retardation caused by maternal fasting. *Endocrinology* 1991; 128:518–25.

27. Fowden AL. The role of insulin in prenatal growth. *J Dev Physiol* 1989; 12:173–82.

28. De Prins F, Van Assche FA. Intrauterine growth retardation and development of endocrine pancreas in experimental rats. *Biol Neonate* 1982; 41:16–21.

29. Van Assche FA, De Prins F, Aerts L, Verjans M. The endocrine pancreas in small or dates infants. *Br J Obstet Gynaecol* 1977; 84:751–3.

30. Garofano A, Czernichow P, Breant B. In utero under-nutrition impairs rat beta-cell development. *Diabetologia* 1997; 40:1231–4.

31. Alvarez C, Martin MA, Goya L et al. Contrasted impact of maternal rat food restriction on fetal endocrine pancreas. *Endocrinology* 1997; 138:2267–73.

32. Swenne I. Glucose-stimulated DNA replication of the pancreatic islets during the development of the rat fetus.

33. Hoet JJ, Dahri S, Reusens B, Remacle C. Do NIDDM and cardiovascular disease originate in utero? In: *Diabetes 1994*. (Elsevier: Amsterdam, 1995) 62–71.

34. Snoeck A, Remacle C, Reusens B, Hoet JJ. Effect of a low protein diet during pregnancy on the fetal rat endocrine pancreas. *Biol Neonate* 1990; 57:107–18.

35. Bennis-taleb N, Remacle C, Hoet JJ, Reusens B. A low protein isocalorific diet during gestation affects brain development and alters permanently cerebral cortex blood vessels in rat offspring. *J Nutr* 1999; 129:1613–19.

36. Barker DJ. The fetal origins of adult disease. *Fetal Matern Med Rev* 1994; 6:71–80.

37. Hales CN, Barker DJ, Clark PM et al. Fetal and infant growth and impaired glucose tolerance at age 64. *Br Med J* 1991; 303:1019–22.

38. Hofman PL, Cutfield WS, Robinson EM et al. Insulin resistance in short children with intrauterine growth retardation. *J Clin Endocrinol Metab* 1997; 82:402–6.

39. Eriksson JG, Forsen T, Tuomilehto J et al. Effects of size at birth and childhood growth on the insulin resistance syndrome in elderly individuals. *Diabetologia* 2002; 45:342–8.

40. Stoffers DA, Zinkin FT, Stanojevik V et al. Pancreatic agenesis attributable to a single deletion in the human IPF-1 coding region. *Nature Genet* 1997; 15:106–10.

41. Hill DJ, Hogg J. Growth factor control of pancreatic β cell hyperplasia. In: (Herington A, ed.) *Clinical Endocrinology and Metabolism*. (Bailliere Tindall: London, 1991) 689–98.

42. Soria B. In vitro differentiation of pancreatic β-cells. *Differentiation* 2001; 68:205–19.

43. Teitelman G. Cellular and molecular analysis of pancreatic islet cell lineage and differentiation. In: (Bardin CW, ed.) *Recent Progress in Hormone Research* (Academic Press: San Diego, 1991) 259–94.

44. Teitelman G. On the origin of pancreatic endocrine cells, proliferation and neoplastic transformation. *Tumor Biol* 1993; 14:167–73.

45. Hill DJ. Fetal programming of the pancreatic β-cells and the implications for postnatal diabetes. *Semin Neonatol* 1999; 4:99–113.

46. Kaung HL. Growth dynamics of pancreatic islet cell populations during fetal and neonatal development of the rat. *Dev Dyn* 1994; 200:163–75.

47. Hellerstrom C, Swenne I, Andersson A. Islet cell replication and diabetes. In: (Lefabvre PJ, Pipeleers DG, eds) *The Pathology of the Endocrine Pancreas in Diabetes*. (Springer-Verlag: Heidelberg, 1988) 141–70.

48. Finegood DT, Scaglia L, Bonner-Weir S. Dynamics of β cell mass in the growing rat pancreas. *Diabetes* 1995; 44:249–56.

49. Scaglia L, Cahill CJ, Finegood DT, Bonner-Weir S. Apoptosis participates in the remodeling of the

endocrine pancreas in the neonatal rat. *Endocrinology* 1997; **138**:1736–41.

50. Petrik J, Arany E, McDonald TJ, Hill DJ. Apoptosis in the pancreatic islet cells of the neonatal rat is associated with a reduced expression of insulin-like growth factor II that may act as a survival factor. *Endocrinology* 1998; **139**: 2994–3004.

51. Hadjivassiliou V, Green MH, James RF et al. Insulin secretion, DNA damage, and apoptosis in human and rat islets of Langerhans following exposure to nitric oxide, peroxynitrite, and cytokines. *Nitric Oxide: Biol Chem* 1998; **2**:429–41.

52. Harrison M, Dunger AM, Berg S et al. Growth factor protection against cytokine-induced apoptosis in neonatal rat islets of Langerhans: role of Fas. *FEBS Lett* 1998; **435**:207–10.

53. Tornehave D, Larsson L-I. Presence of Bcl-Xl during development of the human fetal and rat neonatal endocrine pancreas: correlation to programmed cell death. *Exp Clin Endocrinol Diabetes* 1997; **105**:A27.

54. Edlund H. Transcribing pancreas. *Diabetes* 1988; **47**:817–23.

55. Sander M, German S. The β cell transcription factors and development of the pancreas. *J Mol Med* 1997; **75**:327–40.

56. Madsen OD, Jensen J, Blume N et al. Pancreatic development and maturation of the islet B cell. Studies of pluripotent islet cultures. *Eur J Biochem* 1996; **242**:435–45.

57. Guz Y, Montminy MR, Stein R et al. Expression of murine STF-1, a putative insulin gene transcription factor, in β cells of pancreas, duedenal epithelium and pancreatic exocrine and endocrine progenitors during ontogeny. *Development* 1995; **121**:11–18.

58. Offield MF, Jetton TL, Labosky PA et al. PDX-1 is required for pancreatic outgrowth and differentiation of the rostral duodenum. *Development* 1996; **122**: 983–95.

59. Habener JF, Stoffers DA. A newly discovered role of transcription factors involved in pancreas development and the pathogenesis of diabetes mellitus. *Proc Assoc Am Phys* 1998; **110**:12–21.

60. Sosa-Pineda B, Chowdhury K, Torres M et al. The Pax4 gene is essential for differentiation of insulin-producing β cells in the mammalian pancreas. *Nature* 1997; **386**:399–402.

61. St-Onge L, Sosa-Pineda B, Chowdhury K et al. Pax6 is required for differentiation of glucagon-producing cells in mouse pancreas. *Nature* 1997; **387**:406–8.

62. Sander M, Neubuser A, Kalamaras J et al. Genetic analysis reveals that Pax6 is required for normal transcription of pancreatic hormone genes and islet development. *Genes Dev* 1997; **11**:1662–73.

63. Wells JM, Melton DA. Early mouse endoderm is patterned by soluble factors from adjacent germ layers. *Development* 2000; **127**:1563–72.

64. Arany E, Hill DJ. Ontogeny of fibroblast growth factors in the early development of the rat pancreas. *Pediat Res* 2000; **48**:389–403.

65. Beattie GM, Lappi DA, Baird A, Hayek A. Selective elimination of fibroblasts from pancreatic islet monolayers by basic fibroblast growth factor – saporin mitotoxin. *Diabetes* 1990; **39**:1002–5.

66. Gonzalez AM, Buscaglia M, Ong M, Baird A. Distribution of basic fibroblast growth factor in 18-day rat fetus: localization in the basement membranes of diverse tissues. *J Cell Biol* 1990; **110**:753–65.

67. Gonzalez AM, Hill DJ, Logan A et al. Complementary distribution of fibroblast growth factor-2 (FGF-2) and FGF receptor-1 FGFR1 messenger RNA expression and protein presence in the mid-trimester human fetus. *Pediatr Res* 1996; **39**:375–85.

68. Oberg-Welsh C, Welsh M. Effects of certain growth factors on in vitro maturation of rat fetal islet-like structures. *Pancreas* 1996; **12**:334–9.

69. Goldfarb M. Functions of fibroblast growth factors in vertebrate development. *Cytol Growth Factor Rev* 1996; **7**:311–25.

70. Yi ES, Yin S, Harclerode DL et al. Keratinocyte growth factor induces pancreatic ductal epithelial proliferation. *Am J Pathol* 1994; **145**:80–5.

71. Nguyen HQ, Danilenko DM, Bucay N et al. Expression of keratinocyte growth factor in embryonic liver of transgenic mice causes changes in epithelial growth and differentiation resulting in polycystic kidneys and other organ malformations. *Oncogene* 1996; **12**:2109–19.

72. Bhushan A, Itoh N, Kato S et al. Fgf10 is essential for maintaining the proliferative capacity of epithelial progenitor cells during early pancreatic organogenesis. *Development* 2001; **128**:5109–17.

73. Ferrara N, Houck K, Jakeman L, Leung DW. Molecular and biological properties of the vascular endothelial growth factor family of proteins. *Endocr Rev* 1992; **13**:18–32.

74. Oberg C, Waltenberger J, Claesson-Welsh L, Welsh M. Expression of protein kinases in islet cells: possible role of the Flk–1 receptor for β-cell maturation from duct cells. *Growth Factors* 1994; **10**:115–26.

75. Oberg-Welsh C, Sandler S, Andersson A, Welsh M. Effects of vascular endothelial growth factor on pancreatic duct cell replication and the insulin production of fetal islet-like cell clusters in vitro. *Mol Cell Endocrinol* 1997; **126**:125–32.

76. Lammert E, Cleaver O, Melton D. Induction of pancreatic differentiation by signals from blood vessels. *Science* 2001; **294**:564–7.

77. Sonnenberg E, Meyer D, Weidner KM, Birchmeier C. Scatter factor/hepatocyte growth factor and its receptor, the c-met tyrosine kinase, can mediate a signal exchange between mesenchyme and epithelia during mouse development. *J Cell Biol* 1993; **123**:223–35.

78. Otonkoski T, Cirulli V, Beattie GM et al. A role for hepatocyte growth factor. Scatter factor in fetal mesenchyme-induced pancreatic β cell growth. *Endocrinology* 1996; **137**:3131–9.

79. Garcia-Ocana A, Vasavada RC, Cebrian A et al. Transgenic overexpression of hepatocyte growth factor in the beta-cell markedly improves islet function and islet transplant outcomes in mice. *Diabetes* 2001; **50**:2752–62.

80. Hill DJ. Fetal programming of the pancreatic β cells and the implications for postnatal diabetes. *Semin Neonatol* 1999; **4**:99–113.

81. Whiters DJ, Burks DJ, Towery HH et al. Irs-2 coordinates Igf-1 receptor-mediated β-cell development and peripheral insulin signaling. *Nature Genet* 1999; **23**: 32–40.

82. Hogg J, Hill DJ, Han VKM. The ontogeny of insulin-like growth factor (IGF) and IGF binding protein gene expression in the rat pancreas. *J Mol Endocrinol* 1994; **13**:49–58.

83. Hill DJ, Hogg J, Petrik J et al. Cellular distribution and ontogeny of insulin-like growth factors (IGFs) and IGF binding protein messenger RNAs and peptides in developing rat pancreas. *J Endocrinol* 1999; **160**:305–17.

84. Petrik J, Pell JM, Arany E et al. Overexpression of insulin-like growth factor-II in transgenic mice is associated with pancreatic islet cell hyperplasia. *Endocrinology* 1999; **140**:2353–63.

85. Scaglia L, Cahill CJ, Finegood DT, Bonner-Weir S. Apoptosis participates in the remodeling of the endocrine pancreas in the neonatal rat. *Endocrinology* 1997; **138**:1736–41.

86. Petrik J, Arany E, McDonald TJ, Hill DJ. Apoptosis in the pancreatic islet cells of the neonatal rat is associated with a reduced expression of insulin-like growth factor II that may act as a survival factor. *Endocrinology* 1998; **139**:2994–3004.

87. Hill DJ, Duvillié B. Pancreatic development and adult diabetes. *Pediatr Res* 2000; **48**:269–74.

88. Hill DJ, Strutt B, Arany E et al. Increased and persistent circulating insulin-like growth factor-II in neonatal transgenic mice suppresses developmental apoptosis in the pancreatic islets. *Endocrinology* 2000; **141**:1151–7.

89. Devedjian J-C, George M, Casellas A et al. Transgenic mice overexpressing insulin-like growth factor-II in β cells develop type 2 diabetes. *J Clin Invest* 2000; **105**:731–40.

90. Strutt B, Salih DA, Arany E et al. Over-expression of IGFBP-5 in utero results in altered development of the endocrine pancreas and a reduction in β-cell mass. *Proceedings of the 84th Annual Meeting of the Endocrine Society*, San Francisco, 2002.

91. Lendahl U, Zimmerman LB, McKay RD. CNS stem cells express a new class of intermediate filament protein. *Cell* 1990; **60**:585–95.

92. Hunziker E, Stein M. Nestin-expressing cells in the pancreatic islets of Langerhans. *Biochem Biophys Res Commun* 2000; **271**:16–119.

93. Zulewski H, Abraham EJ, Gerlach MJ et al. Multipotential nestin-positive stem cells isolated from adult pancreatic islets differentiate ex vivo into pancreatic endocrine, exocrine, and hepatic phenotypes. *Diabetes* 2001; **50**:521–33.

94. Joanette E, Arany E, Reusens B, Hill DJ. β-cell precursors are affected by a diet low in protein. In: *Proceedings of the 61st Annual Meeting of the American Endocrine Society*, Denver, 2001, 331.

95. Baumann U, Crosby HA, Ramani P et al. Expression of the stem cell factor receptor c-kit in normal and diseased pediatric liver: identification of a human hepatic progenitor cell? *Hepatology* 1999; **30**:112–17.

96. Wang JF, Hill DJ. Isolation and characterization of homeodomain transcription factor PDX-1 and nestin expressing stem cells from neonatal rat pancreas. *Can J Diabetes Care* 2001; **25**:216.

97. Cecil RL. On hypertrophy and regeneration of the islands of Langerhans. *J Exp Med* 1911; **14**:500–19.

98. Gepts W, de Mey J. Islet cell survival determined by morphology. An immunocytochemical study of the islet of Langerhans in juvenile diabetes mellitus. *Diabetes* 1978; **27 (Suppl 1)**:251–61.

99. Volk BW, Wellman KF. The pancreas in idiopathic diabetes. In: (Volk BW, Arquilla ER, eds.) *The Diabetic Pancreas*, 2nd edn. (Plenum Medical: New York, 1985) 353.

100. Brockenbrough JS, Weir GC, Bonner-Weir S. Discordance of exocrine and endocrine growth after 90% pancreatectomy in rats. *Diabetes* 1988; **37**:232–6.

101. Bonner-Weir S, Baxter LA, Schuppin GT, Smith FE. A second pathway for regeneration of adult exocrine and endocrine pancreas: a possible recapitulation of embryoni development. *Diabetes* 1993; **42**:1715–20.

102. Smith FE, Rosen KM, Vill-Komaroff L et al. Enhanced insulin-like growth factor-I gene expression in regenerating rat pancreas. *Proc Natl Acad Sci USA* 1991; **88**:6152–6.

103. Zangen DH, Bonner-Weir S, Lee CH et al. Reduced insulin, GLUT2, and IDX-1 in β-cells after partial pancreatectomy. *Diabetes* 1997; **46**:258–64.

104. Rosenberg L, Brown RA, Duguid WP. A new model for the development of duct epithelial hyperplasia and the initiation of nesidioblastosis. *J Surg Res* 1983; **35**: 63–72.

105. Rosenberg L, Duguid WP, Vinik AI. The effect of cellophane wrapping of the pancreas in the Syrian golden hamster: autoradiographic observations. *Pancreas* 1989; **4**:31–7.

106. Rafaeloff R, Barlow SW, Rosenberg L, Vinik AI. IGF-II but not IGF-I is involved in islet neogenesis in adult pancreas. *Proceedings of the 54th Annual Meeting of the American Diabetes Association*, Abstracts, 1994.

107. Ilieva A, Yuan S, Wang RN et al. Pancreatic islet cell survival following islet isolation – the role of cellular interactions in the pancreas. *J Endocrinol* 1999; **161**: 357–64.

108. Arany E, Dusky S, Strutt B, Hill DJ. Stem cells and neogenesis in neonatal streptozotocin treated rats. *Proceedings of the 20th Joint Meeting of the British Endocrinology Society*, Belfast, 2001.

109. Arany E, Strutt B, Duvillie B, Hill DJ. Ontogeny of peptide growth factor and transcription factor expression during induced islet cell neogenesis in the neonatal rat pancreas. *Proceedings of the 81th Annual Meeting of the Endocrinology Society*, San Diego, 1999, 2–228.

110. Waguri M, Yamamoto K, Miyagawa J et al. Demonstration of two different processes of β-cell regeneration on a new diabetic mouse model induced by selective perfusion of alloxan. *Diabetes* 1997; **46**: 1281–90.

111. Fernandes A, King, LC, Guz Y et al. Differentiation of new insulin-producing cells is induced by injury in adult pancreatic islets. *Endocrinology* 1997; **138**:1750–62.

112. Guz Y, Nasir I, Teitelman G. Regeneration of pancreatic β cells from intra-islet precursor cells in an experimental model of diabetes. *Endocrinology* 2001; **142**: 4956–68.

113. Reusens B, Dahri S, Snoeck A et al. Long-term consequences of diabetes and its complications may have a fetal origin; experimental and epidemiologial evidence. In: (Cowett RM, ed.) *Diabetes. Nestlé Nutrition Workshop Series 135.* (Raven Press: New York, 1995) 187–98.

114. Cherif H, Reusens B, Ahn MT et al. Effects of taurine on the insulin secretion of fetal rat islets from dams fed a low protein diet. *J Endocrinol* 1998; **159**:341–8.

115. Petrik J, Reusens B, Arany E et al. A low protein diet alters the balance of islet cell replication and apoptosis in the fetal and neonatal rat, and is associated with a reduced pancreatic expression of insulin-like growth factor-II. *Endocrinology* 1999; **140**:4861–73.

116. Joanette E, Arany E, Reusens B, Hill DJ. β-cell precursors are affected by a diet low in protein. *Proceedings of the 61st Annual Meeting of the American Endocrinology Society*, Denver, 2001.

117. Serradas P, Goya L, Lacorne M et al. Fetal insulin and insulin-like growth factor-2 production is impaired in the GK rat model of type 2 diabetes. *Diabetes* 2002; **51**:392–7.

118. Plachot C, Movassat J, Portha B. Impaired beta-cell regeneration after partial pancreatectomy in the adult Goto-Kahizaki rat, a spontaneous model of type II diabetes. *Histochem Cell Biol* 2001; **116**:131–9.

119. Simmons RA, Templeton LJ, Gertz SJ. Intrauterine growth retardation leads to the development of type 2 diabetes. *Diabetes* 2001; **50**:2279–86.

120. Law CM, Egger P, Dada O et al. Body size at birth and blood pressure among children in developing countries. *Int J Epidemiol* 2001; **30**:52–7.

121. Briel G, Gylfe E, Hellman B, Neuhoff V. Microdetermination of free amino acids in pancreatic islets isolated from obese-hyperglycemic mice. *Acta Physiol Scand* 1972; **84**:247–53.

122. Huxtable RJ. Physiological actions of taurine. *Physiol Rev* 1992; **72**:101–63.

123. Cherif H, Reusens B, Dahri S et al. Stimulatory effects of taurine on insulin secretion by fetal rat islets cultured in vitro. *J Endocrinol* 1996; **151**:501–6.

124. Boujendar S, Remacle C, Hill D, Reusens B. Taurine supplementation to the low protein maternal diet restores a normal development of the endocrine pancreas in the offspring. *Diabetologia* 2000; **43 Suppl 1**: A128.

125. Wang JH, Redmond HP, Watson RW et al. The beneficial effect of taurine on the prevention of human endothelial cell death. *Shock* 1996; **6**:331–8.

126. Watson RW, Redmond HP, Wang JH, Bouchier-Hayes D. Mechanisms involved in sodium arsenite-induced apoptosis of human neutrophils. *J Leukoc Biol* 1996; **60**:625–32.

127. Redmond HP, Stapleton PP, Neary P, Bouchier-Hayes D. Immunonutrition: the role of taurine. *Nutrition* 1998; **14**:599–604.

128. Merezak S, Hardikar AA, Yajnik CS et al. Intrauterine low protein diet increases fetal β cell sensitivity to NO and IL-1β: the protective role of taurine. *J Endocrinol* 2001; **171**:299–308.

129. Cherif H, Reusens B, Ahn MT et al. Effect of taurine on the insulin secretion of islets of fetuses from dams fed a low protein diet. *Endocrinology* 1998; **159**:341–8.

18

Pre-implantation embryopathy and maternal diabetes

René De Hertogh, Amaya Leunda Casi, Laurence Hinck

Introduction

The key questions, still largely unsolved, when dealing with diabetic embryopathies are: 'When do they occur?' and 'How?'

Although a generally accepted consensus considers that a diabetic equilibrium close to the physiological situation, obtained before the onset of pregnancy, is the best prerequisite to avoid these embryopathies, it still appears that congenital malformations remain a matter of concern in medical practice.[1-3] The onset of maternal diabetes induced embryo dysmorphogenesis is known to occur very early in pregnancy, between 3 and 7 weeks of gestational age in the human.[4] In accordance with this early occurrence of congenital malformations, many experimental studies in rodents have revealed the high sensitivity of embryos to the teratogenicity of maternal diabetes at the time of organogenesis.[5-7] However, some recent studies have shown that diabetes induced embryopathies in humans were characterized by a high proportion of blastogenic developmental field defects in their pattern of multiple congenital anomalies.[8] This implies that a diabetic insult to the embryo is likely to occur very early in its development, possibly very soon after conception.[8] Both observations, suggesting an early diabetes induced impairment in the embryo development, on the one hand, and a later

disruption of normal differentiation during organogenesis, on the other, are not mutually independent. Indeed, they can be reconciled by the multifactorial/threshold concept, according to which the sensitivity of embryos to teratogenic factors can be influenced by developmental factors that are possibly modified at an early stage.[9] The teratogenic threshold would then be changed, and the proportion of subjects affected by a given teratogenic factor would be raised.

Hence, the answer to the question: 'When does the embryopathy occur?' might involve a time sequence rather than a precise growth age and include a very early step in embryo differentiation. In this respect, the pre-implantation phase appears to be a critical period when the embryo first differentiates into the two essential cell lineages: the trophectoderm (TE), which is at the origin of the placenta, and the inner cell mass (ICM), which contains all the founder cells of the embryo[10] (Fig. 18.1).

The answer to the second question 'How does the embryopathy occur?' also remains largely a matter of debate. This is despite much experimental work and many observations made in this important field, most of which were obtained from post-implantation experimental models.[6,7] The multifactorial aspect of the potential teratogenic agents has been found,[11] and possible mechanisms of cell injury proposed.[7,12] The role of an oxidative stress has

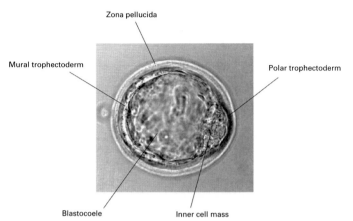

Zona pellucida

Mural trophectoderm

Polar trophectoderm

Blastocoele

Inner cell mass

Figure 18.1. *Mouse pre-implantation blastocyst, with the two cell lineages: the inner cell mass (ICM), at the origin of the embryonic tissues, and the trophectoderm (TE), a single layer of cells at the origin of the placenta. The polar TE is in close contact with the ICM, whilst the mural TE is located distally from the ICM. The inside cavity (the blastocoele) and the outside protective coating of the blastocyst, made of glycoproteins, (the zona pellucida) are also indicated.*

been suggested and is supported by *in vivo* and *in vitro* experiments.[13–16] Expanding on the multifactorial hypothesis of the effect of teratogenic factors at different periods, as mentioned above in the multifactorial/threshold concept, may help to clarify how maternal diabetes in humans induces congenital malformations at much lower levels of metabolic anomalies than those usually found in experimental studies.

The following pages review the major observations related to diabetes induced pre-implantation embryopathies in rodents.

Maternal diabetes and pre-implantation development

Concordant observations made in diabetic rats and mice have shown the deleterious impact of maternal diabetes on pre-implantation embryo development[17] (Table 18.1). Streptozotocin induced diabetic pregnant rats had a 25% decreased implantation rate on day 6 of pregnancy.[18] The number of blastocysts floating in the uterine cavity on day 5 of pregnancy (a few hours before implantation) was similarly decreased by 20%, whereas the number of morulae, in the embryonic stage before the blastocyst stage, was slightly increased.[19] A

negative impact of maternal diabetes on embryo development was further evidenced in the study of blastocysts themselves. Indeed, the total number of cells of those blastocysts was decreased by 15%, the cell deficit being greater in the ICM (20%) than in the TE (12%).[20] In a later study, a similar observation was made in spontaneously diabetic BB rats.[21] In alloxan-diabetic mice, fewer embryos were recovered on day 2 of pregnancy and showed impaired development *in vitro*.[22] Also in mice blastocysts recovered before the time of implantation from diabetic females showed a 10% deficit in total cell number,[23] in agreement with observations made in diabetic rats.

When diabetic rats were treated with insulin during the pre-implantation period (day 1–6 of pregnancy), the development of blastocysts was normalized, thus confirming the specific negative impact of the maternal diabetic environment on embryo development.[24]

Blastocysts from diabetic rats contained a higher proportion of dead cells in the ICM as compared to blastocysts from normal rats. Dead cells showed nuclear fragmentation, suggesting the existence of an apoptotic process.[20] Blastocysts recovered from diabetic rats and transferred on to a fibronectin-coated culture dish to allow *in vitro* attachment, spreading

Species	Parameter	Effect	Reference
Rat	Morphological progression	20% decrease	19
	Average cell number	20% decrease	20,21
	Rate of glucose metabolism	No effect	55
	Rate of implantation	25% decrease	18
	Chromatin degradation index	6-fold increase	45
	Nuclear fragmentation index	5-fold increase	20,45
	Clusterin mRNA expression	1.7-fold increase	45
Mouse	Morphological progression	10–90% decrease	22
	Average cell number	10% decrease	23, 48
	Rate of protein synthesis	35% decrease	23
	Rate of implantation	13% decrease	26
	Chromatin degradation index	6.3-fold increase	46
	Bax mRNA expression	2.5-fold increase	46,47
	Bax protein expression	6.5-fold increase	46,47
	p53 expression		64

Table 18.1.   *Effects of maternal diabetes on rat and mouse blastocyst growth.*

and implantation, displayed growth impairment. A large proportion of those blastocysts failed to maintain a structured ICM at the center of the TE outgrowth, which was smaller and contained fewer nuclei but a higher proportion of giant nuclei, compared to control outgrowths.[25] This observation shows that, after retrieval of the blastocysts from the diabetic milieu, later ICM development remained impaired, and further proliferation and differentiation of the TE was altered. This suggested that pre-implantation embryopathy induced by the diabetic environment could imply post-implantation effects with regard to further embryo development. More direct evidence concerning this was provided by transfer experiments of mouse pre-implantation embryos from diabetic females into normal pseudopregnant recipient females. These experiments demonstrated impaired development of these embryos as well as an increased incidence of fetal malformation, compared to pre-implantation embryos transferred from normal females.[26,27]

Role of glucose

The glucose content of uterine secretions is significantly higher in diabetic mice compared to control mice, and may be considered to be a potential factor implicated in the embryotoxicity of maternal diabetes.[28] Hence, glucose has been used in many *in vitro* studies with rat and mouse embryos (Table 18.2).

The morphological progression of two-cell mouse embryos was retarded when *in vitro* incubation was performed in 53 mM compared to 6 mM glucose.[29] Mouse blastocysts incubated in 17 mM glucose for 72 hours did not develop further, showed an increased rate of degeneration[30] and a decreased rate of *in vitro* attachment.[31] Exposure of rat blastocysts to 17 mM glucose for 24 hours or 48 hours resulted in a 16% and 33% decrease in the number of ICM cells, respectively, compared to embryos incubated in 6 mM glucose.[32] TE cell proliferation was less affected by high glucose concentrations in the culture medium.

Species	Parameter	Effect	Reference
Rat	Average cell number	13–25% decrease	32,50
	Chromatin degradation index	2–3 fold increase	32,50
	Nuclear fragmentation index	3–4 fold increase	32
	Clusterin mRNA expression	2.7 fold increase	32
	Bcl-2 mRNA expression	8 fold increase	49
Mouse	Morphological progression	25–65% decrease	29–31
	Rate of attachment	20% decrease	31
	Rate of implantation	35% decrease	31
	Polyol pathway activity	2.5 fold increase	63
	Krebs cycle activity	2 fold increase	63
	Glycogen content	No effect	63
	Chromatin degradation index	10 fold increase	46
	Bax mRNA expression	2 fold increase	46,47
	Bax protein expression	7.4 fold increase	46,47
	p53 expression		64

Table 18.2. Effects of in vitro *exposure to high glucose concentration on rat and mouse blastocyst growth.*

Other diabetes-linked factors, such as aceto-acetate or β-hydroxybutyrate, added to the culture medium, were found to inhibit the development of mouse embryos, either at the two-cell stage or the blastocyst stage.[33,34] Serum from insulin-dependent diabetic patients added to the culture medium of mouse blastocysts decreased their morphological progression.[35]

Interestingly, high glucose concentrations in the medium increased the occurrence of dead cells in rat blastocysts after 48 hours of culture. Dead cells had the morphological characteristics of apoptotic cells.[32]

Role of tumor necrosis factor-α

The close interplay existing between the pre-implantation embryo and the maternal environment through the uterine milieu is manifold and involves not only metabolic factors, such as glucose or ketones, or hormones like estrogen, progestogen or insulin, but also paracrine or juxtacrine agents such as cytokines.[36] These factors are indeed likely to be disturbed by the diabetic state, and may be involved in diabetic complications.[37]

Tumor necrosis factor (TNF)-α is present in the uterine wall at the time of implantation.[38] Receptors to TNF-α are present on the blasto-cyst, which may then be receptive to the cytokine.[39,40] Indeed, in *in vitro* cultures of normal rat blastocysts, it was shown that TNF-α decreased ICM growth without affecting the TE.[39,40]

TNF-α synthesis was increased in uterine explants from pregnant diabetic rats[41,42] and in primary cultures of uterine cells with high glucose concentrations.[42] Rat blastocysts incu-bated in a culture medium conditioned by uterine explants from diabetic pregnant rats showed a slower ICM growth.[41] This growth inhibition was partly inhibited when TNF-α was neutralized in the medium by specific antibodies or by antisense oligodeoxynucleotides directed against the TNF-α p60 receptor, present on the ICM cells.[43] This suggests that TNF-α secreted in excess by the uterine epithelium from diabetic rats was indeed a factor responsible for the observed blastocyst growth inhibition.

A similar TNF-α induced growth inhibition was observed in mouse blastocysts.[44] Interestingly, when TNF-α treated blastocysts were subsequently transferred to pseudo-pregnant surrogate mothers, a significantly higher rate of resorption was observed on day 15, compared to untreated blastocysts transferred simultaneously in the contralateral uterine horn of the same mother.[44] Moreover, the weight of the surviving fetuses on day 15 was significantly lower for the TNF-α pre-treated as compared to control blastocysts. The 15% weight deficit was observed in the fetuses only, not in the placentae. Hence, post-implantation consequence of a pre-implantation negative impact, likely to occur in diabetic pregnancies, was shown in this model.

Role of apoptosis

In vivo and *in vitro* studies have shown an increased incidence of cell death in the ICM of rat blastocysts obtained either from diabetic mothers or from normal mothers and incubated in the presence of high glucose concentrations (Tables 18.1 and 18.2). Cell death was characterized in both instances by nuclear fragmentation.[20,32] A similar observation was made in blastocysts from spontaneously diabetic BB rats.[21] The occurrence of nuclear chromatin degradation, shown by the TUNEL method, was also increased in the ICM cells of blastocysts from diabetic rats[45] and mice[46] (Fig. 18.2).

In mice, mRNA concentration and protein expression of the pro-apoptotic effector Bax were higher in blastocysts from diabetic animals.[46] Mouse embryos, genetically deficient for this pro-apoptotic effector and recovered from diabetic mothers, had a lower incidence of chromatin degradation than similarly obtained Bax-positive embryos. The Bax null embryos from diabetic mothers also had lower rates of malformation and resorption on day 14 of pregnancy.[47] This suggests that increased apoptosis in the blastocysts might manifest later as increased resorption or malformation, both events observed at an increased rate in diabetic pregnancy.

Transcripts for clusterin, a compound associated with the apoptotic event and supposedly useful in the removal of cellular debris, were twice as high in blastocysts from diabetic rats compared to control embryos.[45] Increased nuclear chromatin degradation, Bax and clusterin expressions were also reported following *in vitro* incubation of rat or mice blastocysts in high concentrations of glucose.[45,46,48] Also, rat blastocysts cultured in 28 mM glucose for 24 hours presented an increased number of cells expressing the anti-apoptotic Bcl-2 mRNA, compared to blastocysts incubated in 6 mM glucose.[49] Inhibition of Bcl-2 expression by anti-sense oligodeoxynucleotide increased the incidence of chromatin degradation in blastocysts incubated in high glucose concentrations.[49] Specific inhibition of two apoptotic effectors, caspase-3 and caspase-activated-deoxyribonuclease (CAD), protected rat blastocysts from the high glucose induced chromatin degradation.[50] Interestingly, Bcl-2 inhibition, on the one hand, and caspase-3 or CAD inhibition on the other, did not influence glucose induced nuclear fragmentation, suggesting that different pathways lead to these two cellular aspects of apoptosis.

From these studies, the hypothesis emerges that glucose induced apoptosis may be at least partly responsible for maternal diabetes-associated malformation or resorption. It may be suggested that a significant loss of key progenitor cells from the ICM may sensitize these embryos from diabetic mothers to later developmental deficiencies. Indeed, previous reports have shown that normal embryogenesis

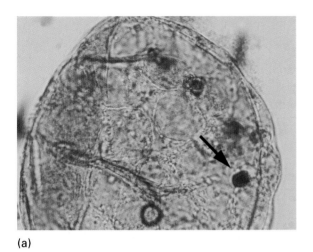
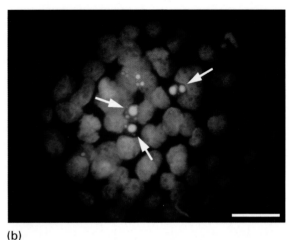

(a) (b)

Figure 18.2. *Identification of nuclear chromatin degradation by the TUNEL method in a rat blastocyst, observed under a visible light microscope* **(a)**. *Nuclei counterstaining with bisbenzimide allows the detection of fragmented nuclei under UV light* **(b)**. *(The scale bar represents 25 μm.)*

can occur only if a sufficient number of functional ICM cells are available.[51]

Role of oxidative stress

Much research, both *in vivo* and on post-implantation embryos *in vitro*, suggests that diabetic embryopathy may result from cellular damage secondary to overproduction and/or decreased inhibition of reactive oxygen species (ROS) in the embryonic cells.[13–16] The origin of ROS may be multiple, and is not precisely defined.

Whether such a mechanism could occur in embryos at the pre-implantation stage has been the subject of some recent investigations. This hypothesis was supported by studies performed by cyclic voltametry on mouse blastocysts cultured in serum from diabetic pregnant women.[52] It was shown that the viability of these blastocysts was decreased as well as the anti-oxidative power of the surviving embryos. Other reports showed that oxidizing agents, such as hydrogen peroxide or diamide, could

trigger cell cycle arrest and apoptosis in mouse zygotes and blastocysts.[53] Hydrogen peroxide has been suggested to be a key mediator of naturally occurring apoptosis in mouse blastocyst.[54] Disruption of this equilibrium by high glucose concentrations could lead to excessive cell damage, inappropriate apoptotic events and impairment of embryo development.

In a direct approach to this hypothesis, mouse blastocysts were incubated in different concentrations of glucose for 24 hours then loaded with dichlorodihydrofluorescein diacetate (DCHFDA) and observed by confocal microscopy. In the presence of an oxidative process within the cell, DCHFDA eventually yields dichlorofluorescein (DCF). The production of DCF is linearly related to the presence of ROS, which can then be quantified through the intensity of the emitted fluorescence. A 2.8-fold increased fluorescence was observed in the ICM region of embryos exposed to 28 mM glucose, compared to 6 mM glucose[48] (Fig. 18.3). The origin of this increased ROS generation by high glucose concentrations is unclear. At the blastocyst stage, embryonic energy metabolism occurs

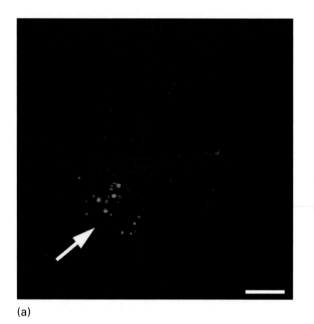

(a)

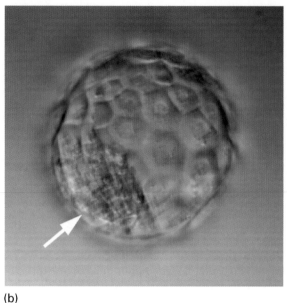

(b)

Figure 18.3. *Reactive oxygen species (ROS) detection and localization in a mouse blastocyst. Three-dimensional reconstitution by confocal laser scanning microscope of a blastocyst loaded with DCHFDA after 24 hours incubation in 28 mM glucose* **(a)***; the ROS induced fluorescent signal is mainly detected in the ICM region of the embryo (arrows), as evidenced by the visible light image of the same embryo* **(b)***. (The scale bar represents 20 µm.)*

mainly through the glycolytic pathway and very little through the Krebs cycle.[48,55] Hence, a substrate overload in the mitochondrial electron transport chain, likely to be at the origin of ROS generation in post-implantation embryos,[14] is less likely to occur at the blastocyst stage, although a transient overload cannot be ruled out. Other mechanisms may be suggested, such as glucose auto-oxidation, glycation processes or disruption of anti-oxidative capacities.

Role of glucose metabolism

Mouse blastocysts depend principally on insulin-independent facilitative glucose transport for glucose supply, but a passive diffusion and an active transport system have also been reported.[56–58] Although an insulin-sensitive glucose transporter, GLUT8,[59] has been recently described in blastocysts, *in vitro* glucose utilization by rat pre-implantation embryos was not increased by the presence of added insulin to the medium.[55]

Recent studies have shown a decreased glucose uptake in mouse blastocysts pre-incubated in high glucose concentrations for 24 hours,[48] and a decreased protein expression and function of the transporter, GLUT1.[47] Blastocysts recovered from diabetic mice showed similarly decreased protein expression and transcript content of GLUT1, -2 and -3.[46] In mouse tropho- blasts[60] and in human term placenta trophoblasts,[61] a downregulation of GLUT1 mRNA and protein expression, with a con-current drop in glucose uptake, have been observed following exposure to high glucose concentrations. It has been suggested that glucose has an auto-regulatory effect on its own transport in human term placenta through the translocation of the transporters from the cell surface to the intracellular compartment.[62] These mechanisms might be considered as protective against the deleterious effects of intracellular glucose accumulation. Such accumulation of glucose or of glucose-derived products has been reported in mouse[63] and rat[55] embryos submitted to high concentrations of glucose *in vitro*.

It has been suggested that the decremental effect of glucose transporters caused by the high concentration on glucose might, however, lower glucose uptake. This could cause intracellular glucose deficiency and energy shortage, eventually leading to genomic damage and apoptosis, through the activation of pathways including p53, Bax and caspases.[47, 64] This interesting, although paradoxical, hypothesis is however difficult to reconcile with previous reports on rat and mouse blastocysts, which show that the main glucose utilization pathway – glycolysis – is saturated at very low extracellular glucose concentrations (< 0.5 mM). Increasing glucose concentration in the medium did allow slow and progressive accumulation of glucose-derived products, possibly in macromolecules, without increasing significantly glucose utilization either through glycolysis or through oxidation.[55,56] Moreover, recent work on mouse blastocysts submitted to high concentrations of glucose *in vitro* has shown that, despite a fourfold reduction in glucose uptake, the amount of glucose taken up by the embryos was still far beyond the saturation capacity of the glycolytic pathway.[48] This seems to rule out, at least in these experimental conditions, that lack of glucose is responsible for intracellular energy shortage. Interestingly, however, the same experimental study showed a 25% decrease in the glycolytic activity of embryos pre-treated with high concentrations of glucose, whilst glucose oxidation, mainly through the pentose phosphate pathway, was unchanged.[48] This apparently specific partial inhibition of glycolysis is thus very unlikely due to the decreased glucose uptake, but could be secondary to oxidative stress; it has indeed been shown that the glycolytic enzyme, glyceraldehydro-3-phosphate dehydrogenase, was inhibited by ROS.[65]

From the above observations it thus appears that high glucose concentrations may cause oxidative stress in the ICM cells, possibly contributing to lower energy production by decreased glycolysis. Thus, decreased glucose uptake may, in some instances, be involved in lower energy production, and contribute to the triggering of the apoptotic events.

Role of fibrobast growth factor-4

Previous observations have shown that TE development of blastocysts recovered from diabetic rats and incubated *in vitro* was impaired.[25] Indeed, outgrowth expansion and differentiation were disturbed, producing a higher proportion of giant cells (Fig. 18.4).

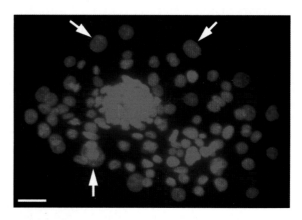

Figure 18.4. *Nuclear staining of a mouse blastocyst expanding over a fibronectin-coated culture substrate. Several giant trophoblast cells (arrows) can be seen at the periphery of the outgrowth. (The scale bar represents 20 μm.)*

Normal mouse blastocysts, incubated in a culture medium containing 17 mM or 28 mM glucose showed similarly an increased outgrowth surface, increased trophoblast nuclear surface and a tendency of higher numbers of giant nuclei.[66, 67]

Experimental data suggest that important regulatory events operate at the surface between ICM cells and the polar TE, in close contact with the ICM (Fig. 18.1). This regulation is necessary in order to prevent these pre-trophoblastic cells from transforming to giant cells, and thereby allowing the maintenance of a sufficient population of diploid cells required for full placental development.[68] Regulatory peptides, belonging to the fibroblast growth factor (FGF) family and produced by the ICM, are suspected to be involved in TE differentiation through a paracrine mechanism.[69]

FGF-4 is expressed in the ICM cells of mouse blastocysts,[69] stimulates TE cell proliferation and represses their differentiation into giant trophoblastic cells.[70] Recent experiments have shown that the ICM from mouse blastocysts, pre-incubated at high glucose concentrations for 24 hours and further incubated for 48 hours in 6 mM glucose, contained 30% less FGF-4 protein than control embryos pre-incubated in 6 mM glucose. The trophoblast outgrowths of these embryos were also 18% larger than those of control embryos.[66, 67] The role of the FGF-4 deficit in the excessive trophoblast surface expansion was strongly suggested by the addition of FGF-4 in the pre-incubation medium. Indeed, mouse blastocysts pre-incubated in high concentrations of glucose with additional FGF-4 showed a normal trophoblast outgrowth, a normal nuclear surface area and a normal giant nuclei index, no different from those of blastocysts pre-incubated in 6 mM glucose.[67]

These observations suggest that the high concentration glucose induced impairment of FGF-4 production by the ICM may contribute to the secondary disturbance of TE growth and differentiation. The diabetes-linked hyperglycemic state may also, through impairment of ICM development and function, disturb TE growth and differentiation, leading to further negative impact on embryo implantation and development.

Conclusions

Diabetic embryopathy and diabetes induced congenital malformations should not be considered to be random events, resulting from the disruption of the normal sequence of differentiation at a critical time of development. A dynamic process involving early and sustained impact of disturbed maternal environment on embryo growth and differentiation might better fit with the clinical and experimental observations so far reported.

Hence, the occurrence of development field defects[8] would imply early events, possibly in the pre-implantation state, and the multifactorial/threshold concept[9] could reconcile and integrate observations made at different steps of embryo development.

For some time, much research performed on post-implantation embryos have convincingly demonstrated the high sensitivity of organogenesis on several diabetes induced metabolic disturbances. Yet, a satisfactory unifying model, taking into account *in vivo* conditions encountered in this physiopathological state, is still lacking. Similarly, the more limited, although clearly confirmed observations made in pre-implantation embryos reviewed above, question an earlier disruptive event in embryo development. This should not be overlooked. As suggested by more recent reports in this field, the high sensitivity of the ICM cells to the diabetic environment and to high glucose levels

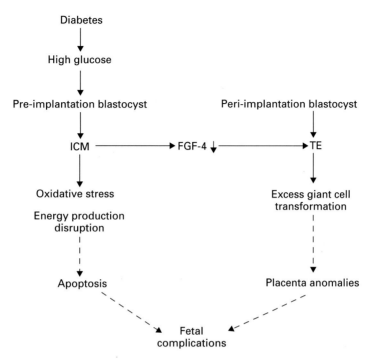

Figure 18.5. *Tentative sequence of events leading from diabetes induced pre-implantation embryo insult to fetal complications. (From Amaya Leunda Casi:* High glucose disturbs different developmental parameters of the mouse blastocyst in vitro, *Thesis, Université Catholique de Louvain, 2001.)*

unavoidably leads to embryo growth distortion, by triggering oxidative stress and possibly a certain degree of energy depletion, leading to apoptosis in these cells (Fig. 18.5). TNF-α, produced by uterine epithelial cells, may be a contributory intermediary factor in this maternal diabetes induced effect. Moreover, abnormal function of the ICM may involve a relative lack of regulatory compounds, like FGF-4, allowing the production of excess giant cells, thereby disrupting trophoblast development and differentiation (Fig. 18.5).

Again, the relevance of these observations to the onset of later congenital malformations is strongly suggested, but deserves more direct evidence. The synergistic effects of both pre- and post-implantation diabetes induced insult to the embryo might, in this respect, be a sound and unifying hypothesis.

References

1. Fuhrman K, Reiher H, Semmler K et al. Prevention of congenital malformations in infants of insulin-dependent diabetic mothers. *Diabetes Care* 1983; **6**:219–23.
2. Mills JL, Knopp RH, Simpson JL et al. Lack of relation of increased malformation rates in infants of diabetic mothers to glycemic control during organogenesis. *N Engl J Med* 1988; **318**:671–6.
3. Kitzmiller JL, Gavin LA, Jovanovic-Peterson L et al. Preconception care of diabetes: glycemic control prevents congenital anomalies. *JAMA* 1991; **265**:731–6.
4. Mills JL, Baker L, Goldman AS. Malformations in infants of diabetic mothers occur before the seventh week. Implications for treatment. *Diabetes* 1979; **28**:292–3.
5. Sadler TW. Effect of maternal diabetes on early embryogenesis:hyperglycemia-induced exencephaly. *Teratology* 1980; **21**:349–56.
6. Eriksson UJ. Congenital malformations in diabetic animal models – a review. *Diabetes Res* 1984; **1**:57–66.
7. Eriksson UJ, Borg LAH, Cederberg J et al. Pathogenesis of diabetes-induced congenital malformations. *Upsala J Med Sci* 2000; **105**:53–84.

8. Martinez-Frias ML. Developmental field defects and associations: Epidemiological evidence of their relationship. *Am J Med Genet* 1994; **49**:45–51.

9. Fraser FC. The multifactorial/threshold concept – uses and misuses. *Teratology* 1977; **14**:267–280.

10. Pampfer S, Vanderheyden I, Michiels B et al. Cell allocation to the inner cell mass and the trophectoderm in rat embryos during in vivo preimplantation development. *Roux's Arch Dev Biol* 1990; **198**:257–263.

11. Reece EA, Homko CJ, Wu Y-K. Multifactorial basis of the syndrome of diabetic embryopathy. *Teratology* 1996; **54**:171–82.

12. Wentzel P, Wentzel CR, Gareskog MB et al. Induction of embryonic dysmorphogenesis by high glucose concentration, disturbed inositol metabolism, and inhibited protein kinase C activity. *Teratology* 2001; **63**:193–201.

13. Eriksson UJ, Borg LAH. Protection by free oxygen radical scavenging enzymes against glucose-induced embryonic malformations in vitro. *Diabetologia* 1991; **34**:325–31.

14. Eriksson UJ, Borg LAH. Diabetes and embryonic malformations: role of substrate-induced free-oxygen radical production for dysmorphogenesis in cultured rat embryos. *Diabetes* 1993; **42**:411–19.

15. Viana M, Herrera E, Bonet B. Teratogenic effects of diabetes mellitus in the rat. Prevention by vitamin E. *Diabetologia* 1996; **39**:1041–6.

16. Zaken V, Kohen R, Ornoy A. Vitamin C and E improve rat embryonic antioxydant defense mechanism in diabetic culture medium. *Teratology* 2001; **64**:33–44.

17. De Hertogh R, Vercheval M, Pampfer S et al. Experimental diabetes interferes with the early development of rat embryo in the pre-implantation period. *Diabetologia* 1989; **32**:480A.

18. De Hertogh R, Vanderheyden I, Glorieux B et al. Oestrogen and progestogen receptors in endometrium and myometrium at the time of blastocyst implantation in diabetic pregnant rats. *Diabetologia* 1989; **32**:568–72.

19. Vercheval M, De Hertogh R, Pampfer S et al. Experimental diabetes impairs rat embryo development during the preimplantation period. *Diabetologia* 1990; **33**:187–91.

20. Pampfer S, De Hertogh R, Vanderheyden I et al. Decreased inner cell mass proportion in blastocysts from diabetic rats. *Diabetes* 1990; **39**:471–6.

21. Lea RG, McCracken JE, McIntyre SS et al. Disturbed development of the preimplantation embryo in the insulin-dependent diabetic BB/E rat. *Diabetes* 1996; **45**:1463–70.

22. Diamond MP, Moley KH, Pellicer A et al. Effects of streptozotocin- and alloxan-induced diabetes mellitus on mouse follicular and early embryo development. *J Reprod Fertil* 1989; **86**:1–10.

23. Beebe LFS, Kaye PL. Maternal diabetes and retarded preimplantation development of mice. *Diabetes* 1991; **40**:457–61.

24. De Hertogh R, Vanderheyden I, Pampfer S et al. Maternal insulin treatment improves preimplantation embryo development in diabetic rats. *Diabetologia* 1992; **35**:406–8.

25. Pampfer S, Wuu Y, Vanderheyden I et al. In vitro study of the carry-over effect associated with early diabetic embryopathy in the rat. *Diabetologia* 1994; **37**: 855–62.

26. Otani H, Tanaka O, Tatewaki R et al. Diabetic environment and genetic predisposition as causes of congenital malformations in NOD mouse embryos. *Diabetes* 1991; **40**:1245–50.

27. Vesela J, Rehac P, Baran V et al. Effects of healthy pseudopregnant milieu on development of two-cell subdiabetic mouse embryos. *J Reprod Fertil* 1994; **100**: 561–5.

28. Nilsson BO, Ostensson CG, Eide S et al. Utilization of glucose by the implanting mouse blastocyst activated by oestrogen. *Endokrinologie* 1980; **76**:82–93.

29. Diamond MP, Moley KH, Logan J et al. Manifestation of diabetes mellitus on mouse follicular and pre-embryo development: effect of hyperglycemia *per se*. *Metabolism* 1990; **39**:220–4.

30. Zusman I, Ornoy A, Yaffe P et al. Effects of glucose and serum from streptozotocin-diabetic and non-diabetic rats on the in vitro development of preimplantation mouse embryos. *Isr J Med Sci* 1985; **21**:359–65.

31. Wordinger RJ, Kell JA. Elevated glucose levels influence in vitro hatching, attachment, trophoblast outgrowth and differentiation of the mouse blastocyst. *Experientia* 1978; **34**:881–2.

32. De Hertogh R, Vanderheyden I, Pampfer S et al. Stimulatory and inhibitory effects of glucose and insulin on rat blastocysts development in vitro. *Diabetes* 1991; **40**:641–7.

33. Zusman I, Yaffe P, Ornoy A. Effects of metabolic factors in the diabetic state on the in vitro development of pre-implantation mouse embryos. *Teratology* 1987; **35**:77–85.

34. Moley KH, Vaughn WK, Diamond MP. Manifestation of diabetes mellitus on mouse preimplantation development: effect of elevated concentration of metabolic intermediates. *Hum Reprod* 1994; **9**:113–21.

35. Zusman I, Yaffe P, Ornoy A. Effects of human diabetic serum on the in vitro development of preimplantation mouse embryos. *Teratology* 1989; **39**:581–9.

36. Tabibzadeh S, Babaknia A. The signals and molecular pathways involved in implantation, a symbiotic interaction between blastocyst and endometrium involving adhesion and tissue invasion. *Hum Reprod* 1995; **10**:1579–602.

37. Pampfer S, De Hertogh R. Preimplantation embryopathy associated with maternal diabetes. *Diabetes Rev* 1996; **4**:90–113.

38. De M, Sanford TR, Wood GW. Expression of interleukin-1, interleukin-6 and tumor necrosis factor-α in mouse uterus during the peri-implantation period of pregnancy. *J Reprod Fertil* 1993; **97**:83–9.

39. Pampfer S, Moulaert B, Vanderheyden I et al. Effect of tumor necrosis factor-α on rat blastocyst growth and glucose metabolism. *J Reprod Fertil* 1994; **101**: 199–206.

40. Pampfer S, Wuu Y, Vanderheyden I et al. Expression of tumor necrosis factor-α receptors and selective effect of TNF-α on the inner cell mass in mouse blastocysts. *Endocrinology* 1994; **134**:206–12.

41. Pampfer S, Vanderheyden I, Wuu Y et al. A possible role for tumor necrosis factor-α in the early embryopathy associated with maternal diabetes in the rat. *Diabetes* 1995; **44**:531–6.

42. Pampfer S, Vanderheyden I, De Hertogh R. Increased synthesis of tumor necrosis factor-α in uterine explants from pregnant diabetic rats and in primary cultures of uterine cells in high glucose. *Diabetes* 1997; **46**: 1214–24.

43. Pampfer S, Vanderheyden I, Vesela J et al. Neutralization of TNF-α action on cell proliferation in rat blastocysts by antisense oligonucleotides directed against TNF-α p-60 receptor. *Biol Reprod* 1995; **52**:1316–26.

44. Wuu Y, Pampfer S, Becquet P et al. Tumor necrosis factor-α decreases the viability of mouse blastocysts in vitro and in vivo. *Biol Reprod* 1999; **60**:479–83.

45. Pampfer S, Vanderheyden I, McCracken JE et al. Increased cell death in rat blastocysts exposed to maternal diabetes in utero and to high glucose or tumor necrosis factor-α in vitro. *Development* 1997; **124**:4827–36.

46. Moley KH, Chi MM, Knudson CM et al. Hyperglycemia induces apoptosis in preimplantation embryos through cell death effector pathways. *Nature Med* 1998; **4**:1421–24.

47. Chi MM, Pingsterhouse J, Carayannopoulos M et al. Decreased glucose transporter expression triggers Bax-dependent apoptosis in the murine blastocyst. *J Biol Chem* 2000; **275**:40252–7.

48. Leunda-Casi A, Genicot G, Donnay I et al. Increased cell death in mouse blastocysts exposed to high D-glucose in vitro: implications of an oxidative stress and alterations in glucose metabolism. *Diabetologia* 2002; **45**:571–9.

49. Pampfer S, Cordi S, Vanderheyden I et al. Expression and role of Bcl-2 in rat blastocysts exposed to high D-glucose. *Diabetes* 2001; **50**:143–9.

50. Hinck L, Van Der Smissen P, Heusterpreute M et al. Identification of caspase-3 and caspase-activated deoxyribonuclease in rat blastocysts and their implication in the induction of chromatin degradation (but not nuclear fragmentation) by high glucose. *Biol Reprod* 2001; **64**:146–53.

51. Snow MH, Aitken J, Ansell JD. Role of the inner cell mass in controling implantation in the mouse. *J Embryol Exp Morphol* 1973; **29**:601–15.

52. Ornoy A, Kimyagarov D, Yaffee P et al. Role of reactive oxygen species in diabetes induced embryotoxicity: studies on pre-implantation mouse embryos cultured in serum from diabetic pregnant women. *Isr J Med Sci* 1996; **32**:1066–73.

53. Liu L, Trimarchi JR and Keefe DL. Thiol oxidation-induced embryonic cell death in mice is prevented by the antioxidant dithiothreitol. *Biol Reprod* 1999; **61**:1162–9.

54. Parchment RE. The implication of a unifying theory of programmed cell death, polyamines, oxyradicals and histogenesis in the embryo. *Int J Dev Biol* 1993; **37**:75–83.

55. Dufrasnes E, Vanderheyden I, Robin D et al. Glucose and pyruvate metabolism in preimplantation blastocysts from normal and diabetic rats. *J Reprod Fertil* 1993; **98**:169–177.

56. Gardner DK, Leese HJ. The role of glucose and pyruvate transport in regulating nutrient utilization by preimplantation mouse embryos. *Development* 1988; **104**:423–9.

57. Gaardner DK, Kaye PL. Characterization of glucose transport in preimplantation mouse embryos. *Reprod Fertil Dev* 1995; **7**:41–50.

58. Chi MM, Manchester JK, Basuray R et al. An unusual active hexose transport system in human and mouse preimplantation embryos. *Proc Natl Acad Sci USA* 1993; **90**:10023–5.

59. Carayannopoulos MO, Chi MM, Pingsterhaus JM et al. Glut-8 is a glucose transporter responsible for insulin-stimulated glucose uptake in the blastocyst. *Proc Natl Acad Sci USA* 2000; **97**:7313–18.

60. Ogura K, Sakata M, Yamagushi M et al. High concentration of glucose decreases glucose transporter-1 expression in mouse placenta in vitro and in vivo. *J Endocrinol* 1999; **160**:443–52.

61. Hahn T, Barth S, Weiss U et al. Sustained hyperglycemia in vitro down-regulates the Glut-1 glucose transport system of cultured human term placenta trophoblast: a mechanism to protect fetal development? *FASEB J* 1998; **12**:1221–31.

62. Hahn T, Hahn D, Blaschitz A et al. Hyperglycemia-induced subcellular redistribution of Glut-1 glucose transporters in cultured human term placenta trophoblast cells. *Diabetologia* 2000; **43**:173–80.

63. Moley KH, Chi MM, Manchester JK et al. Alterations of intraembryonic metabolites in preimplantation mouse embryos exposed to elevated concentrations of glucose: a metabolic explanation for the developmental retardation seen in preimplantation embryos from diabetic animals. *Biol Reprod* 1996; **54**:1209–16.

64. Kleim AL, Chi MM, Moley KH. Hyperglycemia-induced apoptotic cell death in the mouse blastocyst is dependent on expression of p53. *Mol Reprod Dev* 2001; **60**:214–24.

65. Knight RJ, Kofoed KF, Shelbert HR et al. Inhibition of glyceraldehydro-3-phosphate dehydrogenase in post-ischemic myocardium. *Cardiovasc Res* 1996; **32**:1016–23.

66. Leunda-Casi A, De Hertogh R, Pampfer S. Control of trophectoderm differentiation by inner cell mass-derived fibroblast growth factor-4 in mouse blastocysts and corrective effects of FGF-4 on high glucose-induced trophoblast disruption. *Mol Reprod Dev* 2001; **60**:38–46.

67. Leunda-Casi A, De Hertogh R, Pampfer S. Decreased expression of fibroblast growth factor-4 and associated dysregulation of trophoblast differentiation in mouse

blastocysts exposed to high D-glucose in vitro. *Diabetologia* 2001; **44**:1318–25.

68. Pampfer S. Apoptosis in rodent peri-implantation embryos: differential susceptibility of inner cell mass and trophectoderm cell lineages. *Placenta* 2000; **21**(**Suppl A**):S3–S10.

69. Rappolee DA, Basilico C, Patel Y et al. Expression and function of FGF-4 in peri-implantation development in mouse embryos. *Development* 1994; **120**:2259–69.

70. Tanaka S, Kunath T, Hadjantonakis A et al. Promotion of trophoblast stem cell proliferation by FGF-4. *Science* 1998; **282**:2072–5.

19

Fetal oxygenation and mineral metabolism in diabetic pregnancy

Francis B Mimouni, Galit Sheffer-Mimouni

Introduction

The purpose of this chapter is to review two distinct, although in some aspects related, fetal and neonatal outcomes of the pregnancy complicated by diabetes mellitus: (1) fetal oxygenation and (2) fetal-neonatal mineral metabolism. It will be attempted to clarify the pathophysiology of fetal hypoxia in maternal diabetes, and its consequences on the fetus and the newborn. The pathophysiology of neonatal hypocalcemia in the infant of a diabetic mother will then be addressed, and the means to prevent or treat it considered.

Fetal oxygenation in pregnancy complicated by diabetes mellitus

Mechanisms of fetal hypoxia in pregnancies complicated by maternal diabetes

Impaired maternal–fetal oxygen delivery

Oxygen is first transferred from the mother to the placenta, then from the placenta to the fetus. First, the blood oxygen delivery from the **mother to the placenta** will be considered, which is expressed by the Fick equation:

$$V_mO_2 = Hb_m \ X \ Q_m \ X \ (S_aO_2 - S_vO_2)_m$$

where Hb_m is the maternal hemoglobin concentration, Q_m is the intervillous, or placental, blood flow and $(S_aO_2 - S_vO_2)_m$ is the gradient of maternal arterial–venous oxygen saturation.[1] The latter depends upon the arterial and venous oxygen tensions, and the position of the oxyhemoglobin dissociation curve. In pregnancies complicated by diabetes, maternal–placental oxygen transfer may be affected by reduced placental blood flow or changes in oxyhemoglobin dissociation.

Placental blood flow may be reduced by as much as 35–50%, as measured by using diffusible ^{133}Xe or ^{113m}In.[2,3] Although the mechanism of this reduction is not known, it is likely that severe vascular disease may be a contributory factor. Also, Nylund et al[3] found an inverse correlation between maternal glycemia and placental blood flow. In diabetic ketoacidosis, hypovolemia and acidosis itself may further reduce placental blood flow.[4]

In maternal diabetes, the oxyhemoglobin dissociation curve may be affected by glycosylated hemoglobin (HbA1c) having an increased affinity for O_2 oxygen: it has been calculated that an increase in HbA1c of 1% of the total hemoglobin may cause a decrease in $P_{50}O_2$ of c. 0.3 mmHg.[5,6]

Also, in ketoacidosis, the detrimental effect on oxygen release due to a decrease in 2,3-DPG is counteracted by the lower plasma pH (the Bohr effect).[7] However, during the recovery period, plasma pH is corrected within hours, while 2,3-DPG values remain low for days. A subsequent left shift of the oxygen dissociation curve occurs, which may have a significant, deleterious impact on oxygen release. Bellingham et al[7] found that rapid correction of the pH from < 7 to 7.4 resulted in a 70% decrease in red cell oxygen release.

Placental–fetal oxygen transfer (VO_2) is expressed by the Fick diffusion equation:

$$VO_2 = K_pO_2 \times A \, (S_mO_2 - S_fO_2)/L$$

where K_pO_2 is a placental oxygen diffusion constant, A is the villous surface area, ($S_mO_2 - S_fO_2$) is the oxygen saturation gradient between the maternal and fetal placental membranes (which depends upon the oxygen tensions on each side of the placental membranes, as well as on the maternal and fetal oxygen dissociation curves), and L is the average diffusion distance between the maternal and fetal circulation. In a pregnancy complicated by diabetes, placental oxygen transfer may be affected by: (1) the villous surface area (A), which may be reduced by the fact that many villi may be avascular, due to an increase in the incidence of fetal artery thrombosis;[8] (2) the diffusion distance may be significantly increased by the presence of a thickened basement membrane (as demonstrated by electron microscopy[9]) or by the frequent appearance of villous edema.[8]

Impaired fetal oxygen consumption

Many studies of fetal oxygenation have been conducted using the chronically catheterized fetal lamb model. In this model, pregnant sheep are operated upon, and venous and artery catheters are placed in both ewes and their fetuses, and the fetal cardiovascular and metabolic responses to several metabolic imbalances found in uncontrolled diabetes are recorded. Using this model, it has been established that chronic (1 week) fetal hyperglycemia,[10,11] acute (within hours) maternal[12] or fetal[13] hyperketonemia, acute maternal ketoacidemia[14] and fetal hyperinsulinemia[15–18] all lead to fetal hypoxemia and acidosis. In a chronically catheterized fetal lamb model, where maternal diabetes was induced using alloxan, it was possible to replicate the major metabolic and hormonal imbalances of pregnancy in insulin-dependent diabetes mellitus (IDDM): the ewes were hyperglycemic and hypoinsulinemic, and had an increase in blood ketones and glucagon.[19] The fetal lamb, within 1–2 days, became hyperglycemic, hyperketonemic and hyperinsulinemic.[19] Arterial fetal pO_2 dropped sharply, and lactate increased within 1–2 days of alloxan administration.[19] The prevalent theory behind these findings is that in the presence of extra fuels, or of hyperinsulinemia, the metabolic rate of the placenta increases together with the oxygen consumption rate, depriving the fetus of enough oxygen.[20] Hay and co-workers[16–18] demonstrated, using the fetal lamb model, that insulin promotes the entry of glucose, thereby increasing glucose utilization and oxidation rates.

Other factors possibly contributing to fetal hypoxia

In theory, many other factors may also contribute to fetal hypoxia in pregancies complicated by diabetes.

- Hypertension is known to be associated with a reduction in placental blood flow[21] and frequently occurs in advanced diabetes. Furthermore, gestational hypertension is a frequent complication of diabetes in pregnancy[22,23] and is known to be associated with a significant reduction in placental blood flow.[24]

- Maternal diabetic vascular disease also has the potential to reduce utero-placental blood flow.[1]

- Finally, prolonged labor due to fetal dystocia,[25,26] a consequence of fetal macrosomia,[26,27] has the potential to create an additional hypoxic stress on the fetus.

Pathophysiological and clinical consequences of fetal hypoxia in diabetes mellitus

Increased rates of fetal distress and/or neonatal depression

After insulin was introduced in 1921, diabetic women became pregnant in increasing numbers. However, the perinatal mortality was extremely high and remained so until the 1950s, when it still was *c.* 20%. Nearly half of the deaths occurred antenatally.[28] Before 36 weeks gestation, most intrauterine fetal deaths (IUFD) were associated with diabetic ketoacidosis, while after 36 weeks IUFD were often unexplained and somewhat sudden. The series of Kitzmiller et al[29] and Tyson and Hock,[30] both published in the late 1970s, revealed evidence of intrapartum distress and/or low Apgar scores in 25 and 28% of infants, respectively. The most recent large study was published by this group in the late 1980s and found a similar rate of 26.7%.[28] However, in this group's study, intensive fetal monitoring in late pregnancy combined with relatively strict goals of glycemic control allowed fetal distress to be limited in time and/or intensity in most cases, and to maintain low Apgar scores into the mild range of neonatal asphyxia.[28] In this group's series of 160 deliveries, there were only two IUFD, both of which were linked to very poor glycemic control, the presence of pre-eclampsia

and the lack of compliance by the mother with the tests of fetal surveillance that were prescribed.[28] In this study, when the infants with low Apgar scores and/or fetal distress were compared to controls (non-asphyxiated infants), the following significant differences were observed: mothers in the asphyxiated group more often had new-onset nephropathy during pregnancy, and were more often affected by preterm labor.[28] There were no significant differences between the two groups in terms of long-term glycemic control (as assessed by measurements of HbA1c); however, mothers in the asphyxiated group were more often hyperglycemic (> 150 mg/dl) in labor.[28] Asphyxiated infants had higher nucleated red blood cell values (an index of chronic hypoxia) than the controls, but even in infants born without perinatal asphyxia, the mean nucleated red blood cell number was still very high in comparison with a group of normal infants born to mothers without diabetes.[28]

Hematologic consequences

Maternal diabetes during pregnancy has been shown to cause (presumably because of chronic fetal hypoxia) an increase in the production of fetal erythropoietin.[31] In Widness et al's[31] study, mean maternal HbA1c during the last month of pregnancy correlated significantly with fetal umbilical venous erythropoietin at delivery, and amniotic fluid glucose and amniotic fluid insulin also correlated with umbilical venous erythropoietin.[31] This group has shown that maternal concentrations of HbA1 at the time of delivery correlate with neonatal hematocrit at birth.[32] Moreover, neonatal polycythemia is six times more frequent in IDDM mothers than in appropriate matched-pair controls,[33] and circulating nucleated red blood cells are strikingly elevated in IDDM mothers compared to controls.[33,34] The latter finding is also true in infants of gestational diabetic mothers and, interestingly, in large-for-gestational-age infants born to non-diabetic mothers.[35,36] The fetal erythopoietic response to hypoxia may occur at the expense of other bone marrow line cells, as IDDM mothers have decreased platelet counts, which correlate inversely with the circulating nucleated red blood cell counts.[37] Finally, the increased demands for erythropoiesis may deplete iron stores in the fetus of the diabetic mother, who at birth has decreased blood iron and ferritin concentrations, and elevated transferrin and free erythrocyte protoporphyrin concentrations.[38–40] Moreover, it has been suggested that the increase in the red blood cell mass and the increased erythropoietic rate (including in-effective erythropoiesis) may play a role in the neonatal hyperbilirubinemia frequently observed in IDDM mothers.[25,41] Conversely, this group has shown that IDDM mothers whose infants were delivered by Cesarean section had lower hematocrits than those de-livered vaginally, and also had lower rates of hyperbilirubinemia.[25]

Metabolic consequences:
The rates of **neonatal hypoglycemia** may be affected by intrauterine hypoxia through several mechanisms. Firstly, asphyxiated infants fre-quently may develop hypoglycemia, due to increased glucose demands during anerobic metabolism. Also, neonatal polycythemia is a known cause of refractory hypoglycemia, pre-sumably because of increased glucose utilization by the red blood cell mass.[42] This group has shown that polycythemic IDDM patients have rates of hypoglycemia three times higher than non-polycythemic IDDM patients.[33]

Independent from the fact that infants of non-asphyxiated IDDM are at a high risk of **neonatal hypocalcemia** (NHC), asphyxia *per se* adds its own influence on mineral metabolism of the neonate (see below).

Preterm labor of spontaneous occurrence is more prevalent in pregnancies complicated by IDDM, and relates both to poor second trimester glycemic control and urogenital infec-tions.[43] Because of intense fetal surveillance in the modern management of maternal diabetes mellitus, **iatrogenic prematurity** is at times required in order to prevent IUFD:[25,28] the pre-mature infant of the IDDM mother is then exposed to all the risks of prematurity, in par-ticular that of severe respiratory distress syn-drome (RDS).[44–47] This risk may be amplified by the fact that, in poorly controlled diabetes, fetal hyperinsulinism causes a delay in surfac-tant production, placing the infant of an IDDM mother at a higher risk of RDS than one of a non-IDDM mother, at any given gestational age.[44,46] However, it has been demonstrated that adequate glycemic control reduces the risk of RDS to that of the non-diabetic population.[45]

Long-term psychomotor performances of the infants of IDDM mothers
Early studies of the long-term follow-up of infants of IDDM mothers compared early entry to late entry subjects, as it referred to how early in pregnancy diabetic mothers sought perinatal care.[47] Early entry subjects had mothers with lower HbA1c levels than did the mothers of late entry subjects. Both groups were compared with a control group of subjects born to non-diabetic mothers. At 2–3 years of age, early entry subjects were not different from controls, while late entry subjects had lower language measures and a smaller head size, which correlated inversely with HbA1c levels. Although non-controlled and non-randomized, this study favored the theory that poor glycemic control in pregnancy may have an adverse effect on brain development.[47] In another relatively small study, it was shown by Hod et al[48] that at 1 year of age, infants of IDDM mothers had lower average Mental

Developmental and Psychomotor Developmental Indexes than control patients. In a recent study, it was shown that during the neonatal period, infants of IDDM mothers have subtle recognition memory deficits (as tested in the auditory field) compared to healthy controls.[49] Bayley Scales of Infant Development administered at 1 year of age correlated with the neonatal findings.[49] Rizzo et al[50] showed that Mental Development Index scores and Stanford Binet scores correlated inversely with measures of maternal metabolism, in particular third trimester plasma β-hydroxybutyrate and free fatty acid concentrations.[50] These results led Jovanovic-Peterson and Peterson,[51] in an editorial related to Rizzo et al's[50] article, to conclude that the treatment of diabetes of pregnancy is a 'sweet success', but may have a 'bitter aftertaste'.

It is concluded that metabolic imbalances of diabetes have the potential for multiple direct and indirect deleterious effects on fetal oxygenation, a fact that has been verified *in vivo* by cordocentesis.[52] Strict glycemic control, coupled with intensive fetal surveillance, appears to be the mainstay of prevention of these complications.

Disorders of mineral metabolism in infants of IDDM mothers

Decreased bone density

It has been observed that, similar to the results of studies conducted in animals, infants of IDDM mothers have decreased bone densities at birth.[53] Decreased bone densities in infants correlates with decreased bone densities in their mothers, but does not appear to be predictive of their serum Ca.[53] In one study, an index of osteoclastic activity (cord blood telopeptide of Type I collagen) was higher at birth in infants of IDDM mothers than in controls, while an index of bone formation (cord blood propeptide

Type I collagen) was similar.[54] These findings remain to be fully explained.

Neonatal hypocalcemia and hypomagnesemia

Neonatal hypocalcemia (NHC) may occur in infants of IDDM mothers at rates up to 50%.[55] However, over the years, improvements in glycemic control during pregnancy have led to a progressive decrease in the rate, but also in the severity, of NHC. This group and other investigators in Cincinnati conducted a study of NHC in infants of IDDM mothers as part of a Program Project Grant of Diabetes in Pregnancy. In the later years of the study, there were difficulties in recruiting patients due to the fact that NHC had become much rarer, and severe, symptomatic hypocalcemia, rarely seen. Nevertheless, this 15-year study led to a better understanding of NHC in infants of IDDM mothers.

Some risk factors of NHC play a dominant role in the infants of IDDM mothers.[56] Firstly, as mentioned earlier in this chapter, such infants are at a higher risk of developing birth asphyxia, which by itself is a well-known risk factor for NHC.[57] The mechanisms of asphyxia-induced NHC are multiple, and include increased intracellular phosphorus release, usage of sodium bicarbonate to buffer acidosis[58] and stress-induced calcitonin release.[57] Secondly, infants of IDDM mothers are at a higher risk of being born early, either because of iatrogenic prematurity (induced premature delivery because of maternal or fetal reasons)[25,28] or because of a spontaneously occurring preterm labor.[43] Preterm infants have high rates of NHC due to a combination of factors: an increased rate of birth asphyxia; a decreased ability to secrete parathyroid hormone (PTH) in response to induced hypocalcemia;[59,60] sustained calcitonin production in the presence of hypocalcemia;[57] and, maybe also, end-organ resistance to 1,25-$(OH)_2$ cholecalciferol (the most active form of vitamin D).[61] Independent of the asphyxia and the prematurity factor, it appears that magnesium (Mg) deficiency plays an important role in the pathogenesis of NHC in infants of IDDM mothers.[62,63] In poorly controlled IDDM, glycosuria is accompanied by urinary Mg losses, both in non-pregnant and in pregnant patients.[63] Maternal Mg deficiency leads to fetal Mg deficiency, as is evidenced by decreased amniotic fluid Mg concentrations[64] and lower cord blood or neonatal serum Mg concentrations in infants of IDDM mothers.[65,66] It is known that Mg is necessary for the appropriate function of the Mg-dependent adenylate cyclase involved in the secretion of PTH, as well as in the the Mg-dependent adenylate cyclase involved in the action of PTH upon its target cells.[67] Thus, in Mg deficiency, there is a state of functional hypoparathyroidism, combined with end-organ resistance, to PTH. In infants, the PTH response to Mg administration correlates inversely with Mg status: in Mg-replete infants, Mg administration leads to an appropriate negative feedback, and a decrease in PTH production and in serum calcium concentrations. Paradoxically, in Mg-depleted infants, Mg administration leads to an increase in PTH production and in serum calcium concentrations.[67,68] In infants of IDDM mothers, serum calcium concentrations correlate directly with serum Mg concentrations and inversely with maternal HbA1c.[56] Also, such infants have inadequate PTH elevation in response to hypocalcemia.[69,70] Their calcitonin concentrations remain elevated at birth, as in every other normal newborn, but do not appear to play a role in the pathogenesis of NHC.[65,71] This group has shown that a protocol of strict management of diabetes in pregnancy is associated with a reduction in the rate of hypocalcemia.[72] Moreover, in a randomized, blinded, controlled clinical trial, it was shown that prophylactic administration of intramuscular Mg at birth decreased the intensity of the physiologic drop in serum calcium that occurs after birth.[73] However, in this group of very well-controlled diabetic mothers, as stated earlier, NHC was so rare that it was not possible to show that prophylactic Mg therapy decreased the rate of NHC. Thus, while this group recommends screening for hypocalcemia and hypomagnesemia in infants of IDD mothers, ideally at 12–24 hours of life when serum Ca is at its lowest, the routine administration of Mg at birth in such infants is not recommended. Symptomatic hypocalcemia should be treated with calcium salts; Mg salts should be added when hypomagnesemia is also present. The treatment of asymptomatic hypocalcemia is a matter of debate and has been reviewed extensively elsewhere.[74]

References

1. Madsen H. Fetal oxygenation in diabetic pregnancy. With special reference to maternal blood oxygen affinity and its effectors. *Danish Med Bull* 1986; 33:64–74.
2. Pontonnier G, Fournie A, Bertrand JC, Otteni JC. Problems de reanimation pendant la grossesse. In: *Reanimation obstetricale. Raport du XXII e congres national d'anesthesie at reanimation.* (Librairie Arnette: Paris; 1972) 210–12.
3. Nylund L, Lunell N-O, Lewander R et al. Uteroplacental blood flow in diabetic pregnancy: measurement with indium 113m and a computer-linked gamma camera. *Am J Obstet Gynecol* 1982; **144**:298–302.
4. Blechner JN, Stenger VG, Prystowsky H. Blood flow to the human uterus during maternal metabolic acidosis. *Am J Obstet Gynecol* 1975; **121**:789–94.
5. Madsen H, Ditzel J. Changes in red blood cell oxygen transport in diabetic pregnancy. *Am J Obstet Gynecol* 1982; **143**:421–4.
6. Madsen H, Ditzel J. Blood-oxygen transport in first trimester of diabetic pregnancy. *Acta Obstet Gynecol Scand* 1984; **63**:317–20.
7. Bellingham AJ, Detter JC, Lenfant C. The role of hemoglobin affinity for oxygen and red cell 2,3-diphosphoglycerate in the management of diabetic ketoacidosis. *Trans Assoc Am Phys* 1970; **83**:113–20.
8. Fox H. Pathology of the placenta in maternal diabetes mellitus. *Obstet Gynecol* 1969; **34**:792–8.

9. Okudaira Y, Hirota K, Cohen S, Strauss L. Ultrastructure of the human placenta in maternal diabetes mellitus. *Lab Invest* 1966; **15**:910–26.

10. Philips AF, Dubin J, Matty P, Raye JR. Arterial hypoxemia and hyperinsulinemia in the chronically hyperglycemic fetal lamb. *Pediatr Res* 1982; **16**:653–8.

11. Philipps AF, Porte P, Stabinsky S et al. Effects of chronic fetal hyperglycemia upon oxygen consumption in the ovine uterus and conceptus. *J Clin Invest* 1984; **74**:279–86.

12. Miodovnik M, Skillman C, Hertzberg V et al. Effect of hyperketonemia in hypergycemic pregnant ewes and their fetuses. *Am J Obstet Gynecol* 1986; **154**:394–401.

13. Miodovnik M, Lavin JP, Harrington DJ et al. Cardiovascular and biochemical effects of infusion of beta hydroxybutyrate into the fetal lamb. *Am J Obstet Gynecol* 1982; **144**:594–600.

14. Miodovnik M, Lavin JP, Harrington DJ et al. Effect of maternal ketoacidemia on the pregnant ewe and the fetus. *Am J Obstet Gynecol* 1982; **144**:585–93.

15. Milley JR, Rosenberg AA, Philipps AF et al. The effect of insulin on ovine fetal oxygen extraction. *Am J Obstet Gynecol* 1984; **149**:673–8.

16. Hay Jr WW, Meznarich HK. The effect of hyperinsulinaemia on glucose utilization and oxidation and on oxygen consumption in the fetal lamb. *Q J Exp Physiol* 1986; **71**:689–98.

17. Hay Jr WW, Meznarich HK, DiGiacomo JE et al. Effects of insulin and glucose concentrations on glucose utilization in fetal sheep. *Pediatr Res* 1988; **23**:381–7.

18. Aldoretta PW, Carver TD, Hay Jr WW. Ovine uteroplacental glucose and oxygen metabolism in relation to chronic changes in maternal and fetal glucose concentrations. *Placenta* 1994; **15**:753–64.

19. Miodovnik M, Mimouni F, Berk M, Clark KE. Alloxan-induced diabetes mellitus in the pregnant ewe: metabolic and cardiovascular effects on the mother and her fetus. *Am J Obstet Gynecol* 1989; **160**:1239–44.

20. Clark KE, Miodovnik M, Skillman CA, Mimouni F. Review of fetal cardiovascular and metabolic responses to diabetic insults in the pregnant ewe. *Am J Perinatol* 1988; **5**:312–18.

21. Lunnel NO, Nylund LE, Lewander R, Sarby B. Uteroplacental blood flow in preeclampsia. Measurement with indium-113m and a computer-linked gamma camera. *J Exp Clin Hypertens* 1982; **B1**:105–17.

22. Siddiqi T, Rosenn B, Mimouni F et al. Hypertension during pregnancy in insulin-dependent diabetic women. *Obstet Gynecol* 1991; **77**:514–19.

23. Sibai BM, Caritis S, Hauth J et al. Risks of preeclampsia and adverse neonatal outcomes among women with pregestational diabetes mellitus. National Institute of Child Health and Human Development Network of Maternal–Fetal Medicine Units. *Am J Obstet Gynecol* 2000; **182**:364–9.

24. Kaar K, Jouppilka P, Kuikka J et al. Intervillous blood flow in notmal and complicated late pregnancy measured by means of an intervenous 133Xe method. *Acta Obstet Gynecol Scand* 1980; **59**:7–10.

25. Miodovnik M, Mimouni F, Tsang RC et al. Management of the insulin-dependent diabetic during labor and delivery. Influences on neonatal outcome. *Am J Perinatol* 1987; **4**:106–14.

26. Mimouni F, Miodovnik M, Rosenn B et al. Birth trauma in insulin-dependent diabetic pregnancies. *Am J Perinatol* 1992; **9**:205–8.

27. Berk MA, Mimouni F, Miodovnik M et al. Macrosomia in infants of insulin-dependent diabetic mothers. *Pediatrics* 1989; **83**:1029–34.

28. Mimouni F, Miodovnik M, Siddiqi TA et al. Perinatal asphyxia in infants of insulin-dependent diabetic mothers. *J Pediatr* 1988; **113**:345–53.

29. Kitzmiller JL, Cloherty JP, Younger MD et al. Diabetic pregnancy and perinatal mortality. *Am J Obstet Gynecol* 1978; **131**:560–80.

30. Tyson JE, Hock RD. Gestational and pregestational diabetes: an approach to therapy. *Am J Obstet Gynecol* 1976; **125**:1009–27.

31. Widness JA, Teramo KA, Clemons GK et al. Direct relationship of antepartum glucose control and fetal erythropoietin in human type 1 (insulin-dependent) diabetic pregnancy. *Diabetologia* 1990; **33**:378–83.

32. Green DW, Khoury J, Mimouni F. Neonatal hematocrit and maternal glycemic control in insulin-dependent diabetes. *J Pediatr* 1992; **120**:302–5.

33. Mimouni F, Miodovnik M, Siddiqi TA et al. Neonatal polycythemia in infants of insulin-dependent diabetic mothers. *Obstet Gynecol* 1986; **68**:370–2.

34. Green DW, Mimouni F. Nucleated erythrocytes in healthy infants and in infants of diabetic mothers. *J Pediatr* 1990; **116**:129–31.

35. Yeruchimovich M, Mimouni FB, Green DW, Dollberg S. Nucleated red blood cells in healthy infants of women with gestational diabetes. *Obstet Gynecol* 2000; **95**:84–6.

36. Dollberg S, Marom R, Mimouni FB, Yeruchimovich M. Normoblasts in large for gestational age infants. *Arch Dis Child Fetal Neonatal Ed* 2000; **83**:F148–F149.

37. Green DW, Mimouni F, Khoury J. Decreased platelet counts in infants of diabetic mothers. *Am J Perinatol* 1995; **12**:102–5.

38. Chockalingam UM, Murphy E, Ophoven JC et al. Cord transferrin and ferritin values in newborn infants at risk for prenatal uteroplacental insufficiency and chronic hypoxia. *J Pediatr* 1987; **111**:283–6.

39. Georgieff MK, Landon MB, Mills MM et al. Abnormal iron distribution in infants of diabetic mothers: spectrum and maternal antecedents. *J Pediatr* 1990; **117**:455–61.

40. Petry CD, Eaton MA, Wobken JD et al. Iron deficiency of liver, heart, and brain in newborn infants of diabetic mothers. *J Pediatr* 1992; **121**:109–14.

41. Taylor PM, Wolfson JH, Bright NH. Hyperbilirubinemia in infants of diabetic mothers. *Biol Neonat* 1963; 5:289–96.

42. Creswell JS, Warburton D, Susa JB et al. Hyperviscosity in the newborn lamb produces pertubation in glucose homeostasis. *Pediatr Res* 1981; 15:1348–50.

43. Mimouni F, Miodovnik M, Siddiqi TA et al. High spontaneous premature labor rate in insulin-dependent diabetic pregnant women: an association with poor glycemic control and urogenital infection. *Obstet Gynecol* 1988; 72:175–80.

44. Robert MF, Neff RK, Hubbell JP et al. Association between maternal diabetes and the respiratory-distress syndrome in the newborn. *N Engl J Med* 1976; **294**: 357–60.

45. Mimouni F, Miodovnik M, Whitsett JA et al. Respiratory distress syndrome in infants of diabetic mothers in the 1980s: no direct adverse effect of maternal diabetes with modern management. *Obstet Gynecol* 1987; **69**:191–5.

46. McMahan MJ, Mimouni F, Miodovnik M et al. Surfactant associated protein (SAP-35) in amniotic fluid from diabetic and nondiabetic pregnancies. *Obstet Gynecol* 1987; 70:94–8.

47. Sells CJ, Robinson NM, Brown Z, Knopp RH. Long-term developmental follow-up of infants of diabetic mothers. *J Pediatr* 1994; 125:S9–S17.

48. Hod M, Levy-Shiff R, Lerman M et al. Developmental outcome of offspring of pregestational diabetic mothers. *J Pediatr Endocrinol Metab* 1999; 12:867–72.

49. Deregnier RA, Nelson CA, Thomas KM et al. Neurophysiologic evaluation of auditory recognition memory in healthy newborn infants and infants of diabetic mothers. *J Pediatr* 2000; **137**:777–84.

50. Rizzo T, Metzger BE, Burns WJ, Burns K. Correlations between antepartum maternal metabolism and child intelligence. *N Engl J Med* 1991; **325**:911–16.

51. Jovanovic-Peterson L, Peterson CM. Sweet success, but an acid aftertaste? *N Engl J Med* 1991; **325**:959–60.

52. Bradley RJ, Brudenell JM, Nicolaides KH. Fetal acidosis and hyperlacticaemia diagnosed by cordocentesis in pregnancies complicated by maternal diabetes mellitus. *Diabet Med* 1991; **8**:464–8.

53. Mimouni F, Steichen JJ, Tsang RC et al. Decreased bone mineral content in infants of diabetic mothers. *Am J Perinatol* 1988; 5:339–43.

54. Demarini S, Specker BL, Sierra RI et al. Evidence of increased intrauterine bone resorption in term infants of mothers with insulin-dependent diabetes. *J Pediatr* 1995; **126**:796–8.

55. Tsang RC, Chen I, Friedman MA et al. Parathyroid function in infants of diabetic mothers. *J Pediatr* 1975; 86:399–404.

56. Mimouni F, Loughead J, Miodovnik M et al. Early neonatal predictors of neonatal hypocalcemia in infants of diabetic mothers: an epidemiologic study. *Am J Perinatol* 1990; 7:203–6.

57. Venkataraman PS, Tsang RC, Chen IW, Sperling MA. Pathogenesis of early neonatal hypocalcemia: studies of serum calcitonin, gastrin, and plasma glucagon. *J Pediatr* 1987; 110:599–603.

58. Brown DR, Tsang RC, Chen I. Oral calcium supplementation in premature and asphyxiated meonates. *J Pediatr* 1976; 89:973–7.

59. Tsang RC, Chen IW, Friedman MA, Chen I. Neonatal parathyroid function: role of gestational age and postnatal age. *J Pediatr* 1973; 83:728–38.

60. Dincsoy MY, Tsang RC, Laskarzewski P et al. The role of postnatal age and magnesium on parathyroid hormone responses during 'exchange' blood transfusion in the newborn period. *J Pediatr* 1982; 100:277–83.

61. Ravid A, Koren R, Rotem C et al. Mononuclear cells from human neonates are partially resistant to the action of 1,25-dihydroxyvitamin D. *J Clin Endocrinol Metab* 1988; 67:755–9.

62. Cruikshank DP, Pitkin RM, Varner MW et al. Calcium metabolism in diabetic mother, fetus, and newborn infant. *Am J Obstet Gynecol* 1983; **145**:1010–16.

63. Mimouni F, Miodovnik M, Tsang RC et al. Decreased maternal serum magnesium concentration and adverse fetal outcome in insulin-dependent diabetic women. *Obstet Gynecol* 1987; 70:85–8.

64. Mimouni F, Miodovnik M, Tsang RC et al. Decreased amniotic fluid magnesium concentration in diabetic pregnancy. *Obstet Gynecol* 1987; **69**:12–14.

65. Mimouni F, Tsang RC, Hertzberg VS, Miodovnik M. Polycythemia, hypomagnesemia, and hypocalcemia in infants of diabetic mothers. *Am J Dis Child* 1986; 140:798–800.

66. Tsang RC, Strub R, Brown DR et al. Hypomagnesemia in infants of diabetic mothers: perinatal studies. *J Pediatr* 1976; 89:115–19.

67. Shaul PW, Mimouni F, Tsang RC, Specker BL. The role of magnesium in neonatal calcium homeostasis: effects of magnesium infusion on calciotropic hormones and calcium. *Pediatr Res* 1987; 22:319–23.

68. Maggioni A, Orzalesi M, Mimouni FB. Intravenous correction of neonatal hypomagnesemia: effect on ionized magnesium. *J Pediatr* 1998; **132**:652–5.

69. Tsang RC, Chen I, Friedman MA et al. Parathyroid function in infants of diabetic mothers. *J Pediatr* 1975; 86:399–404.

70. Noguchi A, Eren M, Tsang RC. Parathyroid hormone in hypocalcemic and normocalcemic infants of diabetic mothers. *J Pediatr* 1980; 97:112–14.

71. Mimouni F, Loughead JL, Tsang RC, Khoury J. Postnatal surge in serum calcitonin concentrations: no contribution to neonatal hypocalcemia in infants of diabetic mothers. *Pediatr Res* 1990; 28:493–5.

72. Demarini S, Mimouni F, Tsang RC et al. Impact of metabolic control of diabetes during pregnancy on neonatal hypocalcemia: a randomized study. *Obstet Gynecol* 1994; 83:918–22.

73. Mehta KC, Kalkwarf HJ, Mimouni F et al. Randomized trial of magnesium administration to prevent hypocalcemia in infants of diabetic mothers. *J Perinatol* 1998; **18**:352–6.

74. Mimouni F, Tsang RC. Neonatal hypocalcemia: to treat or not to treat? (a review). *J Am Coll Nutr* 1994; **13**:408–15.

20

Clinical and experimental advances in the understanding of diabetic embryopathy

Ulf J Eriksson, Parri Wentzel, Moshe Hod

Introduction

Carbohydrate intolerance is the most common metabolic complication of pregnancy. A review of the literature over the last two decades indicates that the incidence of gestational diabetes mellitus (GDM) varies between 1 and 5%. Between 0.2 and 0.3% of pregnancies occur in women with pregestational diabetes mellitus (preGDM), Types 1 and 2 diabetes and maturity onset diabetes of the young (MODY). When not recognized and treated appropriately, diabetes in pregnancy is associated with high perinatal wastage, congenital anomalies, macrosomia, and neonatal, childhood and adult complications.[1] An increasing body of evidence supports the hypothesis that certain developing tissues and organs in the fetus of the diabetic mother may receive an imprint of the abnormal gestational milieu and that this imprint can have permanent long-range implications for function after birth.

Despite considerable progress in the clinical management of diabetic pregnancy, the prevalence of major congenital malformations is approximately three to five times greater in infants of diabetic mothers than in the offspring of non-diabetic women[2-5] and is presently the most common cause of perinatal death among these infants.[6,7] The infant of the diabetic mother also has increased risk for several neonatal complications, such as macrosomia, hypoglycemia, hypocalcemia, polycythemia and hyperbilirubinemia; up to 25% of such offspring have been reported with these complications. It also appears that early detection and subsequent strict metabolic control of pregnant women with diabetes in pregnancy should decrease the frequency and severity of some of these short- and long-term complications in the offspring of the diabetic mother. The purpose of this chapter is to summarize the current state of knowledge, clinical and experimental, on the advances in the understanding of diabetic embryopathy.

Pathophysiology

Maternal fuels constitute the building blocks for fetal development. Freinkel[8] introduced the concept of 'pregnancy as a tissue culture experience', proposing that the placenta and the fetus develop in an 'incubation medium' that is totally derived from maternal fuels. All these fuels (glucose, amino acids, lipids) traverse the placenta in a concentration-dependent fashion and thus delimit the 'incubation medium' in the fetal circulation. Since all these constituents are regulated by maternal insulin, disturbances in its supply or action will influence the whole nutrient composition to which the fetus is exposed and may lead to fetal hyperinsulinemia (Fig. 20.1). According to Freinkel's hypothesis, described as 'fuel-mediated teratogenesis', the abnormal maternal mixture of metabolites gains access to the developing fetus *in utero*, modifying the phenotypic gene expression in newly forming cells that may, in turn, cause permanent, short- and long-range effects upon the offspring. Accordingly, fetal and neonatal complications occur during the different periods in gestation when the embryo/fetus is exposed to the aberrant fuel mixture.[9–11] Thus, exposure during the early first trimester (organogenesis) can lead to spontaneous miscarriages, early intrauterine growth retardation (IUGR) and organ malformations. During the second trimester, when the formation and development of the brain cells takes place, altered behavioral, intellectual or psychological patterns may occur. During the third trimester, proliferation of fetal adipocytes, muscle cells, pancreatic beta cells and neuroendocrine systems is the basis for the development later in life of obesity and non-insulin-dependent diabetes (NIDDM). Metabolic alterations during parturition are responsible for transient neonatal metabolic complications such as hypoglycemia, hypocalcemia and hypomagnesemia. Fetal hyperinsulinemia leads to a decreased level of arterial oxygen and an increase in the plasma erythropoietin concentration. The chronic hypoxemic state *in utero* may explain some cases of intrauterine fetal death, as well as polycythemia, hyperbilirubinemia and renal vein thrombosis (Fig. 20.2).[8,12]

Clinical studies

One of the most important advancements in the management of diabetic pregnancy was the great effort made to completely prevent the fetal and perinatal complications related to this condition. It was hypothesized that early detection and subsequent strict metabolic control of pregnant diabetic women should prevent the occurrence of most neonatal complications, including congenital malformations. In spite of improvements in the treatment of diabetes in pregnancy, the risk of congenital malformations in offspring of diabetic women remains three to five times higher than in normal pregnancies.[2–5]

Clinical trials (Table 20.1) have demonstrated that preconception care and glycemic control can dramatically lower the rate of congenital malformations in the offspring of diabetic mothers. These studies explored the influence of preconception normoglycemia and postconception strict metabolic control on the prevalence of major congenital anomalies, revealing positive results (reductions in the incidences of major congenital anomalies). The combination of the results of the prospective studies reveals a malformation rate of 2.1% among the offspring of preconception registered and treated mothers, and 9.0% for the postconception group.

There is no specific diabetic embryopathy. Diabetes is associated with a variety of anomalies, mainly cardiovascular, central nervous system (CNS), and musculoskeletal.[13] Most of these are five- to 10-fold more frequent in infants of diabetic mothers (IDM).[7] The malformation considered to be most pathognomic to IDM – caudal regression syndrome or sacral agenesis – is claimed to be 200–400-fold more frequent,[14] but is still very rare among both IDM and non-IDM (Table 20.2).

Most pregnancies are not recognized clinically until ≥ 2 weeks after conception; thus, strict glycemic control is often started after the critical periods of embryogenesis and organogenesis have begun. Intensive blood glucose management initiated in early pregnancy may

Author	Year	Preconception		Postconception		Non-diabetic	
		No. of patients	Major malformations (%)	No. of patients	Major malformations (%)	No. of patients	Major malformations (%)
Pedersen	1979	363	7.4	284	14.1	–	–
Miller	1981	58	3.4	58	22.4	–	–
Fuhrmann	1983	128	0.8	292	7.5	420	1.4
	1984	57	1.8	181	5.0	–	–
Goldman	1986	44	0	31	9.7	–	–
Diep (Mills)	1988	347	4.9	279	9.0	389	2.1
Steel	1989	114	1.8	86	10.5	–	–
Rosenn	1991	28	0	71	1.4	–	–
Kitzmiller	1991	84	1.2	110	10.9	–	–
Cousins	1991	27	0	347	6.6	–	–
Hod	1991	28	3.5	59	6.7	380	1.8
Drury	1992	100	1.0	244	4.1	–	–
Willmote	1993	62	1.6	123	6.5	–	–
Steel	1994	196	1.5	117	12	–	–
TOTAL		**1289**	**2.1**	**2003**	**9.0**	**1189**	**1.7**

Table 20.1. *Prevention of congenital anomalies by preconception care: the influence of strict maternal metabolic control.*

thus be inadequate to prevent adverse pregnancy outcomes.

During intensive insulin therapy in insulin-dependent diabetes mellitus (IDDM) patients, there is a threefold increase in the rate of severe hypoglycemia. The fact that the results of most studies show a comparable rate of congenital malformations between the offspring of IDDM mothers who received intensified periconceptional treatment and controls, suggests that severe hypoglycemia probably does not play an important role in determining the rate of congenital malformations. Despite this exciting possibility of reducing the congenital malformations rate in IDM to that of the non-IDM population, only 30–60% of all women with preGDM are referred to the diabetes-in-pregnancy clinics before conception. A goal of the future is to educate all women with diabetes, and all clinicians that care for women with diabetes, about the necessity of achieving glycemic control before attempting pregnancy.

Folic acid supplementation

Supplementation of folic acid preconceptionally has been shown to reduce the incidence of neural tube defects (NTD). Two large-scale studies assessed these issues recently. The Medical Research Council of Great Britain (MRC) conducted a randomized, controlled multicenter study in patients with prior NTD,[15] while the Hungarian Family Program conducted a randomized, controlled trial evaluating the effect of folic acid supplementation in preventing the first occurrence of NTD.[16] Both studies showed significant reductions in the evidence of NTD in the folic acid supplemented groups,[17] and this pattern has prevailed.[18,19]

Types of major congenital anomalies	Teratological agents
Skeletal and central nervous system	**Excess**
Caudal regression syndrome	Glucose
Neural tube defects	Ketone bodies
Anencephaly	Amino acids (branched chain)
Microcephaly	Somatomedin inhibitors
	Triglycerides
Cardiac	**Deficiency**
Transportation of the great vessels	Glucose
Ventricular septal defects	
Coarctation of the aorta	**Others**
Atrial septal defects	Multifactorial
Cardiomegaly	Genetic predisposition
Renal	**Metabolic consequences**
Hydronephrosis	
Renal agenesis	**Accumulation**
Ureteral duplication	Sorbitol
	Free oxygen radicals
Gastrointestinal	**Deficiency**
Duodenal atresia	Myoinositol
Anorectal atresia	Arachidonic acid
Small left colon syndrome	Zinc
Other	
Single umbilical artery	

Table 20.2. *Diabetic embryopathy types and teratological mechanisms.*

Due to these results, the Centers for Disease Control recommended that all women of childbearing age consume 0.4 mg of folic acid daily. Thus, it seems logical to supplement diabetic patients (*a priori* carrying higher risk for congenital anomalies) with folic acid while preparing them for a planned pregnancy.

Experimental studies

The precise mechanism responsible for abnormal fetal organogenesis in pregnancy complicated by diabetes is unclear. In experimental studies, fuels such as sugars (glucose, galactose, fructose, mannose), ketones, fuel-related modalities such as somatomedin inhibitors, insulin and trace elements, have all been suggested to cause a teratogenic insult to organogenesis (Table 20.2).[20]

Experimental studies have suggested that the major teratogen in diabetic pregnancy is hyperglycemia,[21–24] although other diabetes-related factors may also influence the fetal outcome, e.g. increased levels of ketone bodies,[11,25–29] triglycerides[30,31] and branched chain amino acids.[31,32] Several teratological pathways in the embryonic tissues have emerged, such as alterations in the metabolism of inositol,[33–38] arachidonic acid/prostaglandins,[34,39,40] and reactive oxygen species.[32,41–43] The embryonic formation of sorbitol,[33,35,37,44,45] glycated proteins,[46–48] and the maternal and fetal genotypes,[49–53] are also suggested to influence the complex teratological events in diabetic pregnancy (Table 20.2).

Signal transduction

Cell growth, development and differentiation are controlled by external growth signals, transmitted from the surface of the cell to the nucleus. The plasma membrane lipids, in addition to serving as barriers that separate intracellular from extracellular fluid, are the actual sources of signal molecules (Fig. 20.3). Signal molecules may derive from a variant of a common membrane lipid. Thus, diphosphoinositol is inactivated by esterases that remove the phosphate to yield inositol. This is similar to the activation of the enzyme that hydrolyzes plasma membrane phospholipids to generate arachidonic acid, which is a precursor of signal molecules including the prostaglandins.[12]

The aim is to understand the events involved in signal generation and the many levels at which the perturbation of the signal transduction pathway may result in the loss of control of cell maturation, leading to the development of congenital anomalies. As the mechanisms by which diabetes disrupts normal organogenesis become clearer, it may be possible to reverse them pharmacologically and restore normal organ development.

The polyol pathway and myoinositol

The polyol pathway involves the conversion of glucose into sorbitol. This process is catalyzed by the enzyme aldose reductase, present in most body tissues, which does not usually metabolize glucose because of the high Michaelis constant (K_m) of this substance. In non-compensated diabetes, particularly in tissues that are freely permeable to glucose, sorbitol is produced at an increased rate, and is associated with ocular, neural and renal lesions. The accumulation of sorbitol or, more

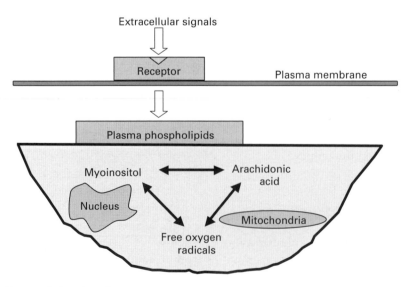

Figure 20.3. *Extracellular signals.*

generally, the increased activity of the polyol pathway, has been convincingly demonstrated to be detrimental to cell function in glucose-permeable tissues. This damage is reversible at first but later progresses to permanent structural derangement.

A hypothesis has been put forward that polyol pathway overactivity is the common denominator of the nephropathy, neuropathy and retinopathy of diabetes by virtue of the compartmental depletion of myoinositol.

Myoinositol is a vital precursor of cell signaling effectors, leading to the formation of phosphoinositides and diacylglycerol (DAG) through the partial hydrolysis of phospholipids. DAG is involved in the maintenance of Na^+/K^+-adenosine triphosphate (ATP)ase activity, as mediated by the enzyme protein kinase C (PKC), which is thought to convert ATPase from the inactive to the active form. ATPase is responsible for pumping Na^+ out of the cell and for Na^+ retention, causing membrane potential alterations, which may be the initial step in the chain of deleterious cell lesions expressed by increased membrane permeability to proteins and other macromolecules.

Aldose reductase inhibitors (ARI) have been used to successfully ameliorate some of the diabetes-related changes in affected tissues without modifying the hyperglycemia.

The presence of the polyol pathway in the early postimplantation embryo has been clearly established, and increases in the sorbitol content of the conceptus have been elicited with hyperglycemia. However, ARI did not diminish the incidence of congenital lesions despite the attenuation in the rise of tissue sorbitol.[44] The glucose-induced increases in sorbitol were accompanied by a fall in the myoinositol content of the conceptus.[38] The changes in myoinositol were inversely proportional to the glucose content of the culture medium and unaffected by two structurally dissimilar ARI.[33]

These findings suggest the possible involvement of myoinositol depletion in the development of dysmorphogenesis in diabetic pregnancy. The high glucose levels cause a decrease in the Na^+-dependent uptake of myoinositol by the embryo.[38,54] The low levels of tissue myoinositol apparently result in a deficient phospholipid turnover,[55] with a reduction in PKC activity[56] and interruption of signal transduction. These results show that addition of myoinositol to the culture medium of embryos reduces the teratogenicity of high glucose concentrations.[34–36,55,56]

Arachidonic acid

Several investigators have suggested that the normal development of a variety of structures, including the palate, mandible, neural tube, genitals and heart, requires phosphatidyl inositol turnover coupled to the arachidonic acid cascade, leading to prostaglandin synthesis. Disruption of this biochemical pathway by hyperglycemia can produce congenital anomalies.

Disturbed metabolism of arachidonic acid and prostaglandins has been found in previous studies of experimental diabetic pregnancies. Addition of arachidonic acid to the culture medium was shown to block the embryonic dysmorphogenesis elicited by high glucose concentrations,[57] a finding that has been repeated[58] and expanded[59] in subsequent studies. Intra- peritoneal injections of arachidonic acid to pregnant diabetic rats diminished the rate of neural tube damage,[57] as did enriching the diet of the pregnant diabetic rats with arachidonic acid,[60,61] thereby indicating disturbance in the arachidonic acid cascade as a consequence of a diabetic environment.[62] Addition of prostaglandin E_2 (PGE$_2$) to the culture medium also blocks glucose-induced teratogenicity *in vitro*,[34,59] as well as maldevelopment of embryos cultured in diabetic serum.[63] Measurements of PGE_2 have indicated that this prostaglandin is decreased in embryos of diabetic rodents during the period of neural tube closure,[64,65] in high-glucose cultured embryos,[65] as well as in the yolk sac of embryos of diabetic women.[66]

Previous studies have shown, however, that the uptake of arachidonic acid by embryonic yolk sacs is increased in a hyperglycemic environment.[40] This finding would preclude an uptake deficiency of arachidonic acid in the conceptus of diabetic pregnancy, a result supported by the demonstration of an unchanged concentration of arachidonic acid in membranes of high-glucose concentration cultured embryos *in vitro*.[67] Recently, however, measurements in day-12 embryos indicate a decreased arachidonic acid concentration in offspring from diabetic rats.[68] From these data, it may be concluded that decreased availability of arachidonic acid and the prostaglandin products of arachidonic acid, is a component of the teratogenicity of diabetic pregnancy.[62]

In a recent *in vitro* study, Wentzel et al[65] found a downregulation of the gene expression of COX-2, the inducible form of the COX enzyme, as well as a growth stimulating hormone (GSH)-dependent enhancement of the conversion of the precursor prostaglandin H_2 (PGH_2) to PGE_2.[65] The PGE_2 concentration of day-10 embryos and membranes was decreased after exposure to high glucose concentration *in vitro* or diabetes *in vivo*. *In vitro* addition of N-acetylcysteine (NAC) to high-glucose concentration cultures restored the PGE_2 concentration.[65] Hyperglycemia/diabetes-induced downregulation of embryonic COX-2 gene expression may be an early event in diabetic embryopathy, leading to lowered PGE_2 levels and dysmorphogenesis. Antioxidant treatment does not prevent the decrease in COX-2 mRNA levels but restores PGE_2 concentrations,[65] suggesting that diabetes-induced oxidative stress aggravates the loss of COX-2 activity.

Culture of rat embryos with COX inhibitors, indomethacin and acetylsalicylic acid, resulted in malformations similar to those caused by high-glucose concentration cultures, a maldevelopment that was blocked by supplementation of arachidonic acid or PGE_2.[59] Addition of superoxide dismutase (SOD) or N-acetylcysteine (NAC) diminished the COX inhibitor-induced dysmorphogenesis, analogous to the effect of the antioxidants on glucose-induced embryonic maldevelopment.[59] This result, together with the finding of diminished glucose-induced embryopathy by addition of arachidonic acid[57–59] and PGE_2,[34,59] suggests crosstalk between teratogenic effects caused by a decreased prostaglandin synthesis and reactive oxygen species (ROS) excess in embryos subjected to a diabetic environment,[20] as well as between inositol and prostaglandins (cf. Fig. 20.4).

Antioxidants

Recent work has suggested that increased embryonic production of ROS[69–73] and/or diminished ROS scavenging capacity[27,49,74–76] are involved in the teratogenic process of diabetic pregnancy. This concept was initially studied in rat embryo culture *in vitro*.[32,41] Supplementing the culture medium with various compounds enhancing the oxygen radical-scavenging capacity of the embryos (SOD,[32,41] catalase,[41] glutathione peroxidase,[41] citiolone,[41] glutathione ester,[74] NAC,[59] and vitamins E and/or C[77]) protected against growth retardation and embryonic malformations induced by increased glucose concentrations. Furthermore, embryos transgenic for the SOD gene, and thereby exhibiting increased activity of SOD, were also protected from the teratogenic effects of high glucose concentrations *in vitro*.[42] Experiments performed *in vivo* have also supported the ROS hypothesis. The

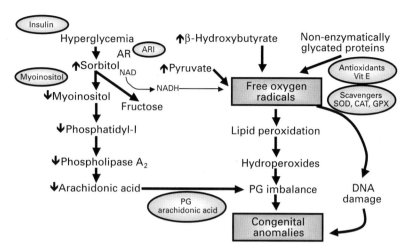

Figure 20.4. *Diabetic embryopathy – a unifying theory.*

concentration of α-tocopherol was reduced and the malonyldialdehyde (MDA):α-tocopherol ratio increased,[78] indicating decreased antioxidant capacity and increased lipid peroxidation/ protein carboxylation in embryos of diabetic rats compared with control embryos.[73] Embryos of diabetic rats showed pronounced morphologic alteration of the mitochondria of the neuroepithelial cells,[79,80] and increased expression of MnSOD,[50] the isoenzyme specific for mitochondria. Pregnant diabetic rats were fed a diet supplemented with the antioxidant butylated hydroxytoluene (BHT). Their offspring were less growth retarded and showed fewer congenital malformations than offspring of diabetic rats without BHT therapy.[43] Subsequently, the outcome of diabetic rodent gestation has been substantially improved by treating the pregnant diabetic animal with several different antioxidants, such as vitamin E,[78,80–83] vitamin C,[84] combinations of vitamin E and C,[85] vitamin E together with arachidonic acid and inositol,[61] glutathione ester,[86] and lipoic acid.[87] These antioxidative agents diminish diabetic embryopathy and improve fetal outcome, often in a dose-dependent fashion (Fig. 20.4).

Thus, it seems that embryos exposed to a diabetic environment show pronounced dysmorphogenesis, which may be induced by enhanced intra-embryonic ROS production. Blocking excess ROS activity may constitute an important therapeutic alternative in the future.

Conclusions

Despite years of meticulous study, a paucity of information still exists regarding the optimal maternal glucose levels that should be aimed for in order to reduce embryonic, fetal and perinatal morbidity, and yet not cause any harm to intrauterine development. Therefore, efforts should be directed towards determining the precise etiology of, and devising strategies for the prevention of, congenital anomalies and most perinatal–neonatal complications accompanying pregnancies of diabetic mothers. Strategies based on the encouraging laboratory evidence of maternal supplementation with folic acid, myoinositol and antioxidants have to be clinically explored. These compounds may serve in the future as a pharmacological prophylaxis against diabetic embryopathy.[88] At the same time, the goal is to encourage the early referral of both pregestational and gestational diabetic women so that tight glycemic control will be instituted at the proper time in order to prevent maternal hyperglycemia complications.

References

1. Pedersen J. *The Pregnant Diabetic and her Newborn. Problems and Management.* (Munksgaard: Copenhagen, 1977.)
2. Kucera J. Rate and type of congenital anomalies among offspring of diabetic women. *J Reprod Med* 1971; 7:61–70.
3. Towner D, Kjos S, Leung B et al. Congenital malformations in pregnancies complicated by NIDDM. *Diabetes Care* 1995; 18:1446–51.
4. von Kries R, Kimmerle R, Schmidt JE et al. Pregnancy outcomes in mothers with pregestational diabetes: a population-based study in North Rhine (Germany) from 1988 to 1993. *Eur J Pediatr* 1997; 156:963–7.
5. Aberg A, Westbom L, Kallen B. Congenital malformations among infants whose mothers had gestational diabetes or preexisting diabetes. *Early Hum Dev* 2001; 61:85–95.
6. Hawthorne G, Robson S, Ryall EA et al. Prospective population based survey of outcome of pregnancy in diabetic women: results of the Northern Diabetic Pregnancy Audit, 1994. *Br Med J* 1997; 315:279–81.
7. Casson IF, Clarke CA, Howard CV et al. Outcomes of pregnancy in insulin dependent diabetic women: results of a five year population cohort study. *Br Med J* 1997; 315:275–8.
8. Freinkel N. Banting lecture 1980. Of pregnancy and progeny. *Diabetes* 1980; 29:1023–35.
9. Buchanan TA, Denno KM, Sipos GF, Sadler TW. Diabetic teratogenesis. In vitro evidence for a multifactorial etiology with little contribution from glucose per se. *Diabetes* 1994; 43:656–60.
10. Wentzel P, Eriksson UJ. Insulin treatment fails to abolish the teratogenic potential of serum from diabetic rats. *Eur J Endocrinol* 1996; 134:439–446.
11. Wentzel P, Thunberg L, Eriksson UJ. Teratogenic effect of diabetic serum is prevented by supplementation of superoxide dismutase and N-acetylcysteine in rat embryo culture. *Diabetologia* 1997; 40:7–14.
12. Hod M. Advances in the understanding of diabetic embryopathy: signal transduction. *Early Preg* 1996; 2:121–8.
13. Martínez-Frias ML. Epidemiological analysis of outcomes of pregnancy in diabetic mothers: identification of the most characteristic and most frequent congenital anomalies. *Am J Med Genet* 1994; 51:108–13.

14. Mills JL. Malformations in infants of diabetic mothers. *Teratology* 1982; 25:385–94.
15. Medical Research Council (MRC). Prevention of neural tube defects: results of the Medical Research Council Vitamin Study. MRC Vitamin Study Research Group. *Lancet* 1991; 338:131–7.
16. Czeizel AE. Prevention of congenital abnormalities by periconceptional multivitamin supplementation. *BMJ* 1993; 306:1645–8.
17. Mills JL, Simpson JL. Prospects for prevention of neural tube defects by vitamin supplementation. *BMJ* 1993; 6:554–8.
18. Lumley J, Watson L, Watson M, Bower C. Periconceptional supplementation with folate and/or multivitamins for preventing neural tube defects. *Cochrane Database Syst Rev* 2001; CD001056.
19. Wald NJ, Law MR, Morris JK, Wald DS. Quantifying the effect of folic acid. *Lancet* 2001; 358:2069–73.
20. Eriksson UJ, Borg LA, Cederberg J et al. Pathogenesis of diabetes-induced congenital malformations. *Upsalon J Med Sci* 2000; 105:53–84.
21. Cockroft DL, Coppola PT. Teratogenic effect of excess glucose on head-fold rat embryos in culture. *Teratology* 1977; 16:141–6.
22. Moley K, Chi M, Manchester J et al. Alterations of intraembryonic metabolites in preimplantation mouse embryos exposed to elevated concentrations of glucose: a metabolic explanation for the developmental retardation seen in preimplantation embryos from diabetic animals. *Biol Reprod* 1996; 54:1209–16.
23. Sadler TW. Effects of maternal diabetes on early embryogenesis. II. Hyperglycemia-induced exencephaly. *Teratology* 1980; 21:349–56.
24. Torchinsky A, Toder V, Carp H et al. In vivo evidence for the existence of a threshold for hyperglycemia-induced major fetal malformations: relevance to the etiology of diabetic teratogenesis. *Early Preg* 1997; 3:27–33.
25. Horton WEJ, Sadler TW. Effects of maternal diabetes on early embryogenesis. Alterations in morphogenesis produced by the ketone body β-hydroxybutyrate. *Diabetes* 1983; 32:610–16.
26. Lewis NJ, Akazawa S, Freinkel N. Teratogenesis from beta-hydroxybutyrate during organogenesis in rat embryo organ culture and enhancement by subteratogenic glucose. *Diabetes* 1983; 32(Suppl 1):11A.
27. Ornoy A, Zaken V, Kohen R. Role of reactive oxygen species (ROS) in the diabetes-induced anomalies in rat embryos in vitro: reduction in antioxidant enzymes and low-molecular-weight antioxidants (LMWA) may be the causative factor for increased anomalies. *Teratology* 1999; 60:376–86.
28. Shum L, Sadler TW. Biochemical basis for D,L,beta-hydroxybutyrate-induced teratogenesis. *Teratology* 1990; 42:553–6.

29. Shum L, Sadler TW. Embryonic catch-up growth after exposure to the ketone body D,L,-beta-hydroxybutyrate in vitro. *Teratology* 1988; 38:369–79.

30. Eriksson RSM, Thunberg L, Eriksson UJ. Effects of interrupted insulin treatment on fetal outcome of pregnant diabetic rats. *Diabetes* 1989; 38:764–72.

31. Styrud J, Thunberg L, Nybacka O, Eriksson UJ. Correlations between maternal metabolism and deranged development in the offspring of normal and diabetic rats. *Pediatr Res* 1995; 37:343–53.

32. Eriksson UJ, Borg LAH. Diabetes and embryonic malformations. Role of substrate-induced free-oxygen radical production for dysmorphogenesis in cultured rat embryos. *Diabetes* 1993; 42:411–19.

33. Hod M, Star S, Passonneau JV et al. Effect of hyperglycemia on sorbitol and myo-inositol content of cultured rat conceptus: failure of aldose reductase inhibitors to modify myo-inositol depletion and dysmorphogenesis. *Biochem Biophys Res Commun* 1986; 140:974–80.

34. Baker L, Piddington R, Goldman A et al. Myo-inositol and prostaglandins reverse the glucose inhibition of neural tube fusion in cultured mouse embryos. *Diabetologia* 1990; 33:593–6.

35. Hashimoto M, Akazawa S, Akazawa M et al. Effects of hyperglycaemia on sorbitol and myo-inositol contents of cultured embryos: treatment with aldose reductase inhibitor and myo-inositol supplementation. *Diabetologia* 1990; 33:597–602.

36. Hod M, Star S, Passonneau J et al. Glucose-induced dysmorphogenesis in the cultured rat conceptus: prevention by supplementation with myo-inositol. *Israel J Med Sci* 1990; 26:541–4.

37. Sussman I, Matschinsky FM. Diabetes affects sorbitol and myo-inositol levels of neuroectodermal tissue during embryogenesis in rat. *Diabetes* 1988; 37:974–81.

38. Weigensberg MJ, Garcia-Palmer F-J, Freinkel N. Uptake of myo-inositol by early-somite rat conceptus. Transport kinetics and effects of hyperglycemia. *Diabetes* 1990; 39:575–82.

39. Pinter E, Reece EA, Leranth CS et al. Yolk sac failure in embryopathy due to hyperglycemia: ultrastructural analysis of yolk sac differentiation associated with embryopathy in rat conceptuses under hyperglycemic conditions. *Teratology* 1986; 33:73–84.

40. Engström E, Haglund A, Eriksson UJ. Effects of maternal diabetes or in vitro hyperglycemia on uptake of palmitic and arachidonic acid by rat embryos. *Pediatr Res* 1991; 30:150–3.

41. Eriksson UJ, Borg LAH. Protection by free oxygen radical scavenging enzymes against glucose-induced embryonic malformations in vitro. *Diabetologia* 1991; 34:325–31.

42. Hagay ZJ, Weiss Y, Zusman I et al. Prevention of diabetes-associated embryopathy by overexpression of the free radical scavenger copper zinc superoxide dismutase in transgenic mouse embryos. *Am J Obstet Gynecol* 1995; 173:1036–41.

43. Eriksson UJ, Simán CM. Pregnant diabetic rats fed the antioxidant butylated hydroxytoluene show decreased occurrence of malformations in the offspring. *Diabetes* 1996; 45:1497–502.

44. Eriksson UJ, Naeser P, Brolin SE. Increased accumulation of sorbitol in offspring of manifest diabetic rats. *Diabetes* 1986; 35:1356–63.

45. Eriksson UJ, Brolin SE, Naeser P. Influence of sorbitol accumulation on growth and development of embryos cultured in elevated levels of glucose and fructose. *Diabetes Res* 1989; 11:27–32.

46. Wolff SP, Jiang ZY, Hunt JV. Protein glycation and oxidative stress in diabetes mellitus and ageing. *Free Rad Biol Med* 1991; 10:339–52.

47. Eriksson UJ, Wentzel P, Minhas HS, Thornalley PJ. Teratogenicity of 3-deoxyglucosone and diabetic embryopathy. *Diabetes* 1998; 47:1960–6.

48. Thornalley PJ. Advanced glycation and the development of diabetic complications. Unifying the involvement of glucose, methylglyoxal and oxidative stress. *Endocr Metab* 1996; 3:149–66.

49. Cederberg J, Eriksson UJ. Decreased catalase activity in malformation-prone embryos of diabetic rats. *Teratology* 1997; 56:350–7.

50. Cederberg J, Galli J, Luthman H, Eriksson UJ. Increased mRNA levels of Mn-SOD and catalase in embryos of diabetic rats from a malformation-resistant strain. *Diabetes* 2000; 49:101–7.

51. Eriksson UJ. Importance of genetic predisposition and maternal environment for the occurrence of congenital malformations in offspring of diabetic rats. *Teratology* 1988; 37:365–74.

52. Otani H, Tanaka O, Tatewaki R et al. Diabetic environment and genetic predisposition as causes of congenital malformations in NOD mouse embryos. *Diabetes* 1991; 40:1245–50.

53. Eriksson UJ, den Bieman M, Prins JB, van Zutphen LFM. Differences in susceptibility for diabetes-induced malformations in separated rat colonies of common origin. *Proceedings of the 4th FELASA Symposium*, Lyon, France. Fondation Marcel Mérieux, 1990;53–7.

54. Strieleman PJ, Connors MA, Metzger BE. Phosphoinositide metabolism in the developing conceptus. Effects of hyperglycemia and scyllo-inositol in rat embryo culture. *Diabetes* 1992; 41:989–97.

55. Strieleman PJ, Metzger BE. Glucose and scyllo-inositol impair phosphoinositide hydrolysis in the 10.5-day cultured rat conceptus: a role in dysmorphogenesis? *Teratology* 1993; 48:267–78.

56. Wentzel P, Wentzel CR, Gareskog MB, Eriksson UJ. Induction of embryonic dysmorphogenesis by high glucose concentration, disturbed inositol metabolism,

and inhibited protein kinase C activity. *Teratology* 2001; 63:193–201.

57. Goldman AS, Baker L, Piddington R et al. Hyperglycemia-induced teratogenesis is mediated by a functional deficiency of arachidonic acid. *Proc Natl Acad Sci USA* 1985; 82:8227–31.

58. Pinter E, Reece EA, Leranth CZ et al. Arachidonic acid prevents hyperglycemia-associated yolk sac damage and embryopathy. *Am J Obstet Gynecol* 1986; 155: 691–702.

59. Wentzel P, Eriksson UJ. Antioxidants diminish developmental damage induced by high glucose and cyclooxygenase inhibitors in rat embryos in vitro. *Diabetes* 1998; 47:677–84.

60. Reece EA, Wu YK, Wiznitzer A et al. Dietary polyunsaturated fatty acid prevents malformations in offspring of diabetic rats. *Am J Obstet Gynecol* 1996; 175:818–23.

61. Reece AE, Wu YK. Prevention of diabetic embryopathy in offspring of diabetic rats with use of a cocktail of deficient substrates and an antioxidant. *Am J Obstet Gynecol* 1997; 176:790–8.

62. Wiznitzer A, Furman B, Mazor M, Reece EA. The role of prostanoids in the development of diabetic embryopathy. *Semin Reprod Endocrinol* 1999; 17:175–81.

63. Goto MP, Goldman AS, Uhing MR. PGE2 prevents anomalies induced by hyperglycemia or diabetic serum in mouse embryos. *Diabetes* 1992; 41:1644–50.

64. Piddington R, Joyce J, Dhanasekaran P, Baker L. Diabetes mellitus affects prostaglandin E2 levels in mouse embryos during neurulation. *Diabetologia* 1996; 39:915–20.

65. Wentzel P, Welsh N, Eriksson UJ. Developmental damage, increased lipid peroxidation, diminished cyclooxygenase-2 gene expression, and lowered PGE2 levels in rat embryos exposed to a diabetic environment. *Diabetes* 1999; 48:813–20.

66. Schoenfeld A, Erman A, Warchaizer S et al. Yolk sac concentration of prostaglandin E2 in diabetic pregnancy: further clues to the etiology of diabetic embryopathy. *Prostaglandins* 1995; 50:121–6.

67. Pinter E, Reece EA, Ogburn PJ et al. Fatty acid content of yolk sac and embryo in hyperglycemia-induced embryopathy and effect of arachidonic acid supplementation. *Am J Obstet Gynecol* 1988; 159:1484–90.

68. Khandelwal M, Reece EA, Wu YK, Borenstein M. Dietary myo-inositol therapy in hyperglycemia-induced embryopathy. *Teratology* 1998; 57:79–84.

69. Lee AT, Plump A, DeSimone C et al. A role for DNA mutations in diabetes-associated teratogenesis in transgenic embryos. *Diabetes* 1995; 44:20–4.

70. Yang X, Borg LAH, Eriksson UJ. Altered metabolism and superoxide generation in neural tissue of rat embryos exposed to high glucose. *Am J Physiol* 1997; 272: E173–E180.

71. Lee AT, Reis D, Eriksson UJ. Hyperglycemia induced embryonic dysmorphogenesis correlates with genomic DNA mutation frequency in vitro and in vivo. *Diabetes* 1999; 48:371–6.

72. Viana M, Aruoma OI, Herrera E, Bonet B. Oxidative damage in pregnant diabetic rats and their embryos. *Free Rad Biol Med* 2000; 29:1115–21.

73. Cederberg J, Basu S, Eriksson UJ. Increased rate of lipid peroxidation and protein carbonylation in experimental diabetic pregnancy. *Diabetologia* 2001; 44:766–74.

74. Trocino RA, Akazawa S, Ishibashi M et al. Significance of glutathione depletion and oxidative stress in early embryogenesis in glucose-induced rat embryo culture. *Diabetes* 1995; 44:992–8.

75. Ornoy A, Kimyagarov D, Yaffe P et al. Role of reactive oxygen species in diabetes-induced embryotoxicity: studies on pre-implantation mouse embryos culture in serum from diabetic pregnant women. *Israel J Med Sci* 1996; 32:1066–73.

76. Menegola E, Broccia ML, Prati M et al. Glutathione status in diabetes-induced embryopathies. *Biol Neonate* 1996; 69:293–7.

77. Zaken V, Kohen R, Ornoy A. Vitamins C and E improve rat embryonic antioxidant defense mechanism in diabetic culture medium. *Teratology* 2001; 64:33–44.

78. Simán CM, Eriksson UJ. Vitamin E decreases the occurrence of malformations in the offspring of diabetic rats. *Diabetes* 1997; 46:1054–61.

79. Yang X, Borg LAH, Eriksson UJ. Altered mitochondrial morphology of rat embryos in diabetic pregnancy. *Anat Rec* 1995; 241:255–67.

80. Yang X, Borg LAH, Simán CM, Eriksson UJ. Maternal antioxidant treatments prevent diabetes-induced alterations of mitochondrial morphology in rat embryos. *Anat Rec* 1998; 251:303–15.

81. Viana M, Herrera E, Bonet B. Teratogenic effects of diabetes mellitus in the rat. Prevention with vitamin E. *Diabetologia* 1996; 39:1041–6.

82. Sivan E, Reece EA, Wu YK et al. Dietary vitamin E prophylaxis and diabetic embryopathy: morphologic and biochemical analysis. *Am J Obstet Gynecol* 1996; 175:793–9.

83. Simán CM, Gittenberger-De Groot AC, Wisse B, Eriksson UJ. Malformations in offspring of diabetic rats: morphometric analysis of neural crest-derived organs and effects of maternal vitamin E treatment. *Teratology* 2000; 61:355–67.

84. Simán CM, Eriksson UJ. Vitamin C supplementation of the maternal diet reduces the rate of malformation in the offspring of diabetic rats. *Diabetologia* 1997; 40: 1416–24.

85. Cederberg J, Siman CM, Eriksson UJ. Combined treatment with vitamin E and vitamin C decreases oxidative stress and improves fetal outcome in experimental diabetic pregnancy. *Pediatr Res* 2001; 49:755–62.

86. Sakamaki H, Akazawa S, Ishibashi M et al. Significance of glutathione-dependent antioxidant system in diabetes-induced embryonic malformations. *Diabetes* 1999; 48:1138–44.

87. Wiznitzer A, Ayalon N, Hershkovitz R et al. Lipoic acid prevention of neural tube defects in offspring of rats with streptozocin-induced diabetes. *Am J Obstet Gynecol* 1999; **180**:188–93.

88. Persson B. Prevention of fetal malformation with antioxidants in diabetic pregnancy. *Pediatr Res* 2001; **49**:742–3.

21

Fetal maturity

Antonio Cutuli, Gian Carlo Di Renzo

Introduction

The immaturity of lung tissue and function leads to an acute progressive breathing failure, the so-called respiratory distress syndrome (RDS). The diabetic pregnancy, and particularly poorly controlled maternal diabetes, represents one of the most important risk condition for RDS. Though the perinatal mortality rate in pregnancies complicated by diabetes has declined, conditions such as congenital malformation, prematurity, hypoglycemia and respiratory distress are still common problems of newborns of diabetic mothers.[1–5]

Despite considerable improvements in neonatal care, the morbidity for respiratory complications such as RDS in the infants of diabetic mothers is considerable, as is the financial burden of the resulting care.[6] According to recent figures, 10–20% of all RDS cases result from elective interference with normal pregnancy. In high-risk pregnancies the planning of the optimal timings of both the therapy and the delivery, and adequate fetal surveillance, is even more critical[7] in improving offspring outcome.[8] Improved outcomes of diabetic pregnancies depend to a large extent on accurate timing of delivery, which is determined by metabolic control, fetal well-being and documentation of fetal lung maturity.

Until recently, RDS was the most common and most serious disease in infants of diabetic mothers. In the 1970s, improved management of diabetic pregnancies resulted in a decline in its incidence from 31 to 3%[8] (Table 21.1).

The observations of Kulovich indicate that a non-diabetic fetus achieves pulmonary maturity at a mean gestational age of 34–35 weeks.[9] By 37 weeks, > 99% of normal newborns have mature lung profiles as assessed by phospholipid assays. In a diabetic pregnancy, however, it is unwise to assume that the risk of respiratory distress has passed until after gestational week 38.5 has been completed.

Clinical studies investigating the effect of maternal diabetes on fetal lung maturation have produced no univocal data. In a series of 805 infants of diabetic mothers delivered over a 10-year period, Robert and Neff[8] found the corrected risk for RDS was nearly six times that for mothers without diabetes mellitus. With the introduction of protocols that emphasize glucose control and antepartum surveillance, RDS has become a less common complication in infants of diabetic mothers.

Several studies agree that, in well-controlled diabetic women delivered at term, the risk of RDS is no higher than that observed in the general population.[10,11]

In conclusion, the risk of hyaline membrane disease at any given gestational age before week 38 is five to six times higher in infants of diabetic mothers than in infants of non-diabetic mothers.

Morbidity	Gestational diabetes (%)	Type 1 diabetes (%)	Type 2 diabetes (%)
Hyperbilirubinemia	29	55	44
Hypoglycemia	9	29	24
Respiratory distress	**3**	**8**	**4**
Transient tachypnea	2	3	4
Hypocalcemia	1	4	1
Cardiomyopathy	1	2	1
Polycythemia	1	3	3

Table 21.1. *Perinatal morbidity in diabetic pregnancies (from the Californian Department of Health Service, 1991).*

Pathophysiology of fetal lung maturation in diabetic pregnancies

Neonatal pulmonary function of the infants of diabetic mothers is suboptimal compared with infants of non-diabetic women matched for gestational age.[10] The mechanism by which maternal diabetes affects pulmonary development remains unknown. An extensive review of the literature confirms that hyperglycemia and hyperinsulinemia are involved in delayed pulmonary maturation, which influences pulmonary surfactant biosynthesis.[12] This may be due to inadequate production of alveolar surfactant or abnormal lung maturation and function.

In vitro studies have documented that insulin can interfere with substrate availability for surfactant biosynthesis. Smith and Giroud[11] demonstrated that when insulin was added to fetal lung cell cultures with cortisol present, steroid-enhanced lecithin synthesis was abolished. Engle and Langan[13] found that higher levels of insulin resulted in diminished glucose and choline uptake by fetal rat type II alveolar cells. Carlson and Smith[14] showed that insulin

blocks cortisol action at the level of the fibroblasts by reducing the production of the fibroblast–pneumocyte factor.

Kulovich and Gluck[9] reported the abnormal timing of phospholipid production in diabetic pregnancy, as indicated by a delay in the appearance of phosphatidylglycerol in the amniotic fluid only in gestational diabetes (White's Class A patients). Smith[15] also postulated that insulin interferes with the normal timing of glucocorticoid-induced pulmonary maturation in the fetus.

Some investigators have disagreed with these findings, reporting that fetal lung maturation occurred later in pregnancies with poor glycemic control regardless of the class of diabetes.[16–20] Bourbon et al[21] proposed that elevated maternal plasma level of myoinositol in diabetic women may inhibit or delay the fetal production of phosphatidylglycerol. In a recent study, Berkowitz et al,[22] in a comparison between gestational diabetic and non-diabetic pregnancies, have also shown that fetal lung maturity does not seem to be significantly delayed in diabetic pregnancies.

It is suspected that neonatal respiratory problems in the these infants have a histologic basis in addition to a biochemical origin. Pinter et al[23] demonstrated decreased fluid clearance and lack of thining of the lung's connective tissue compared with controls in the fetal lung of diabetic rat. Bhavnani et al[24] reported higher lung glycogen levels and reduced pulmonary compliance in offspring of diabetic rabbits compared with controls.

Glucose balance has an effect on the incidence of the hyaline membrane disease. Several studies have attempted to explain the mechanism of hyaline membrane disease. Hawden and Aynsely-Green,[25] in an investigation of type II pneumocytes in rats and rabbits, showed that insulin inhibits the cortisol-dependent production of phosphatidylcholine, apparently as a consequence of the inhibited production of one of the prerequisites of phosphatidylcholine, the fibroblast–pneumocyte factor. In rats, high glucose levels block the transformation of choline to phosphatidylcholine, and butyrate blocks the translation of mRNA into surfactant proteins.

Evaluation of fetal lung maturity

Fetal lung maturity assessment has become a very important tool in the management of high-risk pregnancies, especially diabetic ones. In the past, elective preterm delivery to avoid unexpected intrauterine death was common; a practice which often resulted in a high incidence of neonatal morbidity and mortality (Fig. 21.1). With improvements in glycemic control and better techniques of antepartum surveillance, most patients with diabetes now deliver at term.[26]

In view of the risk of lung immaturity in fetuses of diabetic mothers, the assessment of fetal lung maturity is mandatory.[27] A number of diagnostic methods with high degrees of

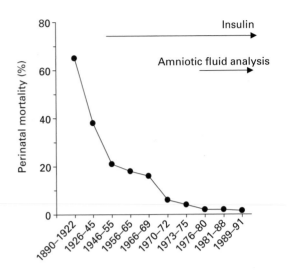

Figure 21.1. *Perinatal mortality after introduction of insulin therapy and amniotic fluid analysis (from Moore[74]).*

accuracy and predictability have been developed and are now available.

Unless excellent gestational dating has been established in a well-controlled patient who has reached 39 weeks gestation, an amniocentesis should be performed before elective delivery to assess fetal pulmonary maturity.

In normal pregnancies, any test of gestational age or general fetal maturation state correlates well with the degree of fetal lung maturity because maturational events are normally linked closely with gestational age. A test of lung maturation in the abnormal pregnancy, such as diabetic one, is not a test of gestational age. A test of fetal lung maturation depends on amniotic fluid composition reflecting the status of the fetal lung (Table 21.2).

Phospholipids

The lecithin–sphingomyelin (LS) ratio was introduced by Gluck et al[28] in 1971. The test depends on the flow of fetal lung fluid into amniotic fluid changing its phospholipid composition. The

Sensitivity	Specificity	False-positive rate	False-negative rate
Ability of test to correctly identify all fetuses at risk for RDS	Ability of test to correctly identify all fetuses not at risk for RDS	Percentage of fetuses identified as being at risk for RDS but do not develop RDS	Percentage of fetuses identified as not being at risk for RDS but do develop RDS

RDS, Resporatory distress syndrome.

Table 21.2. *Accuracy of test for fetal lung maturity.*

result is expressed as the ratio of lecithin (phosphatidylcholine) to sphingomyelin.

Sphingomyelin is a general membrane lipid and is not related to lung maturational events. The sphingomyelin content in amniotic fluid tends to fall from *c.* 32 weeks of gestation to term, whereas the more satured lecithin concentration (a large part from the fetal lung) increases. The LS ratio for normal pregnancies is < 0.5 at 20 weeks, gradually increases to 1.0 at 32 weeks and at *c.* 35 weeks achieves a value of 2.0, correlating it with fetal lung maturity; empirically, RDS is unlikely if the LS ratio is > 2.0.

The evaluation of the LS ratio by chromatography is standardized, and there are reliable methods with sensitivities of 83–97% and specificities of 98%.[29–31] This approach, nevertheless, is not without problems, because of the difficulty of routine activities, it is a difficult test to perform, and specialized laboratory equipment is required.

Many factors can affect the LS ratio, e.g. lecithin is found in many body fluids including blood, vaginal secretions and gastrointestinal fluid, and so the value of LS ratio in diabetic pregnancies has been questioned, where there is an increase in false negative results reaching up to 27% (range 3–27%). Most series, however, report a low incidence of RDS with an LS ratio indicating a mature fetal lung.[32]

Some authors have shown that the LS ratio may not be a reliable indicator of pulmonary maturity in diabetic pregnancies. Those authors affirm that even an LS ratio > 2.0 does not guarantee lung maturation.[9,33] Diabetes may affect the secretion of the fetal lung fluid, resulting in a higher removal of phospholipids from the alveolar lining and in an increased false-negative result rate.[34]

Other authors noted no difference between diabetic patients and controls.[35,36] When maternal diabetes is well controlled during pregnancy, the LS ratio can be used to establish the risk of neonatal RDS.[37,38]

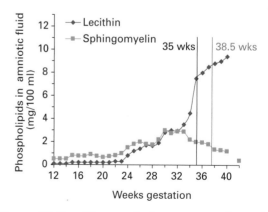

Figure 21.2. *Changes in the concentrations of lecithin and sphingomyelin in amniotic fluid. The vertical lines indicate achieved pulmonary maturity in non-diabetic (left) and diabetic (right) pregnancy.*

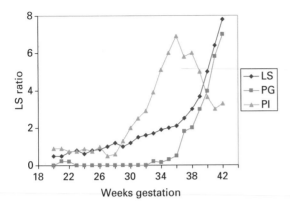

Figure 21.3. *Lecithin–sphingomyelin (LS) ratio, Phosphatidylglycerol (PG) and phosphatidylinositol (PI) in amniotic fluid from normal pregnancies (from Hallman et al[39] and Gluck et al[75]).*

Surfactant of mature lung contains phosphatidylglycerol (PG), which is absent early in gestation and only appears at *c.* 35 weeks of gestation.[39] PG is virtually present only in lung tissue and surfactant. Thus, amniotic fluid contaminated with blood or meconium can be analysed for this substance.[40]

When PG is present, RDS does not occur, except possibly in cases of intrapartum acidemia and hypoxemia or other fetal disease. With trace amounts of PG in amniotic fluid, an incidence of RDS < 1% has been reported.[41] These authors have also confirmed that the addition of detection of PG decreases the rate of false-positives significantly and improves the specificity of the LS ratio.[41]

The appearance of the acidic phospholipid PG may be delayed by fetal hyperinsulinemia and it is associated with an increased incidence of RDS. Although the appearance of PG has been reported to be delayed in pregnancies of diabetic women, it remains a reliable predictor of pulmonary maturity.[42] However, the absence of PG in diabetic pregnancy should not automatically lead to a diagnosis of pulmonary immaturity, since PG fails to appear in 10% of amniotic fluid samples by 40 weeks gestation,[43]

and the presence of PG is reported in only 47% of samples studied for both diabetic and non-diabetic patients with mature LS ratios and gestation of 34 weeks or beyond.

Prior to lung maturation, increases in amniotic fluid phosphatidylinositol (PI) occur from *c.* 26 weeks to 35 weeks. PG appears increasingly in amniotic fluid as the proportion of PI decreases.[39] The lung profile is a test that combines the LS ratio with measurements of the percentage of disaturated (acetone precipitable) lecithin (phosphatidylcholine), PI and PG in the amniotic fluid.[9] The information provided by this profile enhances the accuracy of diagnosing fetal lung maturity and provides further information on lung development. In a small group of cases, the specificity was increased from 69 to 93% by substituting the lung profile for the LS ratio.[29]

The introduction of immunological (Amniostat-FLM) evaluation of PG provides rapid results with minimal requirements for equipment.[44–46] This method has a false-positive rate > 50%. Literature data confirm the use of this approach as a screening test, both for its rapidity and simplicity, particularly for specificity in the case of contamination and/or diabetic patients. The results of PG assay by thin layer chromatography (TLC) and Amniostat-FLM were reported to be concordant in 90–95% of cases.[47]

Proteins

The predominant protein involved in surfactant metabolism is a 35 kDa protein called surfactant-associated protein 35 (SAP–35), a protein that originates from the type II alveolar cells. An increase in amniotic fluid occurs near term and a significant correlation with pulmonary maturity has been noted.[48,49] The measurement of this protein is made simply using an enzyme-linked immunosorbent assay (ELISA) and monoclonal antibodies. Hallman et al[49] used ELISA to predict RDS with an accuracy similar the that of the LS ratio. In high-risk pregnancies, such as diabetes or hypertension, the levels of SAP-35 have less correlation with fetal pulmonary maturity and are probably not reliable in these situations.[49]

Lipids

In amniotic fluid at term cholesterol palmitate is present. Its role is not known but it could serve as a transport mode for palmitic acid which is used in the synthesis of satured phosphatidycholine. A simple method for determining this substance in amniotic fluid using TLC and densitometry has been described.[50] In a small number of patients, levels of cholesterol palmitate were correlated with fetal lung maturity. A similar correlation was not demonstrated in diabetic pregnancies.[51]

Fluorescence polarization

There are at present two systems used to measure fluorescent polarization: the fetal lung maturity assessment (FELMA) microviscometer and the Tdx system. The fluorescent polarization of amniotic fluid is in large part determined by binding of the probe to phospholipid structures and to the predominant protein, albumin.[52] Fluorescence polarization of amniotic fluid is inversely related to the LS ratio.[53,54] The specificity of this method to predict RDS ranges from 50 to 70%.[55,56] The technique is not reliable when amniotic fluid is contaminated by blood or meconium. The fluorescent polarization values are not significantly affected by high-risk pregnancies except for maternal diabetes, which has variable effects on values, and so it is an unreliable indicator of fetal maturity.[57]

In a multicenter study of the TDx system, sensitivity of 96% and a specificity of 88% were obtained with a cut-off value for maturity set at 50 mg/gram (surfactant/albumin value). In this evaluation the corresponding sensitivity and specificity for the LS ratio was 96 and 83%, respectively.[58] In insulin-dependent diabetic patients, a TDx fetal lung maturity, value of at least 70 mg/gram is not associated with RDS requiring intubation.[59,60]

Other tests

A more recently introduced method is evaluation of lamellar body concentrations contained in surfactant secreted by type II pneumocytes, thus lamellar body counts are easy to quantify and require no special instrumentation (Coulter Counter).[61] Cut-off values are ≥ 30.000–35.000/μl, with a sensitivity of almost 100% and a specificity of 96%. Nevertheless, there are no data on the ability of this method to assess fetal lung maturity in diabetic pregnancies.

In the amniotic fluid there are some specific surfactant-associated proteins, such as apoprotein A (SAP-A), which form a complex with dipalmitoilphosphatidylcholine and PG. SAP-A increases in amniotic fluid in parallel with the phospholipids. Several immunological tests are proposed to measure it and enzyme-linked immunoassays have been developed.[62] No data are available regarding its use in diabetic pregnancy.

Caution must therefore be used in planning the delivery of patients with a mature LS ratio and absent PG. The LS ratio can be used to assess fetal lung maturity when glucose levels have been well controlled in a diabetic pregnancy. But when control has been erratic or is difficult to assess, positive PG or high LS ratios (> 2.5) should be used to predict fetal lung maturity.[63]

A study by Piazze et al[64] compared fetal lung maturity as determined by amniotic fluid testing in diabetic pregnancies under euglycemic control with matched controls (Table 21.3). The authors

	Gestation 28–34 weeks			Gestation 35–38 weeks		
	Diabetic pregnancies* (n = 18)	Controls* (n = 18)	P^t	Diabetic pregnancies* (n = 27)	Controls* (n = 27)	P^t
Shake test	2.1:1±1.4	2.6:1±1.1	NS	3.7:1±0.9	3.0±1.2	NS
Planimetric LS ratio	3.0±1.9	2.8±0.9	NS	3.8±1.2	4.6±1.9	NS
Stechiometric LS ratio	5.8±1.7	3.8±1.7	NS	9.8±7.2	8.4±6.6	NS
Phosphatidylglycerol[‡]	33	26	NS	70	79	NS
Lamellar body count (× 10^3/µl)	37.2±38.4	34.2±10.6	NS	45.3±32.7	50.0±32.4	NS

* Values are mean ± standard deviation.
[†] NS, Not significant.
[‡] Percentage of phosphatidylglycerol presence on chromatography.
LS, Lecithin–sphingomyelin.

Table 21.3. Comparison of fetal lung indices between diabetic pregnancies and matched controls (from Piazze et al[64]).

found no statistical difference when comparing fetal lung maturity indices between diabetic pregnancies and controls. Furthermore, comparing Type 1 and Type 2 diabetes with respective controls, the only significant difference found was for a higher proportion of PG present in the Type 2 group than controls (Table 21.4).

Induction of fetal lung maturity

When fetal lungs are immature, the infant will develop RDS, and c. 25% of untreated infants die within 28 days of birth and another 25% will develop chronic lung disease.

	Type 1 Diabetes (IDDM)			Type 2 Diabetes (GDM)		
	IDDM* (n = 19)	Controls* (n = 19)	P^t	GDM* (n = 26)	Controls* (n = 26)	P^t
Shake test	2.6:1±1.4	2.0:1±1.1	NS	4.0:1±0.6	3.0±1.2	NS
Planimetric LS	3.1±1.0	3.3±1.1	NS	3.5±1.4	4.3±2.5	NS
Stechiometric LS	7.6±4.7	6.0±4.4	NS	5.9±3.4	8.8±7.5	NS
Phosphatidylglycerol[‡]	47	42	NS	53	46	0.01
Lamellar body count (× 10^3/µl)	32.0±20.7	34.0±24.0	NS	39.4±30.7	37.1±27.1	NS

* Values are mean ± standard deviation.
[†] NS, Not significant.
[‡] Percentage of phosphatidylglycerol presence on chromatography.
GDM, Gestational diabetes mellitus; IDDM, insulin-dependent diabetes mellitus; LS, lecithin–sphingomyelin.

Table 21.4. Comparison of fetal lung indices between Type 1 and Type 2 diabetic pregnancies, (from Piazze et al[64]).

Since 1972, when Liggins and Howie[65] reported a decrease in RDS in newborns of mothers who had undergone prenatal administration of corticosteroids, several randomized trials have studied whether steroids (or other drugs) can induce and/or improve pulmonary maturity. Many reports have confirmed the original findings that antenatal administration of glucocorticoids to the mother is associated with a statistically significant reduction in the incidence of RDS.[66,67] Almost all of the studies have demonstrated the efficacy of corticosteroid treatment in reducing perinatal morbidity and mortality, as confirmed by a recent meta-analysis on role of corticosteroids to prevent RDS.[68] During the past decade, the strategy for the prevention of RDS has been directed towards the acceleration of fetal lung maturity by administering various hormones to the mother. Currently, glucocorticoids remain the most widely used agents.

Glucocorticoids act by different effects on maturation process:[69]

- prenatal administration significantly increases the content of elastin in the fetal lung;
- as transcriptional activators for the synthesis of SAP (SAP-A and SAP-B);
- on lung fibroblasts, which elaborate the fibroblast–pneumocyte factor that subsequently acts on type II cells and stimulates surfactant synthesis;
- prenatal administration makes the immature lung more responsive to exogenous surfactant;
- stimulate upregulation of corticotropin releasing hormone (CRH) output by the placenta.

Other hormones and drugs have been studied and used for inducing and enhancing fetal lung

Agent	Effect
β-adrenergic agonists	Enhancement of placental transfer of phospholipids from mother to fetus Reduction or suppression of collagen synthesis Augment surfactant release increasing the synthesis of c-adenosine monophosphate (cAMP) by activating adenylcyclase Promote glycogen degradation, essential for the synthesis of phospholipids and for lung growth
Thyrotrophin-releasing hormone	Crossing placenta stimulates thyroid axis and thyroid hormones Additive effect with glucocorticoids on the synthesis of phosphatidylcholine Improvement of lung compliance Enhancement of phospholipid content of the intracellular surfactant
Aminophylline	Stimulation of fetal lung surfactant secretion Crossing placenta and through inhibition of phosphodiesterase, increase the levels of cAMP in fetal lung tissue Acting as a central respiratory stimulant and increasing fetal breathing movements
Inositol	Increasing the synthesis of surfactant phosphotydilglycerol Increasing lung weight, protein and DNA content

Table 21.5. *Action of different substances on fetal lung maturity.*

Clinical recommendations
- All pregnant women between 24 and 34 weeks gestation who are at risk of preterm delivery within 7 days should be considered as candidates for antenatal treatment with a single course of corticosteroids.
- Treatment consists of two doses of 12 mg of betamethasone given intramuscularly 24 hours apart or four doses of 6 mg of dexamethasone given intramuscularly 12 hours apart, as recommended by the consensus panel in 1994. There is no proof of efficacy for any other regimen.
- Because of insufficient scientific data from randomized clinical trials regarding efficacy and safety, repeat courses of corticosteroids should not be used routinely. In general, treatment should be reserved for patients enrolled in randomized controlled trials, several of which are in progress.

What additional information should be obtained?

Research recommendations
- Well-designed randomized clinical trials which are of sufficient power to evaluate efficacy and safety are needed.
- In the light of possible risks, the design of randomized clinical trials should minimize the exposure of mothers and fetuses whilst protecting the integrity of the research design.

What the trials should assess
- clinically important neonatal morbidities, such as respiratory distress syndrome (RDS), chronic lung disease and brain injury;
- clinically important maternal morbidities, such as infection and adrenal suppression;
- the effects of repeat courses of corticosteroids on patterns of fetal and postnatal growth;
- the potential effects of incremental courses on benefits and risks, since the benefits of repeat courses of antenatal corticosteroids are likely to decrease with advancing gestational age;
- the efficacy and safety of rescue therapy;
- the interaction of repeat courses of antenatal corticosteroids with postnatal corticosteroid therapy;
- long-term growth and neuropsychological outcome up to at least school age, using state-of-the-art techniques.

In conclusion
Animal studies should evaluate the pathophysiologic and metabolic mechanisms of potential benefits and risks, including the effects of repeat corticosteroids on central nervous system myelination and brain development.

Box 21.1. National Institute of Health (NIH) guidelines.[70,71]

maturity, such as β-adrenergic agonists, thyroid hormones, aminophylline and inositol (see Table 21.5).

Guidelines produced in US in the 1994 National Institute of Health (NIH) Consensus Statement[70] which was revisited in 2000,[71] to consider the effect of corticosteroids for fetal lung maturations on perinatal outcomes, are summarized in Box 21.1. The guidelines produced by the Royal College of Obstetricians and Gynaecologists about antenatal cortico-steroids to prevent RDS[72] are summarized in Box 21.2.

Effectiveness
- Antenatal corticosteroids are associated with a significant reductions in the rates of respiratory distress syndrome (RDS), neonatal death and intraventricular haemorrhage, although the numbers needing treatment increase significantly after 34 weeks gestation (**evidence level Ia**).
- The cost and duration of neonatal intensive care is reduced following corticosteroid therapy (**evidence level III**).
- The optimal treatment–delivery interval for administration of antenatal corticosteroids is after 24 hours but < 7 days after the start of treatment (**evidence level Ia**).
- The use of antenatal corticosteroids in multiple pregnancies is recommended, but a significant reduction in the rates of RDS has not been demonstrated.
- The use of beta sympathomimetic drugs has been shown to reduce the proportion of women presenting in premature labour, who deliver in the 48 hour period after beginning treatment (**evidence level Ib**).

Safety
- The use of antenatal corticosteroids does not appear to be associated with any significant maternal or fetal adverse effects (**evidence level Ib**).
- The use of antenatal corticosteroids in pregnancies complicated by maternal diabetes mellitus is uncertain.

Repeated doses
- The use of repeated courses of antenatal corticosteroids has not been shown to have any significant advantages (**evidence level III**).

Effectiveness of thyroprophin-releasing hormone (TRH)
- The use of TRH is not recommended in combination with antenatal corticosteroids (**evidence level Ia**).

Indications for antenatal corticosteroid therapy
Every effort should be made to initiate antenatal corticosteroid therapy in women between 24 and 36 weeks gestation with any of the following:
- threatened preterm labour;
- antepartum haemorrhage;
- preterm rupture of the membranes;
- any condition requiring elective preterm delivery.

Contraindications
- Suspected chorioamnionitis;
- tuberculosis;
- porphyria.

Precautions
- Beta sympathomimetics;
- suspected chorioamnionitis;
- repeated dosaging.

Dose and route of administration
- Two doses of betamethasone of 12 mg given intramuscularly 24 hours apart or four doses of dexamethasone of 6 mg given intramuscularly 12 hours apart.

Box 21.2. Royal College of Obstetricians and Gynaecologists' guidelines.[72]

- Phosphatidylglycerol > 3% in amniotic fluid collected from vaginal pool or by amniocentesis;
- completion of 38.5 weeks gestation;
- normal last menstrual period;
- first pelvic examination before 12 weeks to confirm dates;
- sonogram before 20 weeks to confirm dates.

Box 21.3.   Confirmation of fetal maturity before delivery in diabetic pregnancy (adapted from Moore[74]).

Conclusions

If a pregnant woman has poorly controlled diabetes, the infant is at risk for RDS because of delayed lung maturation. The delayed lung maturation includes a delay in the appearance of surfactant and, probably, delayed lung structural maturation as a result of both high insulin and glucose effects on the fetal lung. Concerns about the reliability of the lung maturity test in diabetic pregnancies has decreased as management of the pregnant diabetic has focused on good control of blood glucose levels.[73] Strict blood glucose control should be maintained during pregnancy. A decision about the timing of delivery should be made only when a combination of tests for the prediction of fetal lung maturity have been performed, and confirmed maturity (see Box 21.3).

References

1. Diabetes care and research in Europe: the Saint Vincent declaration. *Diabet Med* 1990; 7:360.
2. Greene MF, Hare JW, Krache M et al. Prematurity among insulin-requiring diabetic gravid women. *Am J Obstet Gynecol* 1989; **161**:106–11.
3. Hanson U, Persson B. Outcome of pregnancies complicated by type 1 insulin-dependent diabetes in Sweden: acute pregnancy complications, neonatal mortality and morbidity. *Am J Perinatol* 1993; **10**:330–3.
4. Landon MB, Gabbe SG, Piana R et al. Neonatal morbidity in pregnancy complicated by diabetes mellitus: predictive value of maternal glycemic profiles. *Am J Obstet Gynecol* 1987; **156**:1089–95.
5. Reece EA, Homko CJ. Infant of the diabetic mother. *Semin Perinatol* 1994; **18**:459–69.
6. Livingstone EG, Herbert WNP, Hage ML. Use of the TDx-FLM assay in the evaluating fetal lung maturity in an insulin-dependent diabetic population. *Obstet Gynecol* 1995; **86**:826–9.
7. Di Renzo GC, Anceschi MM, Guidetti R, Cosmi EV. Requirements of perinatal prevention and treatment of respiratory distress syndrome. *Eur Resp J* 1989; **2 (Suppl 3)**:68s–72s.
8. Robert MF, Neff RK. Association between maternal diabetes and the respiratory distress syndrome in the newborn. *New Engl J Med* 1976; **294**:357–60.
9. Kulovich MV, Gluck CKL. The lung profile: II. Complicated pregnancy. *Am J Obstet Gynecol* 1979; **136**:64.
10. Piper JM, Langer O. Does maternal diabetes delay fetal lung maturity? *Am J Obstet Gynecol* 1993; **168**:783.
11. Bourbon JR, Farrell PM. Fetal lung development in the diabetic pregnancy. *Pediatr Res* 1985; **19**:253–67.
12. Smith BT, Giroud CJP. Insulin antagonism of cortisol action on lecithin synthesis by cultured fetal lung cells. *J Pediatr* 1975; **87**:953–5.
13. Engle M, Langan SM. The effects of insulin and hyperglycemia on surfactant phospholipid biosynthesis in organotypic cultures on type II pneumocytes. *Biochim Biophys Acta* 1983; **753**:6–13.
14. Carlson KS, Smith BT. Insulin acts on the fibroblast to inhibit glucocorticoid stimulation of lung maturity. *J Appl Physiol* 1984; **57**:1577–9.
15. Smith BT. Pulmonary surfactant during fetal development and the neonatal adaptation: hormonal control. In: (Robertson B, Van Golde LMG, Batemburg JJ, eds) *Pulmonary surfactant.* Elsevier: Amsterdam, 1984: 357–81.
16. Ferroni KM, Gross TL, Sokol RJ. What affects fetal pulmonary maturation during diabetic pregnancy? *Am J Obstet Gynecol* 1984; **150**:270.
17. Tyden O, Berne C, Erikkson UJ. Fetal maturation in strictly controlled diabetic pregnancy. *Diabetes Res* 1984; 1:1314.
18. Landon MB, Gabbe SC, Piana R. Neonatal morbidity in pregnancy complicated by diabetes mellitus: predictive

value of maternal glycemic profiles. *Am J Obstet Gynecol* 1987; 156:1089–93.

19. Cunningam MD, Desai NS, Thomson SA. Amniotic fluid phosphatidylglycerol in diabetic pregnancy. *Am J Obstet Gynecol* 1978; 131:712.

20. Ylinen K. High maternal levels of hemoglobin A1c associated with delayed fetal lung maturation in insulin-dependent diabetic pregnancies. *Acta Obstet Gynecol Scand* 1987; 66:263–6.

21. Bourbon JR, Doucet E, Rieutort M. Role of myo-inositol in impairment of fetal lung phosphatidylglycerol biosynthesis in the diabetic pregnancy: physiological consequences of phosphatidylglycerol deficient surfactant in the newborn rat. *Exp Lung Res* 1986; 11:195.

22. Berkowitz K, Reyes C, Saadat P. Comparison of biochemical indices in gestational diabetes and non diabetic pregnancies. *J Reprod Med* 1997; 42:793–800.

23. Pinter E, Peyman JA, Snow K. Effects of maternal diabetes on fetal rat lung ion transport: contribution of alveolar and bronchiolar epithelial cells to Na^+, K^+ ATPase expression. *J Clin Invest* 1991; 87:821–30.

24. Bhavnani BR, Enhorning G, Ekelund L. Maternal diabetes and its effect on biochemical and functional development of rabbit fetal lung. *Biochem Cell Biol* 1988; 66:396–404.

25. Hawdon JM, Aynsley-Green A. Neonatal complications, including hypoglycemia. In: (Dornhorst A, Hadden DR, eds) *Diabetes and Pregnancy: An International Approach to Diagnosis and Management*. (Wiley & Sons: New York, 1996) 303–18.

26. Landon MB, Langer O, Gabbe SG. Fetal surveillance in pregnancies complicated by insulin dependent diabetes mellitus. *Am J Obstet Gynecol* 1992; 167:617.

27. Cosmi EV, Di Renzo GC. Diagnosis of fetal lung maturity. In: (Cosmi EV, Scarpelli EM, eds) *Pulmonary Surfactant System*. (Amsterdam, Elsevier, 1983), 77–98.

28. Gluck L, Kulovisch MV, Boerer Jr RC. Diagnosis of the respiratory distress syndrome by amniocentesis. *Am J Obstet Gynecol* 1971; 109:440.

29. Harvey D, Parkinson C, Campbell S. Risk of respiratory distress syndrome. *Lancet* 1975; 1:42.

30. Kulovich MV, Hallman MB, Gluck L. The lung profile. I. Normal pregnancy. *Am J Obstet Gynecol* 1975; 135:57.

31. Di Renzo GC, Cutuli A, De Graaf O et al. Problematiche diagnostiche nella valutazione della maturità fetale. *Proceedings of the 7th AOGOI Corso di aggiornamento in Medicina Perinatale*, Bormio, 1997, 75–7.

32. Kjos SL, Walther FJ, Montoro M. Prevalence and etiology of respiratory distress in infants of diabetic mothers: predictive value of fetal lung maturation tests. *Am J Obstet Gynecol* 1990; 163:898.

33. Gindes L, Chen R, Perri T et al. Perinatal morbidity in offspring of diabetic mothers. *Israel J Obstet Gynecol* 2002; 12:165–71.

34. Tsai MY, Marshall JG. Phosphatidylglycerol in 261 samples of amniotic fluid from normal and diabetic pregnancies, as measured by one-dimensional thin layer chromatography. *Clin Chem* 1979; 25:682–5.

35. Gluck L, Kulovich MV. Lecithin/sphingomyelin ratios in amniotic fluid in normal and abnormal pregnancy. *Am J Obstet Gynecol* 1973; 115:539:46.

36. Sigh EJ, Mejia A, Zuspan FP. Studies of human amniotic fluid phospholipids in normal, diabetic and drug abuse pregnancy. *Am J Obstet Gynecol* 1974; 119:623–9.

37. Tabsh KMA, Brinkman CR, Bashore RA. Lecithin/sphingomyelin ratio in pregnancies complicated by insulin-dependent diabetes mellitus. *Obstet Gynecol* 1982; 59: 353–8.

38. Farrell PM, Engle MJ, Curet LB. Satured phospholipids in amniotic fluid of normal and diabetic pregnancies. *Obstet Gynecol* 1984; 64:77–85.

39. Hallman M, Kulovich M, Kirkpatrick E. Phosphatidylinositol and phosphatidylglycerol in amniotic fluid: indices of lung maturity. *Am J Obstet Gynecol* 1976; 125:613.

40. Dubin SB. The laboratory assessment of fetal lung maturity. *Am J Clin Pathol* 1992; 97:836.

41. Plauche WC, Faro S. Letellier R. Phosphatidylglycerol and fetal lung maturity. *Am J Obstet Gynecol* 1982; 144:167.

42. Curet LB, Olbson RV, Schneider JM, Zachman RD. Effects of diabetes mellitus on amniotic fluid lecithin/sphingomyelin ratio and respiratory distress syndrome. *Am J Obstet Gynecol* 1979; 135:10–13.

43. Golde SH, Mosley GH. A blind comparison study of the lung phospholipid profile, fluorescence microviscosimetry and the lecithin-sphingomyelin ratio. *Am J Obstet Gynecol* 1980; 126:222.

44. Garite TJ, Yabusaki KK, Moberg LJ. A new rapid slide agglutination test for amniotic fluid phosphatidylglycerol. *Am J Obstet Gynecol* 1983; 147:681–6.

45. Lockitch G, Wittmann BK, Mura SM, Hawkley LC. Evaluation of amniostat-FLM assay for assessment of fetal lung maturity. *Clin Chem* 1984; 159:65–8.

46. Benoit J, Merrill S, Rundell C. An initial clinical trial with both vaginal pool amniocentesis samples. *Am J Obstet Gynecol* 1993; 169:573–6.

47. Saad SA, Fadel HF, Fahmy K et al. The reliability and clinical use of a rapid phosphatidylglycerol assay in normal and diabetic pregnancies. *Am J Obstet Gynecol* 1987; 157:1516–20.

48. McMahon MJ, Mimouni F, Miodovnik M. Surfactant associated protein (SAP-35) in amniotic fluid from diabetic and non dibetic pregnancies. *Obstet Gynecol* 1987; 70:94–8.

49. Hallman M, Arjomaa P, Mizumoto M, Akino T. Surfactant proteins in the diagnosis of fetal lung maturity. *Am J Obstet Gynecol* 1988; 158:531–5.

50. Ludimir J, Alvarez JG, Mennuti MT. Cholesterol palmitate as a predictor of fetal lung maturity. *Am J Obstet Gynecol* 1987; 157:84–8.

51. Ludimir J, Alvarez JG, Landon MB. Amniotic fluid cholesterol palmitate in pregnancies complicated by diabetes mellitus. 1988; **72**:360–2.

52. Tait JF, Franklin RW, Simpson JB, Ashwood ER. Improved fluorescence polarization assay for use in evaluating fetal lung maturity. I. Development of the assay procedure. *Clin Chem* 1986; **32**:248–54.

53. Russell JC. A calibrated fluorescence polarization assay for assessment of fetal lung maturity. *Clin Chem* 1987; **33**:1177–84.

54. Blumenfeld TA, Stark RI, James LS, George JD. Determination of fetal lung maturity by fluorescence polarization of amniotic fluid. *Am J Obstet Gynecol* 1978; **130**:782–7.

55. Golde SH, Vogt JF, Gabbe SG, Cabal LA. Evaluation of the FELMA icroviscometer in predicting fetal lung maturity. *Obstet Gynecol* 1979; **54**:639–42.

56. Ashwood ER, Tait JF, Foerder CA. Improved fluorescence polarization assay for use in evaluating fetal lung maturity. III. *Clin Chem* 1986; **32**:260.

57. Barkau G, Hashiach S, Lanzer D. Detrmination of fetal lung maturity from amniotic fluid microviscosity in high risk pregnancy. *Obstet Gynecol* 1982; **59**:615–23.

58. Russell JC, Cooper CM, Ketchun CH. Multicenter evaluation of TDx test for assessing fetal lung maturity. *Clin Chem* 1980; **35**:1005.

59. Livingston EG, Herbert WN, Hage ML for the Diabetes and Fetal Maturity Study Group. Use of the TDx-FLM assay in evaluating fetal lung maturity in an insulin-dependent diabetic population. *Obstet Gynecol* 1995; **86**:826–9.

60. Tanasijevic MJ, Winkelman JW, Wybenga DR. Prediction of fetal lung maturity in infants of diabetic mothers using FLM S/A and disaturated phosphatidylcholine tests. *Am J Clin Pathol* 1996; **105**:17–22.

61. Ahwood ER, Palmer SE, Taylor JS. Lamellar body counts for rapid feal lung maturity testing. *Obstet Gynecol* 1993; **81**:619.

62. Kuroki Y, Takahashi H, Fukuda Y. Two-site 'simultaneous' immuno-assay with monoclonal antibodies for the determination of surfactant apoproteins in human amniotic fluid. *Pediatr Res* 1985; **19**:1017.

63. Bartelsmeyer JA. Fetal lung maturity. In: (Winn HN, Hobbins JCH, eds) *Clinical Maternal-Fetal Medicine*. (Parthenon Publishers: 2000.)

64. Piazze JJ, Anceschi MM, Maranghi L et al. Fetal lung maturity in pregnancies complicated by insulin-dependent and gestational diabetes: matched cohort study. *Eur J Obstet Gynecol* 1999; **83**:145–50.

65. Liggins GC, Howie RN. A controlled trial of antepartum glucocorticoid treatment for prevention of the respiratory distress syndrome in premature infants. *Pediatrics* 1972; **50**: 515–25.

66. Cosmi EV, Anceschi MM, Piazze Garnica J, Marinoni E. Prevention of fetal and neonatal lung immaturity. In: (Kurjak A, ed.) *Textbook of Perinatal Medicine*. (Parthenon Publishers: 1998.)

67. Di Renzo GC, Anceschi MM, Cosmi EV. Lung surfactant enhancement in utero. *Eur J Obstet Gynecol Reprod Biol* 1989; **32**:1–12.

68. Crowley P. Prophylactic corticosteroids for preterm birth (Cochrane Review). In The Cochrane Library. Oxford. Update Software 2001;3.

69. Anceschi MM, Luzi G, Broccucci L et al. Effects of corticosteroids on fetal lung maturation. In: *The Surfactant System of the Lung*. (MacMillian Press: London, 1991) 23–7.

70. National Health Institute (NIH). Effect of corticosteroids for fetal lung maturation on perinatal outcomes. *NIH Consensus Statement* 1994; **12**:1–24.

71. National Health Institute (NIH). *NIH Consensus Statement* 2000; **17**:1–10. (http://www.nlm.nih.gov/pubs/cbm/cortster.html)

72. Penney DG for the Royal College of Obstetricians and Gynaecologists. Antenatal corticosteroids to prevent respiratory distress syndrome. HYPERLINK: http://www.rcog.org.uk/guidelines/corticosteroids.html

73. Kjos SL, Walther FJ, Montoro M. Prevalence and etiology of respiratory distress in infants of diabetic mothers: predictive value of fetal lung maturation tests. *Am J Obstet Gynecol* 1990; **163**:898–903.

74. Moore TR. Diabetes in pregnancy. In: (Creasy RK, Resnik R, eds) *Maternal Fetal Medicine*, 4th edn. (Saunders: 1999) 964–95.

75. Gluck L, Kulovich MV, Borer RC. The interpretation and significance of the leithin/sphingomyelin ratio in amniotic fluid. *Am J Obstet Gynecol* 1974; **120**:142.

76. Frantz III ID, Epstein MF. Fetal lung development in pregnancies complicated by diabetes. In: (Merkatz IR, Adam PAJ, eds) *The Diabetic Pregnancy: A Perinatal Perspective*. (Grune and Stratton: New York, 1979.)

22

Short-term implications: the neonate

Paul Merlob, Moshe Hod

Introduction

An estimated 0.1–0.5% of all pregnancies are complicated by maternal pregestational diabetes mellitus (Types 1 and 2) and another 1–5% by gestational diabetes (carbohydrate intolerance first recognized during pregnancy).[1,2] The 1988 National Maternal and Infant Health Survey reported a 4% rate of live-birth diabetic pregnancies: 88% gestational diabetes, 8% pregestational Type 2 (non-insulin dependent) and 4% pregestational Type 1 (insulin dependent).[3]

One of the major goals of the Saint Vincent Declaration for Diabetes Care and Research in Europe (1990)[4] was to achieve a pregnancy outcome in diabetic women close to that in non-diabetic women. Thanks to advances in obstetric and neonatologic care, perinatal mortality and neonatal morbidity associated with diabetic pregnancy have been significantly reduced. However, maternal diabetes still poses numerous metabolic, hematologic and anatomic risks to the fetus and the newborn (Fig. 22.1).[1,2,5] Their short-term implications during the first days after birth are discussed in detail in this chapter from a neonatological point of view (macrosomia and congenital malformations are discussed in other chapters).

It should be emphasized that the reported prevalence of short-term neonatal complications of maternal diabetes (pregestational or gestational) varies among different studies, mostly because of the lack of control of confounding variables, such as gestational age, maternal age, parity and body mass index (BMI).[6] Comparative evaluations are further impeded by differences in ethnic origin and socioeconomic status of the study samples, differences in diagnostic criteria, and the type and intensity of interventions during pregnancy.[6]

Neonatal hypoglycemia

Definition

The definition of neonatal hypoglycemia has changed over the past 20 years and still remains elusive. There is no accepted threshold for plasma glucose concentration below which neurologic impairment or injury is inevitable. The cut-off of 44 mg% (2.6 mmol/l) is now currently used as the working definition.[7–9] This 'operational threshold' is not a diagnosis of a disease but an indication for action.[9]

Prevalence

The reported prevalence of neonatal hypoglycemia in diabetic pregnancy varies because of variations in the definition of the disorder; this is in addition to differences in methods of

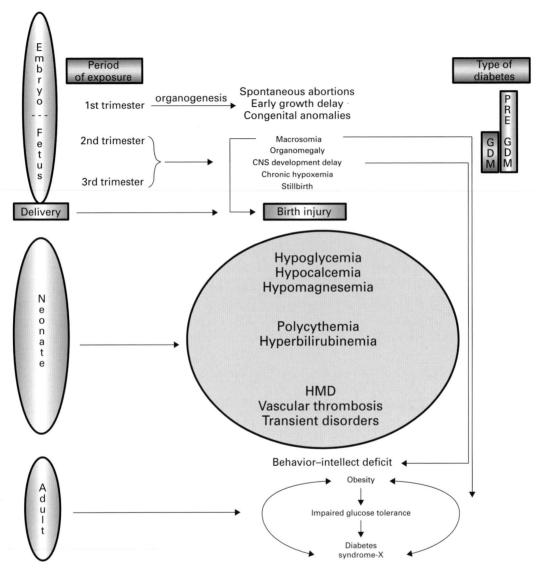

Figure 22.1. *Effects of maternal diabetes on fetus, neonate and adult.*

glucose examination, maternal control of diabetes during pregnancy and labor, and neonatal treatment, particularly feeding. It is not surprising in the light of these great variations that the previous figures for neonatal hypoglycemia in infants of diabetic mothers (IDM) have only historical significance. During the past 10 years, in well-controlled diabetic mothers and using

the 'operational definition' of neonatal hypoglycemia, the prevalence of early neonatal hypoglycemia was still high, particularly in those mothers who were long-standing diabetics. In 2000, Agrawal et al[10] reported 47% prevalence, but they used a threshold of only 2 mmol/l (*c.* 34 mg%). Cordero et al[1] noted a 47% prevalence in macrosomic IDM (Type 1) but only 20% in non-macrosomic infants. In infants of gestational diabetic mothers (IGDM), the rate is *c.* 25%,[10] although some estimates are as high as 40%.[11] In the present authors' population, neonatal hypoglycemia was found in 26.3% of infants whose diabetic mothers maintained strict glycemic control throughout pregnancy and delivery.

Risk factors

The degree of neonatal hypoglycemia in IDM is affected by several maternal and neonatal factors. Early postnatal blood glucose concentrations have been negatively correlated with maternal blood glucose concentrations at delivery and to cord plasma glucose levels. Hypoglycemia did not occur when the maternal blood glucose at delivery was < 7.1 mmol/l (*c.* 120 mg%).[6] Maternal glycemic control during labor and delivery is also important: early postnatal hyperglycemia has been described in infants whose non-diabetic mothers received intravenous (IV) glucose during labor.[6] Neonatal risk factors include perinatal distress, small for gestational age, polycythemia and individual susceptibility.

Etiology

The most accepted explanation for the development of neonatal hypoglycemia in IDM is the Pedersen hypothesis or the maternal hyperglycemia–fetal hyperinsulinemia theory.[5] This hypothesis claims that, even in women under close observation, the episodic diurnal hyperglycemia characteristic of diabetes is the major factor predisposing the fetus to hyperglycemia because of the direct relationship between the maternal and fetal blood glucose concentrations. The fetal hyperglycemia stimulates the release of insulin by fetal islet cells, giving rise to persistent fetal hyperinsulinemia. After birth,

the hyperinsulinemia and inadequate or absent glucose intake leads to neonatal hypoglycemia. Fetal hyperinsulinemia is also associated with suppression of plasma free-fatty-acid levels and hepatic glucose output.

The Pedersen hypothesis has been extended by Freinkel,[12] who examined the role of other nutrients that provide a substrate mixture for the fetus. Freinkel[12] introduced the concept of 'pregnancy as a tissue culture experience', proposing that the placenta and the fetus develop in an incubation medium that is totally derived from maternal fuels. All these fuels (glucose, amino acids, lipids) transverse the placenta in a concentration-dependent fashion and thus delimit the incubation medium in the fetal circulation. Since all these constituents are regulated by maternal insulin, disturbances in its supply or action will influence the whole nutrient composition to which the fetus is exposed and may lead to fetal hyperinsulinemia.

Other hormones may also play a role. Defective counteregulation by catecholamines and/or glucagon (i.e. failure of their release in response to hypoglycemia) results in both increased glucose clearance and diminished glucose production. These, together with the hyperinsulinemia, decrease hepatic production of glucose, increase peripheral glucose uptake and impair lipolysis, resulting in hypoglycemia in the neonate.

Clinical manifestations

The clinical manifestations of neonatal hypoglycemia in IDM and IGDM are not specific, and there is no pathognomonic sign. Symptoms may be neurologic (tremor, jitteriness, high-pitched cry, eye-rolling, convulsions), respiratory signs (cyanosis, tachypnea, apnea), cardiac related (tachycardia, cardiomegaly, cardiac failure), digestive (refusal to feed) or metabolic (hypothermia, sweating), alone or in combination.

However, many infants, even those with very low plasma glucose levels, are asymptomatic, probably because of the initial brain glycogen stores, although the exact biochemistry is still unclear. The characteristics of neonatal hypoglycemia in IDM are: very early onset (first hour after birth); generally asymptomatic, non-recurrent and good response to IV glucose.[9] However, some cases have been reported even after the first 24 hours.[13]

There is no well-defined method for predicting which newborns will have severe hypoglycemia, so all IDM and IGDM must be screened after birth. Blood glucose concentrations should be determined by laboratory measures (stick or glucometer is not reliable for newborns) at 1, 2 and 4 hours after birth, and then again before feeding until stabilization.

Complications

Early diagnosis and prompt and adequate therapy are essential to prevent the late consequences of severe neonatal hypoglycemia in IDM. Studies in both animals and humans clearly show that severe, prolonged neonatal hypoglycemia leads to acute neurologic injury, often with permanent sequelae. The neuropathological findings in hypoglycemic brain damage include acute degeneration of neurons and glial cells throughout the cerebral cortex, especially the occipital lobes.[14] The damage involves layers two and three (in contrast to ischemia, which usually affects pyramidal cells in laminae layers three and five–six).[15] On computerized tomography (CT) and magnetic resonance imaging (MRI), extensive cerebral loss can be seen, most marked in the occipital regions (in contrast to hypoxic–ischemic injuries, in which parasagittal 'watershed' areas are more evident in the frontal and parieto-occipital regions). Long-term follow-up data are still lacking on IDM in general and

asymptomatic hypoglycemic infants in particular. No specific late central nervous system complications have been directly attributed to neonatal hypoglycemia in IDM.

Treatment

The key to the management and treatment of neonatal hypoglycemia is prevention. Feeding should begin as soon as possible after birth. Breast feeding is preferred; for infants with poor sucking, gavage feeding should be provided. If after the initial oral feeding, glucose levels remain < 44 mg%, or if the infant is mildly symptomatic, IV infusion of glucose 10% (6–8 mg/kg/min) should be started. More severe symptomatic neonatal hypoglycemia is treated with infusion of 2 ml/kg/glucose 10% as a bolus administered slowly over a period of 2–4 minutes, followed by continuous IV infusion of glucose 10% (6–8 mg/kg/min). If hypoglycemia persists, higher rates of glucose administration (8–12 mg/kg/min) may be necessary. Once the plasma glucose level stabilizes above 44 mg%, the infusion may be slowly decreased while oral feeding is increased. A prompt response to therapy is good evidence that the hypoglycemia was indeed the cause of the symptoms.

Neonatal hypocalcemia

Definition and prevalence

Hypocalcemia is defined as a serum level of calcium < 8 mg% in the full-term infant and < 7 mg% in the preterm infant, or an ionized calcium level < 0.75–1.1 mmol/l (c. 3–4 mg%). Hypocalcemia occurs frequently in IDM and IGDM, even accounting for perinatal distress, such as asphyxia and/or premature delivery.[16] However, the reported rate of 50% for IDM and 10–20% for IGDM in the first 3 days of life were published before tight glucose control in diabetic pregnancy became the accepted policy. Studies have since shown that the frequency and severity of neonatal hypocalcemia is directly related to the severity of the maternal diabetes,[17] and that the rate can be reduced with strict glycemic control.[18]

Risk factors

Acidosis requiring bicarbonate correction, pregnancy-induced hypertension and oral glucose administration are all potential risk factors for hypocalcemia in IDM.

Etiology

Several explanations for alterations in calcium homeostasis in IDM have been suggested.

- Prolonged functional hypoparathyroidism was proposed as the main explanation for hypocalcemia in IDM. As a result, there is a failure of an appropriate rise in parathyroid hormone (PTH) concentrations in response to hypocalcemia. PTH concentrations are significantly lower in IDM than in infants of non-diabetic mothers during the first 4 days of life, and therefore the PTH response to hypocalcemia occurs later, in the third or fourth day of life.
- Hypomagnesemia may be another explanation for hypocalcemia. It has been suggested that the glucosuria-induced loss in maternal urinary magnesium, and the resulting magnesium deficiency in both mother and fetus, inhibits PTH secretion and leads to hypocalcemia.[17] Pregnant diabetic women had significantly lower serum magnesium concentrations throughout pregnancy than pregnant non-diabetic women.
- Another mechanism that may be at least partially responsible for hypocalcemia is the

physicochemical reaction to hyperphosphatemia during the initial 48 hours after birth. The intense postnatal erythrocyte breakdown increases the serum level of phosphate which, in turn, decreases the calcium ion concentration by both their combination and bone deposition, a process made possible by the inadequate postnatal parathyroid gland response.[19]

- Persistently high levels of calcitonin after birth, possible alterations in vitamin D metabolism and anomalies related to PTH-related protein may also contribute to the complex mechanism of hypocalcemia in IDM.

Clinical manifestations

Clinically, hypocalcemia usually presents between 24 and 72 hours after birth. The minimum calcium level is reached at about the end of the first day (22–26 hours). In general, hypocalcemia is asymptomatic and self-limited. Symptomatic IDM have a high frequency of neuromuscular signs, such as tremor, jitteriness, hyperirritability, hypertonicity, hoarse cry, clonus and also convulsions.

Treatment

Treatment consists of the administration of calcium gluconate 10% per os (0.5–1 g/kg/day) divided into four to six doses. Infants who received glucose infusion for correction of hypoglycemia may be treated with a slow infusion of calcium gluconate 10% (500 mg/kg/day). For more severe symptoms, $MgSO_4$ IM is used. However, in a randomized, controlled trial, Mehta et al[20] demonstrated that the administration of $MgSO_4$ IM to infants of well-controlled diabetic mothers with a cord magnesium level of < 1.8 mg/dl does not reduce the incidence of neonatal hypocalcemia.

If promptly and correctly treated, IDM with hypocalcemia have a good prognosis, even those with convulsions.

Neonatal hypomagnesemia

Definition and prevalence

Neonatal hypomagnesemia is defined as a serum magnesium level of < 1.5 mg/dl (0.62 mmol/l). The frequency and severity of neonatal hypomagnesemia is correlated with the maternal status. A prevalence of up to 37.5% was reported before tight control of maternal diabetes was instituted[21] and recent figures are much lower.

Etiology

Tsang et al[21] observed that decreased serum magnesium in IDM is associated with decreased maternal serum magnesium (due to an increase in renal loss secondary to diabetic glycosuria), in addition to decreased neonatal ionized and total calcium, increased serum phosphate, and decreased parathyroid function. In the diabetic pregnancy, the amniotic fluid magnesium concentrations (which reflect mainly the fetal urine) are significantly lower than in the non-diabetic pregnancy,[22] which demonstrates a state of fetal magnesium deficiency. The fetal hypomagnesemia, in turn, suppresses parathyroid activity, thereby also inducing hypocalcemia.

Clinical manifestations

The clinical manifestations of neonatal hypomagnesemia in IDM (onset in the first 3 days of life) are similar to those of hypocalcemia and consist mostly of neuromuscular hyperexcitability (tremor, jitteriness, hyperactivity, hypertonicity and seizures). However, decreased serum magnesium alone or with decreased ionized or total calcium did not correlate with neuromuscular irritability in these infants. The lack of correlation of these clinical signs with serum levels of magnesium suggests that jitteriness may not be related to hypomagnesemia in IDM. The long-term potential deleterious effects of hypomagnesemia are also unknown.

Treatment

The treatment of hypomagnesemia consists of the administration of $MgSO_4$ IM at a dose of 0.2 ml/kg for 2–3 days, with close monitoring of serum magnesium levels. Maintenance therapy consists of $MgSO_4$ 25% per os at a dose of 0.25 ml/kg/day, diluted to c. 10% concentration, with monitoring of stools (possible diarrhea).

Other metabolic disorders

In addition to disorders of fuel metabolism (glucose, free fatty acids and amino acids), alterations in trace element status also occur in diabetic pregnancy. They are linked to alterations in fetal growth and congenital malformations.

Hyperzincuria

Hyperzincuria is present in Type 1 diabetes. A linear relationship between the magnitude of urinary zinc excretion and the severity of diabetes has been established. However, hyperzincuria is not associated with lower plasma zinc levels. Increased zinc absorption, decreased intestinal zinc excretion or increased tissue catabolism may account for this finding. Studies in diabetic animals have demonstrated reductions in total fetal body zinc concentrations, particularly in the liver, which persisted despite maternal zinc supplementation during pregnancy.[23] The zinc deficiency resulted in a pattern of malformations similar to that seen in human diabetic pregnancy.

Chromium deficiency

Chromium deficiency is associated with Type 1 diabetes and increased chromium losses have been noted in diabetic pregnancy. Treatment with chromium supplementation improves glucose tolerance, insulin levels and serum lipid profiles. Chromium deficiency has been implicated in diabetic teratogenicity (via mediation of glycemic control) as well as cardiovascular disease.[23]

Neonatal erythremia and hyperviscosity

Definition and prevalence

Neonatal erythremia is generally defined as a venous hematocrit > 65%. When time of sampling is taken into account, neonatal polycythemia is diagnosed when venous hematocrit is > 70% at age 2 hours, > 68% at 6 hours and > 65% at 12–18 hours.[24] A venous hematocrit of ≥ 65% has been reported in 20% of IDM[25] and 5% of IGDM[1] during the first days of life. In a prospective study, Mimouni et al[25] reported a prevalence of 29.4% in IDM after excluding possible confounding factors (site of blood sampling, time of sampling, time of cord clamping, gestational age, mode of delivery and asphyxia at birth).

Etiology

Several explanations for the development of neonatal polycythemia in IDM and IGDM have been suggested.

- The main contributory factor is apparently the intrauterine hypoxemia associated with diabetic pregnancy, which causes an increase in erythropoietin production and, thereby, secondary high erythropoiesis. In a study of fetal blood samples obtained by cordocentesis, Salvessen et al[26] noted significantly higher levels of fetal plasma erythropoietin in IDM than in normal controls. There was a significant association between fetal erythropoietin and erythroblast count, and between erythroblasts and hemoglobin levels. Widness et al[27] reported a direct relationship between antepartum maternal glucose control and fetal erythropoietin levels. These authors also found that IDM have increased concentrations of plasma erythropoietin, which were correlated with glucose and insulin levels in the amniotic fluid and cord blood.

- Another explanation involves a change in placento–fetal blood distribution. As a result of intrapartum hypoxia, there is a shift in blood flow between the placental and fetal compartments, so that only 25% of the blood volume remains in the placenta (instead of the usual 35%), with the remainder going to the fetus. This mechanism has not yet been studied in depth, but it is apparently associated with changes in blood vessel resistance.

- Blood viscosity in IDM may be affected by a decrease in fetal erythrocyte deformability due to the different metabolic and hormonal conditions in these babies. This hypothesis has not yet been confirmed.

Clinical manifestations

Clinically, neonatal polycythemia may present as erythrocyanosis, and cardiorespiratory and neurological signs, alone or in combination. In symptomatic infants, neurological signs (jitteriness, irritability, hypertonicity, seizures) and cardiorespiratory signs (tachypnea, cyanosis, respiratory distress, tachycardia, cardiomegaly) are predominant. However, many infants are asymptomatic. The main pathophysiologic problem in neonatal polycythemia is hyperviscosity which, in IDM, leads to decreased blood perfusion, sludging of erythrocytes and increased platelet aggregation – all factors associated with the formation of intravascular thrombi. As a result, vascular thromboses occur in various places in the body: brain, retina, heart, lungs, kidneys (renal vein thrombosis), adrenal glands, and mesenteric (necrotizing enterocolitis) and peripheral vessels.

Treatment

Treatment of neonatal polycythemia (symptomatic or venous hematocrit > 70%) consists of partial dilutional exchange transfusion with albumin 5% or saline. It should be administered as early as possible (preferably 2–4 hours after birth) and with an adequate quantity of albumin or saline to quickly reduce the hematocrit and blood viscosity. There is an urgent need for a double-blind, randomized, controlled study to establish the still controversial indications for dilutional exchange transfusion in asymptomatic polycythemia, and to determine if early diagnosis and treatment prevent serious sequelae later in life.

Neonatal hyperbilirubinemia

Definition and prevalence

Neonatal hyperbilirubinemia is defined as a total serum bilirubin level > 12 mg/dl (205 mmol/l). Indirect neonatal hyperbilirubinemia develops in 20–25% of IDM. The risk is much higher in IDM and IGDM than in infants of non-diabetic mothers.

Etiology

The pathogenesis of neonatal hyperbilirubinemia remains uncertain, although a number of determinant and contributory factors have been suggested.

Determinant factors
* Increased hemoglobin catabolism and, as a result, increased bilirubin production. It was demonstrated in IDM that carbon monoxide production is increased as a result of increased hemoglobin breakdown and bilirubin production.[28]
* The increased rate of erythrocyte breakdown in IDM is probably linked to an altered erythrocyte membrane composition, resulting from changes in maternal fuel availability. As a result, red cell membranes of IDM may be more susceptible to oxidation or physical damage than those of normal infants.
* The increased erythropoietin concentration as a result of *in utero* hypoxemia stimulates the production of erythrocytes.

Contributory factors
* Erythremia, a frequent occurrence in IDM, contributes to neonatal hyperbilirubinemia because it makes more red blood cells available for breakdown.
* Bruising, hematomas or birth trauma secondary to fetal macrosomia will result in resorption of more blood and, thereby, hyperbilirubinemia.
* If enteral feeding is delayed, decreased intestinal motility and increased enterohepatic circulation of bilirubin may also be contributory factors.

Clinical manifestations

Neonatal hyperbilirubinemia is manifested clinically as cutaneous jaundice and, rarely, splenomegaly. It is essential to prevent levels of indirect hyperbilirubinemia that can lead to brain damage. Therefore, all IDM and IGDM need to undergo careful screening of bilirubin levels.

Treatment

Early feeding, correction of metabolic conditions (hypoglycemia, hypoxia, polycythemia) that may exacerbate the hyperbilirubinemia and timely initiation of phototherapy are adequate treatment measures. In the great majority of cases, they may prevent the need for exchange transfusion.

Other hematologic disorders

In addition to the well-known hematologic disorders (polycythemia, hyperbilirubinemia) of IDM, other problems have been observed in individual blood components.

- In a study of 79 IDM, Green and Mimouni[29] observed a significantly higher nucleated red blood cell count than in normal controls. In the absence of hemolysis or blood loss, this finding could be a result of chronic intrauterine hypoxia.
- Relative leukocytosis, a shift to the left and decreased neutrophil chemotaxis have been described.
- Salvessen et al[30] obtained umbilical venous blood within 24 hours of elective delivery from 40 women with diabetic pregnancies at 36–40 weeks gestation. The mean platelet count was significantly lower in the IDM than the corresponding reference values. However, values a little lower than 150,000/mm^3 were observed in only four IDM (10%).
- In IDM, clot formation is facilitated by characteristic abnormalities in the hemostatic mechanism, such as increased platelet aggregation and high fast antiplasmin levels. The reasons for these alterations are not clear.
- IDM who are large for gestational age and have hypoglycemia at birth have a > 90% prevalence of abnormal iron indexes, which include decreased serum ferritin and iron concentrations, and increased total iron-binding capacity and free erythrocyte protoporphyrin concentrations.[31] These abnormalities are associated with elevations in cord blood erythropoietin and hemoglobin concentrations, and may reflect a redistribution of iron from plasma and storage pools into an expanded pool. They are also related to a chronic state of intrauterine hypoxia, most likely a result of fetal hyperglycemia and hyperinsulinism. IDM with abnormal iron indexes at birth require close developmental follow-up because they are at increased developmental risk.[31]

Respiratory distress syndrome

Definition

Respiratory distress syndrome describes a characteristic constellation of clinical (tachypnea, grunting, costal retractions, nasal flares and cyanosis), laboratory (metabolic acidosis and hypoxemia) and radiological (air bronchogram and reticulogranular pattern on chest X-ray) findings. It is caused by deficient surfactant production, which determines decreased lung compliance with resultant hypoxia. Other causes of respiratory distress in IDM are transient tachypnea of the newborn, meconium aspiration syndrome, polycythemia and hypertrophic cardiomyopathy.

Prevalence

Diabetes *per se* predisposes IDM to respiratory distress syndrome. Robert et al[32] found a 5.6-fold higher risk of respiratory distress syndrome in IDM than in infants of non-diabetic mothers when confounding variables were excluded. The overall risk of respiratory distress syndrome has dropped significantly from 31 to 3% with the introduction of strict glucose control during pregnancy and delivery at term or near to term. Nevertheless, it remains a potentially severe complication in preterm infants of diabetic mothers.

Etiology

The increased risk of respiratory distress syndrome in infants born to mothers with uncontrolled or poorly controlled diabetes is due in great part to fetal hyperinsulinemia. Fetal hyperinsulinemia can block the normal enzyme-inducing action of cortisol on the Type 2 fetal pneumocyte production of surfactant, apparently as a consequence of the inhibited production of one of the prerequisites of phosphatidylcholine, fibroblast-pneumocyte factor. Insulin may impair fetal surfactant synthesis by shunting glycerol-β-phosphate toward pyruvate and acetyl-CoA, which decreases its availability for phospholipid biosynthesis. Insulin also seems to interfere with the conversion of phosphatidic acid to phosphatidylglycerol (PG), which has a stabilizing effect on the surfactant. When PG is found in amniotic fluid, respiratory distress syndrome is generally absent. Even in gestational diabetic pregnancies, PG appears later in the amniotic fluid than in normal pregnancies.

Fetal hyperglycemia without hyperinsulinemia may also affect surfactant synthesis. Studies in fetal rat lung explants demonstrated that high glucose concentrations inhibited the incorporation of choline into phosphatidylcholine and that butyrate blocks the transcription of messenger ribonucleic acid (mRNA) for surfactant proteins.[33]

Identification and treatment

The standard methods used to assess antenatal lung maturity may not be applicable to diabetic pregnancy. The lecithin-sphingomyelin (LS) ratio in the amniotic fluid may not accurately predict lung maturity in diabetic pregnancies because respiratory distress syndrome may develop in these offspring despite an LS ratio > 2:0. Kulovitch and Gluck[34] found a significant delay in the appearance of PG that was unrelated to maturation of lecithin. As PG signals final maturation of lung surfactant, once it appears, IDM and IGDM can be delivered safely without risk of respiratory distress syndrome. Therefore, in the event of elective delivery before 38–39 weeks, fetal lung maturity must be documented by amniocentesis, by either the presence of PG (1% risk of respiratory distress syndrome), or an LS ratio ≥ 2:0 (3% risk of respiratory distress syndrome).[35] These tests are unnecessary beyond 38–39 weeks gestation in women with good glycemic control, when the risk of respiratory distress syndrome approaches that of the normal population.[36] To minimize respiratory complications in IDM, obstetricians should aim to deliver each infant as close to term as possible (provided that fetal well-being is assured and there are no other antenatal complications), to allow delivery to occur after spontaneous onset of labor (to avoid transient tachypnea) and to prescribe antenatal steroid treatment for mothers who may deliver before term.

Ventricular septal hypertrophy

Definition

Ventricular septal hypertrophy is defined as a septal thickness of more than two standard deviations (2 SD) above the normal mean. Septal size during diastole increases in a linear and statistically significant fashion from the twentieth week of gestation to term.[37] In IDM, however, cardiac hypertrophy develops late in gestation (at 34–40 weeks), even in the presence of good glycemic control.[38]

Prevalence

Veille et al,[37] in a study of 64 pregnant women with diabetes, recorded a 75% rate of septal hypertrophy. However, this high prevalence may apply only to patients with less than optimal glucose control. In the present authors' diabetic population with strict glycemic control, ventricular septal hypertrophy was noted in only 7.5% of IDM. Ventricular septal hypertrophy is more prevalent in macrosomic than in normal-sized infants (8.3 versus 1.8%). Mehta et al[39] found that IGDM had significantly lower left ventricular dimensions during systole and diastole than healthy infants. They also exhibited altered diastolic filling patterns despite the absence of left ventricular or septal hypertrophy, indicating poor myocardial relaxation or decreased passive compliance of the ventricular myocardium. All these IGDM were asymptomatic; however, if exposed to significant stress, they could be at risk of higher morbidity.

Etiology

Cardiac hypertrophic changes can occur in IDM as a result of the fetal hyperinsulinemic state acting on insulin or insulin-like growth factor (IGF)-II receptors, which are present in high densities in the heart, particularly in the intraventricular septum.[40] The fetal insulin stimulation leads to an increase in myocardial nuclei, cell number and fibers, and, thereby, septal hypertrophy, with decreased left ventricular function and left ventricular outflow

obstruction.[1] Echocardiography suggests a left ventricular obstruction to blood outflow caused by the opposition of the thickened interventricular septum to the atrioventricular valves during systole. On non-invasive Doppler ultrasonography, there is a strong negative correlation between septal thickness and cardiac output.

Clinical manifestations

Most infants with ventricular septal hypertrophy are asymptomatic. The septal thickness is detected only by echocardiography and electrocardiography, because cardiomegaly and septal hypertrophy *per se* do not necessarily translate into poor myocardial function. A small number of infants may have left outflow obstruction severe enough to cause left ventricular failure. In these cases, there may be cardiac insufficiency and signs of respiratory distress, such as tachypnea, tachycardia, increased oxygen consumption and defective feeding.

Treatment

Ventricular septal hypertrophy usually resolves spontaneously after 3–6 months without sequelae (no permanent effects on the myocardium). Infants with obstructive heart failure should be treated with propranolol (not digoxin!) and supportive care; those who survive the initial period with medical management will also show spontaneous improvement in the hypertrophy.

Ovarian cyst

Prevalence and type

Ovarian cysts are common in the general neonatal population. Using three-dimensional ultrasound, Cohen et al[41] noted an 84% rate of ovarian cysts in consecutive infants aged 1 day to 24 months: the prevalence is even higher in IDM. Antenatal sonographic detection of ovarian cysts and polyhydramnios should raise a suspicion of maternal diabetes.[42]

There are different histological types of neonatal ovarian cysts but the most frequent are follicular cysts.

Etiology

The exact etiology of ovarian cysts is unknown, but it probably involves an endocrinological disturbance (imbalance) of the ovarian anterior pituitary axis, with excessive stimulation of the fetal ovary by placental and maternal hormones. Elevated circulating estradiol levels in neonatal ovarian cysts was recently demonstrated by Arisaka et al.[43] The high rate of ovarian cysts in IDM is presumably due to hypersecretion of the placental human chorionic gonadotropin (HCG) or increased permeability of the placenta to HCG.

Clinical manifestations

Clinically, ovarian cysts appear as a smooth, non-tender and freely movable mass in the lower abdomen, usually unilaterally. They measure a few millimeters to > 20 cm in diameter. Polyhydramnios is observed in 5–12% of cases and is presumed to result from the mass compressing the small intestine.

Complications

In the absence of complications, ovarian cysts usually involute or regress spontaneously. There are three types of complications: primary, secondary and maternal. Primary complications are torsion, hemorrhage or rupture. Torsion has been noted in 42% of patients, often with asymptomatic cysts detected antenatally. Large cysts may cause secondary complications, such as incarceration into an inguinal hernia, bowel or urinary tract obstruction, or thorax compression. Maternal complications are polyhydramnios and vaginal dystocia with cyst rupture.

Treatment

In IDM, treatment of ovarian cysts depends largely on cyst size, sonographic characteristics, and potential risks of complications. Single ovarian cysts < 4 cm in diameter can be followed expectantly by serial ultrasound scans, as they usually regress spontaneously. Ovarian cysts with a diameter > 5 cm should be treated. Management options include cystectomy, laparoscopic needle aspiration or laparoscopy. Very large cysts may require intrauterine aspiration to reduce the risk of secondary pulmonary hypoplasia. When surgery is performed, it is important to preserve as much gonadal tissue as possible and, if practical, merely to remove the cyst.

Small left colon

Definition

Neonatal small left colon is a functional transient disease that produces the typical signs and symptoms of a low intestinal obstruction. It was first described by Davis et al[44] in 1974, in 20 full-term infants with symptoms and signs of a low colonic obstruction and a barium enema picture of a uniformly narrowed colon from anus to splenic flexure (caliber < 1 cm), with an abrupt transition at the splenic flexure to a dilated right colon. The small colon had smooth margins without the usual tortuosity and was smaller than normal. Eight of these newborns (40%) were IDM. Further investigation of 12 asymptomatic IDM yielded six (50%) with the same colon configuration.

Etiology

The etiology of neonatal small left colon is unknown, but it may involve neurohumoral imbalances between the autonomic nervous system and glucagon. Fetal and neonatal hypoglycemia is associated with significant hyperglucagonemia with a resultant inhibition of left colon activity.[45] Presumably, the immature intramural ganglion cells are unable to respond to sympathetic stimulation (secondary to hypoglycemia), thereby compounding the ileus.[46] Other suggested causes of *in utero* neonatal small left colon are hypermagnesemia (after maternal $MgSO_4$ treatment), immaturity of the myenteric plexus in the left bowel wall and maternal ingestion of psychotropic drugs.

Clinical manifestations

Clinically, neonatal small left colon occurs in the first 24–48 hours after birth with abdominal distension and delayed passage of meconium. The diagnosis is based on radiographic findings observed after water-soluble contrast enema, as described by Davis et al.[44] The infant can retain the contrast medium for 24–48 hours. Neonatal small left colon is considered to have a benign course. The prognosis is good in the absence of complications. The colon returns to its normal size after 5–7 days, either spontaneously or after repeated daily saline enemas. Neonatal small left colon should be distinguished from Hirschprung's disease (congenital megacolon), which has a different prognosis and requires different treatment.

Complications

Complications are usually seen in severe cases (hypoglycemic cardiomyopathy, cyanosis and persistent fetal circulation shortly after birth), and include cecal or ileal perforations and intussusception.

Treatment

Treatment is conservative, except when complications are present. Water-soluble contrast enema examination, done for diagnosis in newborns who develop clinical signs and symptoms of colon obstruction, is also therapeutic.[44] Repeated daily saline enemas have a permanent curative effect.

Strict glycemic control and short-term neonatal complications

It was hypothesized that the early detection (preconception) of maternal diabetes, with subsequent normoglycemia before conception and strict metabolic control during pregnancy, could prevent the occurrence of most short-term neonatal complications, including congenital malformations.[47,48] Fuhrman et al,[47] in a prospective controlled study, tried to verify this hypothesis and showed a statistically significant reduction in the prevalence of congenital malformations in the strict metabolic control group. Another 12 similar prospective studies in the world literature have explored the incidence of preconception normoglycemia and postconception strict glycemic control on the prevalence of major congenital malformations, and some of them on short-term neonatal complications.[48] A significant reduction in neonatal morbidity, particularly severe disorders such as respiratory distress syndrome and major malformations, has been reported; nevertheless, rates remain twice those seen in the general population. Also, short-term neonatal complications cannot be completely prevented. The studies reported to date on the effectiveness of treatment of gestational diabetes on perinatal outcomes have been contradictory, and their results have been inconsistent and subject to

Implication	Definition	Prevalence (%)
Macrosomia	> 4000 gram	13.7
Hypoglycemia	< 44 mg%	26.3
Hypocalcemia	< 8 mg% in full-term infant	
	< 7 mg% in preterm infant	7.5
Polycythemia	> 70% (at 2–4 hours)	
	> 68% (at 6 hours)	7.5
	> 65% (at > 12 hours)	
Hyperbilirubinemia	> 12 mg%	19.4
Thrombocytopenia	< 150,000	5.0
Respiratory distress	Clinical findings plus blood	
syndrome	gases plus chest X-ray	3.7
Ventricular septal	Echocardiography	
hypertrophy	Septal thickness > 2 SD	7.5

Table 22.1. *Neonatal short-term implications of 160 mothers with very strict control of pregestational diabetes.*

methodological flaws. In 160 diabetic women treated and followed at the Diabetes and Pregnancy Center, Perinatal Division, Rabin Medical Center, during the period 1998–2000, the present authors' group were able to reduce, but not completely exclude, short-term neonatal complications (Table 22.1). However, it is important to emphasize that almost all neonatal complications of maternal diabetes can be efficiently reduced, or at least can be detected very early, and treated promptly, thus avoiding later consequences. In the future, other methods and therapeutic measures will be necessary in order to fulfill the goal of the Saint Vincent Declaration, i.e. to achieve a pregnancy outcome in the diabetic woman close to that of the non-diabetic woman.

Breastfeeding and maternal diabetes

Almost nothing has been written about the role of breastfeeding in IDM and IGDM. There is no contraindication to breastfeeding in these infants and diabetic women should have the same opportunity to breastfeed as women without diabetes.

The milk composition of diabetic mothers is not significantly different from that of the non-diabetic population in total nitrogen, lactose, fat and calories, given the wide variations normally found in control subjects.[49] The only differences reported are a slightly elevated sodium level (140 versus 100 μg/gram) and a significantly higher glucose concentration.[49] A lower fat content and higher concentrations of polyunsaturated fatty acids have also been found.

Although maternal hypoglycemia does not cause a reduction in the breast milk lactose level, it does lead to increased secretion of epinephrine, which inhibits milk production and the ejection reflex. In addition, elevated acetone levels can be expressed in breast milk, placing stress on the newborn liver.[49] As a result, the diabetic mother should be well instructed in order to achieve the right adjustment of diabetes to lactation, and to understand the issues of diet and insulin. These problems are not related to breastfeeding *per se* but to the overall management of diabetes.

Establishing very early breastfeeding is paramount, since colostrum, like breast milk, provides a generous concentration of glucose. The most important factor in success is the time lapse from birth to the first feeding. Furthermore, the duration of lactation is inversely related to the delay in first feeding. Therefore, good hospital management is critical to successful lactation in diabetic mothers. Intensive-care hospitalization should be kept to a minimum (to avoid mother–infant separation), and a breast pump and other assistance should be provided by the staff in order to maximize the chances of successful long-term breastfeeding.

References

1. Cordero L, Treuer SH, Landon M, Gabbe SG. Management of infants of diabetic mothers. *Arch Pediatr Adolesc Med* 1998; **152**:249–54.

2. Hod M, Merlob P, Friedman S et al. Prevalence of congenital anomalies and neonatal complications in the offspring of diabetic mothers in Israel. *Isr J Med Sci* 1991; **27**:498–502.

3. Engelgau MM, Herman WH, Smith PJ et al. The epidemiology of diabetes and pregnancy in the U.S. *Diabetes Care* 1995; **18**:1029–33.

4. Diabetes Care and Research in Europe. The Saint Vincent Declaration. *Diabetic Med* 1990; **7**:360.

5. Merlob P, Reisner SH. Fetal effects from maternal diabetes. In: (Buyse ML, ed) *Birth Defects Encyclopedia*, 1st edn. (Blackwell Scientific Publications Inc: Cambridge, 1990) 700–2.

6. Persson B, Hanson U. Neonatal morbidities in gestational diabetes mellitus. *Diabetes Care* 1998; **21**: B79–B84.

7. Koh THHG, Aynsley-Green A, Tarbit M, Eyre JA. Neural dysfunction during hypoglycemia. *Arch Dis Child* 1998; **63**:1353–58.

8. Lucas A, Morley R, Cole T. Adverse neurodevelopmental outcome of moderate neonatal hypoglycemia. *Br Med J* 1988; **297**:1304–8.

9. Cornblath M, Ichord R. Hypoglycemia in the neonate. *Semin Perinatol* 2000; **24**:136–49.

10. Agrawal RK, Lui K, Gupta JM. Neonatal hypoglycemia in infants of diabetic mothers. *J Paediatr Child Health* 2000; **36**:354–6.

11. Hagay Z, Reece EA. Diabetes mellitus in pregnancy. In: (Reece EA, Hobbins JC, eds) *Medicine of the Fetus and Mother*, 2nd edn. (Lippincott-Raven: Philadelphia, 1999) 1055–91.

12. Freinkel N. Banting Lectures 1980: of pregnancy and progeny. *Diabetes* 1980; **29**:1023–35.

13. Schwartz R, Teramo KA. Effects of diabetic pregnancy on the fetus and newborn. *Semin Perinatol* 2000; **24**:120–35.

14. Anderson JM, Milner RDG, Strich SJ. Effects of neonatal hyperglycemia on the nervous system: a pathological study. *J Neurol Neurosurg Psychiatry* 1967; **30**: 295–310.

15. Banker BQ. The neuropathological effects of anoxia and hypoglycemia in the newborn. *Dev Med Child Neurol* 1967; **9**:544–50.

16. Tsang RC, Kleinman LI, Sutherland JM, Light IJ. Hypocalcemia in infants of diabetic mothers. *J Pediatr* 1972; **80**:384–95.

17. Reece EA, Homko CJ. Infant of diabetic mother. *Semin Perinatol* 1994; **18**:459–69.

18. Demarini S, Mimouni F, Tsang RC et al. Impact of metabolic control of diabetes during pregnancy on neonatal hypocalcemia: a randomized study. *Obstet Gynecol* 1994; **83**:918–22.

19. Merlob P, Amir J. Pathogenesis of hypocalcemia in neonatal polycythemia. *Med Hypothesis* 1989; **30**: 49–50.

20. Mehta KC, Kalkwarf HJ, Mimouni F et al. Randomized trial of magnesium administration to prevent hypocalcemia in infants of diabetic mothers. *J Perinatol* 1998; **18**:352–6.

21. Tsang RC, Strub R, Brown DR et al. Hypomagnesemia in infants of diabetic mothers: perinatal studies. *J Pediatr* 1976; **89**:115–19.

22. Mimouni F, Miodovnik M, Tsang RC et al. Decreased amniotic fluid magnesium concentration in diabetic pregnancy. *Obstet Gynecol* 1987; **69**:12–14.

23. Meyer BA, Palmer SM. Pregestational diabetes. *Semin Perinatol* 1990; **14**:12–23.

24. Shohat M, Reisner SH, Mimouni F, Merlob P. Neonatal polycythemia: II. Definition related to time of sampling. *Pediatrics* 1984; **73**:11–13.

25. Mimouni F, Miodovnik M, Siddiqi TA et al. Neonatal polycythemia in infants of insulin-dependent diabetic mothers. *Obstet Gynecol* 1986; **68**:370–2.

26. Salvessen DR, Brudenell JM, Snijders RJM et al. Fetal plasma erythropoietin in pregnancies complicated by maternal diabetes mellitus. *Am J Obstet Gynecol* 1993; **168**:88–94.

27. Widness JA, Teramo KA, Clemons GK et al. Direct relationship of antepartum glucose control and fetal erythropoietin in human type I (insulin-dependent) diabetic pregnancy. *Diabetologia* 1990; **33**:378–93.

28. Stevenson DK, Bartoletti AL, Ostrander CR, Johnson JD. Pulmonary excretion of carbon monoxide in the human

infant as an index of bilirubin production. II. Infants of diabetic mothers. *J Pediatr* 1979; **94**:956–8.

29. Green DW, Mimouni F. Nucleated erythrocytes in healthy infants and in infants of diabetic mothers. *J Pediatr* 1990; **116**:129–31.

30. Salvessen DR, Brudenell MJ, Nicolaides KH. Fetal polycythemia and thrombocytopenia in pregnancies complicated by maternal diabetes mellitus. *Am J Obstet Gynecol* 1992; **166**:1287–92.

31. Amarnath UM, Ophoven JJ, Mills MM et al. The relationship between decreased iron stress, serum iron and neonatal hypoglycemia in large-for-date newborn infants. *Acta Paediatr Scand* 1989; **78**:538–43.

32. Robert MF, Neff RK, Hubbell JP et al. Association between maternal diabetes and the respiratory distress syndrome in the newborn. *N Engl J Med* 1976; **294**: 357–60.

33. Gewold IH. High glucose causes delayed fetal lung maturation in vitro. *Exp Lung Res* 1993; **19**:619–30.

34. Kulovitch MV, Gluck L. The lung profile. II. Complicated pregnancy. *Am J Obstet Gynecol* 1979; **135**:64–70.

35. Hallman M, Teramo K, Kankaanpää K et al. Prevention of respiratory distress syndrome: current view of fetal lung maturity studies. *Ann Clin Res* 1980; **12**:36–44.

36. Ojomo EO, Coustan DR. Absence of evidence of pulmonary maturity at amniocentesis in term infants of diabetic mothers. *Am J Obstet Gynecol* 1990; **163**:954–7.

37. Veille JC, Sivakoff M, Hanson R, Fanaroff AA. Interventricular septal thickness in fetuses of diabetic mothers. *Obstet Gynecol* 1992; **79**:51–4.

38. Weber HS. Cardiac growth in fetuses of diabetic mothers with good metabolic control. *J Pediatr* 1991; **118**:103–7.

39. Mehta S, Nuamah I, Kalhan S. Altered diastolic function in asymptomatic infants of mothers with gestational diabetes. *Diabetes* 1991; **40**:56–60.

40. Breitwesser JA, Meyer RA, Sperling MA et al. Cardiac septal hypertrophy in hyperinsulinemic infants. *J Pediatr* 1980; **96**:530–9.

41. Cohen JL, Shapiro MA, Mandel FS, Shapiro ML. Normal ovaries in neonates and infants: a sonographic study of 77 patients 1 day to 24 months old. *Am J Roentgenol* 1993; **160**:583–6.

42. Nguyen KT, Reid RL, Sauerbrei E. Antenatal sonographic detection of a fetal theca lutein cyst: a clue to maternal diabetes mellitus. *J Ultrasound Med* 1986; **5**:665–7.

43. Arisaka O, Kanazawa S, Ohyama M et al. Elevated circulating estradiol level in neonatal ovarian cyst. *Arch Pediatr Adolesc Med* 1999; **153**:1202–3.

44. Davis WS, Allen RP, Favara BE, Slovis TL. The neonatal small left colon syndrome. *Am J Roentgenol* 1974; **120**:322–9.

45. Philippart AI, Reed JO, Georgeson KE. Neonatal small left colon syndrome. *J Pediatr Surg* 1975; **10**:733–40.

46. Stewart DR, Nixon W, Johnson DG, Condon VR. Neonatal small left colon syndrome. *Ann Surg* 1977; **186**:741–5.

47. Fuhrmann K, Reiher H, Semmler K et al. Prevention of congenital malformations in infants of insulin-dependent diabetic mothers. *Diabetes Care* 1983; **6**:219–23.

48. Hod M, Merlob P. A meta-analysis of perinatal complications of maternal diabetes. Can they be prevented? *Early Preg: Biol Med* 1996; **2**:15–17.

49. Lawrence RA. *Breast-Feeding: A Guide for the Medical Profession*, 5th edn. (Mosby Publishers Inc: New York, 1999).

23

Long-term implications: child and adult

Dana Dabelea, David J Pettitt

Introduction

Exposure to the diabetic intrauterine milieu during gestation has long been recognized to have important consequences for the fetus and the newborn. However, it is only recently that long-term effects of such exposure on the child, adolescent and young adult offspring of the diabetic mother have been acknowledged. It is becoming increasingly clear that the effects of the diabetic intrauterine environment extend beyond those apparent at birth.

The long-term changes that may result from development in a diabetic intrauterine environment can be divided into three categories:

- *Anthropometric*: growth rates for both weight and height are excessive during the latter stages of gestation, and also during childhood and early adulthood, resulting in the development of *macrosomia, overweight* and *obesity*.
- *Metabolic*: glucose homeostasis is deregulated and glucose tolerance is more likely to be abnormal than that observed in offspring of non-diabetic women, resulting in the development of *impaired glucose tolerance (IGT)* and *diabetes mellitus*.
- *Neurological and psychological*: offspring of high-risk pregnancies often have neurological deficits, which are usually relatively

minor but which may be significant; psychological and intellectual development may also be affected.

Obesity

Pima Indian study

The offspring of women with diabetes during pregnancy are not only more likely to be large newborns but also tend to be more obese during childhood and adolescence. The data from the longitudinal follow-up of offspring of diabetic Pima Indian women demonstrate this clearly.[1–6] Fig. 23.1 shows data on Pima Indians who were examined at birth and then followed up during childhood.[1] The offspring of diabetic women are larger for gestational age at birth

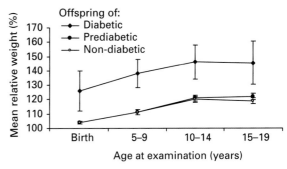

Figure 23.1. *Mean relative weight for height in offspring by age and mother's diabetes. Reprinted with permission from Pettitt et al.[1]*

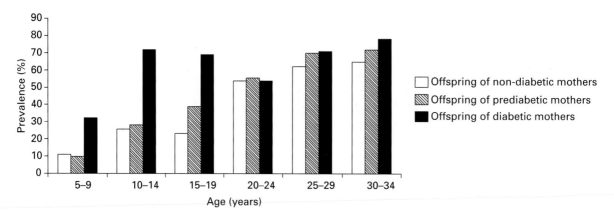

Figure 23.2. *Prevalence of severe obesity (weight ≥ 140% of standard weight for height) in offspring by age and mother's diabetes. Reprinted with permission from Dabelea et al.[7]*

and at every age before 20 years of age they are heavier for height than are the offspring of prediabetic women, i.e. women who developed diabetes only after the child was born, or of non-diabetic women. Relative weight in these latter two groups is similar. Fig. 23.2 shows the prevalence of severe obesity,[7] defined as a weight ≥ 140% of the standard weight for height. After 20 years of age, the differences between the offspring of diabetic women and the other two groups are much less, reflecting the high rates of obesity that are present in this population regardless of the intrauterine environment.[8] However, it is important to bear in mind that, at older ages, the obese offspring of the diabetic women are likely to have been obese much longer than the obese offspring of the non-diabetic and prediabetic women. As duration of obesity is a risk factor for diabetes in this population,[9] this will inevitably increase the risk for developing diabetes in the offspring of diabetic women.

From the data presented in Fig. 23.1, it is not clear whether the diabetic intrauterine environment leads to childhood obesity directly or simply results in a large birthweight that in turn leads to the childhood obesity. However, from

Fig. 23.3 it can be seen that in the subset of the population that had a normal birthweight, the large size at birth was not a pre-requisite for childhood obesity.[3] Even these normal birthweight offspring of the diabetic women were heavier by 5–9 years of age than the offspring of non-diabetic and prediabetic women.

The comparison between offspring of diabetic and prediabetic women is an attempt to control for any potential association between a genetic predisposition to obesity and a genetic predisposition to diabetes. However, the ideal

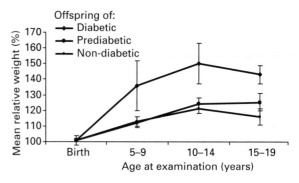

Figure 23.3. *Mean relative weight for height in offspring by age and mother's diabetes in normal birth weight offspring (birth weight = 90–109% of the median weight for gestational age). Reprinted with permission from Pettitt et al.[3]*

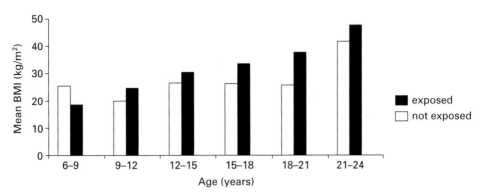

Figure 23.4. *Mean BMI by age in siblings exposed and not exposed to a diabetic intrauterine environment. Reprinted with permission from Dabelea et al.[10]*

way to approach this question is to examine sibling pairs in which one sibling is born before and one born after the onset of their mother's diabetes. Fig. 23.4 shows the results of such an analysis.[10] The mean body mass index (BMI) in the 62 siblings born after the onset of the mother's diabetes, i.e. the offspring of the diabetic women, was significantly higher than among the 121 siblings who were born before the onset of the mother's diabetes and who were therefore not exposed to diabetes *in utero.*

There is some suggestion that relative hyperinsulinemia may be a precursor to childhood obesity. At 5–9 years of age, Pima offspring of women with diabetes or IGT during pregnancy have higher fasting insulin concentrations than the offspring of women with better glucose tolerance during pregnancy.[5] Although this difference is no longer apparent at older ages, a follow-up of children and adolescents found that the fasting insulin concentration at 5–9 years of age was significantly correlated with the rate of weight gain during follow-up.[11]

Diabetes in Pregnancy Center, Chicago, study

The Diabetes in Pregnancy Center at Northwestern University in Chicago is the other

longitudinal study that has reported excessive growth in the offspring of women with diabetes during pregnancy.[12,13] In this study, amniotic fluid insulin was collected at 32–38 weeks of gestation. At 6 years of age there was a significant association between the amniotic fluid insulin and childhood obesity, as estimated by the symmetry index. The insulin concentrations in 6-year-old children who had a symmetry index < 1.0 (86.1 pmol/l) or between 1.0 and 1.2 (69.9 pmol/l) were only half of the concentrations measured in the more obese children who had a symmetry index > 1.2 (140.5 pmol/l; $P < 0.05$ for each comparison).

Children who were born during this study were examined at birth, at 6 months and annually to 8 years of age.[13] The symmetry index, which was normal at 1 year of age, deviated increasingly from the norm during follow-up, so that by the age of 8 the mean symmetry index was almost 1.3, i.e. the children were, on average, 30% heavier than expected for their height.

This study has added unique insight into the causes of excessive growth and provides evidence that the diabetic intrauterine environment plays an important role. Amniotic fluid insulin is of fetal origin and is directly correlated to the amount of fetal insulin produced.

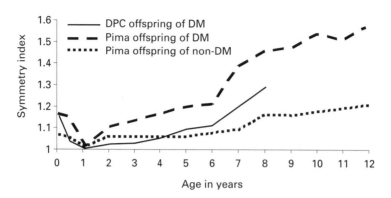

Figure 23.5. *Symmetry index by age in offspring of diabetic mothers (DM) from the Diabetes in Pregnancy Center (DPC), Pima offspring of DM and and Pima offspring of non-DM. Reprinted with permission from Pettitt.*[15]

Fetal insulin, in turn, is correlated with the amount of the circulating glucose, which is of maternal origin and is directly correlated with the mother's diabetes control. Thus, this study demonstrates a direct correlation between an objective measure of the diabetic intrauterine environment and the degree of obesity in children and adolescents.[14]

Although the two studies detailed above are of very different design and the patient populations are quite different, the effect on the offspring is similar. Fig. 23.5 shows the age-specific symmetry index in offspring from both studies.[5,13,15] From birth to 8 years of age, the offspring of diabetic women from the Diabetes in Pregnancy Center, Chicago, while less obese than the Pima Indian offspring of diabetic women, have a steady increase in their mean symmetry index that parallels that seen in the Pima Indians. After 5 years of age, the symmetry index in the Chicago group exceeds that in the Pima Indian children whose mothers did not have diabetes during pregnancy.

Other studies

Freinkel,[16] in his 1980 American Diabetes Association Banting Lecture, summarized the evidence available at that time, before the data from the longitudinal studies described above were available. In this classic paper, he postulated that permanent changes in habitus or anthropometric modifications in the offspring of diabetic women should be expected.

Most studies have not systematically included a longitudinal follow-up from birth of the offspring of diabetic women, but many provide evidence that these offspring are prone to obesity. In 1959, Hagbard et al[17] reported the stature of 239 children with an average age of 5 who were born after the onset of their mothers' diabetes and 68 with an average age of 16 who were born before the onset of their mothers' diabetes. Since the two groups of children were of quite different ages, each was compared with age-appropriate normal data. Those born after the mothers got diabetes were significantly shorter and significantly heavier than normal for their age, while those born before the onset of the mother's diabetes showed no deviation from normal.

Cummins and Norrish[18] reported the heights and weights of 50 4–13-year-old offspring of diabetic women. The children tended to be tall and heavy, with 68% being above the 50th percentile for height and 70% being above the 50th percentile for weight. In addition, there was an excess of children with excessive weight for height – 32% were above the 90th percentile for weight while only 20% were over the 90th percentile for height.

Vohr et al[19] examined 7-year-old offspring of diabetic and control women, and found that the offspring of diabetic women were significantly more likely to be have a weight to height index > 1.2. Most of these heavy children had been large for gestational age at birth, probably indicating poor diabetes control during pregnancy.

Gerlini et al[20] looked at the heights and weights of infants of diabetic mothers at birth, during the first year of life and annually up to age 4. They found that by the age of 4, the children of mothers with poor metabolic control during pregnancy were significantly heavier and had a significantly higher weight to height ratio than the offspring of women who had been well controlled. The difference was smallest at 6 months and increased progressively during the 4 years of observation. Interestingly, the differences were larger in the female offspring.

Many previous studies of obesity in offspring have not specified the type of diabetes, have used mixed samples, or have limited the data to offspring of women with either gestational or Type 2 diabetes. Recently, Weiss et al[21] studied the offspring of women with Type 1 diabetes and reported that they have a significantly higher BMI and symmetry index than the offspring of control women. These measures of obesity were significantly correlated with fasting and post-load blood glucose.

Impaired glucose tolerance and diabetes mellitus

Pima Indian study

Among the Pima Indians of Arizona, the population with the highest reported prevalence and incidence of Type 2 diabetes in the world, individuals at particular risk include those whose parents developed diabetes at an early age[22] and those whose mothers had diabetes during pregnancy.[23] For more than 30 years, Pima Indian women have had oral glucose tolerance tests during pregnancy as well as on a routine basis *c.* every 2 years. Consequently, extensive maternal diabetes information based on glucose data rather than on assessment of family history of diabetes is available for offspring of women who had diabetes before or during pregnancy (diabetic mothers), as well as of those who developed diabetes only after pregnancy (prediabetic mothers) or remained non-diabetic.

Fig. 23.6 shows the prevalence of Type 2 diabetes by age group in offspring of diabetic, prediabetic and non-diabetic mothers.[7] Between the ages of 5–9 and 10–14, diabetes was almost exclusively present among the offspring of diabetic women. In all age groups there was significantly more diabetes in the offspring of diabetic women than in those of prediabetic and non-diabetic women, and there was only a small difference in diabetes prevalence between offspring of prediabetic and non-diabetic women. The small difference may be due to differences in the genes inherited from the mothers, while the large difference in prevalence between the offspring of diabetic and prediabetic mothers, which have presumably inherited the same genes from their mothers, is the consequence of exposure to the diabetic intrauterine environment.[24] These differences persisted after adjusting for the presence of diabetes in the father, age at onset of diabetes in either parent and obesity in the offspring.

A significant correlation between the 2-hour post-load plasma glucose in 15–24-year-old Pima women and their mother's 2-hour glucose during pregnancy has also been described,[5] suggesting that the diabetic intrauterine environment has effects on the offspring's plasma

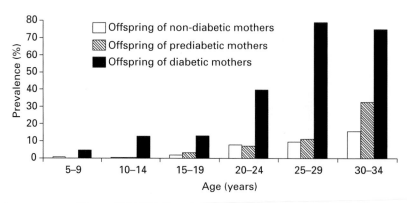

Figure 23.6. *Prevalence of Type 2 diabetes, by mother's diabetes during and following pregnancy, in Pima Indians 5–34 years of age. Reprinted with permission from Dabelea et al.[7]*

glucose that are in addition to genetic or other familial effects.

The congenital effects acquired during development *in utero* may be confounded by genetic factors. Women who develop diabetes at an early age might carry more susceptibility genes than those who develop the disease later in life and, therefore, they might transmit greater genetic susceptibility to their offspring. Thus, the greater frequency of diabetes in the offspring of diabetic pregnancies might be due to greater genetic susceptibility in such offspring. To determine the role of exposure to the diabetic intrauterine environment that is in addition to genetic transmission of susceptibility, the prevalence of Type 2 diabetes was compared in Pima Indian siblings born before and after their mother developed diabetes.[10] The selection of nuclear families for study was based on having at least one sibling born before and at least one born after the mother was diagnosed with Type 2 diabetes. Nineteen families with 58 siblings and 28 sib-pairs, discordant both for diabetes and for diabetes exposure, were informative for the analysis. In 21 of the 28 sib-pairs, the diabetic sibling was born after mother's diabetes and in only

seven of the 28 pairs was the diabetic sibling born before [odds ratio (OR) 3.0, $P < 0.01$; Fig. 23.7]. In contrast, among 84 siblings and 39 sib-pairs from 24 families of diabetic fathers, the risk for Type 2 diabetes was similar in the sib-pairs born before and after father's diagnosis of diabetes (Fig. 23.7). It is evident that, within the same family, siblings born after mother's diagnosis of diabetes have a much greater risk of developing diabetes at an early age than siblings born before the diagnosis of diabetes in the mother. Since siblings born before and after carry a similar risk of inheriting the same susceptibility genes, the different risk reflects the effect of intrauterine exposure to hyperglycemia. Since these differences were not seen in the families of diabetic fathers, it is unlikely that these findings are due to cohort or birth order effects.

In Pima Indian children of 5–19 years of age, the prevalence of Type 2 diabetes has increased two- to threefold over the past 30 years.[25] The percentage of children who have been exposed to diabetes *in utero* has also increased significantly over the same time period, which is associated with a doubling of the amount of diabetes in children that may be

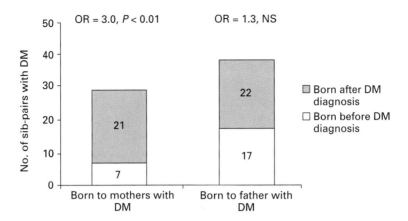

Figure 23.7. *Pima Indian sib-pairs discordant for diabetes and exposure to diabetes in utero. Reprinted with permission from Dabelea et al.[10]*

attributed to this exposure (from 18.1% in 1967–1976 to 35.4% in 1987–1996). The 'epidemic' of Type 2 diabetes in Pima Indian children was almost entirely accounted for, statistically, by the increase in exposure to diabetes during pregnancy and the increase in obesity. Exposure to intrauterine maternal hyperglycemia was the strongest single risk factor for Type 2 diabetes in Pima Indian youth (OR 10.4, $P < 0.0001$).

Diabetes in Pregnancy Center, Chicago, study

This follow-up study enrolled offspring of women with pregestational diabetes (both insulin and non-insulin dependent) and gestational diabetes from 1977 to 1983. Plasma glucose and insulin were measured both fasting and after a glucose load yearly from 1.5 years of age in offspring of diabetic mothers and once between the ages of 10 and 16 in control subjects.[26] On their most recent evaluation (12.3 years of age), offspring of diabetic mothers had a significantly higher prevalence of IGT than the age and sex-matched control group (19.3 versus 2.5%; Fig. 23.8), and two

female offspring had developed Type 2 diabetes, at ages of 7 and 11. Interestingly, in this cohort, the predisposition to IGT was associated with maternal hyperglycemia, regardless of whether it was caused by gestational diabetes or pre-existing insulin-dependent or non-insulin-dependent diabetes. Moreover, excessive insulin secretion *in utero*, assessed by the amniotic fluid concentration measured at 32–38 weeks gestation, was a strong predictor of IGT in childhood.

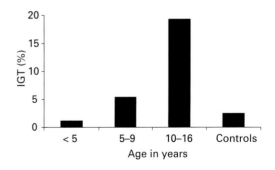

Figure 23.8. *Prevalence of IGT in offspring of diabetic mothers in three age groups and in control subjects (between the ages of 10 and 16). Reprinted with permission from Silverman et al.[26]*

Other studies

Most,[27–32] although not all,[33–35] family studies have shown a greater transmission of Type 2 diabetes to offspring from mothers than from fathers with Type 2 diabetes. Both genetic and environmental effects have been advanced to explain this excess maternal transmission.

A higher frequency of maternal than of paternal transmission of diabetes has been demonstrated in GK rats.[36] In these rats the diabetic syndrome is produced by strepotozotocin injection or glucose infusion. They do not have any genetic predisposition for diabetes, nor can their diabetes be classified as Type 1 or 2. These studies have demonstrated that hyperglycemia in the mother during pregnancy leads to IGT, and decreased insulin action and secretion in adult offspring.[37–42]

The mechanisms by which exposure to diabetes *in utero* increases the risk of IGT and Type 2 diabetes are still uncertain. Several studies performed in newborns of diabetic mothers have shown an enhanced insulin secretion to a glycemic stimulus in these neonates[43,44] and, accordingly, Van Assche and Gepts[45] and Heding et al[46] described hyperplasia of the beta cells in newborns of diabetic mothers. Whether this is a transient phenomenon, as suggested by Isles et al,[47] or leads to IGT later in life when insulin resistance becomes important, is still uncertain. Impaired insulin secretion[48,49] has also been proposed as a possible mechanism. Among 104 normal glucose-tolerant Pima Indian adults, insulin secretion rates were lower in individuals whose mothers had developed diabetes before the age of 35 compared with those whose parents remained non-diabetic until the age of 49. The acute insulin response was *c.* 40% lower in individuals whose mothers had diabetes during pregnancy than in those whose mothers developed diabetes at an early age but after the birth

of the subject.[50] These results suggest that exposure to the diabetic intrauterine environment is associated with impaired insulin secretion. Based on the observation made in rats and supported by the Pima Indian findings, it may be hypothesized that exposure to hyperglycemia during critical periods of fetal development 'programs' the developing pancreas in a way that leads to a subsequent impairment in insulin secretion.

Is the situation different if the mother has Type 1 diabetes? There is a two- to fivefold higher risk for Type 1 diabetes in offspring of fathers than in offspring of mothers with Type 1 diabetes.[51] There are several possible explanations for this finding:[24] genetic transmission with differential susceptibility (imprinting) depending on which parent supplies the predisposing genes; true maternal protection against Type 1 diabetes in offspring; increased perinatal mortality of babies who have inherited the susceptibility genes for Type 1 diabetes from their mothers. In the cohort of adolescent offspring of diabetic mothers followed by Silverman et al,[26] however, the predisposition to IGT was only associated with maternal hyperglycemia, and not with the type of diabetes in the mother. Moreover, the prevalence of IGT was similarly increased in infants (1–4 years of age) and children (5–9 years of age) of mothers with pregestational Type 1 diabetes and in those of mothers with gestational diabetes.[52]

The metabolic effects of the diabetic intrauterine environment on the fetus might be similar regardless of whether the mother has Type 1 or 2 diabetes. Recent data suggest that effects of maternally-transmitted diabetes genes may be modified by congenital influences in both Type 1 and 2 diabetes, although perhaps in a different direction. A recent report from the Framingham Offspring Study[53] showed that paternal and maternal Type 2 diabetes conferred equivalent risks for offspring Type 2 diabetes. Offspring of diabetic mothers with an age of onset < 50 years of age, however, had an increased risk for both Type 2 diabetes and IGT compared with offspring of diabetic fathers. Based on comparable effect sizes among maternal and paternal Type 2 diabetes, the authors concluded that fathers may transmit unique genetic factors of similar strength to maternal environmental effects. An association between paternal, but not maternal, Type 2 diabetes, low birth weight and Type 2 diabetes was recently reported in Pima Indian offspring.[54] Using family-based association methods in parent–offspring trios with Type 2 diabetes, Huxtable et al[55] reported a relationship between the insulin gene and Type 2 diabetes that was mediated exclusively through paternally transmitted class III variable number tandem repeat (VNTR) alleles.

Neurological and psychological development

Reports of long-term neurological deficits in the offspring of diabetic mothers include impaired visual motor function, Erb's palsy, seizure disorders, cerebral palsy, mental retardation, speech disturbances, reading difficulties, behavior disturbances and deafness.[56–65] Mechanisms potentially involved in the occurrence of such problems are: birth trauma, especially trauma to the head and neck because of large infant size and shoulder dystocia;[66] prolonged, severe neonatal hypoglycemia, which may damage the central nervous system with potentially permanent deficits;[67,68] neonatal hyperbilirubinemia, which leads to kernicterus;[59] abnormal fuel metabolism during gestation, which may cause long-term aberrations in neurological and psychological development.

Major neurological dysfunction has been related to uncontrolled severe diabetes in pregnancy.[60] However, even in the newborn offspring of women with well-controlled diabetes, Rizzo et al[63] found a significant inverse correlation between maternal blood glucose concentrations during pregnancy and newborn behavior. A correlation between acetonuria during pregnancy and diminished intelligence quotients (IQ) in the offspring of diabetic mothers has been reported in at least two studies.[60,69] In one of these studies, birthweight was also predictive of IQ, with smaller infants at birth having lower IQ scores at 5 years of age.[60] However, Rizzo et al[64] found no correlation between maternal acetonuria and the child's IQ, but they did report an inverse correlation between maternal second trimester β-hydroxybutyrate concentrations and the offspring's mental development index scores at 2 years of age. The mothers of these children had well-controlled diabetes during pregnancy and only infrequent acetonuria.

The offspring of the 1977–1983 gravida enrolled in the Diabetes in Pregnancy Center, Chicago, follow-up study[14] were longitudinally followed to make inferences concerning the behavioral and intellectual influences of intrauterine exposure to diabetes. Direct correlations between mild maternal ketonemia in the second and third trimesters and poorer performances on the Mental Development Index of the Bayley Scales of Infant Development at 2 years of age, on the Stanford-Binet Intelligence Scales at 3–5 years of age,[64] and on the Bruininks-Oseretsky Test of Motor Proficiency at 6–9 years of age[70] were found. The associations between exposure to maternal diabetes *in utero* and psychomotor and cognitive functions in childhood were independent of socioeconomic status and ethnicity, and were similar regardless of the gestational or pregestational maternal diabetes status. Moreover, they were not explained by perinatal morbidities occurring more frequently in newborns born to mothers with diabetes.

Blood glucose control throughout gestation may prevent neurological problems in the offspring of diabetic women.[68,59] Sells et al[71] compared neurodevelopment through 36 months of age in offspring of women with Type 1 diabetes and control infants. Infants of mothers with tight glycemic control during pregnancy had similar neurological test results to the control infants, while offspring of mothers with poorer glycemic control during pregnancy scored less well on tests of language development.

Acknowledgements

We would like to thank Dr Bernard L Silverman for his thoughtful review of this manuscript.

References

1. Pettitt DJ, Baird HR, Aleck KA, et al. Excessive obesity in offspring of Pima Indian women with diabetes during pregnancy. *N Engl J Med* 1983; 308:242–5.
2. Pettitt DJ, Bennett PH, Knowler WC et al. Gestational diabetes mellitus and impaired glucose tolerance during pregnancy: long-term effects on obesity and glucose tolerance in the offspring. *Diabetes* 1985; 34(Suppl 2): 119–22.
3. Pettitt DJ, Knowler WC, Bennett PH et al. Obesity in offspring of diabetic Pima Indian women despite normal birthweight. *Diabetes Care* 1987; 10:76–80.
4. Pettitt DJ, Knowler WC. Diabetes and obesity in the Pima Indians: a cross-generational vicious cycle. *J Obesity Weight Regulation* 1988; 7:61–75.
5. Pettitt DJ, Bennett PH, Saad MF et al. Abnormal glucose tolerance during pregnancy in Pima Indian women: long-term effects on the offspring. *Diabetes* 1991; 40 (Suppl 2):126–30.
6. Dabelea D, Pettitt DJ. Intrauterine diabetic environment confers risks for type 2 diabetes mellitus and obesity in the offspring, in addition to genetic susceptibility. *J Pediatr Endocrinol Metab* 2001; 14:1085–91.
7. Dabelea, D, Knowler WC, Pettitt DJ. Effect of diabetes in pregnancy on offspring: follow-up research in the Pima Indians. *J Matern–Fetal Med* 2000; 9:83–8.
8. Price RA, Charles MA, Pettitt DJ, Knowler WC. Obesity in Pima Indians: large increases among post-world war II birth cohorts. *Am J Physical Anthropol* 1993; 92:473–9.
9. Everhart JE, Pettitt DJ, Bennett PH, Knowler WC. Duration of obesity increases the incidence of NIDDM. *Diabetes* 1992; 41:235–40.
10. Dabelea D, Hanson RL, Lindsay RS et al. Intrauterine exposure to diabetes conveys risks for type 2 diabetes and obesity: a study of discordant sibships. *Diabetes* 2000; 49:2208–11.
11. Odeleye OE, de Courten M, Pettitt DJ, Ravussin E. Fasting hyperinsulinemia is a predictor of increased body weight gain and obesity in Pima Indian children. *Diabetes* 1997; 46:1341–5.
12. Metzger BE, Silverman BL, Freinkel N et al. Amniotic fluid insulin concentration as a predictor of obesity. *Arch Dis Child* 1990; 65:1050–2.
13. Silverman BL, Rizzo T, Green OC et al. Long-term prospective evaluation of offspring of diabetic mothers. *Diabetes* 1991; 40 (Suppl 2):121–5.
14. Silverman BL, Rizzo TA, Cho NH, Metzger BE. Long-term effects of the intrauterine environment: the Northwestern University Diabetes in Pregnancy Center. *Diabetes Care* 1998; 21 (suppl 2):B142–B149.
15. Pettitt DJ. Summary and comment of Silverman BL, Rizzo T, Green OC et al. Long-term prospective evaluation of offspring of diabetic mothers, *Diabetes* 1991; 40 (Suppl 2):121–5. *Diabetes Spectrum* 1992; 5:39–40.
16. Freinkel N. Banting Lecture 1908: of pregnancy and progeny. *Diabetes* 1980; 29:1023–35.
17. Hagbard L, Olow I, Reinand T. A follow-up study of 514 children of diabetic mothers. *Acta Paediatr* 1959; 48:184–97.
18. Cummins M, Norrish M. Follow-up of children of diabetic mothers. *Arch Dis Child* 1980; 55:259–64.
19. Vohr BR, Lipsitt LP, Oh W. Somatic growth of children of diabetic mothers with reference to birth size. *J Pediatr* 1980; 97:196–9.
20. Gerlini G, Arachi S, Gori MG et al. Developmental aspects of the offspring of diabetic mothers. *Acta Endocrinol* 1986; (Suppl 277):150–5.
21. Weiss PAM, Scholz HS, Haas J et al. Long-term follow-up of infants of mothers with type 1 diabetes. *Diabetes Care* 2000; 23:905–11.
22. Hanson RL, Elston RC, Pettitt DJ et al. Segregation analysis on non-insulin-dependent diabetes mellitus in Pima Indians: evidence for a major gene effect. *Am J Hum Genet* 1995; 57:160–70.
23. Pettitt DJ, Aleck KA, Baird HR et al. Congenital susceptibility to NIDDM: role of intrauterine environment. *Diabetes* 1988; 37:622–8.
24. Pettitt DJ. Diabetes in subsequent generations. In: (Dornhorst A, Hadden DR, eds) *Diabetes and Pregnancy: an International Approach to Diagnosis and Management.* (John Wiley & Sons Ltd: Chichester, 1996) 367–76.
25. Dabelea D, Hanson RL, Bennett PH et al. Increasing prevalence of type 2 diabetes in American-Indian children. *Diabetologia* 1998; 41:904–10.

26. Silverman BL, Metzger BE, Cho NH, Loeb CA. Impaired glucose tolerance in adolescent offspring of diabetic mothers. *Diabetes Care* 1995; **18**:611–17.

27. Dorner G, Mohnike A. Further evidence for a predominantly maternal transmission of maturity-onset type diabetes. *Endokrinologie* 1976; **68**:121–4.

28. Alcolado JC, Alcolado R. Importance of maternal history of non-insulin-dependent diabetic patients. *Br Med J* 1991; **302**:1178–80.

29. Thomas F, Balkau B, Vauzelle-Kervroedan F, Papoz L, for the CODIAB–INSERM–ZENECA Study Group. Maternal effect and familial aggregation in NIDDM: the CODIAB Study. *Diabetes* 1994; **43**:63–7.

30. Young CA, Kumar S, Young MJ, Boulton AJ. Excess maternal history of diabetes in Caucasians and Afro-origin non-insulin-dependent diabetic patients suggests dominant maternal factors in disease transmission. *Diabetes Res Clin Pract* 1995; **28**:47–9.

31. Groop L, Forsblom C, Lehtovirta M et al. Metabolic consequences of a family history of NIDDM (the Botnia Study): evidence for sex-specific parental effects. *Diabetes* 1996; **45**:1585–93.

32. Karter AJ, Rowell SE, Ackerson LM et al. Excess maternal transmission of type 2 diabetes: the Northern California Kaiser Permanente Diabetes Registry. *Diabetes Care* 1999; **22**:938–43.

33. Mitchell BD, Kammerer CM, Reinhart LJ et al. Is there an excess in maternal transmission of NIDDM? *Diabetologia* 1995; **38**:314–17.

34. Viswanathan M, McCarthy MI, Snehalatha C et al. Familial aggregation of type 2 (non-insulin-dependent) diabetes mellitus in south Indians: absence of excess maternal transmission. *Diabet Med* 1996; **13**:232–7.

35. McCarthy M, Cassell P, Tran T et al. Evaluation of the importance of maternal history of diabetes and of mitochondrial variation in the development of NIDDM. *Diabet Med* 1996; **13**:420–8.

36. Gauguier D, Nelson I, Bernard C et al. Higher maternal than paternal inheritance of diabetes in GK rats. *Diabetes* 1994; **43**:220–4.

37. Bihoreau MT, Ktorza A, Kinebanyan MF, Picon L. Impaired glucose homeostasis in adult rats following intrauterine exposure to mild hyperglycemia during late gestation. *Diabetes* 1986; **35**:979–84.

38. Gauguier D, Bihoreau MT, Ktorza A et al. Inheritance of diabetes mellitus as consequence of gestational hyperglycemia in rats. *Diabetes* 1990; **39**:734–9.

39. Aerts L, Van Assche FA. Is gestational diabetes an acquired condition? *J Dev Physiol* 1979; **1**:219–25.

40. Aerts L, Van Assche FA. Endocrine pancreas in the offspring of rats with experimentally induced diabetes. *J Endocrinol* 1981; **88**:81–8.

41. Aerts L, Sodoyez-Goffaux F, Sodoyez JC et al. The diabetic intrauterine milieu has a long-lasting effect on insulin secretion by B cells and on insulin uptake by target tissues. *Am J Obstet Gynecol* 1988; **259**:1287–92.

42. Grill V, Johansson B, Jalkanen P, Eriksson UJ. Influence of severe diabetes mellitus early in pregnancy in the rat: effects on insulin sensitivity and insulin secretion in the offspring. *Diabetologia* 1991; **34**:373–8.

43. Gentz J, Lunell NO, Olin P et al. Glucose tolerance in overweight babies and infants of diabetic mothers. *Acta Paediatr Scand* 1967; **56**:228–9 (letter).

44. Pildes PS, Hart RJ, Warrner R, Cornblath M. Plasma insulin response during oral glucose tolerance tests in newborns of normal and gestational diabetic mothers. *Pediatrics* 1969; **44**:76–83.

45. Van Assche FA, Gepts W. The cytological composition of the foetal endocrine pancreas in normal and pathological conditions. *Diabetologia* 1971; **7**:434–44.

46. Heding LG, Perrson B, Strangenberg M. β-cell function in newborn infants of diabetic mothers. *Diabetologia* 1980; **19**:427–30.

47. Isles TE, Dickson M, Farquhar JW. Glucose toleance and plasma insulin in newborn infants of normal and diabetic mothers. *Acta Paediatr Scand* 1968; **57**:460–1.

48. Hultquist GT, Olding LB. Pancreatic-islet fibrosis in young infants of diabetic mothers. *Lancet* 1975; **2**: 1015–18.

49. Wilson CA, Weyer C, Knowler WC, Pratley RE. Acute insulin secretion is impaired in adult offspring of diabetic pregnancies. *Diabetes* 1999; **48** (**Suppl 1**):A300.

50. Gautier JF, Wilson C, Weyer C et al. Low acute insulin secretory responses in adult offspring of people with early onset type 2 diabetes. *Diabetes* 2001; **50**:1828–33.

51. Warram JH, Krolewski AS, Gottlieb MS, Kahn CR. Differences in risk of insulin-dependent diabetes in offspring of diabetic mothers and diabetic fathers. *N Engl J Med* 1984; **311**:149–52.

52. Plagemann A, Harder T, Kohlhoff R et al. Glucose tolerance and insulin secretion in children of mothers with pregestational IDDM or gestational diabetes. *Diabetologia* 1997; **40**:1094–100.

53. Meigs JB, Cupples AL, Wilson PWF. Parental transmission of type 2 diabetes. The Framingham Offspring Study. *Diabetes* 2000; **49**:2201–7.

54. Lindsay RS, Dabelea D, Roumain J et al. Type 2 diabetes and low birth weight: the role of paternal inheritance in the association of low birth weight and diabetes. *Diabetes* 2000; **49**:445–9.

55. Huxtable SJ, Saker PJ, Haddad L et al. Analysis of parent–offspring trios provides evidence for linkage and association between the insulin gene and type 2 diabetes medated exclusively through paternally transmitted class III variable number tandem repeat alleles. *Diabetes* 2000; **49**:126–30.

56. Yssing M. Long-term prognosis of children born to mothers diabetic when pregnant. In: (Camerini-Davalos RA, Cole HS, eds) *Early Diabetes in Early Life*. (Academic Press: San Diego, 1975) 575.

57. Drorbaugh JE, Moore DM. The effect of maternal diabetes on development of central nervous system function

in the child. In: (Moghissi KS, ed) *Birth Defects and Fetal Development: Endocrine and Metabolic Factors.* (Charles C Thomas: Springfield, IL, 1974) 106.

58. Pedersen J. Future years of surviving babies. In: (Pedersen J, ed.) *The Pregnant Diabetic and Her Newborn*, 2nd edn. (Munksgaard: Copenhagen, 1977) 233.

59. Cowett RM, Schwartz R. The infant of the diabetic mother. *Pediatr Clin N Am* 1982; **29**:1213–16.

60. Stehbens JA, Baker GL, Kitchel M. Outcome at ages 1, 3, and 5 years of children born to diabetic women. *Am J Obstet Gynecol* 1977; **127**:408–13.

61. Persson B, Gentz J. Follow-up of children of insulin-dependent and gestational diabetic mothers. *Acta Paediatr Scand* 1984; **73**:349–53.

62. Naeye RL, Chez RA. Effects of maternal acetonuria and low pregnancy weight gain on children's psychomotor development. *Am J Obstet Gynecol* 1981; **139**:189–94.

63. Rizzo T, Freinkel N, Metzger BE et al. Correlations between antepartum maternal metabolism and newborn behavior. *Am J Obstet Gynecol* 1990; **163**:1458–64.

64. Rizzo T, Metzger BE, Burns WJ, Burns K. Correlations between antepartum maternal metabolism and intelligence of offspring. *N Engl J Med* 1991; **325**:911–16.

65. Hadden DR, Byrn E, Trotter I et al. Physical and psychological health of children of type 1 (insulin-dependent) diabetic mothers. *Diabetologia* 1984; **26**:250–5.

66. Dor N, Mosberg H, Stern W et al. Complications in fetal macrosomia. *N Y State J Med* 1984; **84**:302–4.

67. Knobloch H, Sotos JF, Sherard Jr ES et al. Prognostic and etiologic factors in hypoglycemia. *Pediatrics* 1967; **70**:876–8.

68. Pildes RS. Infants of diabetic mothers. *N Engl J Med* 1973; **289**:902–5.

69. Churchill JA, Berendes HW, Newmore J. Neuropsychological deficits in children of diabetic mothers. *Am J Obstet Gynecol* 1969; **105**:257–60.

70. Rizzo TA, Dooley SL, Metzger BE et al. Prenatal and perinatal influences on long-term psychomotor development in offspring of diabetic mothers. *Am J Obstet Gynecol.* 1995; **173**:1753–58.

71. Sells CJ, Robinson NM, Brown Z, Knopp RH. Long term developmental follow-up of infants of diabetic mothers. *J Pediatr* 1994; **125**:S9-S17.

24

Growth and neurodevelopment of children born to diabetic mothers and to mothers with gestational diabetes mellitus

Asher Ornoy

Introduction

It is well known that diabetes during pregnancy may be associated with an increased rate of spontaneous abortions, intrauterine death and congenital anomalies among the offspring.[1–8] This increase is directly related to the severity of the disease, especially to the blood levels of glycosylated hemoglobin (HbA1c).[3,7,8] The reduction in the prevalence of congenital anomalies among offspring of mothers with pregestational diabetes mellitus (PGDM) observed over recent years is directly related to the improvement of glycemic control in early pregnancy. However, even in well-treated diabetic pregnant women, the rate of congenital anomalies is still significantly higher than in the general population.[2,5] No increase in congenital anomalies was observed among children born to mothers with gestational diabetes mellitus (GDM).

In addition, growth disturbances are relatively common among offspring of diabetic mothers. In severe and uncontrolled PGDM, intrauterine growth retardation is often found, especially in mothers with diabetic nephropathy.[9] In well-controlled diabetes or GDM, macrosomia is the more common growth disturbance.[9]

Many studies have assessed the postnatal development of children born to diabetic mothers, using a variety of age-appropriate psychometric tests, and the findings correlated with the degree of glycemic control and the onset of diabetes (whether pregestational or gestational). In this chapter these issues will be addressed and detailed results of the present author's developmental follow-up studies will be reported.

The effects of diabetes on intrauterine growth

Growth disturbances in infants of diabetic mothers

General comments

In 1967 Pedersen[9] summarized the literature on birthweight, length, organ size and body composition, as well as the state of maturity, of infants born to mothers with PGDM. In addition to newborns with appropriate-for-gestational-age (AGA) birthweights, many infants had increased adipose tissue and were overweight (macrosomic). In addition, he also pointed out that in PGDM women with nephropathy, infants may also suffer from intrauterine growth restriction and are small for gestational age (SGA). The fetus responds to maternal hyperglycemia by hyperinsulinemia and enhanced growth, thus reducing his/her hyperglycemia. Farquar[10] described in detail the appearance of macrosomic infants born to diabetic mothers and their prognosis. He vividly described these newborns as 'plump, sleek, liberally coated with vernix caseosa, full faced and phletoric'. He also commented that 'they commonly exceed the mean body weight and crown heel length, and resemble each other.'[10] Farquar[10] also described a variety of perinatal complications and increased neonatal mortality in these infants, as well as placental enlargement and insufficiency. Morbidity and mortality was higher in SGA infants of diabetic mothers when compared to the AGA and macrosomic infants. On follow up, Farquar[10] did not find exceptional differences in the weight and height of these children in comparison to control children of similar ages.

The role of insulin in fetal growth

The outcome of children of diabetic mothers has significantly improved since the 1960s, when many studies were published. However, even in well-controlled diabetic mothers, 15–45% of newborns are overweight.[11] Silverman et al[12] found that mean amniotic fluid insulin concentrations were more than twice the control levels in fetuses of mothers with PGDM and GDM. Similarly, high amniotic fluid insulin levels were observed in obese children by Mezger et al.[13] As fetal hyperinsulinemia is known to occur in diabetic pregnancies, and hyperinsulinemic fetuses are often, or become, macrosomic, this is an expected result of maternal diabetes.[12] Hyperinsulinemia would affect the size of insulin responsive tissues such as adipose tissue more than other organs; indeed, adipose tissue is increased in infants of diabetic mothers. Carpenter et al[14]

examined second-trimester amniotic fluid insulin levels in 247 pregnancies at 14–20 weeks of pregnancy. They found that high amniotic fluid insulin levels were associated with the subsequent development of gestational diabetes. In gravidas with abnormal oral glucose challenge tests, high amniotic fluid insulin levels were associated with fetal macrosomia. They deduced from their findings that maternal glucose intolerance during pregnancy may have already affected fetal insulin production by the second trimester of pregnancy.

Role of glucose

Mello et al[15] found that infants born to mothers with PGDM with glucose blood levels 95 mg% throughout pregnancy had children with normal birthweights, while mothers with higher blood glucose levels in the second and third trimesters of pregnancy had a high proportion of macrosomic infants. Moreover, in the Tri-Hospital GDM study in Toronto,[16] children born to untreated borderline GDM mothers had increased rates of macrosomia, while Simmons and Robertson[17] found that insulin treatment in women with GDM reduced the incidence of obesity in their offspring.

Romon et al[18] found that the incidence of fetal macrosomia in infants of 99 mothers with GDM could be reduced if there was an adequate daily intake of carbohydrates (250 gram/day) and a reduction in fat intake. According to Pedersen,[9] high maternal glucose levels in diabetic pregnant mothers are found to increase the transplacental passage of nutrients to the fetus, hence resulting in macrosomia. To further study the role of maternal blood glucose levels during pregnancy on fetal growth, Scholl et al[19] studied the influence of maternal blood glucose levels in non-diabetic women on the birthweight of their offspring. They found that mean weight of newborns increased by 50 grams with maternal blood levels of 99–130 mg% and by 200 grams if blood levels were > 130 mg%. However, higher maternal blood glucose levels were associated with a higher rate of pregnancy complications. On the other hand, maternal hypoglycemia is associated with reduced birthweight of term infants.[20] All the studies described here emphasize repeatedly the importance of good glycemic control during pregnancy.

Blood leptin levels and fetal weight

Leptin, the product of the obesity gene *ob/ob* is a 167 amino acid peptide produced and released by adipose tissue.[21] Secretion of leptin is highly correlated with body fat mass and adipocyte size.[21,22] Circulating leptin levels are increased in obese children and adults. As leptin is known to interact with insulin and insulin-like growth factors, several recent studies have investigated the relation between leptin, insulin and weight at birth.[21,22] A direct correlation was indeed observed between cord levels of leptin and insulin with birthweight. Marchini et al[22] found high leptin levels in cord blood of macrosomic infants, implying that leptin levels are related to the nutritional status during fetal development. These studies rapidly led to very recent studies on infants born to mothers with PGDM or GDM.[23–25] Lepercq et al[23] found increased leptin, c-peptide and insulin levels in cord blood of macrosomic newborns of mothers with Type 1 PGDM in comparison to similar infants born with a normal birthweight. Similar findings were observed by Tapanainen et al,[24] who also concluded that leptin may be involved in the increased accumulation of adipose tissue found in infants of diabetic mothers. In that study the cord levels of leptin in newborns of mothers with GDM were intermediate between the levels in infants of mothers with PGDM and controls. Similar results were

obtained regarding insulin blood levels. In another recent study, Hytinantti et al[25] found that the increased blood leptin levels observed in newborn infants of PGDM mothers were reduced in the third day of life to resemble control values, implying that the high fetal leptin levels in maternal PGDM are apparently a result of the influence of disturbed glucose metabolism on feto-placental leptin metabolism. However, these studies are not sufficient to elucidate a specific role, if there is one, of leptin, in the etiology of diabetes-induced fetal macrosomia.

Low birthweight

In the pre-insulin era, most infants of diabetic mothers were of low birthweight (LBW) due to maternal starvation, which was then the method used to reduce serum glucose levels and avoid intrauterine fetal death.[11] With the introduction of insulin, fetal weight improved and overweight is often observed at birth. Since then, LBW in infants of mothers with PGDM is usually a sign of severe diabetic vascular complications, and is observed in increasing frequencies in women with PGDM and hypertension, renal disease or in malformed infants.[9,11,26]

LBW is a risk factor for a variety of diseases, including hypertension, cardiovascular diseases and diabetes.[27,28] With better treatment of PGDM and improved pregnancy outcome, most LBW infants are born to mothers with diabetic complications and the offspring may well be subjected to associated later disease(s).[28] As pregnant diabetic women tend to develop thiamine deficiency – a vitamin important for glucose oxidation, insulin production and cell growth – it may be pertinent to advise dietary supplementation of this substance to diabetic women during pregnancy, as this may at least improve fetal growth in growth-retarded fetuses.[29]

Follow-up studies of weight and height in children of diabetic mothers

SGA infants

In a recent study published by Biesenbach et al,[26] 10 children of mothers with PGDM and nephropathy were compared to 30 children of mothers with PGDM without nephropathy. In the first group, birthweight was significantly reduced (2250 versus 3554 grams) and 5 infants had birthweights < 2400 grams. Prematurity was increased to 60% in the first group, with no premature infants in the second group. At follow-up at 3 years of age, 6 of the 10 children from the first group had body weights below the 50th percentile and 5 had heights below the 50th percentile, with none in the second group. Language development in the children of the first group was also delayed and they had more infectious diseases.[26]

AGA or macrosomic infants

In a follow-up study on infants of diabetic mothers, Silverman et al[12] found that the higher the birthweight of infants born to mothers with GDM and PGDM observed in their series, the higher was their amniotic fluid insulin. Birthweight was above the 90th percentile for gestational age in > 50% of the newborns in their series, gradually disappeared. At 1 year, body weight was similar to that known for the general population of children at that age.[12] Overweight then reappeared after the age of 5, and at age 8 > 50% of the boys had body weights at or above the 90th percentile. A similar trend was observed in the girls – at 8 years of age almost 50% had weights had above the 90th percentile. The heights of boys and girls at 8 years of age was also significantly higher than in the comparison control group. Similar results were reported by Metzger et al[13] and Rizzo et al[30,31] in their studies on children born to

diabetic mothers. In an earlier study published by Amendt et al,[32] on children born to diabetic mothers with birthweights ≥ 4000 grams, the authors found that at school age these children were taller and heavier than controls. In another study, Seidman et al[33] found that children with high birthweights tended to be overweight and taller as adolescents. However, in macrosomic offspring of diabetic mothers this trend did not reach statistical significance, perhaps due to the small size of the group.[33] In another study, it was observed that macrosomic infants, not necessarily of diabetic mothers, also tended to be taller and heavier as adults.[34]

The present author's group has studied the weight and height of children between the ages of 6 and 12 born to women with PGDM or GDM.[35–37] The children weighed more than age and socioeconomic status (SES)-matched control children; there was no correlation between birthweight and the weight at examination. There was no significant difference between the diabetic groups of children and the controls in average height and head circumference measurements. Overweight became more pronounced in the older children (between the ages of 9 and 12): the number of children born to mothers with PGDM who had a body weight in the 90th percentile was four times higher than in the age-appropriate controls (Table 24.1).

Effects of diabetes on postnatal development

Summary of the literature

Intellectual development

The development of children born to diabetic mothers over the past 30 years was considered by several investigations. Churchill et al[38] were apparently the first to describe, in 1969, the finding of lower intelligence quotient (IQ) scores

	Control		PGDM mothers		GDM mothers	
	Mean	SD	Mean	SD	Mean	SD
Birthweight (grams)	3381*	582	3528	645	3348	676
Head circumference (percentile)	48	24	47	24	47	22
Height (percentile)	44	30	45	23	49	25
Weight (percentile)	44	30†	57	32	68	27

* Mean ± SD.
† Significantly lower than PGDM or GDM mothers, $P < 0.05$.

Table 24.1. Comparison of physical evaluations between control children and children born to pregestational diabetic (PGDM) mothers and to mothers with gestational diabetes mellitus (GDM) (from Ornoy et al,[37] with permission).

in children born to diabetic mothers with acetonuria, while children born to diabetic mothers without acetonuria functioned normally. No effect of insulin treatment on the IQ of the offspring was noted, and there was no correlation of the IQ with the duration of maternal diabetes. In the same year Schulte et al[39] published their study on the neurological development of newborn infants born to diabetic mothers. They found longer rapid eye movement (REM) sleep time in these newborns in comparison to controls. Stehbens et al[40] examined children born to diabetic mothers at 1, 3 and 5 years of age: the SGA children born to diabetic mothers had lower IQ scores in comparison to controls. Similarly, Petersen et al[41] found that SGA children of diabetic mothers had lower verbal performance at 5 years of age, but the children who had not suffered from growth retardation *in utero* were normal. Cummins and Norrish[42] did not find differences in IQ scores of children born to diabetic mothers at 4.25–13.5 years of age as compared to controls, and Person and Gentz[43] found no differences in these measures at 5 years of age. Rizzo et al[30] did not find developmental delay in children born to diabetic mothers or to mothers with GDM, but did find

an inverse correlation between maternal blood β-hydroxybutyrate levels and IQ scores for these children. In a later study, Rizzo et al[31] evaluated psychomotor development of children between the ages of 6 and 9, and found a significant negative correlation between maternal second and third trimester β-hydroxybutyrate levels and performance on the Bruininks–Oseretzki test, which measures fine and gross motor abilities. Yamashita et al[44] prospectively evaluated the development of 33 children born to diabetic mothers in comparison to 34 control children. They found significantly lower scores on the Tanaka–Binet intelligence test. These investigators did not find any correlation between the IQ of the child and the HbA1c blood levels during pregnancy. This was in contrast to the findings by Sells et al[45] who reported an inverse correlation between maternal HbA1c levels during pregnancy of diabetic women and the development of their offspring.

In contrast to these reassuring studies, Kimmerle et al[46] studied the development of 36 children born to mothers with PGDM and nephropathy (White's class F), 10 of them having renal failure. They found reduced birthweights and a high rate of prematurity, as has also been observed by others.[9,26] The children had a neuro-developmental examination at 0.4–10 years of age, using either the Denver Developmental Test (up to 6 years of age) or, in older children, evaluating the achievements at school. Twenty-seven children were developmentally normal, 7 had moderate to severe developmental retardation, 1 had severe motor impairment and 1 died at a young age. Kizmiller et al[47] also found that two of 24 children born to mothers with PGDM and nephropathy suffered at 8–35 months of age from developmental retardation. Bloch-Petersen et al[48] also found that children born to diabetic mothers with LBW or prematurely had, at 4–5 years of age, an increased risk of poor developmental performance. These results show that in mothers with poor diabetic control during pregnancy and severe complications, the long-term developmental outcome of the offspring may be impaired, emphasizing the importance to avoid LBW and prematurity in diabetic pregnancies. It is, however, possible that the majority of the developmental problems in these children are attributed to prematurity and intrauterine growth restriction, as these problems are also common among premature infants of non-diabetic mothers.

Fine neurological dysfunction

All of the studies described raise the possibility that children born to diabetic mothers suffer from slight neurological damage that does not necessarily affect their scores in IQ tests. This may express itself in fine neuropsychological abilities and in ages later than those studied previously.

Various investigators have addressed the question of possible brain damage induced by diabetic metabolic factors during the second half of pregnancy, such as occurs in GDM. This issue has important clinical implications since GDM that develops exclusively in the second half of pregnancy may cause significant metabolic

dysfunction; hence, this may lead to an increase in the rate of developmental disorders. This increase is anticipated because the major developmental events of the cerebral cortex occur during the second half of pregnancy.[49]

Children born after high-risk pregnancies tend to show developmental delay, learning difficulties at school and a high rate of inattention and hyperactivity [attention deficit disorder (ADD)], although predictors of individual outcome are difficult.[50] *The American Psychiatric Association Diagnostic and Statistical Manual of Mental Disorders – IV (DSM-IV)*[51] indicates that ADD is associated with a variety of behavioral problems, although intellectual ability in such children is usually within the normal range.[51,52] It is accepted that various maternal factors, such as exposure to high levels of opiates or severe environmental deprivation,[53] as well as disturbances in glucose metabolism, may delay maturation of the fetal brain. With age and the provision of an appropriate environment, postnatal brain maturation may become normal.

Several of the developmental studies performed on children born to diabetic mothers were also carried out at an early school age – a stage when ADD can be diagnosed. However, the issue whether diabetes may affect the prevalence of ADD, and hence school performance, was rarely discussed. The present author's group has performed a series of follow-up studies on school-age children to specifically address these issues.[35–37]

Developmental studies

The purpose of the present author's group's studies was to assess the development of early school-age children born to mothers with PGDM or GDM in comparison to pair-matched controls, using a number of cognitive, sensory, motor, behavioral and neurological tests. It was also intended to correlate the neurological function of these children to the degree of metabolic dysfunction observed in the diabetic mothers.

Subjects and methods of study

The development of early school-age children born to mothers with PGDM or GDM to age-matched control children was compared using a number of developmental criteria.

Subjects

The sample consisted of: (1) 57 children (49% girls), born to 48 Type 1 and Type 2 diabetic mothers; (2) 32 children (41% girls) born to 32 women with GDM; and (3) 57 control children (44% girls) born to 57 non-diabetic healthy mothers. (Note: there was one set of triplets and seven sets of twins in the research group). The children were pair-matched on age, SES (based on parental education and occupation), gestational age, birth order and family size. None of the control mothers had GDM. All children were born between 1982 and 1987 at the Sheba Medical Center, Tel Hashomer, near Tel-Aviv, where the mothers with PGDM or GDM were also followed up and managed for diabetes with the goal of achieving optimum glycemic control. All of the children studied in regular schools. Only children born after 34 weeks of gestation participated in the study. (Details of the groups and the methods used are described elsewhere.[35–37])

Testing procedures

The following tests were administered to each participating child:[35–37]

- A complete physical and neurological examination.

- The Touwen and Prechtl neurological examination for children with minor neurological dysfunction.
- Evaluation of the cognitive score using the Wechsler Intelligence Scales for Children Revised (WISC-R, 1974) and the Bender Visual Gestalt test.
- The Pollack Taper test, which is designed to assess attention deficits. The child is asked to repeat a specific sequence of light blinks and auditory taps presented by the tester; the number, sequence and duration of these stimuli is adapted to the child's age. Children with ADD tend to obtain lower scores than children with normal attention spans. The higher the score, the better is the child's attention to rhythmic stimuli.
- Bruininks–Oseretsky Motor Development test. This test examines fine and gross motor development of children between the ages of 4.5 and 14.5.
- Southern California Integration test, for the evaluation of children's sensory functioning. This test includes three subtests: manual form perception (MFP), finger identification (FI) and localization of tactile stimuli (LTS).
- The Conner's Abbreviated Parent–Teacher's Questionnaire for the study of hyperactivity and inattention, which is administered to the parents. In this subjective test, the higher the score, the more hyperactivity and attention problems (i.e. ADD) in the child.[35–37,52]

Maternal state of diabetes control in the PGDM and GDM women

The medical files of all diabetic mothers and of the mothers with GDM were examined for the evaluation of the degree of diabetes control. The clinical details in the diabetic mothers included the time of pregnancy when tight control of diabetes started, the stage of diabetes for each woman (White's stages), and the presence of hypertension, retinopathy, nephropathy or neuropathy of diabetes. The laboratory examinations performed included pre- and postprandial glucose blood levels, performed up to six times a day by the pregnant women, using a glucometer and urine examination for acetonuria.

For each woman with PGDM the following were calculated: (1) average blood glucose levels, counting the number of cases of hypoglycemia (<60 mg/dl) or hyperglycemia; (2) the complications of diabetes according to White's classification; (3) the average percentage of HbA1c (available for only 19 women with PGDM). These variables were correlated with the results of the developmental assessments of the children.

Statistical evaluation

Research and control groups were compared by paired *t*-tests for each dependent variable. For comparison of the groups on the Touwen and Prechtl neurological examinations, the Wilcoxon matched-pair signed-ranks test was used. The Pearson correlation was calculated between the metabolic findings of the diabetic mothers and the scores on the neurodevelopmental tests of their children.[54] The correlation was calculated for each trimester of pregnancy and then for the entire period of pregnancy.

Results

Birthweight, perinatal complications and physical parameters at examination

Table 24.1 shows the results of birthweight and physical examination at school in the various groups of children. The children were examined at 6–12 years of age. The average birthweight of the children born to PGDM mothers was 3528 grams, of the children born to women with GDM 3254 grams and of the controls 3381 grams (Table 24.1). The differences between the groups were not statistically significant. Body weight was increased in the children born to diabetic mothers in comparison to controls.

Cognitive and neurological functions

Table 24.2 shows the results of the WISC-R and Bender tests for the diabetic and control group children. No differences were found between the two groups of children for the WISC-R scores, but the Bender scores of the children born to mothers with GDM were slightly lower than in the controls (Table 24.2).

Results of the neurological and the motor assessments of the children are given in Table 24.3. Children born to mothers with

Test	Control		PGDM mothers		GDM mothers	
	Mean	SD	Mean	SD	Mean	SD
IQ	118.5[†]	11	117.7	12	113.5	14.3
Verbal	114.4	12	112.4	12	108.0	11.5
Performance	119.7	11.5	120.4	19	116.0	16.0
Bender (%)	48.6	26.5	48.0	24	32.0[‡]	27.0

* Wechsler Intelligence Scales for Children Revised.
[†] Mean ± SD.
[‡] Significantly lower than controls, $P < 0.05$.

Table 24.2. Comparison of cognitive scores using the WISC-R* and Bender Visual Gestalt tests of control children and those born to pregestational diabetic (PGDM) and gestational diabetic (GDM) mothers (from Ornoy et al,[37] with permission).

PGDM or GDM had significantly lower scores on the Bruininks–Oseretsky fine and gross motor scores as compared to controls.

No differences between the children of either diabetic group or the control group were observed in any of the three subtests of the Southern California Integration test (MFP, FI and LTS) that were designed to reflect sensory – motor functioning (results not shown). Children born to mothers with PGDM, but not those with GDM, had a significantly higher number of soft neurological signs in the Touwen and Prechtl examination (Table 24.3). A higher score is indicative of a larger number of soft neurological deficiencies, also implying more children with ADD and/or hyperactvity.[35,36,52]

Attention functioning

There was a marked difference on the Pollack Taper test between the control group children and the children born to mothers with either PGDM or GDM, the average score of these latter children being lower than in controls (Table 24.3).

Table 24.3 also reveals that children born to mothers with PGDM obtained higher scores on the Conner's Abbreviated Parent–Teacher's Questionnaire in comparison to controls, indicating more hyperactivity and inattention; however, the differences in the scores were not statistically significant. When the number of children having 15 or more failure points was compared among the groups, it was significantly higher in both research group children in comparison to controls (results not shown).

Correlation between neurodevelopmental assessment and severity of PGDM

Table 24.4 presents the correlation between the results of the neurodevelopmental assessments and the severity of maternal glucose impairment only in offspring of mothers with PGDM, as indicated by glucose blood levels, urinary acetone and the percentage of HbA1c. A negative correlation was found between the percentage of HbA1c and the scores on the Bender Gestalt test, as well as the total motor scores on the Bruininks–Oseretsky test, indicating that

Test	Controls		PGDM mothers		GDM mothers	
	Mean	SD	Mean	SD	Mean	SD
Bruininks, total	138*	21[†]	129	20	121	27
Bruininks, gross motor	60.8	12[†]	57	11	57	15
Bruininks, fine motor	62.5	9[†]	58	10	49	11
Touwen and Prechtl (no. of failure signs)	4.00[‡]		8.45		4.8	
Pollack	28.9	5.7[†]	24.3	11.2	24.3	11
Conners	7.7	4.3	9.1	4.8	7.4	6.3

* Mean±SD.
[†] Significantly higher than in children born to mothers with PGDM or GDM, $P < 0.05$.
[‡] Significantly lower than children born to mothers with PGDM, $P < 0.05$.

Table 24.3. Comparison of motor development (Bruininks–Oseretzky), and neurological and behavioral evaluation (Touwen and Prechtl, Pollack, and Conners) in control children and those born to mothers with pregestational diabetes mellitus (PGDM) or gestational diabetes mellitus (GDM) (from Ornoy et al,[37] with permission).

Neurological test	Maternal blood glucose (n = 47)	Glycosylated hemoglobin (HbAlc) (n = 19)	Acetonuria (n = 46)	Glycemic control: White's class (n = 53)
Touwen and Prechtl	−0.07	0.03	0.15	0.00
IQ (general)	0.27*	−0.07	0.01	−0.03
Bender	0.32*	−0.50*	0.06	0.00
Bruininks (general motor)	0.10	−0.41*	−0.31*	−0.08
Bruininks (gross motor)	0.03	0.33*	−0.27*	0.02
Bruininks (fine motor)	0.19	−0.41*	−0.26*	−0.13
MFP‡ (sensory)	0.04	0.31	−0.10	−0.31*
FI§ (sensory)	0.09	−0.11	−0.35*	−0.10
LTS″ (sensory)	0.11	−0.14	−0.05	−0.29*
Conners	0.08	0.07	0.17	−0.03
Pollack	−0.12	−0.25	0.07	0.04

* A significant positive or negative (−) correlation ($P < 0.05$)
† The correlations were calculated using Pearsons's correlations.
‡ Manual form perception.
§ Finger identification.
″ Localization of tactile stimuli.

Table 24.4. *Correlation between maternal glycemic control and the results of the neurodevelopmental assessment in the children born to mothers with pregestational diabetes (PGDM) (from Ornoy et al,[37] with permission).*

sensory–motor function of children born to diabetic mothers tends to be lower with higher HbA1c levels. A similar negative correlation was found between positive urinary acetone and the motor ability of the children (Table 24.4); the higher the acetonuria, the lower were the total motor scores on the Bruininks test.

A negative correlation was found between the percentage of HbA1c and the Pollack Taper test, indicating that a high percentage of HbA1c was related to poorer attention ability. However, due to the small number of women where HbA1c was measured ($n = 19$), this correlation was not statistically significant. Surprisingly there was a positive correlation between the glucose blood levels and the results of the Bender test and those of IQ on the WISC-R test. The correlation between maternal hyperglycemia and maternal education was found to be positive, indicating that maternal education may be the factor responsible for the high WISC-R and Bender–Gestalt scores in the children of these mothers.

No correlation was found between the medical status (i.e. hypoglycemia, increased or decreased birthweight) of the newborn infants and outcome of any of the associated variables in the children born to women with PGDM or GDM. This emphasizes again the importance of the environment of the child in the development of its intellectual capacity, as observed in several other studies of high-risk infants.

Conclusions

Children born to diabetic mothers are often macrosomic, especially if maternal hyperglycemia occurs during the second and third trimesters of pregnancy. In mothers with PGDM and nephropathy or other vascular complications, many infants are born prematurely and SGA. On follow-up, the macrosomic children tend to normalize their weight and height within the first year of life, but there is a strong tendency for increased weight and height to reappear at early school age, which persists into adolescence and adulthood. Children born SGA tend to be smaller for at least the first several years of life.

In well-controlled diabetes in pregnancy, the intellectual function of the offspring is usually within normal limits. However, fine and gross motor abilities, attention span and activity levels are impaired among children born to diabetic mothers and to mothers with GDM when compared to matched controls. In some studies the differences compared to controls are larger in children between the ages of 5 and 8, and the differences are reduced in older children. Intellectual impairment is commonly observed among children born to PGDM mothers with vascular complications and nephropathy, and many of them are also born prematurely and are SGA.

Children born to diabetic mothers may be able to compensate for their slight neurological impairment and their daily function may be normal. However, when coping with complex motor or intellectual tasks, they may have difficulty in performing adequately.

It is possible that the diabetic metabolic abnormalities during pregnancy delay brain maturation and therefore fine neurological functions are impaired at a young age. Advancement in age will enable full functional recovery, providing that the child is raised in an environment that is optimal for growth and development.

The effects of maternal diabetes on development may result from the adverse effects of metabolic diabetic factors (i.e. hyperglycemia and hyperketonemia) mainly during the second half of pregnancy, when higher functions of the brain develop. Indeed, the severity of the effects in children born to PGDM mothers inversely correlate with the degree of glycemic control, and in children of PGDM mothers with vascular complications, developmental impairment seems to be most severe. These results emphasize the importance of good glycemic control throughout pregnancy in diabetic mothers and not just in the first trimester, which is the commonly advised practice.

References

1. Eskes TKAB, Mooij PNM, Steegers-Theunissen RpyM et al. Pregnancy care and prevention of birth defect. *J Perinatol Med* 1992; 20:253–65.
2. Hod M, Diamant YZ. The offspring of a diabetic mother – short and long range implications. *Israel J Med Sci* 1992; 28:81–6.
3. Miller E, Hare JW, Cloherty JP et al. Elevated maternal hemoglobin Alc in early pregnancy and major congenital anomalies in infants of diabetic mothers. *N Engl J Med* 1981; 304:1331–4.
4. Mills JL, Baker L, Goldman AS. Malformations of infants of diabetic mothers occur before the 7th gestational week: implications for treatment. *Diabetes* 1979; 28:292–3.
5. Mills JL, Knopp RH, Simpson JL et al. NIHHD and diabetes in early pregnancy study: lack of relation of increased malformation rates in infants of diabetic mothers to glycemic control during organogenesis. *N Engl J Med* 1991; 318:671–6.
6. Miodovnik M, Mimouni F, St. John Dignan P. Major malformations in infants of IDDM women: vasculopathy and early first-trimester poor glycemic control. *Diabetes Care* 1988; 11:713–18.
7. Cordero L, London MB. Infants of the diabetic mother. *Diabetes Preg* 1993; 20:635–48.
8. Leslie RDG, Pyke DA, John PN, White JM. Hemoglobin Alc in diabetic pregnancy. *Lancet* 1978; ii:958–62.
9. Pedersen J. *The Pregnant Diabetic and Her Newborn: Problems and Management.* (Williams & Wilkins Company: Baltimore, 1967.)
10. Farquhar JW. The child of the diabetic woman. *Arch Dis Child* 1959; 34:76–96.
11. Moore TR. Fetal growth in diabetic pregnancy. *Clin Obstet Gynecol* 1997; 40:771–86.

12. Silverman BL, Landsberg L, Metzger BE. Fetal hyperinsulinism in offspring of diabetic mothers. *Ann NY Acad Sci* 1993; **699**:36–45.

13. Metzger BE, Silverman B, Freinkel N et al. Amniotic fluid insulin as a predictor of obesity. *Arch Dis Child* 1990; **65**:1050–2.

14. Carpenter MW, Canick JA, Hogan JW, et al. Amniotic fluid insulin at 14–20 weeks gestation: association with later maternal glucose intolerance and birth macrosomia. *Diabetes Care* 2001; **24**:1259–63.

15. Mello G, Parretti E, Mecacci F et al. What degree of maternal control in women with type I diabetes is associated with normal body size and proportions in full-term infants? *Diabetes Care* 2000; **23**:1494–8.

16. Sermer M, Naylor CD, Farine D et al. The Toronto tri-hospital gestational diabetes project preliminary review. *Diabetes Care* 1998; **2**:B33.

17. Simmons D, Robertson S. Influence of maternal insulin treatment of the infants of women with gestational diabetes. *Diabet Med* 1997; **14**:762–5.

18. Romon M, Nuttens MC, Vambergue A et al. Higher carbohydrate intake is associated with decreased incidence of newborn macrosomia in women with gestational diabetes. *J Am Diet Assoc* 2000; **101**:897–902.

19. Scholl TO, Sowers MF, Chen X, Lenders C. Maternal glucose concentration influences fetal growth, gestation, and pregnancy complications. *Am J Epidemiol* 2001; **154**:514–20.

20. Caruso A, Paradisi G, Ferrazzani S et al. Effect of maternal carbohydrate metabolism of fetal growth. *Obstet Gynecol* 1998; **92**:8–12.

21. Wiznitzer A, Furman B, Zuili I et al. Cord leptin levels and fetal macrosomia. *Obstet Gynecol* 2000; **96**:707–13.

22. Marchini G, Fried, G, Ostlund E, Hagenas L. Plasma leptin in infants: relations to birth weight and weight loss. *Pediatrics* 1998; **101**:429–32.

23. Lepercq J, Taupin P, Dubois-Laforgue D et al. Heterogeneity of fetal growth in type I diabetic pregnancy. *Diabetes Metab* 2001; **27**:339–44.

24. Tapanainen P, Leinonen E, Ruokonen A, Knip M. Leptin concentration are elevated in newborn infants of diabetic mothers. *Horm Res* 2001; **55**:185–90.

25. Hytinantti TK, Juntunen M, Kiostinen HA et al. Postnatal changes in concentrations of free and bound leptin. *Arch Dis Child Fetal Neonatal Ed* 2001; **85**:F123–F126.

26. Biesenbach G, Grafinger P, Zazgornik J, Stoger H. Perinatal complications and three year follow up of infants of diabetic mothers with diabetic nephropathy stage IV. *Renal Failure* 2000; **22**:573–80.

27. Erickson J, Forsen T, Tuomilehto J et al. Fetal and childhood growth and hypertension in adult. *Hypertension* 2000; **36**:790–7.

28. Barker DJ. Maternal nutrition, fetal nutrition, and disease in later life. *Nutrition* 1997; **13**: 807–13.

29. Bakker SJ, ter Maaten JC, Gans RO. Thiamine supplementation to prevent induction of low birth weight by conventional therapy for gestational diabetes mellitus. *Med Hypotheses* 2000; **55**:88–90.

30. Rizzo TA, Metzger BE, Burns WJ, Burns K. Correlations between antepartum maternal metabolism and intelligence of offspring. *N Engl J Med* 1991; **325**:911–16.

31. Rizzo TA, Dooley SL, Metzger BE et al. Prenatal and perinatal influences on long-term psychomotor development in offspring of diabetic mothers. *Am J Obstet Gynecol* 1995; **173**:1753–8.

32. Amendt P, Michaelis D, Hildman W. Clinical and metabolic studies in children of diabetic mothers. *Endocronologie* 1976; **67**:351–61.

33. Seidman DS, Laor A, Stevenson DK et al. Macrosomia does not predict overweight in late adolescence in infants of diabetic mothers. *Acta Obstet Gynecol Scand* 1998; **77**:58–62.

34. Mikulandra F, Gryuric J, Banovic I et al. The effect of high birth weight (400 g or more) on the weight and height of adult men and women. *Coll Antropol* 2000; **24**:133–6.

35. Ornoy A, Ratzon N, Greenbaum C, et al. Neuro-behaviour of school age children born to diabetic mothers. *Arch Dis Child* 1998; **79**:F94–F99.

36. Ornoy A, Wolf A, Ratzon N et al. Neurodevelopmental outcome at early school age of children born to mothers with gestational diabetes. *Arch Dis Child* 1999; **81**:F10–F14.

37. Ornoy A, Ratzon N, Greenbaum C et al. School-age children born to mothers with pregestational or gestational diabetes exhibit a high rate of inattention and fine and gross motor impairment. *J Pediatr Endocrinol Metab* 2001; **14**:681–9.

38. Churchill JA, Berendes HW, Nemore J. Neuropsychological deficits in children of diabetic mothers: a report from the collaborative study of cerebral palsy. *Am J Obstet Gynecol* 1969; **105**: 257.

39. Shulte FJ, Michalis R, Nolte R et al. Brain and behavioral maturation in newborn infants of diabetic mothers. *Neuropediatrics* 1969; **1**:24–55.

40. Stehbens JA, Baker GL, Kitchell M. Outcome at age 1,3 and 5 years of children born to diabetic women. *Am J Obstet Gynecol* 1977; **127**:408–15.

41. Petersen BM, Pedersen SA, Greisen G et al. Early growth delay in diabetic pregnancy: relation to psychomotor development at age 4. *Br Med J* 1988; **296**:598–600.

42. Cummins M, Norrish M. Follow-up of children of diabetic mothers. *Arch Dis Child* 1980; **55**:259–64.

43. Person B, Gentz J. Follow-up of children of insulin-dependent and gestational diabetes mothers. *Acta Pediatr Scand* 1984; **73**:349–358.

44. Yamashita Y, Kawano Y, Kuriya N et al. Intellectual development of offspring of diabetic mothers. *Acta Paediatr* 1996; **85**:1192–6.

45. Sells CJ, Robinson NM, Brown Z, Knopp RH. Long-term developmental follow-up of infants of diabetic mothers. *J Pediatr* 1994; **125**:S9–S17.

46. Kimmerle R, Zab RP, Cupisti S et al. Pregnancies in women with diabetic nephropathy: long-term outcome for mother and child. *Diabetologia* 1995; **38**:227–35.

47. Kizmuller JL, Brown ER, Phillippe M et al. Diabetic nephropathy and perinatal outcome. *Am J Obstet Gynecol* 1981; **149**:741–52.

48. Bloch-Petersen M. Status at 4–5 years in 90 children of insulin-dependent diabetic mothers. In: (Stowers, Sutherland HW, eds) *Carbohydrate Metabolism in Pregnancy and the Newborn*. (Springer: New York, 1989) 354–61.

49. Ornoy A. Is the developing brain responsive to external stimulation? In: (Tamir D, ed.) *Stimulation and Intervention in Infant Development*. (Freund's Publishing House Ltd: UK, 1986) 316–18.

50. Acardo PJ, Blondis TA, Whitman BY. Disorders of attention and activity level in a referral population. *Pediatrics* 1990; **85**:426–31.

51. American Psychiatric Association. *American Psychiatric Association Diagnostic and Statistical Manual of Mental Disorders*, 4th edn. (American Psychiatric Association: Washington, DC, 1994).

52. Ornoy A, Ariel L, Tenenbaum A. Inattention, hyperactivity and speech delay at 2–4 years of age as a predictor for ADD-ADHD syndrome. *Israel J Psychiatry* 1993; **30**:155–63.

53. Ornoy A, Michailevskaya V, Lukashov I et al. The developmental outcome of children born to heroin dependent mothers raised at home or adopted. *Child Abuse Neglect: Int J* 1996; **20**:385–96.

54. Beyer BH. *Handbook of Tables for Probability and Statistics*, 2nd edn. (The Chemical Rubber Co.: New York, 1968).

25

Management of gestational diabetes mellitus

Massimo Massi-Benedetti, Marco Orsini Federici, Gian Carlo Di Renzo

Diabetes and pregnancy

Global fetal and infant loss, perinatal mortality, neonatal mortality, and malformations rates are significantly greater if the mother is diabetic compared with the non-diabetic population.[1] Studies conducted by Casson et al[2] confirm that among unselected populations of women with insulin-dependent diabetes mellitus (IDDM), pregnancy loss remains significantly higher than in the normal population. The diagnosis of congenital anomalies is also more accurate in infants of diabetic mothers, since they are more carefully looked for in respect to control infants and because of the more frequent autoptic evaluation due to the higher mortality rate.[3] Consolidated experiences clearly correlate fetal and maternal complications to the degree of metabolic control during pregnancy, indicating without a doubt the need for effective metabolic and obstetrical management of women with different degrees of alteration of the glucose homeostasis during pregnancy.

Gestational diabetes mellitus

Diagnosis

Approximately 7% of all pregnancies are complicated by GDM, resulting in > 200,000 cases annually in the US and in Europe. The prevalence may range from 1 to 14% of all pregnancies, depending on the population studied and the diagnostic tests adopted.[4]

Risk factors for GDM are well known and their presence allows the identification of three risk categories: **high risk**, characterized by marked obesity, diabetes in first-degree relatives, a history of glucose intolerance, previous infants with macrosomia, current glycosuria; **average risk**, inclusive of women that fit neither the low- or high-risk categories; **low risk**, including women < 25 years of age, a normal weight before pregnancy, a member of an ethnic group with a low prevalence of GDM, with no known diabetes in first-degree relatives, and no history of abnormal glucose tolerance, nor of poor obstetric outcome.[5]

Risk assessment for GDM should be undertaken at the first prenatal visit. Women with clinical characteristics consistent with a high risk of GDM should undergo glucose testing as soon as is feasible. A fasting plasma glucose level > 126 mg/dl (7.0 mmol/l) or a casual plasma glucose > 200 mg/dl (11.1 mmol/l) meets the threshold for the diagnosis of diabetes and if confirmed on a subsequent day rules out the need for any glucose challenge. In the absence of this degree of hyperglycaemia, the screening for GDM in women with high-risk characteristics should be performed according to two different possible procedures:

the one-step procedure and the two-step procedure. The one-step procedure consists of a diagnostic oral glucose tolerance test (OGTT) performed on all subjects, while the two-step procedure consists of a 50 gram glucose challenge test (GCT) followed by a diagnostic OGTT in those meeting the threshold value in the GCT (see Chapter 13).

Women at average risk should be evaluated at 24–28 weeks of gestation; even for this category of women both procedures are indicated and in case of negative results testing should be repeated later. In the case of low-risk women, profile blood glucose testing is not routinely required; a fasting plasma glucose measurement between 24 and 28 weeks of gestation has been considered sufficient.[5] However, in 1998 Carr et al[6] demonstrated that using the risk-category approach to select the screening strategies meant that 44–53% of GDM cases went undiagnosed.

Monitoring and therapy

Once diagnosis of GDM has been confirmed, the woman should be closely monitored until the early postpartum period. The general goal of therapeutic interventions in GDM is to achieve and maintain blood glucose as near to normal as possible in order to reduce morbidity and mortality of the mother, and of the fetus newborn.

In order to provide a care of high quality, a multidisciplinary team approach is essential, inclusive of the diabetologist, the diabetes-specialized nurse, the dietician, the obstetrician, the midwife and the neonatologist.[7]

Metabolic surveillance needs to be rather strict, with frequent reviews every 1–2 weeks, either directly or by phone contact,[7] with the target to detect and prevent hyperglycaemia. Daily self-blood glucose monitoring (SBMG) appears to be superior to intermittent office monitoring of plasma glucose.[8] For women treated with insulin, various evidence indicates that postprandial monitoring is superior to preprandial monitoring. De Veciana et al[9] showed that postprandial glucose measurements are significantly better at predicting lower daily insulin doses and glycosylated haemoglobin (HbA1c) levels, a reduced risk for Caesarean section, large-for-gestational-age infants and neonatal hypoglycaemia.

Urine glucose monitoring is not useful in GDM as it does not allow for fine tuning of therapy and can be an unreliable indicator of metabolic control due to the changes of the renal glucose threshold occurring during pregnancy. HbA1c levels should be evaluated every 4–6 weeks.

Follow-up at a diabetes clinic should be performed monthly until week 28 of gestation, fortnightly until week 36 and weekly until term.[10] Additional clinic visits should be programmed if the need arises. Maternal surveillance should include monitoring of blood pressure and of urinary protein excretion to detect hypertensive disorders. Urine ketones should be evaluated every morning during the first trimester, as ketone levels can be useful in detecting insufficient caloric or carbohydrate intake in women treated with a restricted caloric intake. Special attention should be paid to the evaluation of the presence and the evolution of diabetes complications. A urine test inclusive of culture should be done fortnightly, and serum creatinine, microalbuminuria and proteinuria every trimester. Eyes must be examined during the first trimester and successively as the need arises. An electrocardiogram (ECG) should be evaluated at the first clinic visit.

All women with GDM should receive nutritional counselling by a dietician. The first therapeutic step recommended is the individualization of medical nutrition therapy (MNT) depending on maternal weight and height.

MNT should include the provision of adequate calories and nutrients to meet the needs of pregnancy, and should be consistent with the target defined for maternal blood glucose. Non-caloric sweeteners may be used in moderation.[11]

The daily energy intake recommended for women with an ideal weight in the normal range is 30 kcal/kg of the ideal weight; for obese women 20–25 kcal/kg of the ideal weight, and for underweight women 40 kcal/kg of the ideal weight. For obese women [body mass index (BMI) > 30 kgram/m^2], a 30–33% caloric restriction (to *c.* 25 kcal/kg actual weight per day) has been shown to reduce hyperglycaemia and plasma triglycerides with no increase in ketonuria.[12] Meals should be constituted of 50–60% of carbohydrates (breakfast < 45%, lunch 55% and dinner 50%), 25–30% of lipids and 10–20% of proteins.

Caloric intake should be modified if the woman undertakes physical activity. In the case of moderate exercise lasting 30–60 minutes and a starting blood glucose of 100–160 mg/dl (5.5–8.8 mmol/l), an increased intake of 15 gram of carbohydrates is suggested. If the starting blood glucose is between 161 and 250 mg/dl (8.9–13.9 mmol/l) the amount of carbohydrate intake is not to be changed. In the presence of frank hyperglycaemia [blood glucose > 250 mg/dl (13.9 mmol/l)] with ketonuria, exercise should not be performed until normalization of metabolic control.[13]

The increase in weight during pregnancy should depend on the pregestational weight. Women with a BMI < 19.8 should have a weight increase of 12.5–18 kg; with a BMI between 19.5 and 25, a weight increase of 11.5–16 kg; and in the case of overweight women, i.e. BMI > 25, the weight increase should be 7–11.5 kg.[14]

Insulin is the pharmacologic therapy that has most consistently been shown to reduce fetal morbidities when added to MNT. Selection of pregnancies for insulin therapy can be based on the level of maternal glycaemia with or without assessment of fetal growth characteristics. When maternal glucose levels are used, insulin therapy is recommended when MNT fails to maintain SBGM at the following levels: fasting blood glucose ≤ 105 mg/dl (5.8 mmol/l) or 1-hour postprandial blood glucose ≤ 155 mg/dl (8.6 mmol/l) or 2-hour postprandial blood glucose ≤ 130 mg/dl (7.2 mmol/l).

Measurement of the fetal abdominal circumference early in the third trimester can be considered another indicator to define the need to start insulin therapy. In 1998, Buchanan et al[15] tested the utility of this approach to drive therapy choice. They proposed the following decisional cascade: diet therapy as the first approach with fasting blood glucose evaluation every 2 weeks; if fasting blood glucose is > 105 mg/dl (5.8 mmol/l), insulin should be started; if fasting blood glucose remains below this threshold until 29–33 weeks gestation, insulin should not be prescribed; thereafter fetal ultrasound could be used to define the need for insulin therapy (see Chapter 27). If the abdominal circumference is below the 70th percentile then diet therapy alone should be continued. If the abdominal circumference is above the 70th percentile then insulin therapy should be started independently of the glycaemic values.[15]

Human insulin should be used when insulin is prescribed, however, purified insulin of animal origin can be prescribed if human insulin is not available. The generally suggested starting dose is 0.7 U/kg of body weight. The doses and timing of the insulin regimen should thereafter be guided by the SBGM levels, with particular attention paid to the insulin adjustment in the second and third trimesters. In fact, from weeks 20 and 32 of gestation there is a physiological progressive increase in insulin requirement up to 50% of the initial dose.[16] The use of insulin analogues has not been adequately tested in GDM. In 1998, a study by Jovankovic et al[17] demonstrated that insulin lispro was able to improve postprandial glucose without increasing immunogenecity, reducing one of the major concerns for the utilization of insulin analogues in pregnancy. However, the position statement published in 2002 by the American Diabetes Association (ADA)[18] suggests caution in the utilization of insulin analogues until more evidence on the safety of their use during pregnancy is available.

The most effective insulin regimen for insulin therapy during pregnancy consists of four injections per day. In 1999, Nachum et al[19] compared the twice-daily insulin injection regimen versus the four-daily in a cohort of more than 400 pregnant women with diabetes. They showed that the four-daily insulin injection regimen improved metabolic control and perinatal outcomes more than the twice-daily injection regimen. Moreover, the intensified therapy did not increase the risk of hypoglycaemia in the mothers.

A higher risk of hypoglycaemia with intensified insulin therapy can be observed during the first trimester of gestation when there is an increase of passive diffusion of glucose across the placenta and an impaired counter-regulation response.

Continuous subcutaneous insulin infusion (CSII) therapy, through the utilization of insulin pumps, could represent an optimal means to improve metabolic control with a reduction in the risk of hypoglycaemia in diabetic pregnant women. Several studies have shown a better or at least equal efficacy of CSII in metabolic control than the optimized multiple-daily injection regimen with a reduction of mild and severe hypoglycaemic episodes, provided that correct criteria have been used for the selection of the candidates for CSII.[20,21]

Oral glucose-lowering agents have generally not been recommended during pregnancy. However, one randomized, unblinded clinical trial compared the use of insulin and glyburide in women with GDM who were not able to meet glycaemic goals on MNT.[22] Treatment with either agent resulted in similar perinatal outcomes. All patients were beyond the first trimester of pregnancy at the initiation of therapy. Although very promising, glyburide is not approved by the Food and Drug Administration (FDA) for the treatment of gestational diabetes; further studies are needed in a larger patient populations to establish its safety. Research is underway in this respect (Langer, personal communication).

Programmes of moderate physical exercise have been shown to lower maternal glucose concentrations in women with GDM. In fact, physical exercise can improve unsatisfactory metabolic control in diabetic pregnant women on diet therapy alone. Controversial results about safety of exercise for the fetus have been reported. Some authors demonstrated an exercise-induced fetal bradycardia,[23] while others did not find cardiac effects in the fetus deriving from the mother's exercise.[24] Same antithetic results were also shown with regard to the uterine activity that was found to be increased by some authors[25] but not affected by exercise in others.[26]

Physical exercise with utilization of upper body muscles was demonstrated to be safer than exercise involving lower body muscles.[27] However, physical exercise that can increase blood pressure needs to be avoided because of the risk of pre-eclampsia in GDM patients. Although the impact of exercise on neonatal complications awaits to be defined through rigorous clinical trials, the beneficial glucose-lowering effects warrant a recommendation that women without medical or obstetrical contraindications be encouraged to start or continue a programme of moderate exercise as a part of treatment for GDM. Jovanovic[28] suggested light exercise of at least 20 minutes daily three times per week.

Increased surveillance for pregnancies at risk for fetal demise is appropriate, particularly when fasting glucose levels exceed 105 mg/dl (5.8 mmol/l) or pregnancy progresses past term. The initiation, frequency and specific techniques used to assess fetal well-being will depend on the cumulative risk the fetus bears from GDM and any other concomitant medical/obstetric condition. Assessment for asymmetric fetal growth by ultrasonography, particularly in the early third trimester, may aid in identifying fetuses that can benefit from maternal insulin therapy (see Chapters 27 and 30).

The timing of the beginning and the frequency of fetal monitoring depends on the presence of complications of the pregnancy such as pre-eclampsia, hypertension, antepartum haemorrhage and fetal growth retardation. The intensity and the type of monitoring should be dictated by the severity of the obstetric complication. Ultrasonography should be considered at around week 24 to detect abnormalities of fetal growth and signs of polyhydramnios.[9] Ultrasonography has also been proposed as a more accurate method of estimation of fetal weight. Unfortunately, the reported mean error ranges from 300 to 550 grams (11.6–19.4 oz) (see Chapter 30).[29]

Delivery

GDM is not an indication for delivery by Caesarean section nor for delivery before 38 completed weeks of gestation. The prolongation of the gestation beyond 38 weeks increases the risk of fetal macrosomia without reducing Caesarean section rates, so that delivery during the 38th week has been recommended unless obstetric considerations dictate otherwise.[9]

The main objectives during labour are to maintain normal glycaemic values, adequate hydration and caloric intake.[30,31] If women are only on a diet therapy, it is suggested to avoid breakfast on the morning when the delivery is planned. During delivery, an intravenous infusion of saline solution at the speed of 100–150 ml/hour and regular glucose monitoring are advised.

In the case of women on insulin treatment it has to be considered that labour determines a reduction of insulin need and an increase of caloric necessity. The day before labour women should follow their usual insulin and diet regimen with an injection at bedtime of intermediate insulin adjusted to produce a satisfactory fasting blood glucose. The morning of the delivery women should not receive either breakfast nor a rapid-acting insulin bolus. An intravenous insulin infusion of 1–2 U of short-acting insulin/hour together with a 5% glucose solution or a saline solution at 100–150 ml/hour is recommended. Blood glucose should be evaluated every hour and the insulin infusion should be adjusted in order to obtain a glycaemic target of between 70 and 130 mg/dl (3.8–7.2 mmol/l). During delivery, insulin infusion should be suspended while glucose infusion and glucose monitoring should be continued.

The neonates of mothers with GDM or with pregestational diabetes are at the same risk for complications, particularly those infants born macrosomic (birthweight > 4000 grams).[32] A paediatrician experienced in resuscitation of the newborn should be present whether delivery is vaginal or by Caesarean section. As soon as the infant is born, the following actions are mandatory:

- early clamping of the cord, i.e. within 20 seconds of delivery, to avoid erythrocytosis;

- evaluate vital signs; Apgar scores at 1 and 5 minutes;
- clear oropharynx and nose of mucus; later empty the stomach – be aware that stimulation of the pharynx with the catheter may lead to reflex bradycardia and apnoea;
- avoid heat loss, keep neonate warm, transfer to incubator pre-warmed to 34°C;
- perform a preliminary physical examination to detect major congenital malformations;
- monitor heart and respiratory rates, colour, and motor behaviour for at least the first 24 hours after birth;
- start early feeding, preferably breast milk, at 4–6 hours after delivery: aim at full caloric intake (125 kcal/kg/24 hours) at 5 days, divided into six to eight feeds a day;
- promote early infant–parent relationship (bonding).

The neonate is usually best cared for in specialized neonatal units. Interference with the infant should be minimal. The neonate should be observed closely after delivery for respiratory distress. Capillary blood glucose should be monitored at 1 hour of age and before the first four breast feedings (and for up to 24 hours in high-risk neonates). Currently, some amperometric blood glucose meters are acceptable for use in neonates, provided that suitable quality-control procedures and operator training are in place. A neonatal blood glucose level < 36 mg/dl (2.0 mmol/l) needs to be verified by repeat testing (laboratory verification is preferred but should not delay the initiation of treatment). Levels < 36 mg/dl (2.0 mmol/l) should be considered abnormal and treated. If the baby is obviously macrosomic, calcium and magnesium levels should be checked on day 2.[9] Breastfeeding, as always, should be encouraged in women with GDM.[18]

Postpartum maternal follow-up

Women with GDM have an increased risk of developing diabetes, usually Type 2, after pregnancy. Obesity and other factors that promote insulin resistance appear to enhance the risk of Type 2 diabetes after GDM, while markers of islet-cell-directed autoimmunity are associated with an increase in the risk of Type 1 diabetes.[33,34] ADA advices a reclassification of the maternal glycaemia at 6 weeks after delivery. If the blood glucose levels are normal, another evaluation should be done after 3 years. In the case of impaired fasting glucose (IFG) or impaired glucose tolerance (IGT), glucose testing is advised every year. These patients should be placed on an intensive MNT, and on an individualized exercise regimen due to their very high risk of developing diabetes.[35] Medications that provoke insulin resistance should be avoided if possible. Patients should be educated on symptoms of hyperglycaemia and they should be advised to seek medical attention should they develop such symptoms.[36] They should also be educated on the need for family planning to assure optimal glycaemic control from the start of any subsequent pregnancy. Offspring of women with GDM are at increased risk of obesity, glucose intolerance and diabetes in late adolescence and young adulthood.[14]

Pregestational diabetes

Preconceptional care of women with diabetes

Elements of an organized programme for preconceptional care are best based on the various published clinical trials that have been successful in preventing excess spontaneous abortions and major malformations in IDDM.[3,37,38]

Preconceptional care is also provided on the basis of a cost–benefit analysis.

The model for diabetes preconception and early pregnancy health care includes four main elements: (1) education of the patient about the interaction between diabetes, pregnancy and family planning; (2) education in diabetes self-management skills; (3) physician-directed medical care and laboratory testing; and (4) counselling by a mental health professional, when indicated, to reduce stress and improve adherence to the diabetes treatment plan.[36]

The desired outcome of the preconception phase of care is to lower HbA1c values to a level associated with optimal development during organogenesis. Epidemiological studies indicate that HbA1c test values up to 1% above normal are associated with rates of congenital malformations and spontaneous abortions that are not greater than rates in non-diabetic pregnancies. However, rates of each complication continue to decrease with even lower HbA1c test levels. Thus, the general goal for glycaemic management in the preconception period and during the first trimester should be to obtain the lowest HbA1c test level possible without undue risk of hypoglycaemia in the mother. To obtain these values, there is need for: an appropriate meal plan, SBGM, self-administration of insulin and self-adjustment of insulin doses, treatment of hypoglycaemia (patient and family members), incorporation of physical activity, and development of techniques to reduce stress and cope with denial.[36]

A complete anamnesis is imperative before planning for pregnancy. This should include, but not be limited to: questioning for duration and type of diabetes (Type 1 or Type 2); acute complications, including a history of infections, ketoacidosis and hypoglycaemia; chronic complications, including retinopathy, nephropathy, hypertension, atherosclerotic vascular disease, and autonomic and peripheral neuropathy; diabetes management, including insulin regimen, prior or current use of oral glucose-lowering agents, SBGM regimens and results, MNT, and physical activity; concomitant medical conditions and medications, e.g. thyroid disease (in particular for patients with Type 1 diabetes), menstrual/pregnancy history; contraceptive use and support system, including family and work environment.[36] To minimize the occurrence of malformations, standard care for all women with diabetes who have child-bearing potential should include: (1) counselling about the risk of malformations associated with unplanned pregnancies and poor metabolic control; (2) use of effective contraception at all times, unless the patient is in good metabolic control and actively trying to conceive;[36] (3) integration of the patient into the management of her condition; (4) identification and treatment of complications of diabetes such as retinopathy, nephropathy and hypertension.[39]

Diabetic retinopathy, nephropathy, autonomic neuropathy (especially gastroparesis) and coronary artery disease (CAD) can be affected by or can affect the outcome of pregnancy. Thus, physical examination should give particular attention to: blood pressure measurement, including testing for orthostatic changes; dilated retinal examination by an ophthalmologist or other eye specialist knowledgeable about diabetic eye disease; cardiovascular examination for evidence of cardiac or peripheral vascular disease – if found, patients should have screening tests for CAD before attempting pregnancy to assure that they can tolerate the increased cardiac demands; and a neurological examination, including examination for signs of autonomic neuropathy.

Laboratory evaluation should focus on assessment and detection of diabetic complications that may affect or be affected by pregnancy: serum creatinine and urinary excretion of total protein and/or albumin (albumin: creatinine ratio or 24-hour excretion rate). Patients with protein excretion > 190 mg/24 hours have been shown to be at increased risk for hypertens- ive disorders during pregnancy. Patients with protein excretion > 400 mg/24 hours are also at risk for intrauterine growth retardation during later pregnancy. No specific treatments are indicated but patients should be counselled about these risks. Since patients should not take angiotensin-converting enzyme (ACE) inhibitors during pregnancy, these assessments should be carried out after cessation of these drugs.

Women with incipient renal failure (serum creatinine > 265.2 µmol/l or creatinine clearance < 50 ml/minute) should be counselled that pregnancy may induce a permanent worsening of renal function in > 40% of patients. In subjects with less severe nephropathy, renal function may worsen transiently during pregnancy, but permanent worsening occurs at a rate no different from the background. Therefore, it should not serve as a contraindication to conception and pregnancy. As mentioned above, the presence of proteinuria > 190 mg/24 hours before or during early pregnancy is associated with a tripling of the risk of hypertensive disorders in the second half of pregnancy. ACE inhibitors for treatment of microalbuminuria should be discontinued in women who are attempting to become pregnant.

The presence of autonomic neuropathy, particularly manifested by gastroparesis, urinary retention, hypoglycaemic unawareness or orthostatic hypotension, may complicate the management of diabetes in pregnancy. These complications should be identified, appropriately evaluated and treated before conception. Peripheral neuropathy, especially compartment syndromes such as carpal tunnel syndrome, may be exacerbated by pregnancy.

Measurement of serum thyroid stimulating hormone and/or free thyroxin level in women with Type 1 diabetes should be performed because of the 5–10% coincidence of hyper- or hypothyroidism; other tests may follow as indicated by physical examination or patient history.

Successful preconception care programmes have used the following pre- and postprandial glycaemic goals: **before meals** – capillary whole-blood glucose 70–100 mg/dl (3.9–5.6 mmol/l), or capillary plasma glucose 80–110 mg/dl (4.4–6.1 mmol/l) at 2 hours; **after meals** – capillary whole-blood glucose < 140 mg/dl (< 7.8 mmol/l) at 2 hours, or capillary plasma glucose < 155 mg/dl (< 8.6 mmol/l) at 2 hours.[14] The treatment plan should be implemented and HbA1c levels monitored at 1–2 week intervals until stable. Then, the patient should be counselled about the risk associated with her HbA1c level. If she does not achieve a low-risk level of < 1% above the upper limit of normal, modification of the treatment regimen should considered, including addition of postprandial glucose monitoring.[7] Glycaemic goals may need to be modified according to the patient's recognition of hypoglycaemia and risk of severe neuroglycopenia. Outpatient management is the appropriate forum for achieving preconception glycaemic goals.

Once the patient has achieved stable glycaemic control (assessed by the HbA1c test) as good as can be achieved, then she can be counselled about the risk of malformations and spontaneous abortions. If the risk, as well as the status of maternal diabetic complications and any coexisting medical conditions are acceptable, then contraception can be discontinued. If conception does not occur within 1 year, the patient's fertility should be assessed.

Metabolic monitoring during pregnancy

Metabolic and weight targets for diabetic pregnant women are similar to those presented for the GDM patient. Close attention should be paid to the management of insulin doses, considering that during pregnancy insulin needs progressively increase from the first to the third trimester, and that it inversely reduces in the immediate postpartum period. Therefore, educational support for self-management, both for the home SBGM and for the insulin self-adjustment, are very important.

Moreover, a strict control of blood pressure should be guaranteed. According to the recent classification by the fifth report of the Joint National Committee (JNCV),[40] four levels of blood pressure control are defined. The first stage corresponds to blood pressures of 140–159/90–99 mmHg and indicate the lowest degree of severity. However, due to the fact that diabetic pregnant women have a higher risk of hypertensive disorder, some authors suggest starting antihypertensive treatment when blood pressure levels are > 135/85 mmHg. The contraindication of ACE-inhibitor treatment during pregnancy has to be reinforced due to the higher risk of fetal malformation. Diuretics and beta blockers should also be avoided during pregnancy.

One of the greatest risks for the diabetic mother is the worsening of a pre-existing diabetic retinopathy. In the case of development of proliferative lesions, laser treatment can be used during pregnancy.

Hospitalization is not an elective choice for pregnant women with diabetes but it should be considered in cases of severe complications like ketoacidosis, hypoglycaemic coma or pre-eclampsia.

Also, Caesarean sections should be avoided whenever possible. However, Caesarean sections are recommended in the following cases: pre-eclampsia, fetal malformations, abnormal fetal presentation, advanced aged mother and previous Caesarean section(s).

References

1. Hawthorne G, Robson S, Ryall EA et al. Prospective population based survey of outcome of pregnancy in diabetic women: results of the Northern Diabetic Pregnancy Audit, 1994. *Br Med J* 1997; **315**:279–81.

2. Casson IF, Clarke CA, Howard CV et al. Outcomes of pregnancy in insulin dependent diabetic women: results of a five year population cohort study. *Br Med J* 1997; **315**:275–8.

3. Kitzmiller JL, Buchanan TA, Kjos S et al. Pre-conception care of diabetes, congenital malformations, and spontaneous abortions. *Diabetes Care* 1996; **19**:514–41.

4. King H. Epidemiology of glucose intolerance and gestational diabetes in women of child bearing age. *Diabetes Care* 1998; **21** (**Suppl 2**):B9–B13.

5. Metzger BE, Coustan DR. Summary and recommendations of the Fourth International Workshop–Conference on Gestational Diabetes Mellitus. The Organizing Committee. *Diabetes Care* 1998; **21** (**Suppl 2**):B161–B167.

6. Carr SB. Screening for gestational diabetes mellitus. *Diabetes Care* 1998; **21** (**Suppl 2**):B14–B18.

7. International Diabetes Federation – European Region. *Guidelines for Diabetes Care. A Desktop Guide to Type 2 Diabetes Mellitus.* (Walter Wirtz Druck & Verlag, editors; Germany, 1998).

8. Homko CJ, Sivan E, Reece EA. Is self-monitoring of blood glucose necessary in the management of gestational diabetes mellitus? *Diabetes Care* 1998; **21** (**Suppl 2**):B118–B122.

9. De Veciana M, Major CA, Morgan MA et al. Postprandial versus preprandial blood glucose monitoring in women with gestational diabetes mellitus requiring insulin therapy. *N Engl J Med* 1995; **333**:1237–41.

10. Hoffman L, Nolan C, Wilson JD et al. Gestational diabetes mellitus – management guidelines. The Australasian Diabetes in Pregnancy Society. *Med J Aust* 1998; **169**:93–7.

11. American Diabetes Association. Gestational diabetes mellitus. *Diabetes Care* 2001; **24** (**Suppl 1**):77.

12. Franz MJ, Horton ES, Bantle JP et al. Nutrition principles for the management of diabetes and related complications (technical review). *Diabetes Care* 1994; **17**:490–518.

13. Luke B, Murtaugh MA. Dietetic treatment. In: (Reece EA, Coustan DR, eds) *Diabetes Mellitus in Pregnancy.* (Churchill Livingstone: New York 1998).

14. Lapolla A, Botta RM, Vitacolonna E. Diabete in gravidanza. *Il Diabete* 2001; **13**:269–83.

15. Buchanan TA, Kjos Sl, Schafer U et al. Utility of foetal measurements in the management of gestational diabetes mellitus. *Diabetes Care* 1998; **21** (**Suppl 2**):B99–B106.

16. Langer O. Maternal glycaemic criteria for insulin therapy in gestational diabetes mellitus. *Diabetes Care* 1998; **21** (**Suppl 2**):B91–B98.

17. Jovanovic L, Ilic SS, Gutierrez M, Bastyri EI. Insulin lispro improves postprandial glucose without increased immunogenecity or hypoglycaemia in gestational diabetic women. *Diabetes* 1998; **47(Suppl 1)**:A49.

18. American Diabetes Association. Gestational diabetes mellitus. *Diabetes Care* 2002; **25**:S94–S96.

19. Nachum Z, Ben-Shlomo I, Weiner E, Shalev E. Twice daily versus four times daily insulin dose regimens for diabetes in pregnancy: randomised controlled trial. *Br Med J* 1999; **319**:1223–7.

20. Simmons D, Thompson CF, Conroy C, Scott DJ. Use of insulin pumps in pregnancies complicated by Type 2 diabetes and gestational diabetes in a multiethnic community. *Diabetes Care* 2001; **24**:2078–82.

21. Carta Q, Meriggi E, Trossarelli GF et al. Continuous subcutaneous insulin infusion versus intensive conventional insulin therapy in type I and type II diabetic pregnancy. *Diabetes Metab* 1986; **12**:121–9.

22. Langer O, Conway DL, Berkus MD et al. A comparison of glyburide and insulin in women with gestational diabetes mellitus. *N Engl J Med* 2000; **343**:1134–8.

23. Jovanovic L, Kessler A, Peterson GM. Human maternal and fetal response to graded exercise. *J Appl Physiol* 1985; **56**:1719–22.

24. Collings C, Curet IB. Fetal heart rate response to maternal exercise. *Am J Obstet Gynecol* 1985; **151**:498–501.

25. Erkkola R. The physical work capacity of the expectant mother and its effect on pregnancy, labor and newborn. *Int J Gynecol Obstet* 1976; **14**:153–9.

26. Veille JC, Hohimer RA, Burry K, Speroff L. The effect of exercise on uterine activity in the last eight weeks of pregnancy. *Am J Obstet Gynecol* 1985; **151**:727–30.

27. Durak EP, Jovanovic-Peterson L, Peterson CM. Comparative evaluation of uterine response to exercise on five aerobic machines. *Am J Obstet Gynecol* 1990; **162**:754–6.

28. Jovanovic L. American Diabetes Association's Fourth International Workshop–Conference on Gestational Diabetes Mellitus: Summary and Discussion. Therapeutic interventions. *Diabetes Care* 1998; **21 (Suppl 2)**: B131–B137.

29. Zamorski MA, Biggs WS. Management of suspected foetal macrosomia. *Am Fam Phys* 2001; **63**:302–5.

30. Coustan DR. Delivery time, mode and management. In: (Reece EA, Coustan DR, eds) *Diabetes Mellitus in Pregnancy*. (Churchill Livingstone: New York, 1998).

31. Hod M, Bar J, Peled Y et al. Antepartum management protocol. Timing and mode of delivery in gestational diabetes. *Diabetes Care* 1998; **21 (Suppl 2)**: B113–B117.

32. Persson B, Hanson U. Neonatal morbidities in gestational diabetes mellitus. *Diabetes Care* 1998; **21 (Suppl 2)**:B79–B84.

33. Dalfrà MG, Lapolla A, Masin M et al. Antepartum and early post-partum predictors of type 2 diabetes development in women with gestational diabetes mellitus. *Diabetes Metab* 2001; **27**:675–80.

34. Dornhorst A, Rossi M. Risk and prevention of type 2 diabetes in women with gestational diabetes. *Diabetes Care* 1998; **21 (Suppl 2)**:B43–B49.

35. American Diabetes Association. Report of the Expert Committee on the diagnosis and classification of diabetes mellitus. *Diabetes Care* 2002; **25(Suppl 1)**:S5–S20.

36. American Diabetes Association. Preconception care of women with diabetes. *Diabetes Care* 2002; **25 (Suppl 1)**:S82–S84.

37. Rosenn B, Miodovnik M, Combs CA et al. Glycaemic thresholds for spontaneous abortion and congenital malformations in insulin-dependent diabetes mellitus. *Obstet Gynecol* 1994; **84**:515–20.

38. Willhoite MB, Bennert HW, Palomaki GE et al. The impact of preconception counselling on pregnancy outcomes. The experience of the Maine Diabetes in Pregnancy Program. *Diabetes Care* 1993; **16**:450–5.

39. Elixhauser A, Weschler JM, Kitzmiller JL et al. Cost–benefit analysis of preconception care for women with established diabetes mellitus. *Diabetes Care* 1993; **16**:1146–57.

40. Joint National Committee. The Fifth Report of the Joint National Committee on Detection and Treatment of High Blood Pressure. *Arch Intern Med* 1993; **153**:154.

26

Nutritional management in diabetic pregnancy: a time for reason not dogma

Anne Dornhorst, Gary Frost

Introduction

The nutritional management of a diabetic pregnancy is controversial. To date there have been too few clinical studies of sufficient quality assessing different nutritional managements on pregnancy outcomes in diabetic women to provide evidence-based guidelines. All too often women with Type 1 diabetes and gestational diabetes mellitus (GDM) are considered together, when in fact their nutritional needs are different and should be considered separately. The lack of nutritional evidence-based studies has resulted in diametrically opposed views being expressed in the literature, as exemplified by some experts advocating high-carbohydrate/low-fat diets, while others favour low-carbohydrate/high-fat diets, when in reality there is not enough evidence to support either. As more definitive dietetic studies are awaited, a non-dogmatic approach to the nutritional management of the diabetic pregnant woman needs to be adopted, emphasizing those areas where evidence allows consensus while acknowledging those areas of uncertainty. There is now good animal evidence for a link between maternal nutrition in pregnancy and fetal programming. Animal studies have shown that small manipulations of maternal nutrition can have long-term detrimental metabolic

effects for the progeny. While these studies provide plausible explanations for human epidemiological studies linking maternal diet with adult diseases, more importantly, and worryingly, these animal studies highlight the potential harm that could be done to the future health of children by imposing radical changes to the macronutrient composition of the maternal diet in pregnancy. It will be important in the future that advice on nutritional interventions in pregnancy should receive the same critical scrutiny and appraisal as that given to all pharmaceutical products.

Scope of this chapter

In this chapter the general principles of nutrition in pregnancy are covered briefly before concentrating on how these principles may need to be adapted in the presence of diabetes. In particular, the different challenges facing the nutritional management of a Type 1 diabetic mother, than one with Type 2 diabetes or GDM, will be highlighted. Those topics of nutritional management that are most controversial will be focused on. These include the role of energy restriction in the overweight diabetic women, the merits of favouring carbohydrate or fat as the major dietary macronutrient and the potential of manipulating dietary micronutrients to reduced diabetic teratogenesis. The concerns of giving dietetic advice in pregnancy that is fundamentally different from that given outside pregnancy will also be considered. Finally, the potential of delaying the progression to diabetes following GDM, through dietary advice given at the time of pregnancy, will be discussed.

Principles of nutritional management for a non-diabetic pregnancy

- The energy content of the diet should ensure that the energy costs of pregnancy and lactation are met, without causing unnecessary weight gain either intra- or postpartum.
- Vitamin and mineral intakes should meet recommended daily allowances for pregnancy. A balanced diet usually provides all the vitamins and minerals required with the exception of folate. Prior to conception and during the first 12 weeks of pregnancy the folate intake should be increased to minimize the risk of neural tube defects, this can be achieved by consuming a folate-rich diet plus an additional daily 400 µg folic acid supplement.[1] Many women require iron supplements during pregnancy and lactation, while adolescent pregnancies should receive calcium supplements. Women with poor sunlight exposure and low calcium intakes may also need calcium and vitamin D supplements.[2,3]
- Certain foods that carry a potential risk of infection or others which are potentially toxic should be avoided. Such foods include: raw meat with the risk of toxoplasmosis; soft and mould-ripened cheeses, and

pates with the small risk of listeria infections. Supplements of vitamin A should not be given due to the association of excess vitamin A levels with facial deformities.[2] Alcohol should be minimized or withdrawn altogether due to its association with fetal developmental problems.[4]

Principles of nutritional management for a diabetic woman in pregnancy

- Dietary advice throughout pregnancy needs to focus on optimizing glycaemic control, avoiding large fluctuations of blood glucose, especially in the postprandial period, while avoiding ketosis, and minimizing the risk of hypoglycaemia in those women taking insulin.
- The energy content and the mixture of nutrients in the diet must be sufficient to allow normal fetal growth throughout pregnancy while avoiding accelerated fetal growth patterns. Limiting unnecessary weight gain in already obese diabetic women must be balanced against compromising fetal growth and development, and inducing ketosis.
- Folic acid supplementation is particularly important early in a diabetic pregnancy due to the increased risk of spina bifida and other neural tube malformations in such pregnancies. Higher dose folic acid supplements, 5 mg daily, are often recommended despite any evidence of abnormal folate metabolism in pregnant diabetic women.[5]
- Women with GDM need to be given dietary and lifestyle advice at the end of pregnancy that will minimize their future risk of Type 2 diabetes and cardiovascular disease.

Energy requirements in pregnancy

As a consequence of metabolic adaptation in pregnancy, the dietary increase required to meet the energy requirements of pregnancy are extremely modest. In the West, a well-nourished woman will need to increase her food intake by only 200 kcal/day (0.8 MJ/day) above her estimated average requirements (EAR) for only the last trimester. These figures on energy requirements form the basis of the current UK Department of Health official dietary reference values for pregnancy.[6] The American recommendations are slightly higher than those for the UK, being an extra 300 kcal/day during both the second and third trimesters.[7]

During pregnancy energy is required for the synthesis of the fetal–placental unit and maternal tissues that together result in a 15–26% increase in the metabolic rate.[8] The total calculated energy cost of pregnancy was derived theoretically 40 years ago; it was confirmed more recently using modern physiological techniques to be 85,000 kcal (336 MJ), or an extra 285 kcal/day (1.2 MJ/day).[9–11] Interestingly, in well-nourished women, longitudinal nutritional studies show that only 20% of the pregnancy energy requirements are accounted for by an increase in dietary intake.[11,12] Despite this many dietary recommendations today still reflect the assumption that the earlier energy costs of pregnancy need to be covered by an increase in dietary intake.[13]

The study of human anthropology has shown that maternal physiology is highly adaptable. This allows reproduction to continue during periods of extreme food deprivation or physical activity.[12] Under adverse environmental conditions human pregnancies can usually conserve sufficient energy to support a fetus to term, by reducing maternal adipose deposition and diet-induced thermogenesis, and by decreasing physical activity.[8,11,14,15] If calorie restriction is further compromised, maternal basal metabolic rate may also fall in the first half of pregnancy.[12] A 20% reduction in maternal physical activity will itself meet the total energy costs of most pregnancies.[9] In women with high physical expenditure before pregnancy a decrease in physical activity during pregnancy will contribute to these energy costs.[11,17]

In conclusion, the energy requirements in pregnancy in well-nourished women are extremely modest, which is reflected by the American recommendations of an additional food intake of 300 kcal/day (1.2 MJ/day) during the second and third trimesters,[7] and the UK recommendations of 200 kcal/day (0.8 MJ/day) in the third trimester only. As many diabetic women are obese with adequate pre-pregnancy adipose stores to sustain a complete pregnancy and the period of lactation, a theoretical question arises as to whether any increase in maternal fat stores are required for these women in pregnancy.

Influence of obesity and excessive weight gain on pregnancy outcome

Women with GDM and Type 2 diabetes are usually obese. Both obesity and diabetes are independent risk factors for many of the same adverse pregnancy outcomes; those for obesity are listed in Box 26.1.[18,19] There is a suggestion that when obesity and diabetes coexist then their effects on pregnancy outcome may not only be additive but also synergistic. Epidemiological studies have demonstrated a synergistic interaction between obesity and diabetes in terms of congenital abnormalities.[20,21] Why obesity is associated with congenital

Worsening glucose tolerance
Increased hypertension
Increased Caesarean deliveries
Higher incidence of anaesthetic and postoperative complications
Increased perinatal morbidity and mortality (including stillbith)
Lower Apgar scores
Macrosomia (although fewer small-for-gestational-age infants)
Delivery at or before 32 weeks gestation
Increased non-chromosomal congenital birth defects (orofacial clefts; club foot; cardiac septal and neural defects)
Long-term obesity in the child and worsening obesity in the mother

Box 26.1.   Obesity associated adverse pregnancy outcomes.

abnormalities is currently unknown; however, any influence obesity may have on diabetic malformation rates is important, as potentially weight reduction in obese women prior to conception could help to reduce congenital abnormalities.[22] The majority of women with pre-existing Type 2 diabetes or those who develop GDM are obese [body mass indexes (BMI) > 30 kg/m^2], as are a much smaller percentage of women with Type 1 diabetes. Ideally, the nutritional management of these obese diabetic women should start before pregnancy with a supervised controlled weight-reducing diet. As soon as a pregnancy has been confirmed a daily calorie intake needs to be calculated on an individual basis for all obese women to help minimize unnecessary weight gain and accelerated fetal growth, while ensuring that optimal glycaemic control is achieved without hypoglycaemia or ketosis.

Case for energy restriction in obese diabetic woman

As mentioned above, human metabolism in pregnancy is highly efficient at conserving energy in pregnancy, by a combination of limiting maternal fat deposition, curtailing physical activity and reducing postprandial thermogenesis. Studies in very obese non-diabetic women (BMI > 35 kg/m^2) have shown infant birthweights are not compromised when women gain no or little weight in pregnancy.[23] Similarly, women with BMI > 30 kg/m^2 but < 35 kg/m^2 who experience no net weight gain after pregnancy do not appear to experience any increase in perinatal morbidity. Despite large epidemiological studies to this effect, the standard weight-gain recommendation of pregnancy provided by the Institute of Medicine in 1990[24] suggests that even the most obese women should gain at least the weight to cover the products of conception (Table 26.1). These recommendations have subsequently been endorsed by the American College of Obstetrics and Gynecology[25] and the American Diabetic Association.[26] However, the appropriateness of these figures have been questioned by others, and there is a need for large-scale randomized trials to assess the short-term and longer term impact of limiting weight gain in pregnancy in overweight and obese women.[25,26]

If a women remains weight neutral throughout pregnancy, a degree of calorie restriction during pregnancy will have occurred and she will lose weight at delivery. There are genuine

Pre-pregnancy BMI (kg/m²) category	Total weight gain (kg)	Weight gain (kg/4 weeks) in 2nd and 3rd trimesters
Underweight (BMI < 19.8)	12.7–18.2	2.3
Normal (BMI 20.1–26.0)	11.4–15.9	1.8
Overweight (BMI 26.1–29.0)	6.8–20.4	1.2
Obesity (BMI > 29.0)	> 6.8	0.6
Twin	15.9–20.4	2.7

Table 26.1. Recommended total weight gain ranges for pregnant women by pregnancy body mass index (BMI) (with permission from Institute of Medicine[24]).

and well-founded concerns regarding the long-term effect of maternal calorie restriction on infant psychological and physical development, as well as long-term metabolic effects on carbohydrate metabolism. Dutch infants born during the 5 month 1994–1995 famine to previously well-nourished women who in late pregnancy had access to only 800 kcals/day were thinner at birth and at 18 years of age, but were otherwise healthy. However, 40 years on these same infants had a higher than expected incidence of glucose intolerance and diabetes[27] and the females were more obese.[28] The epidemiological studies of Baker and co-workers,[29–31] showing an association between thin infants at birth and a future increased adult risk of diabetes and cardiovascular disease, provides supporting evidence that calorie restriction to the point that fetal growth is compromised is to be avoided. Calorie restriction also predisposes to fasting ketosis that is more exaggerated in pregnancy and occurs earlier. Increased maternal ketonaemia, with raised plasma β-hydroxybutyrate and free fatty acid levels, has been associated with lower intelligence scores in the offspring at 2–5 years of age and poor fetal neurophysiological development.[32–34] The degree of maternal ketosis, if any, that can be induced through calorie restriction that poses

no risk to the neurophysiological development of the child is not known.

To what extent and to what degree one should actively promote calorie restriction to obese pregnant women with GDM or Type 2 diabetes remains a major area of controversy surrounding the nutritional management of diabetic pregnancies. The necessary randomized trials with long-term follow-up have not yet been done. It is likely that obese women with GDM can be calorie restricted more safely than similarly obese but not diabetic women, as glucose intolerance in pregnancy is associated with higher hepatic glucose outputs and this will help to protect against diet-induced ketosis.[35–37] Meanwhile, ketosis due to calorie restriction can be reduced with frequent small meals containing slowly absorbed carbohydrates. Such snacks promote an attenuated insulin response that delays lipolysis and ketogenesis between meals in non-diabetic patients.[38]

In a study carried out by this group modest calorie restriction was implemented in obese GDM women (20–25 kcal/kg/day) from 24 weeks gestation; a reduction in the incidence of large-for-gestational-age (LGA) infants below that of obese glucose tolerant non-dieted controls was shown. In this study the 28-weeks-to-term weight gain in the women with GDM was half that of the controls (1.7±1.6 versus 4.1±3.1 kg).[39] This degree of calorie restriction has been reported to be associated with an improvement in glycaemic control.[36]

Extrapolating from large epidemiological studies, the present authors support limiting weight gain in all obese GDM pregnancies to the bottom rather than the top of that recommended for non-diabetic pregnancies. The present authors advocate that on present epidemiological evidence there is no clinical reason why women with a pre-pregnancy BMI > 35 kg/m² should be set any minimum weight-gain target. Ideally, some of these women could remain weight neutral in pregnancy and be given dietary advice to have frequent small meals containing slowly absorbed carbohydrates to prevent ketosis, with regular fetal ultrasound performed to ensure that fetal growth is not compromised. Adopting an approach of mild calorie restriction in overweight and obese women will help towards achieving no overall weight gain postpartum. A slightly greater degree of calorie restriction is probably safe in morbidly obese woman, which could potentially lead to weight loss after pregnancy. In the present authors' practice an individual's energy requirement is calculated using their pre-pregnancy weight: the resting energy expenditure is established using Schofield's formula[40] and a physical activity ratio of 1.6 is employed. To this is added 200 kcal for the energy requirements for the third trimester. If a mild degree of negative energy balance is required then 500 kcal is subtracted from this calculated daily energy requirement to provide the total energy for the diet.

There is a clear need for controlled studies looking at the influence of mild to moderate calorie restriction on fetal growth and early childhood development. With the rising epidemic of childhood obesity and adolescent diabetes the influence, if any, of maternal weight and weight gain, as a contributing factor to these statistics needs to be examined.

Factors influencing glycaemic control during a diabetic pregnancy

The nutritional advice for all pregnant diabetic women should be aimed at achieving euglycaemia while avoiding hypoglycaemia and ketosis. Many of the clinical problems of a diabetic pregnancy are directly attributable to maternal hyperglycaemia and the accompanying fetal hyperinsulinaemia. In early pregnancy hyperglycaemia is a key factor in the pathogenesis of congenital abnormalities; in later pregnancy it is a major determinant of accelerated fetal growth, stillbirth, and neonatal hypoglycaemia and hypocalcaemia. Although euglycaemia is strived for in all diabetic pregnancies its achievement in Type 1 and, to a lesser extent, Type 2 diabetic women is rarely possible due to the multiple factors that influence fasting and postprandial blood glucose values. These factors are listed in Box 26.2, which includes the physiological changes of pregnancy, the presence of comorbidities, changes in lifestyle, insulin treatment and finally the diet itself. The extent to which dietary manipulation interacts with these other variables to influence glycaemic control will differ between individuals and will change during the duration of the pregnancy. In women with Type 1 diabetes the interaction between dietary factors, insulin adjustments and blood glucose are so interdependable that it is unwise to consider any one without the others. Therefore, it follows that all diets should be adapted on an individual basis and be flexible enough to adjust to the expected and unexpected changes encountered during pregnancy.

Physiological changes of pregnancy
Increased insulin resistance
Increased hepatic glucose output
Increased tendency to ketosis
Gastric stasis
Lactation

Comorbidities
Hyperemesis gravidarum
Autonomic dysfunction with impaired hypoglycaemic awareness
Acid reflux
Intercurrent illness

Changes in lifestyle
Reduction in physical activity

Insulin treatment
Type and frequency of insulin
Mode of delivery

Dietary factors
Changes in appetite
Meal frequency and timing
Meal composition
Glycaemic index

Box 26.2. Factors influencing glycaemic control during a diabetic pregnancy.

Factors influencing glycaemic exposure of the fetus

Maternal glucose is the predominant fetal fuel substrate. Reducing maternal hyperglycaemia reduces fetal exposure to glucose, as glucose crosses the placenta in a concentration-dependent manner using specific glucose transporters.[41] Feto-placental growth is highly dependent on maternal substrate delivery along with placental-bed blood flow.[42] While severe and prolonged reductions in maternal substrate delivery result in a reduced fetal growth rate and birthweight, the reverse of chronic over-exposure, as occurs with maternal hyper-glycaemia, results in accelerated fetal growth rate and birth size.[43,44] As maximal maternal–fetal glucose transfer occurs postprandially, nutritional management needs to target the postprandial glycaemic response. In the third trimester the 1 hour postprandial glucose value, rather than the premeal glucose value, is a strong predictor of infant birthweight in women with Type 1 diabetes, with a continuum of risk of an infant > 90% seen above a blood glucose level of > 7.3 mmol/l.[45,46] It is therefore rational that treatment interventions should target glucose concentrations at this time. In women with GDM adjusting treatment to the 1 hour postprandial reading is more effective at limiting accelerated fetal growth than trying to lower fasting glucose values.[47]

There are basically two dietary means by which postprandial glucose excursions can be attenuated: firstly by limiting overall dietary carbohydrate at the expense of increasing dietary fat; and secondly by increasing the use of low glycaemic index carbohydrates. Both of these approaches need to be critically assessed together with a more detailed analysis of the type, as well as the absolute amount, of dietary carbohydrate and fat that is associated with the most favourable metabolic response.

Case for and against a relatively high-fat/low-carbohydrate diet

Postprandial glucose is a reflection of both the quantity and type of carbohydrate in the meal, and food preparation and physiological functions, such as the rate of gastric emptying, enzymic digestion and finally the rate of intestinal absorption (Box 26.3). The type of dietary carbohydrate varies between populations and cultures. For example, in rural Africa dietary carbohydrate comprises of low glycaemic starches and soluble non-starch polysaccharides that give a much lower glycaemic response than the dietary carbohydrate obtained from highly processed foods and soft drinks consumed in industrialized Western countries.[48] This difference helps to explain why healthy non-obese African women consuming traditional diets do not invariably experience a deterioration in their glucose tolerance during pregnancy, despite dietary carbohydrate forming > 60% of their diet.[49] While the glycaemic index of carbohydrates are likely to be highly relevant in diet-controlled women with GDM, for women with Type 1 diabetes the impact dietary carbohydrate has on the glycaemic response is less, provided that the premeal insulin is adjusted proactively in anticipation of the carbohydrate content.[50]

A pragmatic approach to limiting the postprandial glucose response is to restrict all forms of dietary carbohydrate. This is most easily achieved by replacing the energy content of the carbohydrate in the diet with fat. The current guidelines of the American Diabetic Association[51] endorse limiting carbohydrate to 40–45% of the total energy content while increasing dietary fat to 40%. This advice is based on a few clinical studies in obese women with GDM rather than of Type 1 diabetic women. In one study, improved glycaemic control and a reduced risk of delivering a LGA

Amount of carbohydrate
Type of sugar (glucose, fructose, sucrose, lactose)
Nature of the starch (amylose, amylopectin, resistant starch)
Cooking and food processing (degree of starch gelatinization, particle size, cellular form)
Food structure
Other food components (fat and natural substances that slow digestion – lectins, phytates, tannins, and starch–protein and starch–lipid combinations)
Fasting and preprandial glucose concentrations
Severity of glucose intolerance
The second meal, or lente effect, and the timing of the daily intake

Box 26.3. Factors influencing the glycaemic response to food (adapted from Franz et al,[53] with permission).

infant was shown when 21 obese GDM, predominately Hispanic women, consumed < 42% of their calorie intake as carbohydrate as opposed to 21 similarly obese GDM women taking > 45% but < 50% dietary carbohydrate in the second half of pregnancy.[52] In an earlier study on 14 obese women with GDM, in the third trimester the carbohydrate content of the meal was shown to be correlated with the 1 hour postprandial glucose, such that to maintain a 1 hour postprandial capillary blood value < 7.8 mmol/l the carbohydrates at breakfast needed to be < 45%, < 55% at lunch and 50% at dinner. In this small study it was calculated that to drop the 1 hour postprandial blood glucose to < 6.7 mmol the carbohydrate content of breakfast, lunch and dinner would need to fall to 33, 45 and 40%, respectively.[46] It remains unproven as to whether similar proportions for meal carbohydrate are safe in Type 1 diabetic mothers in whom the possibility of hypoglycaemia increases with increasingly tight glycaemic control.

One important question to answer is if dietary carbohydrate is to be reduced and dietary fat increased, which type of fat should be advocated: saturated fat (SF), polyunsaturated fatty acids (PUFA), monounsaturated fatty acids (MUFA) or *n*-3 polyunsaturated fatty acids? Any advantage of a low carbohydrate high fat diet on glycaemic control needs to be considered against any adverse effect this type of diet may have on other metabolic parameters, such as insulin resistance or hypertriglyceridaemia.

Metabolic effects of dietary fats in pregnancy

Reducing the intake of SF and cholesterol in the diet is central to the nutritional management of diabetes, and the current evidence-based recommendation is that SF intake be < 10% of the total energy intake for the nongravid diabetic subject.[53] If one was to advocate an increase in the SF dietary content during a diabetic pregnancy, for woman with an already increased risk of heart disease, there would need to be clear evidence for its superior benefits over other alternative nutrients.

Under test-meal conditions women with GDM have been shown to have lower 3 hour glycaemic and insulin responses to a breakfast containing SF than to an equivalent isocaloric breakfast containing MUFA.[54] This type of clinical study involving test meals performed on small numbers, in this case only 10 women, are subject to overinterpretation, as they may not give an accurate metabolic picture to what would happen over the duration of a pregnancy if this type of meal was consumed on an habitual basis. Test meals fail to take into account any potential effects they may have on the metabolic responses of subsequent meals, or the overall effect such meals may have on appetite, nausea and total calorie intake. Differences in gastric emptying time may explain some of the observed differences in the glycaemic and insulin responses between the SF and MUFA test meals. Even if a high SF breakfast was to benefit the glycaemic response mid-morning, a time of the day recognized as being particularly difficult to control in diabetic pregnancies, advocating a high SF meal needs to be considered in the light of epidemiological evidence that severe hyperemesis gravidarum is increased 5.4-fold for each 15 grams per day increase in dietary saturated fat.[55] In addition, if women with GDM were to continue on a high-fat diet after pregnancy they would be increasing their risk of having GDM again in a subsequent pregnancy.[56] On the basis of the human data available, advising a diet with a SF intake > 10% in the nutritional management of diabetic pregnancies is premature, especially as the long-term effects on the children are not known and similar diets in animal studies suggest high SF diets in pregnancy can promote cardiovascular disease in the progeny.[57,58]

The adult female offspring of pregnant rats fed a diet high in SF, 20% of total energy, for 10 days prior to, throughout pregnancy and during weaning, develop a more athrogenic lipoprotein profile than offspring of controlled rats receiving a normal pregnancy diet consisting of 4% fat. Furthermore, the offspring of rats fed the high SF diet also had a marked reduction in the content of arachidonic and docosahexaenoic acids in the fatty acid compositions of their aortas.[57] Similar high-fat diets given to pregnant rats have been shown to lead to vascular dysfunction in the young adult offspring, with the greasest changes seen in the offspring of diabetic rats.[58]

The possibility of long-term adverse effects from a maternal high SF diet on fetal programming have not been evaluated in human pregnancies, but given the overwhelming evidence linking SF intake to future cardiovascular disease, such diets should not be advocated as there are alternative dietary means available to reduce postprandial hyperglycaemia.

Increasing the PUFA content of the diet while ensuring a high PUFA:SF ratio provides a potentially safe alternative approach to reducing dietary carbohydrate in pregnancy. In a large epidemiological studies involving non-diabetic pregnancies, the habitual intake of PUFA correlated with the degree of glucose tolerance observed in pregnancy, such that women with a high content of PUFA in the diet were protected against developing GDM.[59] In this study 8002 consecutive pregnant women in Shanghai, China, were stratified into tertiles according their PUFA dietary intakes; the incidence of abnormal glucose tolerance in pregnancy was observed to be 70, 54 and 44% in the low, middle and upper tertiles, respectively.

A decreased PUFA intake, whether expressed as %kcal, % of total fat, or fat kcal was an independent predictor of glucose intolerance, as was a low dietary PUFA:SF ratio.[59] How transferable the findings of this epidemiological study conducted in China are to women in the West is unknown. In China, women eat and prepare traditional meals in their homes using soybean and vegetable oils as the food sources of PUFA, while in the West, unlike China, PUFA intake is correlated with SF intake. It is therefore possible that similar high PUFA intakes in the West would not give similar protection against GDM or deteriorating glucose intolerance due to an accompanying rise in SF intake.

Outside pregnancy MUFA diets have been associated with favourable metabolic changes, including improved insulin resistance and serum triglyceride levels.[60] When either high-carbohydrate diets or MUFA-enriched diets replace SF, reductions in plasma low-density lipoprotein (LDL) cholesterol have been reported.[61] There is, however, concern that when high-MUFA diets are eaten *ad libitum* outside of a study setting, overall energy intake increases resulting in weight gain.[62] Recently, a small Danish study failed to show any improvement in insulin sensitivity in the third trimester of pregnancy when women with GDM ate high-MUFA diets compared with high-carbohydrate diets, although the high-MUFA diets did seem to have a favourable effect on blood pressure.[63] Further metabolic studies with diets enriched with MUFA are required before any firm recommendations on the use of MUFA in pregnancy can be made.

Long-chain *n*-3 fatty acids (omega-3 fatty acids) are found in fish and fish oils, and recently, their consumption in early pregnancy has been shown to be protective against low birthweights and preterm deliveries in a Swedish prospective cohort study of 8729 pregnant women.[64] Increasing the dietary intake of *n*-3 PUFA in Type 2 diabetic subjects has been shown to have some favourable metabolic effects, e.g. including lowering serum triglycerides, however, this benefit may be counteracted by an accompanying rise in plasma LDL cholesterol.[65,66] Other food sources of *n*-3 PUFA include flaxseed and flaxseed oil, canola oil, soybean oil, and nuts. General population studies suggest that foods containing *n*-3 fatty acids, specifically eicosapentaenoic acid and docosahexaenoic acid, may be cardioprotective.[67,68] Therefore, there are potential benefits in increasing dietary long-chain *n*-3 fatty acids for diabetic pregnant women that warrant further evaluation.

As the evidence for a precise SF:PUFA:MUFA:fish oil ratio is not known for pregnancy, a pragmatic view would be to reflect the recommendations for diabetes and coronary heart disease aiming for a SF:PUFA:MUFA ratio 1:1:1 with the specific advice to eat oily fish three times a week.[69]

Is there an optimal macronutrient mix of dietary carbohydrate and fat?

In Western societies with high consumptions of highly processed foods, glycaemic control deteriorates in women with GDM when the carbohydrate content of the diet contributes > 45% of the total energy.[52] This finding is a reflection of the type rather than the quantity of carbohydrate: when the carbohydrate is not highly processed but has a low glycaemic index, a diet can comprise of up to 60% of its total energy as carbohydrate without any detrimental effect on glucose tolerance.[49,70] British guidelines, like those from Europe, differ from American advice in actively encouraging diets to contain

> 45% of their energy intake in the form of low glycaemic carbohydrates.[69,71] Low-glycaemic-index carbohydrates diets appear in non-diabetic women to improve postprandial glycaemia while limiting overall fat intake and excessive weight gain.[72] Low-glycaemic-index diets have also been reported to reduce insulin sensitivity in both pregnant and non-pregnant individuals.[49,70,73] Indeed, women on a traditional African diet which is very high in carbohydrate, consisting of predominately slowly absorbed starches and non-soluble polysaccharides, show no deterioration in their glucose tolerance during pregnancy.[70]

One could argue the striking increase in insulin resistance and fall in glucose tolerance in pregnancy is a function of a Western diet rather than a physiological inevitability, and if Western women adopted more traditional low-glycaemic diets there would be less insulin resistance and glucose tolerance in pregnancy. In support of this is that birthweights have been reported to be lower in women who eat a diet containing low- rather than high-glycaemic carbohydrates.[44] Therefore, there are good theoretical reasons why obese women with GDM should be encouraged to avoid carbohydrates in the form of rapidly absorbed sugars in favour of slowly absorbed starches and soluble non-starch polysacarides, such as those present in pulses, vegetables, whole fruits, oats and barley.[48] Due to the greater satiety of low-glycaemic-index carbohydrates as compared to refined sugars it is often difficult for women to adhere to a diet with > 50% of the total energy intake in the form of low-glycaemic carbohydrates.

An added advantage of the more slowly absorbed low-glycaemic-index diets is that this form of carbohydrate ensures a more attenuated and more prolonged glycaemic response postprandially, which helps mitigate against preprandial hypoglycaemia and ketosis in women on insulin.[74,75] These types of carbohydrates are particularly well suited for women with Type 1 diabetes (see below).

Specific nutritional problems related to women with Type 1 diabetes

Women with Type 1 diabetes pose particular diet management problems in pregnancy and this is especially so when diabetic complications are present. The complications of a diabetic pregnancy all increase with increasing duration of diabetes: in clinical practice there are now many older pregnant women with Type 1 diabetes, as more women defer their first pregnancy until after establishing their own careers, and by this time many women will have had diabetes for > 25 years. The rise in prevalence of Type 1 diabetes in children under the age of 5[76] will further contribute to the increase in duration of diabetes seen in the Type 1 antenatal population. The complexity of diabetic complications encountered in the Type 1 diabetic women who actually become pregnant has also increased, reflecting advances in the management of renal disease, transplant medicine and infertility treatment. The nutritional management of all these women needs to be highly adaptable to the many different medical complications that may be encountered.

Pregnancy poses a serious risk to the Type 1 diabetic mother, particularly in those with a long duration of diabetes. Although maternal mortality has fallen to between 0.1 to 0.5%, it remains significantly higher than for non-diabetic pregnancies. In the UK, over half of all maternal diabetic deaths in the past 10 years have been attributable to hypoglycaemia,[77-80] a similar finding has been reported for Type 1 diabetic women in Finland, with many of these events occurring at the end of the first trimester

in women with a long duration of diabetes.[81] As the clinicians strive for greater glycaemic control in the first trimester, sound dietary advice to avoid hypoglycaemia is essential. A number of factors are thought to contribute to the increased risk of hypoglycaemia in pregnancy that appear to be more severe in the first 20 weeks of gestation.[82] The importance of regular meals and snacks containing carbohydrate between meals is essential. The best educational model to put this across is still a matter of debate, as there is no randomized controlled trial evidence on this subject. Whether there is an advantage of a system of formal carbohydrate exchanges over advice that focuses more on a general message is not known. Evidence from the Diabetic Control and Complication Trial would suggest that different people respond to different education messages; therefore, agreeing the way to teach is possibly the most important aspect.[83] This is important, as many manufacturing companies recommend exchange systems without an evidence base. It is this group's practice to establish a regular eating pattern of three meals and and three snacks, all of which contain carbohydrate to provide a suitable substrate around which the insulin can be adjusted for. A major problem occurs when patients try to control their blood glucose by changing their eating pattern rather than their insulin dose. This group use low-glycaemic-index carbohydrates both for meals and snacks to reduce hypoglycaemic episodes, an approach which has been shown to be useful in non-pregnant Type 1 diabetes subjects.[74,75]

Ketoacidosis is another potentially fatal condition in Type 1 diabetic pregnancies. The tendency to early ketosis is due to the metabolic changes of accelerated starvation, and respiratory alkalosis can result in its development over a few hours at relatively low maternal blood glucose levels.[84,85] An important contributing factor in the development of ketoacidosis in pregnancy is a reduced calorie intake due to nausea, often accompanied by a decrease in insulin dosage. Episodes of ketosis can be minimized in Type 1 diabetes by encouraging regular carbohydrate input as described above. If nausea prevents women form eating solid foods most women can manage to drink sufficient volumes of sweetened liquids taken hourly to prevent ketoacidosis. Hospital admission is required when a Type 1 diabetic woman is unable to maintain an adequate calorie intake to prevent ketosis due to nausea or vomiting.

Protein requirement in pregnancy

Dietary protein makes up 15–20% of the total calorie intake of the Western diet and appears to vary little in life. Protein requirements in pregnancy are the same in diabetic and non-diabetic women. The current recommended protein requirement is 0.75 gram/kg a day plus an additional 10 grams a day.[53] While a lot is written and known about the consequences of protein malnutrition, both in pregnancy and outside, little is known on the long-term effects of a high-protein diet. One solutions to reducing total carbohydrate and SF in the diet of pregnant mothers would be to increase dietary protein, and this possibility should be addressed. Although the effects of dietary protein on the regulation of energy intake and satiety have not been well studied in the test-meal situation, high protein meals appear to increase satiety.[86]

The use of high-protein/low-carbohydrate diets in pregnancy have been associated historically with low birthweights and poor maternal weight gain, as observed in the relatively prosperous Motherwell and Wishaw District of Scotland from 1938 to 1977, when all pregnant women were advised to consume a high-protein/low-carbohydrate diet, with no specific instruction to reduce their energy intake.[87] The babies born to primigravidae during this period in Motherwell were, when compared to babies born to primigravidae mothers from neighbouring Aberdeen, who received no dietary advice, on average 400 grams lighter for gestational age, 2940 versus 3393 grams. The typical Aberdeen primigravidae diet at this time consisted of 54% carbohydrate, 34% fat and 12% protein, with a total daily calorie intake in the second trimester of 2500 kcal, which compared with the Motherwell mother's diet of c. 34% carbohydrate, 42% fat and 24% protein. In the few Motherwell pregnant women who had their daily calorie intake calculated, this was significantly less (1465 kcal), despite the dietary instructions only focusing on limiting carbohydrate and increasing dietary protein. The Motherwell experience of blanket dietary advice given to a generation of pregnant women in the belief that it may reduce the incidence of pre-eclampsia provides further evidence of the need for long-term controlled nutritional studies before advocating radical changes to the diet.

Dietary supplements including antioxidants

Hyperglycaemic-induced malformations of rat embryos involves reactive oxygen species: experimentally reducing oxygen-radical-related tissue damage decreased malformation rates under experimental conditions.[88] Vitamin E is a lipophilic antioxidant that interferes with the chain reaction of lipid peroxidations; vitamin C is a hydrophilic molecule that can scavenge several radicals, among them the hydroxyl radical. Both vitamins E and C have been shown to decreases diabetic fetal malformation rates in rat embryos.[89] The possibility that diets enriched with antioxidant vitamins may reduce malformations in human diabetic pregnancies has as yet to be demonstrated.

Lipid peroxidation and oxygen-radical-related tissue damage has been implicated in the pathophysiology of pre-eclampsia; lower plasma vitamin E and C values have been observed in pre-eclamptic women as compared to normotensive pregnant controls.[90] It has been suggested that in pre-eclampsia these vitamins may be utilized more quickly to counter-act free-radical-mediated cell disturbances. Early trials with dietary supplementation of vitamin C (1000 mg/day) and vitamin E (400 IU/day) have shown a possible beneficial effect on the prevention of pre-eclampsia in high-risk groups, including diabetic women.[91]

The role of antioxidant vitamin supplementation in diabetic pregnancies needs further evaluation before being universally recommended to all diabetic pregnant women.

Long-term consequences from the nutritional management of diabetic pregnancies

There is increasing evidence emerging that growth-promoted infants of poorly controlled diabetic mothers become more obese and insulin resistant around the time of puberty compared to infants born to diabetic mothers who were better controlled in pregnancy, and that these children have metabolic risk factors for future Type 2 diabetes.[92] High aminotic fluid insulin levels in Type 1 diabetic pregnancies are correlated with metabolic markers of insulin resistance in the children in adolescent life.[92] Follow-up data of Pima Indian children of women with Type 2 diabetes and GDM also highlight how maternal hyperglycaemia predisposes to future obesity and diabetes in the children.[93,94] These studies on children of diabetic mothers highlights the public health importance of aggressively managing maternal hyperglycaemia. A diet that helps reduce post-prandial glucose levels is therefore central to this management.

The follow-up studies of offspring of diabetic rodents fed high-fat diets implicated in premature vascular disease raises the potential concern that high-fat diets in human pregnancies may also be associated with accelerating vascular disease in the children. In Western society, increasing dietary fat to limit total carbohydrate intake to < 45% of energy by promoting dietary MUFA, PUFA and *n*-3 long-chain fatty acids without increasing total SF or total calories needs to be shown to be feasible outside the clinical research setting. Changing the source of maternal dietary carbohydrate from highly processed sugars to those with a lower glycaemic index may prove a practical and valuable means of limiting maternal–fetal transfer of glucose without increasing, or limiting, overall calories or compromising future cardiovascular risk. Again, although on theoretical grounds this approach appears to be attractive, the adherence to high-carbohydrate/low-glycaemic diets that allow dietary SF to remain < 10% needs to be demonstrated, and assessed along with short- and long-term follow-up studies of the children. Such diets would potentially allow 60–70% of the energy of the diet to come from carbohydrate and MUFA sources, with *c*. 10% from PUFA and < 10% from SF and from protein.

Nutritional intervention following GDM to limit the progression to Type 2 diabetes

Women who have GDM are at increased risk of future diabetes and long-term cardiovascular disease. The recent publication of the Diabetic Prevention Program Research Group[95] provides conclusive evidence that lifestyle changes encompassing dietary advice, weight loss and exercise can reduce the rate of progression from impaired glucose tolerance to Type 2 diabetes. The possibility of further limiting this progression in high-risk women with previous GDM by the addition of pharmaceutical agents, such as metformin or a thiozolidinidione, need to be further evaluated.[96] In the meantime, all women with previous GDM should receive lifestyle advice, along the lines given by the Diabetic Prevention Program Research Group.[97] This advice should aim for c. 7% weight loss in obese women and c. 150 minutes of physical activity a week. Women should be encouraged to make dietary changes so that their habitual diets contain plenty of fresh fruit and vegetables, are low in fat and low in carbohydrates with a high glycaemic index; these types of diets have been shown by large epidemiological studies to reduce the long-term risk of Type 2 diabetes.[98–100] Given the risk of diabetes in the children of the women with previous GDM, healthy lifestyle changes should be encouraged in the family as a whole. How best these necessary lifestyle changes can be achieved in a community setting outside a large intervention trial, and without the high intensity individual contact with health personnel that a trial setting provides, still needs to be researched.

Conclusions

The optimal composition of the diet for diabetic women has not been validated in controlled clinical trials. As maternal nutrition can influence the future health of the child, fundamental changes to the macronutrient composition of the maternal diet should be resisted without considering their potential long-term consequences.

Women with Type 1 diabetes pose different nutritional and clinical challenges to obese women with GDM, and too rigid a prescriptive diet for women with Type 1 diabetes is potentially dangerous. The general nutritional advice for all diabetic pregnancies, however, remains the same, i.e. to achieve euglycaemia while minimizing the risk of hypoglycaemia and ketosis. Diets need to target postprandial glucose excursions as hyperglycaemia at this time is linked to abnormal accelerated fetal growth. Limiting overall dietary carbohydrate at the expense of increasing dietary fat may have short-term benefits on postprandial blood glucose but its long-term influence on vascular disease in the children needs to evaluated first. Increasing the use of low-glycaemic-index carbohydrates provides an alternative nutritional means of reducing postprandial glycaemia without increasing the maternal fat content of the diet.

The potential benefits on pregnancy outcome of enriching the maternal diet with MUFA, PUFA and 3-omega fatty acids all require further studies, preferably controlled randomized ones.

There are theoretical reasons why the use of antioxidant vitamin supplements early in pregnancy may lessen the risk of congenital malformation in diabetic pregnancies and further studies evaluating their use should be undertaken. The use of these same vitamins in reducing the incidence of pre-eclampsia in high-risk diabetic pregnancies appears promising and warrants further clinical studies.

Postpartum, all women with GDM should receive lifestyle advice aimed at reducing their long-term risk of developing Type 2 diabetes.

The nutritional management of the diabetic pregnancy needs to receive the same critical scientific scrutiny as other treatment modalities.

It is only when this has been done that will be sufficient clinical studies to support evidence-based nutritional guidelines for the management of such pregnancies.

References

1. The Medical Research Council (MRC) Vitamin Research Study Group. *Prevention of neural tube defects: the results of the Medical Research Council Vitamin Study*. (MRC: 1991.)

2. The Chief Medical Officer. *Vitamin A and Pregnancy*. (Department of Health United Kingdom, HMSO: London, 1993.)

3. Daaboul J, Sanderson S. Vitamin D deficiency in pregnant and breast-feeding women and their infants. *J Perinatol* 1997; **17**:10–14.

4. Janerich DT. Alcohol and pregnancy. An epidemiologic perspective. *Ann Epidemiol* 1990; **1**:179–85.

5. Kaplan JS, Iqbal S, England BG et al. Is pregnancy in diabetic women associated with folate deficiency? *Diabetes Care* 1999; **22**:1017–21.

6. Committee on Medical Aspects of Food Policy. *Dietary Reference Values for Food Energy and Nutrients for the United Kingdom*. (Her Majesty's Stationary Office: London, 1991.)

7. Food and Nutrition Board. *Recommended Daily Allowances*, 10th edn. (National Accademy: Washington, DC, 1989) 59–62.

8. Butte NF, Hopkinson JM, Mehta N, et al. Adjustments in energy expenditure and substrate utilisation during late pregnancy and lactation. *Am J Clin Nutr* 1999; **69**:299–307.

9. Hytten F, Leitch I. *The Physiology of Human Pregnancy*. (Blackwell Scientific: Oxford, 1964.)

10. Hytten FF. Clinical physiology in obstetrics. In: (Hytten E, Chamberlain G, eds) *Nutrition*. (Blackwell Scientific: Oxford, 1980.)

11. Kopp-Hoolihan LE, van Loan MD, King JC. Longitudinal assessment of energy balance in well nourished, pregnant women. *Am J Clin Nutr* 1999; **69**:697–704.

12. Durnin J. Energy requirements of pregnancy: an integrated study in five countries. Background and methods. *Lancet* 1987; **ii**:895–7.

13. Institute of Medicine. *Nutrition During Pregnancy: Weight Gain and Nutritional Supplements*. (National Academy Press: Washington, DC, 1990.)

14. Illingsworth PJ, Jung RT, Howie PW. Reduction in post-prandial energy expenditure during pregnancy. *Br Med J* 1987; **294**:1573–6.

15. Poppitt SD, Prentice AM, Jequier E et al. Evidence of energy sparing in Gambian women during pregnancy: a longitudinal study using whole-body calorimetry. *Am J Clin Nutr* 1993; **57**:353–64.

16. Poppitt SD, Prentice AM, Goldberg GR, Whitehead RG. Energy-sparing strategies to protect human fetal growth. *Am J Obstet Gynecol* 1994; **171**:118–25.

17. Lawrence M, Whitehead RG. Physical activity and total energy expenditure of child-bearing Gambian village women. *Eur J Clin Nutr* 1987; **42**:145–60.

18. Galtier-Dereure F, Boegner C, Bringer J. Obesity and pregnancy: complications and cost. *Am J Clin Nutr* 2000; **71**:1242–8.

19. Cnattingius S, Bergström R, Lipworth L, Kramer MS. Prepregnancy weight and the risk of adverse pregnancy outcomes. *N Engl J Med* 1998; **338**:147–52.

20. Watkins ML, Botto L. Maternal Prepregnancy Weight and Congenital Heart Defects in the Offspring. *Epidemiology* 2001; **12**:439–46.

21. Moore L, Singer M, Bradlee ML et al. A prospective study of the risk of congenital defects associated with maternal obesity and diabetes mellitus. *Epidemiology* 2000; **11**:689–94.

22. Baeten J, Bukusi E, Lambe M. Pregnancy complications and outcomes among overweight and obese nulliparous women. *Am J Public Health* 2001; **91**:436–40.

23. Bianco A, Smilen S, Davis Y et al. Pregnancy outcome and weight gain recommendations for the morbidly obese woman. *Obstet Gynecol* 1998; **91**:97–102.

24. Food and Nutrition Board. Weight gain. In: *Nutrition During Pregnancy*. (National Academy of Sciences: Washington, DC, 1990).

25. Feig D, Naylor CD. Eating for two: are guidelines for weight gain during pregnancy too liberal? *Lancet* 1998; **351**:1054–5.

26. Schieve L, Cogswell M, Scanlon K. An empiric evaluation of the Institute of Medicine's pregnancy weight gain guidelines by race. *Obstet Gynecol* 1998; **91**: 878–84.

27. Ravelli ACJ, van der Meulen JHP, Michels RP et al. Glucose tolerance in adults after prenatal exposure to famine. *Lancet* 1998; **351**:173–7.

28. Ravelli AC, van Der Meulen JH, Osmond C et al. Obesity at the age of 50 y in men and women exposed to famine prenatally. *Am J Clin Nutr* 1999; **70**:811–16.

29. Barker DJP. Fetal growth and adult disease. *Br J Obstet Gynaecol* 1992; **99**:275–6.

30. Barker DJP. Fetal origins of coronary heart disease. *Br Heart J* 1993; **69**:195–6.

31. Barker DJP, Hales CN, Fall CHD et al. Type 2 (non-insulin-dependent) diabetes mellitus, hypertension and hyperlipidaemia (syndrome X: relation to reduced fetal growth. *Diabetologia* 1993; **36**:62–7.

32. Churchill JA, Berendez HW, Nemore J. Neuro-psychological deficits in children of diabetic mothers. *Am J Obstet Gynecol* 1966; **105**:257–68.

33. Rizzo T, Metzger BE, Burns WJ, Burns K. Correlation between antepartum maternal metabolism and intelligence of offspring. *N Engl J Med* 1991; **325**:408–13.

34. Rizzo T, Dooley B, Metzger N et al. Prenatal and peri-natal influences on long-term psychomotor development in offspring of diabetic mothers. *Am J Obstet Gynecol* 1995; **173**:1753–8.

35. Buchanan TA, Metzger BE, Freinkel N. Accelerated starvation in late pregnancy: a comparison between obese normal pregnant women and women with gestational diabetes. *Am J Obstet Gynecol* 1990; **162**:1015–20.

36. Knopp RH, Magee MS, Raisys V, Benedetti T. Metabolic effects of hypocaloric diets in management of gestational diabetes. *Diabetes* 1991; **40**:165–71.

37. Catalano PM, Huston L, Amini SB, Kalhan SC. Longitudinal changes in glucose metabolism during pregnancy in obese women with normal glucose tolerance and gestational diabetes mellitus. *Am J Obstet Gynecol* 1999; **180**:903–16.

38. Wolever TM, Bentum-Williams A, Jenkins DJ. Physiological modulation of plasma free fatty acid concentrations by diet. Metabolic implications in non-diabetic subjects. *Diabetes Care* 1995; **18**:962–70.

39. Dornhorst A, Nicholls JSD, Probst F et al. Calorie restriction for the treatment of gestational diabetes. *Diabetes* 1991; **40**:161–4.

40. Schofield WN, Schofield C, James WPT. Basal metabolic rate review and prediction, together with annotated of source material. *Hum Nutr Appl Nutr* 1985; **39C**:5–96.

41. Gaither K, Quraishi AN, Illsley NP. Diabetes alters the expression and activity of the human placental GLUT1 glucose transporter. *J Clin Endocrinol Metab* 1999; **84**:695–701.

42. Schwartz R, Susa J. Fetal macrosomia – animal models. *Diabetes Care* 1980; **3**:430–2.

43. Langer O, Levy J, Brustman L et al. Glycemic control in gestational diabetes mellitus – how tight is tight enough: small for gestational age versus large for gestational age? *Am J Obstet Gynecol* 1989; **161**:646–53.

44. Clapp J. Maternal carbohydrate intake and pregnancy outcome. *Proc Nutr Soc* 2002; **61**:45–50.

45. Combs CA, Gunderson E, Kitzmiller JL et al. The relationship of fetal macrosomia to maternal postprandial glucose control during pregnancy. *Diabetes Care* 1992; **15**:1251–7.

46. Jovanovic-Peterson L, Peterson CM, Reed GF et al. Maternal postprandial glucose levels and infant birth weight: the Diabetes in Early Pregnancy Study Group. *Am J Obstet Gynecol* 1991; **164**:103–11.

47. DeVeciana M, Major CA, Morgan MA. Postprandial versus preprandial glucose monitoring in women with gestational diabetes mellitus requiring insulin therapy. *N Engl J Med* 1995; **333**:1237–41.

48. Frost G, Dornhorst A. The relevance of the glycaemic index to our under standing of dietary carbohydrates. *Diabet Med* 2000; **17**:336–45.

49. Fraser R, Ford F, Lawrence G. Insulin sensitivity in third trimester pregnancy. A randomized study of dietary effects. *Br J Obstet Gynaecol* 1988; **95**:223–9.

50. Rabasa-Lhoret R, Garon J, Langelier H et al. Effects of meal carbohydrate content on insulin requirements in type 1 diabetic patients treated intensively with the basal-bolus (ultralente-regular) insulin regimen. *Diabetes Care* 1999; **22**:667–73.

51. American Diabetes Association (CADA): Nutritional management. In: (ADA, ed) *Medical Management of Pregnancy Complicated by Diabetes*. (ADA Inc: Virginia, 1995) 47–56.

52. Major C, Henry M, De Veciana M, Morgan M. The effects of carbohydrate restriction in patients with diet-controlled gestational diabetes. *Obstet Gynecol* 1998; **91**:600–4.

53. Franz MJ, Bantle JP, Beebe CA et al. Evidence-based nutrition principles and recommendations for the treatment and prevention of diabetes and related complications. *Diabetes Care* 2002; **25**:148–98.

54. Ilic S, Jovanovic L, Pettitt D. Comparison of the effect of saturated and monounsaturated fat on postprandial plasma glucose and insulin concentration in women with gestational diabetes mellitus. *Am J Perinatol* 1999; **16**:489–95.

55. Signorello L, Harlow B, Wang S, Erick M. Saturated fat intake and the risk of severe hyperemesis gravidarum. *Epidemiology* 1998; **9**:636–40.

56. Moses RG, Shand JL, Tapsell LC. The recurrence of gestational diabetes: could dietary differences in fat intake be an explanation? *Diabetes Care* 1997; **20**:1647–50.

57. Ghosh P, Bitsanis D, Ghebremeskel K et al. Abnormal aortic fatty acid composition and small artery function in offspring of rats fed a high fat diet in pregnancy. *J Physiol* 2001; **533**:815–22.

58. Kucera J. Rate and Type of congenital anomalies among offspring of diabetic women. *J Reprod Med* 1971; **7**:61–70.

59. Wang Y, Storlien L, Jenkins A et al. Dietary variables and glucose tolerance in pregnancy. *Diabetes Care* 2000; **23**:460–4.

60. Georgopoulous A, Bantle JP, Noutsou M et al. Differences in the metabolism of postprandial lipoproteins after a high-monounsaturated-fat versus a high-carbohydrate diet in patients with Type 1 diabetes mellitus. *Arterioscler Thromb Vasc Biol* 1998; **18**:773–82.

61. Garg A, Bantle JP, Henry RR et al. Effects of varying carbohydrate content of diet in patients with non-insulin dependent diabetes mellitus. *J Am Med Ass* 1994; **271**:1421–8.

62. Yu-Poth S, Zhao G, Etherton T et al. Effect of National Cholesterol Education Program's Step 1 and Step 11 dietary intervention programs of cardiovascular disease risk factors; a meta-analysis. *Am J Clin Nutr* 1999; **69**:632–46.

63. Lauszus F, Rasmussen O, Henriksen J et al. Effect of a high monounsaturated fatty acid diet on blood pressure and glucose metabolism in women with gestational diabetes mellitus. *Eur J Clin Nutr* 2001; **55**:436–43.

64. Olsen SF, Secher NJ. Low consumption of seafood in early pregnancy as a risk factor for pretem delivery: prospective cohort study. *Br Med J* 2002; **324**:447–50.

65. Glauber H, Wallace P, Griver K, Brechtel G. Adverse metabolic effect of omega-3 fatty acids in non-insulin-dependent diabetes mellitus. *Ann Intern Med* 1988; **108**: 663–8.

66. Westerveld HT, deGraaf JC, van Breugel HH et al. Effects of low-dose EPA-E on glycemic control, lipid profile, lipoprotein (a), platelet aggregation, viscosity, and platelet and vessel wall interaction in NIDDM. *Diabetes Care* 1993; **16**:683–8.

67. de Lorgeril M, Salen P, Martin JL et al. Mediterranean diet, traditional risk factors, and the rate of cardiovascular complications after myocardial infarction: final of the Lyon Diet Heart Study. *Circulation* 1999; **99**:733–5.

68. Daviglus ML, Stamler J, Orencia AJ et al. Fish consumption and the 30-year risk of fatal myocardial infarction. *N Engl J Med* 1997; **336**:1046–53.

69. Lean MEJ, Brenchley S, Connor H et al. Dietary recommendations for people with diabetes: an update for the 1990s. Nutrition subcommittee of the British Diabetic Association's Professional Advisory Committee. *Diabet Med* 1992; **9**:189–202.

70. Fraser RB. The normal range of OGTT in the African female: pregnant and non-pregnant. *East Africa Med J* 1981; **58**:90–4.

71. Ha KK, Lean MEJ. Recommendations for the nutritional management of patients with diabetes mellitus. *Eur J Clin Nutr* 1998; **52**:467–81.

72. Clapp J. Effect of dietary carbohydrate on the glucose and insulin response to mixed caloric intake and exercise in both nonpregnant and pregnant women. *Diabetes Care* 1998; **21**:B107–B12.

73. Frost G, Leeds A, Dornhorst A. Insulin sensitivity in women at risk of coronary heart disease and the effect of a low glycaemic diet. *Metabolism* 1998; **47**: 1245–51.

74. Gilbertson HR, Brand-Miller JC, Thorburn AW et al. The effect of flexible low glycemic index dietary versus measured carbohydrate exchange diets on glycemic control in children with type 1 diabetes. *Diabetes Care* 2001; **24**:1137–43.

75. Giacco R, Parillo M, Rivellese AA et al. Long-term dietary treatment with increased amounts of fibre-rich low-glycemic index natural foods improves blood glucose control and reduces the number of hypoglycemic events in type 1 diabetic patients. *Diabetes Care* 2000; **23**:1461–6.

76. Gardner SG, Bingley PJ, Sawtell PA et al. Rising incidence of insulin dependent diabetes in children aged under 5 years in the Oxford region: time trend analysis. *Br Med J* 1997; **315**:713–17.

77. Chief Medical Officer. *The Report on the Confidential Enquiries into Maternal Deaths 1997–1999*. (Her Majesty's Stationary Office: London, 2000.)

78. Chief Medical Officer. *The Report on the Confidential Enquiries into Maternal Deaths 1994–1996*. (Her Majesty's Stationary Office: London, 1998.)

79. Chief Medical Officer. *The Report on the Confidential Enquiries into Maternal Deaths 1991–1993*. (Her Majesty's Stationary Office: London, 1996.)

80. Chief Medical Officer. *The Report on the Confidential Enquiries into Maternal Deaths 1988–1990*. (Her Majesty's Stationary Office: London, 1994.)

81. Leinonen PJ, Hilesmaa VK, Teramo KA. Maternal mortality in Type 1 diabetes. *Diabetes Care* 2001; **24**:1501–2.

82. Heller SR. Hypoglycaemia and pregnancy. In: (Frier BM, Fisher BM, eds) *Hypoglycaemia in Clinical Diabetes* (John Wiley & Sons: Chichester, UK, 1999) 243–60.

83. Anderson RM, Fitzgerald JT, Oh MS. The relationship between diabetes-related attitudes and patients' self-reported adherence. *Diabetes Educator* 1993; **19**: 287–92.

84. Cullen MT, Reece EA, Homko CJ, Sivan E. The changing presentations of diabetic ketoacidosis during pregnancy. *Am J Perinatol* 1996; **13**:449–51.

85. Ramin KD. Diabetic ketoacidosis in pregnancy. *Obstet Gynecol Clin N Am* 1999; **26**:481–8.

86. Hill AJ, Blundell JE. Macronutrients and satiety: the effects of high-protein or high-carbohydrate meal on subjective motivation to eat and food preferences. *Nutr Behav* 1986; **3**:133–44.

87. Kerr JF, Cambell-Brown BM, Johnstone FD. A study of the effect of a high protein low carbohydrate diet on birthweight on an obstetric population. In: (Sutherland HW, Stowers JM, eds) *Carbohydrate Metabolism in Pregnancy and the Newborn 1978*. (Springer-Verlag: Berlin, 1979) 518–34.

88. Zaken V, Kohen R, Ornoy A. Vitamins C and E improve rat embryonic antioxidant defense mechanism in diabetic culture medium. *Teratology* 2001; **64**: 33–44.

89. Cederberg J, Siman C, Eriksson U. Combined treatment with vitamin E and vitamin C decreases oxidative stress and improves fetal outcome in experimental diabetic pregnancy. *Pediatr Res* 2001; **49**:755–62.

90. Kharb S. Vitamin E and C in preeclampsia. *Eur J Obstet Gynecol Reprod Biol* 2000; **93**:37–9.

91. Chappell LC, Seed PT, Briley AL et al. Effect of antioxidants on the occurrence of pre-eclampsia in women at increased risk: a randomised trial. *Lancet* 1999; **354**: 810–16.

92. Weiss PA, Scholz HS, Haas J et al. Long-term follow-up of infants of mothers with type 1 diabetes: evidence

for hereditary and nonhereditary transmission of diabetes and precursors. *Diabetes Care* 2000; **23**:905–11.

93. Dabelea D, Pettitt DJ, Hanson RL et al. Birth weight, type 2 diabetes, and insulin resistance in Pima Indian children and young adults. *Diabetes Care* 1999; **22**:944–50.

94. Dabelea D, Hanson RL, Lindsay RS et al. Intrauterine exposure to diabetes conveys risks for Type 2 diabetes and obesity: a study of discordant sibships. *Diabetes* 2000; **49**:2208–11.

95. Diabetes Prevention Program Research Group. Reduction in the incidence of type 2 diabetes with lifestyle intervention or metformin. *N Engl J Med* 2002; **346**:393–403.

96. Buchanan TA, Xiang AH, Peters RK et al. *Response of pancreatic [beta]-cells to improved insulin sensitivity in women at high risk for type 2 diabetes.* Diabetes 2000; **49**:782–8.

97. Diabetes Prevention Program Research Group. The Diabetes Prevention Program (DDP). *Diabetes* 1997; **46**:138A.

98. Salmeron J, Manson JE, Stampfer J et al. Dietary fibre, glycemic load, and risk of non-insulin-dependent diabetes mellitus in women. *J Am Med Ass* 1997; **277**:472–7.

99. Salmeron J, Ascherio A, Rimm EB et al. Dietary fiber, glycemic load, and risk of NIDDM in men. *Diabetes Care* 1997; **20**:545–50.

100. Marshall JA, Bessesen DH, Hamman RF. High saturated fat and low starch and fibre are associated with hyperinsulinaemia in a non-diabetic poulation: the San Luis Valley Study. *Diabetologia* 1997; **40**:430–8.

27

Insulin therapy in pregnancy

John L Kitzmiller, Lois Jovanovic

Introduction

Before the advent of insulin, few diabetic women lived to childbearing age. Before 1922, fewer than 100 pregnancies in diabetic women were reported, and most likely these women had Type 1 and not Type 2 diabetes.[1] Even with this assumption, these cases of diabetes and pregnancy were associated with a > 90% infant mortality rate and a 30% maternal mortality rate. As late as 1980, physicians were still counseling diabetic women to avoid pregnancy. This philosophy was justified because of the poor obstetric history in 30–50% of diabetic women. Improved infant mortality rates finally occurred after 1980, when treatment strategies stressed better control of maternal plasma glucose levels, and once self-blood glucose monitoring (SBGM) and hemoglobin A1c (HbA1c) became available. As the pathophysiology of pregnancy complicated by diabetes has been elucidated, and as management programs have achieved and maintained near normoglycemia throughout pregnancy complicated by Type 1 diabetes, perinatal mortality rates have decreased to levels seen in the general population. This chapter is intended to help the clinician understand the increasing insulin requirements of pregnancy, and to design treatment protocols to achieve and maintain normoglycemia throughout pregnancy.

Glucose toxicity and the role of postprandial hyperglycemia

If the mother has hyperglycemia, the fetus will be exposed to either sustained hyperglycemia or intermittent pulses of hyperglycemia; both situations prematurely stimulate fetal insulin secretion. Fetal hyperinsulinemia may cause increased fetal body fat (macrosomia) and, therefore, a difficult delivery, or cause inhibition of pulmonary maturation of surfactant and, therefore, respiratory distress of the neonate. The fetus may also have decreased serum potassium levels caused by the elevated insulin and glucose levels, and may therefore have cardiac arrhythmias. Neonatal hypoglycemia may cause permanent neurological damage.

There is also an increased prevalence of congenital anomalies and spontaneous abortions in diabetic women who are in poor glycemic control during the period of fetal organogenesis, which is nearly complete by 7 weeks postconception. Thus, a woman may not even know she is pregnant at this time. It is for this reason that prepregnancy counseling and planning is essential in women of childbearing age who have diabetes. Because organogenesis is complete so early on, if a woman presents to her health care team and announces that she has missed her period by only a few days, if the blood glucose levels are immediately normalized then there is still is a chance to prevent cardiac anomalies, although the neural tube defects are already 'set in stone' by the time the first period is missed. These findings emphasize the importance of glycemic control at the earliest stages of conception.[2–4] Ideally, if a diabetic woman plans her pregnancy, then there is time to create algorithms of care that are individualized and a woman can be given choices. When a diabetic woman presents in her first few weeks of pregnancy, there is no time for individualization, but rather rigid protocols must be urgently instituted to provide optimal control within 24–48 hours.

After the period of organogenesis, maternal hyperglycemia interferes with normal fetal growth and development during the second and third trimesters.[5] The maternal postprandial glucose level has been shown to be the most important variable to impact on the subsequent risk of neonatal macrosomia.[6–8] The fetus thus is 'overnourished' by the peak postprandial glucose level.[9] This peak response occurs in > 90% of woman at 1 hour after beginning a meal. Therefore, 1 hour after beginning a meal the glucose level needs to be measured and treatment designed to maintain this blood glucose in the normal range. Studies have shown than when the postprandial glucose levels are maintained from the second trimester onward to < 120 mg/dl 1 hour after beginning a meal, then the risk of macrosomia is minimized.[8]

Diabetogenic forces of normal pregnancy increase insulin requirements[10]

The fetal demise associated with pregnancy complicated by Type 1 diabetes seems to arise from glucose extremes. Elevated maternal plasma glucose levels should always be avoided, because of the association of maternal hyperglycemia with subsequent congenital malformation and spontaneous abortions.[2,5] To achieve normoglycemia, a clear understanding of 'normal' carbohydrate metabolism in pregnancy is paramount. Thus, the amount of insulin required to treat Type 1 diabetic women throughout pregnancy needs to be sufficient to compensate for: (1) increasing caloric needs; (2) increasing adiposity; (3) decreasing exercise; and (4) increasing anti-insulin or diabetogenic hormones of pregnancy.

The major diabetogenic hormones of the placenta are human chorionic somatomammotropin (hCS), previously referred to as human placental lactogen (hPL), estrogen and progesterone. Also, serum maternal cortisol levels (both bound and free) are increased. In addition, at the elevated levels seen during gestation, prolactin has a diabetogenic effect.[10]

The strongest insulin antagonist of pregnancy is hCS. This placental hormone appears in increasing concentrations beginning at 10 weeks of gestation. By 20 weeks of gestation, plasma hCS levels are increased 300-fold, and by term the turnover rate is c. 1000 mg/dl. The mechanism of action whereby hCS raises plasma glucose levels is unclear, but probably originates from its growth hormone-like properties. hCS also promotes free fatty acid (FFA) production by stimulating lipolysis, which promotes peripheral resistance to insulin.

Placental progesterone rises 10-fold above non-pregnant levels and is associated with an insulin increase in normal healthy pregnant women by two- to fourfold.

Most of the marked rise of serum cortisol during pregnancy can be attributed to the increase of cortisol-binding globulin induced by estrogen. However, free cortisol levels are also increased. This increase potentiates the diurnal fluctuations of cortisol with the highest levels occurring in the early morning hours.

The rising estrogen levels also trigger the rise in pituitary prolactin early in pregnancy. Prolactin's structure is similar to a growth hormone and at concentrations reached by the second trimester (> 200 ng/ml) prolactin can affect glucose metabolism. Although there are no studies that have examined prolactin alone as an insulin antagonist, there is indirect evidence that suppressing prolactin in gestational diabetic women with large doses of pyridoxine improves glucose tolerance.

In addition to the increasing anti-insulin hormones of pregnancy, there is also increased degradation of insulin in pregnancy caused by placental enzymes comparable to liver insulinases. The placenta also has membrane-associated insulin-degrading activity. Concomitant with the hormonally induced insulin resistance and increased insulin degradation, the rate of disposal of insulin slows. The normal pancreas can adapt to these factors by increasing the insulin secretory capacity. If the pancreas fails to respond adequately to these alterations then gestational diabetes mellitus (GDM) results. In a woman with Type 1 diabetes, her insulin requirement will rise progressively. Failure to increase her insulin doses appropriately will result in increasing hyperglycemia.[10]

Rationale for the use of human insulin during pregnancy

Although controversial, the rate of complications in pregnancies of diabetic women has been tied to the metabolic control of maternal glucose.[1-5] Perhaps the debate remains because some reports claim that neonatal complications occur in spite of excellent metabolic control, although there fail to measure postprandial glucose levels.[11,12] Postprandial glucose control has been suggested as key to neonatal outcome for the pregnant woman with either Type 1 diabetes or GDM.[6-8] Alternatively, some have suggested that neonatal morbidity is secondary to the variability of maternal serum glucose and the presence of antibodies to insulin.[13] Placental transfer of insulin complexed with immunoglobulin has also been associated with fetal macrosomia in mothers with near-normal glycemic control during gestation. Menon et al[13] reported that antibody-bound insulin transferred to the fetus was proportional to the concentration of antibody-bound insulin measured in the mother. Also, the amount of antibody-bound insulin transferred to the fetus correlated directly with macrosomia in the infant and was independent of maternal blood glucose levels. In contrast, Jovanovic et al[14] discovered only improved glucose control, as evidenced by lower postprandial glucose excursions, but not lower insulin antibody levels, correlated with lower fetal weights. They showed that insulin antibodies to exogenous insulin do not influence infant birthweight.

Recently, it has been reported that insulin lispro, an analog of human insulin with a peak insulin action achieved within 1 hour after injection, significantly improves the postprandial glucose levels in non-pregnant diabetic patients.[15]

Because normoglycemia is important in the treatment of pregnant diabetic women, the use of insulin analogs would appear beneficial in the care of these women if the safety profile can be documented. This review presents the reports that studied the safety and efficacy of insulin analogs in pregnancy, and offers an opinion as to the utility of insulin analogs for treatment of the diabetes during pregnancy.

Concern about anti-insulin antibody formation during pregnancy

Anti-insulin antibodies that cross the placenta may contribute to hyperinsulinemia *in utero* and thus potentiate the metabolic aberrations in the fetus. Although insulin does not cross the placenta, antibodies to insulin do cross the placenta and may bind fetal insulin; this necessitates the increased production of free insulin to re-establish normoglycemia. Thus, the anti-insulin antibodies may potentiate the effect of maternal hyperglycemia to produce fetal hyperinsulinemia. Human and highly purified insulins are significantly less immunogenic than mixed beef–pork insulins.[16] Human insulin treatment has been reported to achieve improved pregnancy and infant outcome compared to using highly purified animal insulins.[14] Recently, the insulin analog lispro (which has the amino acid sequence in the beta chain reversed at positions B28 and B29) has been reported to be more efficacious than human regular insulin to normalize the blood glucose levels in GDM women. This insulin rapidly lowered the postprandial glucose levels, thereby decreasing the HbA1c levels, with fewer hypoglycemic episodes and without increasing the anti-insulin antibody levels.[17] Although the safety and efficacy of insulin lispro in the treatment of Type 1 and Type 2 diabetic women throughout pregnancy is not yet established, the following discussion helps the clinician decide if the newer insulin's benefit outweighs any risks.

Use of insulin lispro in pregnancies complicated by diabetes

Postprandial glucose control in the patient with GDM is important to neonatal outcome.[6–8] The Diabetes in Early Pregnancy (DIEP) Study identified 28.5% of infants from diabetic mothers who were > 90th percentile in infant birthweights.[8] The birthweight in this 28.5% correlated positively with fasting blood glucose and HbA1c. When adjusted for fasting blood glucose and HbA1c, the non-fasting blood glucose concentration in the third trimester was an even stronger predictor of infant birthweight and fetal macrosomia. Combs et al confirmed these findings, as they associated macrosomia with higher postprandial glucose concentrations obtained between weeks 29 and 32 of gestation. In addition, they described a higher risk of small-for-gestational-age (SGA) infants in those with lower [< 130 mg/dl (7.2 mmol/l)] 1 hour postprandial glucose levels. De Veciana et al[6] described improved fetal outcome and less risk of neonatal hypoglycemia, macrosomia and Cesarean delivery in patients who managed GDM by controlling 1 hour postprandial glucose concentrations than in those who managed by only the preprandial glucose concentrations. Therefore, insulin lispro, an analog of human insulin that possesses unique properties, which may make it a valuable therapeutic option in the treatment of GDM and the prevention of neonatal complications. First, the rapid absorption of insulin lispro from the subcutaneous site allows for a faster insulin peak concentration versus regular human insulin.[18] This effect more closely mimics the physiologic first-phase insulin release and results in lower postprandial glucose concentrations, and may lead to improved postprandial coverage.[15] In addition, insulin lispro is known to upregulate insulin receptors.[19,20] In the present authors' study,[17] the postprandial glucose response to the test meal was more frequently within the normal glucose range after a standardized dose of insulin lispro as compared with regular human insulin. Second, the elimination of insulin from the venous space is the same as with regular human insulin, but the faster absorption of insulin lispro allows both the glucose-lowering effect and the patient's exposure to insulin to be less, which may result in a diminished antibody response. Certainly, in clinical trials there has not been any increase in antibody response associated with insulin lispro use.[15,18,19] Since placental transfer of insulin occurs when it is complexed with immunoglobulin, the lack of insulin lispro-induced antibody formation could be expected to result in little, if any, placental transfer of insulin lispro to the neonate, as was demonstrated in the present authors' study. Thus, the overall decrease in circulating insulin as lispro, plus the lower immunogenic response of lispro, leads to less maternal antibody formation and, therefore, less insulin transfer to the fetus with a reduction in risk for physical malformations.[17,21] Menon et al[13] attempted to link maternal antibody formation to negative fetal outcomes. Careful review of the paper reveals, instead, better overall control of maternal hyperglycemia with attendant reductions in fetal macrosomia. This may have ultimately diminished the risk of neonatal complications, including macrosomia. Previous investigations have demonstrated that birthweight could be normalized with regular human insulin.[22–24] This aggressive therapeutic intervention may explain the apparent lack of macrosomia in both patient groups. No differences in fetal parameters, as would be expected in the clinical setting where euglycemia is a goal of therapy, reduce risk to the fetus.

Although the present authors were interested in the metabolic effects of insulin lispro in GDM women, the primary concern was safety, specifically the risk of hypoglycemia, hyperglycemia and antibody production that might cause the insulin to cross the placenta to the fetal side. In the study, 42 GDM women were randomized to receive regular human insulin or insulin lispro prior to consuming a test meal.[17] Throughout the remainder of gestation, subjects received pre-meal insulin lispro or regular human insulin (with and without basal insulin), and performed blood glucose monitoring before and after each meal. During the test meal, the areas under the glucose curve (AUGC), and those for insulin and C-peptide levels, were significantly lower in the insulin lispro group. The incidence of postprandial hyperglycemia (> 120 mg/dl) was significantly lower in the lispro group. Overall metabolic control also improved significantly in the insulin lispro group, which showed the greatest absolute decrease in HbA1c levels as compared to the regular human group. The reduction from baseline HbA1c concentrations at 6 weeks was statistically significant for the insulin lispro group but not for the regular human insulin group.[17]

Most importantly, because safety was considered to be a critical issue, it was pleasing to see a significant reduction in hypoglycemic episodes with the insulin lispro group. To determine the immunologic effects of insulin lispro compared with regular human insulin, three different types of antibodies were studied: (1) lispro-specific antibodies; (2) regular-specific antibodies; and (3) cross-reactive antibodies. Levels of all three antibodies were evaluated at the time of enrollment, 6 weeks after enrollment, at delivery (both in the maternal serum and the umbilical cord blood) and at the postpartum follow-up visit in maternal serum. At each evaluation point, antibody levels in both study groups were within the reference range. No statistically significant differences were seen between the insulin lispro and regular human insulin groups.

To determine whether the absence of cord insulin lispro was due to lack of placental transfer or to undetectable insulin concentrations in the mothers, the last 10 subjects in the study were infused with either high-dose regular human insulin or high-dose insulin lispro during labor and delivery. Subjects were infused with high-dose glucose to maintain blood glucose levels in the normal range. Using a sensitive lispro assay, it was not possible to detect insulin lispro in the umbilical cord blood.[17]

Conclusions from the study are that those women with GDM who are not optimally managed with diet and exercise need insulin therapy. Insulin lispro causes fewer hypoglycemic events than human regular insulin and it attenuates a greater postprandial response than regular human insulin. Furthermore, the antibody levels in lispro insulin are not increased over those seen with regular human insulin. Insulin lispro, to the best of the present authors' knowledge, does not cross the placenta to the fetus and, therefore, may be considered a treatment option in patients with GDM.

Theoretical risks of the use of insulin analogs during pregnancy complicated by pregestational diabetes

Possible effects of insulin lispro on the fetus

Diamond and Kormas[25] first questioned the safety of using insulin lispro during pregnancy in 1997. They reported on two patients who used insulin lispro during pregnancies and deliveries. One of these pregnancies was terminated at 20 weeks gestation and the second pregnancy resulted in a seemingly healthy infant after an elective Cesarean delivery, but who subsequently died unexpectedly 3 weeks later. Both infants were discovered to have congenital abnormalities, which led the authors to question whether insulin lispro might have teratogenic effects on the fetus, in which case it should not be used during pregnancy. The report raises concerns about insulin lispro use during pregnancy, yet it does not provide conclusive evidence that insulin lispro was responsible for the malformations of the infants mentioned. In fact, there is sufficient reason to doubt that insulin lispro was to blame, since these isolated case reports were not part of a study and there was no control group. Therefore, the findings should stimulate initiation of clinical trials testing the safety of insulin lispro during pregnancy and not be taken as evidence that it is unsafe.

Despite the opinion of Diamond and Kormas[25] that poor glycemic control was not responsible for the abnormalities of the infants in the cases described above, there is insufficient evidence to support this claim. The letter reports that HbA1c levels were determined every 3 months and that both women had values < 7% at each test. However, an HbA1c of 7% may be associated with an increased risk of fetal malformations. Since organogenesis is complete within the first 7 weeks of pregnancy,[26] and women tend to improve their glycemic control as the pregnancy progresses, an HbA1c measured at 3 months of pregnancy is a poor reflection of the mother's blood glucose levels at conception and during the critical first organogenic weeks of pregnancy.

The report also indicated that both women maintained a mean blood glucose level of

< 108 mg/dl. A pregnant woman's target blood glucose should be < 90 mg/dl fasting and < 120 mg/dl postprandially.[27] If the women measured their fasting blood glucose only, the reported mean is obviously too high. If postprandial measurements were also taken into account, the mean is still too high, although less so. These women would be categorized as being at high risk for bearing infants with malformations.

Throughout pregnancy, the second mother was being treated for hypertension and if the malformations were due to a medication it is perhaps unfair to single out insulin lispro. In spite of the medication used, the malformations reported are more indicative of poor glycemic control: situs inversus, one of the abnormalities in the first infant, occurs almost exclusively in children of diabetic mothers.[28]

During the initial clinical trials testing insulin lispro, pregnant women were excluded. However, some participants became pregnant unexpectedly during the trials and 19 infants were born by these mothers who were using insulin lispro. Of these births, one child had a right dysplastic kidney but the other 18 were healthy.[29]

Jovanovic et al[17] studied the immunologic effects of insulin lispro versus regular human insulin when used during GDM. Umbilical cord blood was analyzed for traces of insulin lispro, but none was found. This is true for the women who received their last dose of lispro hours prior to delivery and for the four women who received lispro during delivery. This outcome suggests that insulin lispro does not cross the placenta. Although these findings emanate from studies in GDM, there is no reasonable basis that a study done with pregnant Type 1 women would generate different results. Currently, there is a large multicenter trial to observe the safety and efficacy of insulin lispro in pregnancies complicated by Type 1 diabetes.

Possible effects of insulin lispro on the mother

There are three situations in life in which rapid normalization of blood glucose levels increase the risk for deterioration of diabetic retinopathy: puberty, pregnancy and rapid normalization of blood glucose levels. If two of these events occur in the same patient, the risk for retinopathy progression is potentiated.[30,31] All three situations are associated with increased serum concentrations of growth-promoting factors.[32] It is hypothesized that when the blood glucose level is rapidly decreased, there is increased retinal extravasation of serum proteins. If there is a concomitant increase in the concentration of serum growth-promoting factors, a predisposed retina may deteriorate.

Pregnancy *per se* is the most frequently reported situation in which rapid normalization of blood glucose is associated with deterioration of retinal status. Normal pregnancy is associated with high concentrations of many growth-promoting factors.[33–36] Hill et al[34] reported that a potent mitogen and angiogenic factor normally absent from the adult circulation become detectable by 14 weeks of gestation and is maximal at 22–32 weeks of gestational. A placental growth hormone variant had been found to increase throughout pregnancy, along with hCS and prolactin.[35] Maternal insulin-like growth factor (IGF)-1 production has also been shown to increase significantly above non-pregnant levels.[34] It is well known that diabetes mellitus is associated with perturbations of growth hormone IGF-1 in cases of poor metabolic control.[37]

Kitzmiller et al[38] have suggested that treatment with insulin lispro during pregnancies complicated by diabetes may be associated with acceleration of diabetic retinopathy. If treatment with lispro insulin did play a role in the rapid deterioration of retinopathy in the case reports, it most likely was not mediated by IGF-1 activity of lispro. Human insulin binds to the IGF-1 receptor with an affinity of 0.1–0.2% that of IGF-1. A comparison of insulin lispro and human insulin was made to determine the relative IGF-1 receptor binding affinity in human placenta membranes, skeletal muscle, smooth muscle cells and mammary epithelial cells. Insulin lispro had a slightly higher affinity for the human placenta membranes when compared with human insulin (1.3 times greater than human insulin). No other differences were observed in any other cell lines. Despite the suggested increased affinity, it should be noted that the absolute affinity for the IGF-1 receptor is extremely low for both insulin lispro and human insulin. Concentrations > 1000 times above the normal physiologic range are needed to reach 50% receptor binding. IGF-1 is a much larger protein chain than insulin and there is a 49% homology between human insulin and IGF-1. The reversal of the B28 and B29 amino aids in insulin lispro increases this homology to 51%, because of the analogous position in the IGF molecule. It has been shown that insulin lispro has the same affinity for the IGF-1 receptor as does human insulin; also, the dissociation kinetics of insulin lispro on the insulin receptor are identical to those of insulin, indicating that insulin lispro should have no excess mitogenic effect via either the IGF-1 or the insulin receptor.[39,40] Patients in the Kitzmiller reports[36] all had elevated levels of IGF-1 due to poor control of their diabetes and due to pregnancy *per se*, independent of the possible IGF-1 activity of lispro. However, anecdotal cases can never be used to infer a cause–effect relationship. In controlled clinical trials of > 2000 patients with insulin lispro, no significant differences in retinopathy were observed, but there were no pregnant women in this trial.[15]

The factors that emerge as the independent risk factors for retinopathy progression include: elevated HbA1c at baseline, duration of diabetes, significant proteinuria (> 300 mg/24 hours), pregnancy and rapid normalization of blood glucose (in < 14 weeks). In fact, the strongest risk factor for retinopathy progression, independent of baseline retinal status, is baseline elevation of HbA1c associated with a rapid decline to normal. Of 14 patients who were treated with insulin lispro during pregnancy, described by Kitzmiller et al,[38] 11 had risk factors, including evidence of baseline retinopathy, which have been associated with progression to proliferative retinopathy during pregnancy. Of concern are the three patients said to have no retinopathy on first examination during pregnancy. Kitzmiller et al[38] state: if there is no retinopathy during the first trimester of a pregnancy complicated by diabetes, progression to proliferative retinopathy needing laser therapy is rare, however, many of the cited references above emphasize that baseline elevation of glucose associated with rapid normalization can accelerate retinopathy. Phelps et al[41] clearly showed that deterioration of retinopathy correlated significantly with the levels of plasma glucose at entry and with the magnitude of improvement in glycemia during the first 6–14 weeks after entry. Although the 13 patients with no retinopathy at baseline did not progress to proliferative retinopathy, one did develop moderate hemorrhages, exudates and intraretinal microaneurysms (IRMA). Of their 20 patients with initial background retinopathy, two progressed to proliferative retinopathy. Laatikainen et al[42] confirmed that the decrease in HbA1c levels was most rapid in the two patients with the worst progression. They concluded that a rapid near normalization of glycemic control during pregnancy could accelerate the progression of retinopathy in poorly controlled diabetic patients. The DIEP Study[31] reported that the 10.3% of diabetic women who progressed, despite no retinopathy at baseline, had an initial glycohemoglobin elevation standard deviations (SD) above the mean of a normal population [risk progression 40%, odds ratio (OR) 2.4]. Independent of retinal status, the DIEP study also reported that duration of diabetes increased the risk of progression such that after 6 years duration of diabetes the OR was 3.0, by 11–15 years it was 9.7 and > 16 years it was 15.0, but hyperglycemia was a stronger risk factor. Additional evidence has been reported by the Diabetes Control and Complications Trial (DCCT).[43] In the conventional care group who became pregnant (n = 135), and thus had immediate intensification of glucose control, 47% worsened their retinal status and the OR for progression by the second trimester was 2.6 compared to diabetic women in the conventional group who did not become pregnant. In order to compare the HbA1c levels reported by the DCCT trial[43] to other published reports, the approximate equivalent baseline HbA1c levels, using the DCCT normal range, is 7.1, 9.8 and 9.5%, respectively. In addition, the rate of fall of the HbA1c level in the three case reports was faster than the reported rate of fall associated with deterioration of retinal status.

There is one case report in the literature which clearly shows that the combination of pregnancy and rapid normalization of severe hyperglycemia is sufficient to 'explode' a previously normal retina. Hagay et al[44] reported a case of a woman with no previously documented hyperglycemia who presented at 8 weeks of gestation with an HbA1c level of 16% and her ophthalmic examination was reported to be 'completely normal'. She was treated with intensive insulin therapy and at 12 weeks her HbA1c level was 5.9%. By the second trimester she had severe bilateral proliferative diabetic retinopathy needing photocoagulation.

In the three patients with no retinopathy at the start of pregnancy who progressed to proliferative retinopathy, each woman had at least three risk factors (an elevated HbA1c level at baseline into the highest risk category followed by rapid normalization of blood glucose, duration of diabetes > 6 years and pregnancy), and one had an additional risk factor of proteinuria. Of note, two of the three patients reported above had Type 2 diabetes. If they were of Asian descent, they had an added risk. In a report by Omori et al,[45] studying Japanese pregnant diabetic women, the prevalence of retinopathy was 34.4% in their Type 2 diabetic population. In addition, the prevalence of proliferative retinopathy was as high in the Type 2 women as in the Type 1 pregnant women, despite the shorter duration of documented diabetes in their Type 2 patients. Need for photocoagulation occurred in 50% of their Type 2 pregnant diabetic women patients with greater than background retinopathy at the beginning of pregnancy.

If insulin lispro did play a role in the progression of retinopathy, it is more likely that the insulin lispro facilitated the rapid normalization of the blood glucose levels. In pregnant diabetic patients, it has been shown that insulin lispro improves glucose control and thus significantly lowers the HbA1c level compared to patients who are administered human regular insulin.[17,29] There is danger in normalizing blood glucose quickly, regardless of the type of insulin used, in pregnant women with a long duration of diabetes and elevated HbA1c levels in the first trimester, in those with proteinuria and perhaps those with Type 1 diabetes.

Busy clinics may have a decreased ability to examine retinae thoroughly. Mild background retinopathy may be missed, even in the best of settings. Any retinopathy increases the risk, especially if the blood glucose level is elevated. Rather than recommending angiography to all women before each pregnancy is planned, in the case of no retinopathy seen on retinal examination, it is prudent to improve the glucose control slowly. These case reports reinforce the need to intensify preconceptional care programs to allow the luxury of slowly normalizing the blood glucose and to plan the pregnancy only after the blood glucose levels have been stabilized in the normal range for at least 6 months.[46–48] If a patient presents pregnant, with high HbA1c levels, regardless of the retinal status, as suggested by these cases, then a retinal specialist needs to be on the team, be vigilant and treat any developing angiopathy while the blood glucose is normalized.

If an insulin analog was available that was not immunogenic and had the rapid action of insulin lispro but had less IGF-1 activity than human insulin, then even if there was no proof that the IGF-1 activity of the insulin plays a role in the acceleration of diabetic retinopathy when the blood glucose level is normalized quickly, such an insulin would become the treatment of choice. Insulin aspart, an insulin analog that has been shown to produce a peak blood level at 40 minutes and lowers postprandial glucose levels significantly better than human insulin, has only 69% the IGF-1 activity of human insulin. However, use of insulin aspart in pregnancy must await the results of ongoing clinical trials in pregnancy to prove that insulin aspart does not cause an IgG response and does not cross the placenta.

Long-acting insulin analogs have only recently been used in clinical practice. The first clinically available long-acting insulin analog is insulin glargine. Insulin glargine has a glycine substitution in the alpha chain at the 21 position and two glargines attached to the beta-chain terminal at position 30. It is soluble insulin and has been shown to provide peakless, sustained and predictable 24 hour action. There are no clinical trials using insulin glargine in pregnancy. Of note, insulin glargine has a sixfold increase in IGF-1 activity as compared to human insulin. Another insulin analog that is currently in clinical trials is insulin detemir. Here again there are no trials using this insulin in pregnancy, but the studies show that detemir has the same IGF-1 activity as human insulin.

The clinician has to keep in mind that the most important concern is to safely normalize the maternal blood glucose. Before 1985, impure animal insulin was used, with a result that the IgG antibody levels rose the longer the women were treated. After 20 years of diabetes, women had antibody levels > 10,000. Purified human insulin has been available for >15 years, so there is a new generation of Type 1 diabetic women who have never been treated with animal insulins, and thus have negligible antibodies. Before giving these women insulin analogs it must be proved that: (1) they do not cause an immunologic response; (2) they do not cross the placenta; (3) they do not increase the risk of congenital anomalies or spontaneous abortions; and (4) they do not significantly increase the serum IGF-1 levels or accelerate diabetic retinopathy.

Definition of normoglycemia based on infant outcome

Previously, glucose control and targets for treatment were based on clinical judgment and concern for hypoglycemia. In fact, most clinicians preferred to maintain hyperglycemia rather than increase the risk of a hypoglycemic reaction. As tools and techniques improved to achieve near-normal glucose levels during pregnancy, the emphasis has changed to strive for the degree of maternal metabolic control that is associated with normal body size and proportions in full-term infants. Mello et al[49] published their study in which they investigated the anthropomorphic characteristics of 98 full-term singleton infants born to 98 women with Type 1 diabetes. They reported that those women who had a mean daily blood glucose level < 95 mg/dl had normal infants, whereas the women with mean blood glucose levels > 95 mg/dl delivered infants with an increased prevalence of being large for gestational age, with a significantly greater ponderal index and thoracic circumference with respect to the control group. Others have confirmed that overall mean glucose levels of < 95 mg/dl can avoid alterations in fetal growth.[5]

Jovanovic et al[50] studied 52 Type 1 diabetic women and found that when the mean blood glucose was maintained between 80 and 84 mg/dl, the outcome of pregnancy was normal. Langer et al[51] assessed the relationship between optimal levels of glycemic control and perinatal outcome in a prospective study of 334 GDM women and found that when the mean glucose levels were < 86 mg/dl, this group had a significantly higher prevalence of small-for-gestational age infants. In contrast, when the mean glucose levels were >105 mg/dl, there was a 20% prevalence of large-for-gestational-age infants. Hellmuth et al[52] found that the frequency of hypoglycemia, especially nocturnal hypoglycemia, was seen with a prevalence of 37% in the first trimester of pregnancies treated with intensified insulin therapy. Sacks et al[53] studied 48 Type 1 and 113 Type 2 diabetic women during pregnancy; they found that the mean glucose levels were higher in the Type 1 patients and at least one daily glucose level was < 50 mg/dl during 19% of observational days compared to only 2% of days in the Type 2 group. Rosenn et al[54] and Rosenn and Miodovnik[55] published papers on the topic of the increased risk of hypoglycemia during pregnancies complicated by diabetes. They found that at least 40% of mothers reported hypoglycemia during pregnancy. Clinically significant hypoglycemia requiring assistance from another person occurred in 71% of the 84 women studied, with a peak incidence occurring between 10 and 15 weeks of gestation. They did not observe any increase in embryopaqthy. Jovanovic et al[56] then published the first trimester insulin requirements of women studied in the DIEP Study. They showed that there was a drop in insulin requirements during weeks 8–11 of gestation, which was seen in all Type 1 diabetic women whose glucose concentrations were insensitively managed. The majority of the insulin requirement drops were seen in the overnight period. It was concluded that the insulin doses needed to be decreased for the overnight insulin requirement to prevent nocturnal hypoglycemia during the late first trimester.

Insulin requirements

Type 1 diabetic women must increase their insulin dosage to compensate for the diabetogenic forces of normal pregnancy. However, the exact patterns of insulin dosage increase is still controversial. Many observers have detected a decline in insulin requirement late in the first trimester of diabetic pregnancies. Jorgen Pedersen, the father of the study of diabetes in pregnancy, was among the first to observe that first trimester hypoglycemia was a symptom of pregnancy and that it was common knowledge among the physicians of the day. Pedersen wrote, 'Those physicians who manage diabetic women should be particularly alert for hypoglycemia in women who have recently become pregnant. About the 10th week of gestation there is an improvement in glucose tolerance manifesting itself as insulin coma, milder insulin reaction or an improvement in the degree of compensation. When a reduction in insulin dosage is called for it amounts to an average of 34%.' Indeed, he even claimed, 'Once in a while pregnancy may be diagnosed on account of inexplicable hypoglycemic attacks.' In a total of 26 cases of insulin coma, all of the cases in his series occurred in months 1–4 of gestation, with the majority occurring at months 2–3. He also noted that by late gestation, regardless of the metabolic control and duration of diabetes, average daily insulin requirements increased twofold from earlier in pregnancy.

Early first trimester overinsulinization might explain a later first trimester drop in insulin requirement. One example of this effect may be the significantly greater weight gain seen in the first trimester by diabetic women compared to healthy non-diabetic women. Perhaps the drive to increase caloric intake to prevent hypoglycemia in the first trimester may have been the cause of the first trimester excessive weight gain in the diabetic women compared to the controls.

On the other hand, others have not seen the first trimester decrease in insulin requirement. There are also reports of rising insulin requirement in the first trimester. The present authors have described the insulin requirements during pregnancy of a population of well-controlled Type 1 diabetic women which possibly lends credence to the notion that first trimester overinsulinization may be the cause of the hypoglycemia seen by some workers in the first trimester. In addition, together with the DIEP Study Group, the present authors have analyzed the insulin requirement and substratified based on degree of glucose control in the first trimester.[56] The weekly insulin requirement (as units/kg/day) were examined in the first trimester of diabetic women in the DIEP Study

with accurate gestational dating, regular glucose monitoring, daily insulin dose recording and monthly glycohemoglobin measurements. In pregnancies that resulted in live-born, term, singleton infants, a significant increase in mean weekly dosage was observed in weeks 3–7 ($P < 0.001$), followed by a significant decline in weeks 8–15 ($P < 0.001$). The Friedman non-parametric test localized significant changes to the interval between weeks 7–8 and weeks 11–12. To determine if prior poor glucose control exaggerated these trends, the women were divided based on their glycohemoglobin values: < 2 SD above the mean of a normal population (Group 1), 2–4 SD (Group 2) and > 4 SD (Group 3) at baseline. Late first trimester declines in dosage were statistically significant in Group 2 ($P = 0.002$) and in Groups 2 and 3 together ($P = 0.003$). Similarly, women with body mass index (BMI) > 27.0 had a greater initial insulin rise and then fall compared to leaner women. Observations in the DIEP Study cohort disclosed a mid-first trimester decline in insulin requirement in insulin-dependent, diabetic pregnant women. Possible explanations include overinsulinization of previously poorly controlled diabetes and a transient decline in progesterone secretion during the late first trimester luteo-placental shift in progesterone secretion.

Clinicians should anticipate a reduction in insulin requirement in the 4 week interval between weeks 8 and 12 of gestation. Based on these studies of well-controlled diabetic women, an algorithm for care and an insulin requirement protocol has been created, based on gestational week and the woman's current pregnant body weight. The total daily dose of insulin in the first trimester (weeks 5–12) insulin requirement is 0.7 units/kg/day; in the second trimester (weeks 12–26) the insulin requirement is 0.8 unit/kg day; in the third trimester (weeks 26–36) the

Time	Fraction of total daily insulin dose (I*)	
	NPH (50% of I)	Regular or lipro or aspart insulin (50% of I)
Pre-breakfast	1/6I	4/20I (or 0.20I)
Pre-lunch		3/20I (or 0.15I)
Pre-dinner	1/6I	3/20I (or 0.15I)
Bedtime	1/6I	

* I = 0.7 units times the present pregnant weight (in kg) for weeks 1–12; I = 0.8 units times the present pregnant weight (in kg) for weeks 12–26; I = 0.9 units times the present pregnant weight (in kg) for weeks 26–36; I = 1.0 units times the present pregnant weight (in kg) for weeks 36–40.

Table 27.1. *Initial calculation of insulin therapy for pregnancy.*

insulin requirement is 0.9 units/kg/day; and at term (weeks 36–40) the insulin requirement is 1.0 units/kg/day (Table 27.1). The insulin needs to be divided throughout the day to provide the basal need (the dose of insulin that keeps a woman normal in the fasting state) and meal-related need. When multiple insulin injections are

used to provide the basal need, NPH insulin is preferred because it has a more predictable absorption pattern than lente or ultralente insulin. Also, the recently developed long-acting insulin analogs (insulin glargine or insulin determir) have not yet been proven to be safe or efficacious in pregnancy.

Preferred use of NPH is to give one sixth of the total daily dose of insulin (I) as morning, dinner and bedtime injections (i.e. NPH dose equals 50% of daily dose divided into three equal injections of NPH given every 8 hours, or at 8 am, 4 pm and 12 midnight; Table 27.1).

The other half of the total daily insulin dose should be a short-acting insulin (human regular, insulin lispro or insulin aspart) given before each meal to control postprandial glycemia (Table 27.1). This dose of short-acting insulin can be given using the insulin infusion pump or by multiple doses of subcutaneously injected insulin (Tables 27.1–27.3).

The meal-related insulin dose [one half of the total daily insulin requirement (0.5I)] is divided such that 40% of the meal-related dose is given to cover breakfast and the remaining 60%

Period	Basal requirement (B*) hourly infusion rate	Rationale
Midnight to 4 am	50% less basal (B/24 × 0.5)	Maternal cortisol at nadir
4 am to 10 am	50% more basal (B/24 × 1.5)	Highest level of maternal cortisol
10 am to noon	Basal (B/24)	

* B = 0.5I (the total daily insulin) or an hourly rate of B/24.
To refine basal settings, have the patient perform self-blood glucose monitoring at the end of each period to determine whether adjustments are needed. For instance, at the 4 am test, the blood glucose level should be 60–90 mg/dl; if blood glucose level is out of this range, dial up or down insulin in increments of 0.10 units/hour. (Consider using 0.1 units/kg as NPH insulin at bedtime to prevent diabetic ketoacidosis secondary to needle slippage; then decrease the overnight basal from 4 am to 10 am by 0.02 units/kg/hour.)

Table 27.2. *Basal insulin pump program (using human regular, insulin lispro or insulin aspart).*

Pre-meal basal glucose (mg/dl)	Compensatory insulin[†]
< 60	Meal-related insulin dose minus 3% I
61–90	Meal-related insulin dose – no adjustment necessary
91–120	Meal-related insulin dose plus 3% I
> 121	Meal-related insulin dose plus 6% I

* Human regular insulin or insulin lispro or insulin aspart.
[†] Meal-related insulin is half the total daily insulin dose (I), such that 40% of the dose is at breakfast, 30% is at lunch and 30% is at dinner.

Table 27.3. *Pre-meal sliding scale dose calculation using rapid-acting insulin.**

is left to cover the lunch and dinner meals (Table 27.1). The exact division of this meal-related insulin dose depends on the size of the woman's lunch versus her dinner. Breakfast necessitates the majority of the meal-related dose because the diurnal variation in cortisol levels is potentiated by pregnancy.

Compensatory doses to adjust for high or low glucose levels are calculated as 3% of the total daily insulin requirement. Clinicians should note that hyperglycemia would occur if the patient used only insulin lispro or insulin apart for the meal-related needs, and if the woman goes a long time between meals. The dose of NPH insulin may not be sufficient to prevent an escape of the blood glucose before the next dose of insulin is given. To prevent this escape of blood glucose when >3 hours elapses between injections of the rapid-acting insulin analogs of lispro or aspart, the patient should add 3% of her total daily insulin requirement as regular human insulin to the lispro injection to extend the effectiveness of the short-acting component.

Insulin infusion pumps

Insulin infusion pumps have been used for treatment for over two decades.[57] However, the data on the safety and efficacy of insulin pumps in pregnancy complicated by diabetes are still in infancy. Kitzmiller et al[58] showed that insulin pump therapy did improve glucose control and minimized clinically significant hypoglycemic events to 2.2/week. Coustan et al[59] then reported a randomized clinical trial of insulin pump therapy versus conventional therapy in pregnancies complicated by diabetes. They showed that there were no differences between the two treatment groups with respect to outpatients mean glucose levels, symptomatic hypoglycemia or HbA1c levels. They concluded that excellent diabetes control can be achieved with both insulin infusion pumps and with multiple injections of insulin. Carta et al[60] also performed a randomized trial of continuous subcutaneous insulin infusion versus intensive conventional insulin therapy in Type 1 and Type 2 diabetic pregnant women. They reported that there were no significant differences in mean insulin requirements at the different stages of gestation and that perinatal outcome was satisfactory in both groups, however, in their study, control of fetal growth was better with interfiled convention therapy compared to fetal growth in the pump group. Mancuso et al[61] studied the efficacy of the insulin pump in the home treatment of pregnant diabetic women. They reported that seven Type 1 diabetic women using the pump delivered term infants and had no macrosomia or neonatal problems along with normal glucose tolerance tests at two years of life. Potter et al[57] studied continuous insulin infusion in the third trimester of eight pregnancies complicated by diabetes. Compared to historical controls, they concluded that diurnal variations of blood glucose concentrations were dampened. Leveno et al[62] performed a case-controlled trial of insulin pump therapy versus literature intensified conventional therapy, and observed no significant differences between the groups for glucose control, cost and complications. They concluded that insulin pumps were not acceptable to all pregnant diabetic women and that such therapy may not be necessary to improve pregnancy outcome. Caruso et al[63] treated 12 poorly controlled pregnant diabetic women with insulin infusion pumps and showed that glucose levels could be quickly normalized with a remarkable decrease in variation of glucose excursions. In addition, they showed that amniotic fluid insulin, glucose and C-peptide levels were normal, and none of the infants were macrosomic or had any neonatal problems. They concluded that insulin infusion pump therapy was highly effective compared to intensified conventional treatment. In a nested case–control study, Simmons et al[64] utilized insulin pumps in pregnancies complicated by Type 2 diabetes and GDM in a multiethnic community, and showed in 30 women that none experienced severe hypoglycemia and 79% had improved glycemic control within 1–4 weeks. Mothers using the pump had greater insulin requirements and greater weight gain. Although their infants were more likely to be admitted to the special care unit, they were not heavier nor did they have more hypoglycemic events than control subjects. Jensen et al[65] reported their series using insulin infusion pump therapy ($n = 11$) in the preconceptional treatment period in Type 1 diabetic women compared to women treated with conventional therapy ($n = 9$). Two infants born of mothers treated with conventional therapy exhibited early group delay, whereas all 11 infants born of mothers treated with pump therapy were normal; there were no malformations in either group. Gabbe et al[66] published a series of 24 Type 1 diabetic patients and reported no difference in the groups of women treated with pump compared with those treated with intensified insulin therapy for episodes of hypoglycemia, costs, complication, glycemic control or in pregnancy outcome. The advantages seen were all postpartum because those women who were on the pump into their postpartum period sustained better glucose control than those who were on intensified insulin therapy during pregnancy. The conclusion drawn from this review of the literature on using insulin pump therapy in pregnant women with diabetes is that pump therapy is not necessary in order to achieve and maintain optimal control (Table 27.4); however, five of the 10 papers suggest that insulin pump therapy has an advantage over intensified multiple injections of insulin. In addition, only 155 patients were reported in these 10 trials and in all but one paper the women had their pump therapy started in the second or third trimester (Table 27.4).

Insulin algorithms for continuous insulin infusion pump therapy in pregnancy

The basal need is usually 50% of the total daily insulin dose (0.5I) and may be delivered using a constant infusion pump (Table 27.2) or by multiple doses of intermediate-acting insulin (Table 27.1). When using a constant infusion pump the basal need is calculated as an hourly rate (Table 27.2) and is delivered such that the calculated rate (0.5I or total dose over 24 hours divided by 24) is given between 10 am and midnight. The rate is cut in half (i.e. 0.5I divided by 24 times 0.5) from midnight to 4 am, and increased by another 50% (i.e. 0.5I divided by 24 times 1.5) to counteract the morning rise of cortisol levels that are potentiated during pregnancy.

Author and year (reference)	No. on CSII*	Trimester or weeks gestation	Type of DM†	Type of trial/comments
Potter et al 1980 (57)	8	Third	1	Longitudinal/improved
Kitzmiller et al 1985 (58)	24	5–10	1	Longitudinal/no difference
Coustan et al 1986 (59)	22	Second and third	1	Randomized/no difference
Carta et al 1986 (60)	14	First	1	Case–control/improved
Mancuso et al 1986 (61)	12	Third	1	Longitudinal/improved
Jensen et al 1986 (65)	9	Before and all trimesters	1	Case–control
Caruso et al 1987 (63)	12	Third	1	Longitudinal/improved
Leveno et al 1988 (62)	11	Second and third	1	Self-selection/no difference
Gabbe et al 2001 (66)	23	Second, third and postpartum	1	Only postpartum improved
Simmons et al 2002 (64)	30	Second	GDM‡ and 2	Equal

* Continuous subcutaneous insulin infusion.
† Diabetes mellitus.
‡ Gestational diabetes mellitus.

Table 27.4. *Review of the literature on using insulin infusion pump therapy in pregnancies complicated by diabetes.*

Also, low-dose NPH before bedtime has been used by some clinicians to prevent the possible occurrence of diabetic ketoacidosis if the needle slips out of position during the overnight period. This dose of NPH insulin needs to be sufficient to provide protection from ketosis, or 0.1 units of NPH times the weight of the women in kilograms. Then the overnight basal insulin needs to be decreased to allow for the NPH dose. The 4 am to 10 am basal insulin should thus be adjusted downward by 0.02 units/kg/hour.

Insulin and glucose treatment during labor

With improvement in antenatal care, intrapartum events play an increasingly crucial role in the outcome of pregnancy. The artificial beta cell may be used to maintain normoglycemia during labor and delivery, but normoglycemia can be maintained easily by subcutaneous injections. Before active labor, insulin is required, and glucose infusion is not necessary to maintain a blood glucose level of

70–90 mg/dl. With the onset of active labor, insulin requirements decrease to zero and glucose requirements are relatively constant at 2.5 mg/kg/minute. From these data, a protocol for supplying the glucose needs of labor has been developed.[67]

The goal is to maintain the maternal plasma glucose between 70 and 90 mg/dl. In cases of the onset of active spontaneous labor, insulin is withheld and an intravenous (IV) dextrose infusion is begun at a rate of 2.55 mg/kg/minute. If labor is latent, normal saline is usually sufficient to maintain normoglycemia until active labor begins, at which time dextrose is infused at 2.55 mg/kg/minute. Blood glucose is then monitored hourly and if it is < 60 mg/dl then the infusion rate is doubled for the subsequent hour. If the blood glucose rises to > 120 mg/dl, 2–4 units of regular insulin are given IV each hour until the blood glucose level is 70–90 mg/dl. In the case of an elective Cesarean section, the bedtime dose of NPH insulin is repeated at 8 am on the day of surgery and every 8 hours if the surgery is delayed. A dextrose infusion may be started if the plasma glucose level falls to < 60 mg/dl, and 2–4 units of regular insulin given IV every hour if the blood glucose rises to > 120 mg/dl.[67]

Insulin and glucose requirements postpartum

Maternal insulin requirements usually drop precipitously postpartum, possibly for 48–96 hours. Insulin requirements should be recalculated at 0.6 units/kg based on the postpartum weight and should be started when the 1 hour postprandial plasma glucose value is > 150 mg/dl or the fasting glucose level is > 100 mg/dl. The postpartum caloric requirements are 25 kcal/kg/day, based on the postpartum weight. For women who wish to breastfeed, the calculation is 27 kcal/kg/day and insulin requirements are 0.6 units/kg/day. The insulin requirement during the night drops dramatically during lactation, owing to the glucose siphoning into the breast milk. Thus, the majority of the insulin requirement is needed during the daytime to cover the increased caloric needs of breastfeeding. Normoglycemia should especially be prescribed for nursing diabetic women, because hyperglycemia elevates milk glucose levels.[68]

Conclusions

With the advent of tools and techniques to maintain normoglycemia before, during and between all pregnancies complicated by diabetes, infants of diabetic mothers now have the same chances of good health as those infants born to the non-diabetic woman. Animal and human studies clearly implicate glucose as the teratogen. These studies, and others, emphasize the need for preconceptional programs and the need for support systems to facilitate the maintenance of normoglycemia throughout pregnancy. The morbidity and subsequent development of the infant of the diabetic mother is associated with hyperglycemia. Therefore, the goal of insulin therapy is to achieve and maintain normoglycemia before, during and after all pregnancies complicated by diabetes.

References

1. Pedersen J. Course of diabetes during pregnancy. *Acta Endocrinol* 1952; 9:342–7.
2. Mills JL, Knopp RH, Simpson JL et al. Lack of relation of increased malformation rates in infants of diabetic mothers to glycemic control during organogenesis. *N Engl J Med* 1988; 318:671–6.
3. Mills JL, Simpson JL, Driscoll SG et al. Incidence of spontaneous abortion among normal women and insulin-

dependent diabetic women whose pregnancies were identified within 21 days of conception. *N Engl J Med* 1988; 319:1617–23.

4. Mills JL, Fishl AR, Knopp RH et al. Malformations in infants of diabetic mothers: problems in study design. *Prev Med* 1983; 12:274–86.

5. Jovanovic L, Peterson CM, Saxena BB et al. Feasibility of maintaining normal glucose profiles in insulin-dependent pregnant diabetic women. *Am J Med* 1980; 68:105–12.

6. DeVeciana M, Major CA, Morgan MA et al. Postprandial versus preprandial blood glucose monitoring in women with gestational diabetes mellitus requiring insulin therapy. *N Engl J Med* 1995; 333:1237–41.

7. Combs CA, Gunderson E, Kitzmiller JL et al. Relationship of fetal macrosomia to maternal postprandial glucose control during pregnancy. *Diabetes Care* 1992; 15:1251–7.

8. Jovanovic L, Peterson CM, Reed GF et al. Maternal postprandial glucose levels and infant birth weight: the Diabetes In Early Pregnancy Study. *Am J Obstet Gynecol* 1991; 164:103–11.

9. Jovanovic L. What is so bad about a big baby? *Diabetes Care* 2001; 24:1317–18 (editorial).

10. Knopp RH. Hormone mediated changes in nutrient metabolism in pregnancy: a physiological basis for normal fetal development. In: (Jacobsen MS, Rees JM, Golden NH, Irwin CE, eds) *Adolescent Nutritional Disorders: Prevention and Treatment.* (New York Academy of Sciences: New York, 1997) 251–71.

11. Knight G, Worth RC, Ward JD. Macrosomia despite well-controlled diabetic pregnancy. *Lancet* 1983; 2:1431.

12. Visser GHA, van Ballegooie E, Slutter WJ. Macrosomia despite well-controlled diabetic pregnancy. *Lancet* 1984; 1:284–5.

13. Menon RK, Cohen RM, Sperling MA et al. Transplacental passage of insulin in pregnant women with insulin-dependent diabetes mellitus. Its role in fetal macrosomia. *N Engl J Med* 1990; 323:309–15.

14. Jovanovic L, Kitzmiller JL, Peterson CM. Randomized trial of human versus animal species insulin in diabetic pregnant women: improved glycemic control, not fewer antibodies to insulin, influences birth weight. *Am J Obstet Gynecol* 1992; 167:1325–30.

15. Anderson Jr JH, Brunelle RL, Koivisto VA et al. Reduction of postprandial hyperglycemia and frequency of hypoglycemia in IDDM patients on insulin-analog treatment. *Diabetes* 1997; 46:265–70.

16. Fineberg SE, Rathbun MJ, Hufferd S et al. Immunologic aspects of human proinsulin therapy. *Diabetes* 1988; 37:276–80.

17. Jovanovic L, Ilic S, Pettitt DJ et al. The metabolic and immunologic effects of insulin lispro in gestational diabetes. *Diabetes Care* 1999; 22:1422–6.

18. Fineberg NS, Fineberg SE, Anderson JH et al. Immunologic effects of insulin lispro [Lys(B23), Pro

(B29) human insulin in IDDM and NIDDM patients previously treated with insulin. *Diabetes* 1996; 45:1750–4.

19. Jehle PM, Fussgaenger RD, Kunze U et al. The human insulin analog insulin lispro improves insulin binding on circulating monocytes of intensively treated insulin dependent diabetes mellitus patients. *J Clin Endocrinol Metab* 1996; 81:2319–27.

20. Jehle PM, Fussgaenger RD, Seibold A et al. Pharmacodynamics of insulin lispro in 2 patients with type II diabetes mellitus. *Int J Clin Pharmacol Ther* 1996; 34:498–503.

21. Balsells M, Corcoy R, Mauricio D et al. Insulin antibody response to a short course of human insulin therapy in women with gestational diabetes. *Diabetes Care* 1997; 20:1172–5.

22. Jovanovic L, Bevier W. The Santa Barbara County Health Care Services Program: birth weight change concomitant with screening for and treatment of glucose-intolerance of pregnancy: a potential cost-effective intervention. *Am J Perinatol* 1997; 14:221–8.

23. Jovanovic L, Druzin M, Peterson CM. Effect of euglycemia on the outcome of pregnancy in insulin-dependent diabetic women as compared with normal control subjects. *Am J Med* 1981; 71:921–7.

24. Jovanovic L, Peterson CM. Rationale for prevention and treatment of glucose-mediated macrosomia: a protocol for gestational diabetes. *Endocr Pract* 1996; 2:118–29.

25. Diamond T, Kormas N. Possible adverse fetal effects of insulin lispro. *N Engl J Med* 1997; 337:1009.

26. Mills JL, Baker L, Goldman A. Malformations in infants of diabetic mothers occur before the seventh gestational week: implications for treatment. *Diabetes* 1979; 23:292.

27. Jovanovic L. Role of diet and insulin treatment of diabetes in pregnancy. *Clin Obstet Gynecol* 2000; 43:46–51.

28. Kucera J. Rate and type of congenital anomalies among offspring of diabetic mothers. *J Reprod Med* 1971; 7:61–4.

29. Anderson J, Bastyr E, Wishner K. Response to Diamond and Kormas. *N Engl J Med* 1997; 337:1009–12.

30. Jovanovic L. Retinopathy risk: what is responsible? Hormones, hyperglycemia, or humalog? *Diabetes Care* 1999; 22:846–50.

31. Chew EY, Mills JL, Metzger BE et al. National Institute of Child Health and Human Development Diabetes in Early Pregnancy Study: metabolic control and progression of retinopathy: the Diabetes In Early Pregnancy Study. *Diabetes Care* 1995; 18:631–7.

32. Merimee TJ, Zapf J, Froesch ER. Insulin-like growth factors: studies in diabetics with and without retinopathy. *N Engl J Med* 1983; 309:527–31.

33. Larinkari J, Laatikainen L, Ranta T. Metabolic control and serum hormone levels in relationship to retinopathy in diabetic pregnancy. *Diabetologia* 1982; 22:327–31.

34. Hill DJ, Clemmons DR, Riley SC et al. Immunohistochemical localization of insulin like growth factors

and IGF binding proteins-1, -2, and -3 in human placenta and fetal membranes. *Placenta* 1993; **14**:1–12.

35. MacLeod JN, Worsley I, Ray Y et al. Human growth hormone variant is a biologically active somatogen and lactogen. *Endocrinology* 1991; **128**:1298–302.

36. Gluckman PD. The endocrine regulation of fetal growth in late gestation: the role of insulin-like growth factors. *J Clin Endocrinol Metab* 1995; **80**:1047–50.

37. Holly JMP, Amiel SA, Sandhu RR et al. The role of growth hormone in diabetes mellitus. *J Endocrinol* 1988; **118**:353–64.

38. Kitzmiller J, Main E, Ward B et al. Insulin lispro and the development of proliferative diabetic retinopathy during pregnancy. *Diabetes Care* 1999; **22**:874.

39. DiMarchi RD, Chance RE, Long HB et al. Preparation of an insulin with improved pharmacokinetics relative to human insulin through consideration of structural homology with insulin-like growth factor-1. *Horm Res* 1994; **41**(Suppl 2):93–6.

40. Llewelyn J, Slieker LJ, Zimmermann JL. Pre-clinical studies on insulin lispro. *Drugs Today* 1998; **34** (**Suppl C**):11–21.

41. Phelps RL, Sakol L, Metzger BE et al. Changes in diabetic retinopathy during pregnancy: correlations with regulation of hyperglycemia. *Arch Ophthalmol* 1986; **104**:1806–10.

42. Laatikainen L, Teramo K, Hieta-Heikurainen H et al. A controlled study of the influence of continuous subcutaneous insulin infusion treatment on diabetic retinopathy during pregnancy. *Acta Med Scand* 1987; **221**:367–76.

43. Lachin J, Clearly P, and the DCCT Research Group. Pregnancy increases the risk of complication in the DCCT. *Diabetes* 1998; **47** (**Suppl 1**):1091.

44. Hagay ZJ, Schachter M, Pollack A, Ley R. Case report: development of proliferative retinopathy in a gestational diabetes patient following rapid metabolic control. *Euro J Obstet Gynecol Reprod Biol* 1994; **57**:211–13.

45. Omori Y, Minei S, Tamaki T et al. Current status of pregnancy in diabetic women. A comparison of pregnancy in IDDM and NIDDM mothers. *Diabetes Res Clin Pract* 1994; **24**:S273-S278.

46. Ylinen K, Aula P, Stenman U-H et al. Risk of minor and major fetal malformations in diabetics with high haemoglobin A_{1c} values in early pregnancy. *Br Med J* 1984; **289**:345–6.

47. Hanson U, Persson B, Thunell S. Relationship between haemoglobin A_{1c} in early type 1 (insulin-dependent) diabetic pregnancy and the occurrence of spontaneous abortion and fetal malformation in Sweden. *Diabetologia* 1990; **33**:100–4.

48. Greene MF, Hare JW, Cloherty JP et al. First-trimester hemoglobin A_1 and risk for major malformation and spontaneous abortion in diabetic pregnancy. *Teratology* 1989; **39**:225–31.

49. Mello G, Paretti E, Mecacci F et al. What degree of maternal metabolic control in women with type 1 diabetes is

associated with normal body size and proportions in full-term infants? *Diabetes Care* 2000; **23**:1494–8.

50. Jovanovic L, Druzin M, Peterson CM. Effect of euglycemia on the outcome of pregnancy in insulin-dependent diabetic women as compared with normal control subjects. *Am J Med* 1981; **71**:921–7.

51. Langer O, Levy J, Brustman L et al. Glycemic control in gestational dietbes: how tight is tight enough: small for gestational age versus large for gestational age? *Am J Obstet Gynecol* 1989; **161**:646–53.

52. Hellmuth E, Damm P, Molsted-Pedersen L, Bendtson I. Prevalence of nocturnal hypoglycemia in the first trimester of pregnancy in patients with insulin treated diabetes mellitus. *Acta Obste Gynecol Scand* 2000; **79**:3–5.

53. Sacks DA, Chen W, Greenspoon JS, Wolde-Tsadik. Should the same glucose values be targeted for type 1 as for type 2 diabetics in pregnancy? *Am J Obstet Gynecol* 1997; **177**:113–19.

54. Rosenn BM, Miodovnik M, Holcberg G et al. Hypoglycemia: the price of intensified insulin therapy for pregnant women with insulin-dependent diaebtes mellitus. *Obstet Gynecol* 1995; **85**:417–22.

55. Rosenn BM, Miodovnik M. Glycemic control in the diabetic pregnancy: is tighter always better? *J Matern Fetal Med* 2000; **9**:29–34.

56. Jovanovic L, Mills Jl, Knopp RH et al, and the National Institute of Child Health and Human Development – Diabetes in Early Pregnancy Study Group. Declining insulin requirement in the late first trimester of diabetic pregnancy. *Diabetes Care* 2001; **24**:1130–6.

57. Potter JM, Beckless JP, Cullen DR. Subcutaneous insulin infusion control of blood glucose concentration in diabetics in third trimester of pregnancy. *Br Med J* 1980; **26**:1099–101.

58. Kitzmiller JL, Younger MD, Hare JW et al. Continuous subcutaneous insulin therapy during early pregnancy. *Obstet Gynecol* 1985; **66**:606–11.

59. Coustan DR, Reece A, Sherwin RS et al. A randomized clinical trial of the insulin pump versus intensive conventional therapy in diabetic pregnancies. *J Am Med Assoc* 1986; **255**:631–5.

60. Carta O, Meriggi E, Trossarelli GF et al. Continuous subcutaneous insulin infusion versus intensive conventional insulin therapy in type 1 and type 2 diabetic pregnancy. *Diabetes Metab* 1986; **12**:121–9.

61. Mancuso S, Caruso A, Lanzone A et al. Continuous subcutaneous insulin infusion in pregnant diabetic women. *Acta Endocrinol* 1986; (**Suppl**) 277:112–16.

62. Leveno KJ, Fortunato SJ, Raskin P et al. Continuous subcutaneous insulin infusion during pregnancy. *Diabetes Res Clin Pract* 1988; **4**:257–68.

63. Caruso A, Lanzone V, Massidda M et al. Continuous subcutaneous insulin infusion in pregnant diabetic patients. *Prenatal Diag* 1987; **7**:41–50.

64. Simmons D, Thompson CF, Conroy C, Scott DJ. Use of insulin pumps in pregnancies complicated by type 2

diabetes and gestational diabetes in a multiethnic community. *Diabetes Care* 2002; **24**:2078–82.

65. Jensen BM, Kuhl C, Petersen LM et al. Preconceptional treatment with insulin infusion pumps in insulin-dependent diabetic women with particular reference to prevention of congenital malformations. *Acta Endocrinol* 1986; **(Suppl) 277**:81–5.

66. Gabbe SG, Holing E, Temple P, Brown ZA. Benefits, risks, costs, and patient satisfaction associated with insulin pump therapy for the pregnancy complicated by type 1 diabetes mellitus. *Am J Obstet Gynecol* 2000; **182**:1283–91.

67. Jovanovic L, Peterson CM. Insulin and glucose requirements during the first stage of labor in insulin-dependent diabetic women. *Am J Med* 1983; **75**:607–12.

68. Jovanovic L (editor-in-chief). *Medical Management of Pregnancy Complicated by Diabetes*. (American Diabetes Association, Inc.: Alexandria, 1993) (revised 1995 and 2000).

28

Use of oral hypoglycemic agents in pregnancy
Oded Langer

Introduction

Gestational diabetes mellitus (GDM) continues to be a major public health problem for the mother and unborn fetus, with an estimated incidence of 3–10%, depending upon geographic location, affecting at least 105,000–350,000 women annually in the United States. The cornerstone of treatment is diabetic diet and when dietary modifications do not control maternal glycemia, insulin therapy is initiated. The administration of short- and long-acting insulin will be required in 20–60% of pregnancies that are complicated by GDM in order to maintain adequate glycemic control. Based on its high efficacy (50–80% will achieve good glycemic control), and its inability to cross the placenta by itself and reach the fetus because of its molecular size, insulin has remained the drug of choice.[1]

Bauman and Yallow,[2] however, confirmed that insulin can readily cross the placenta as insulin antibody complexes, while the results of Menon et al[3] correlated insulin antibody passage rates with macrosomia. Therefore, these findings regarding the safety of insulin therapy need to be addressed. Moreover, the introduction of new insulin analogs (e.g. lispro) requires further investigation to rule out stimulation of antibody production that may assist insulin transfer through the placenta. In

addition, insulin is inconvenient and expensive, which makes this factor of even greater concern in developing countries. Therefore, a continuous search for a safe and effective alternative to insulin therapy has been an ongoing challenge. The use of oral hypoglycemic agents in non-pregnant Type 2 diabetics has become the standard of care in the United States (US) to help patients maintain the tight glucose control that lowers their risk for microvascular complications.[4,5] The prevalence of GDM varies in direct proportion to the prevalence of Type 2 diabetes in a given population or ethnic group. In the US, the prevalence rate ranges from 1 to 14%.[6] Among different ethnic groups, both forms have been diagnosed in varying rates. Both Type 2 diabetes and GDM are heterogeneous disorders whose pathophysiology is characterized by peripheral insulin resistance, impaired regulation of hepatic glucose production and declining beta-cell function. It has become the prime objective for treatment of both pregnant and non-pregnant diabetic patients to optimize the glycemic profile. Insulin and the oral hypoglycemic agents were all designed to reduce the level of glycemia.[7–10] Although paucity of information exists on the efficacy of the use of oral hypoglycemic agents in pregnancy, and therefore its restricted role in the management of GDM in the US, both glyburide and metformin have been widely prescribed in Europe and in South Africa without reported adverse side effects to the fetus.[11–22] It is only recently in the US that consideration of the use of oral hypoglycemic agents in pregnancy has even become 'debatable' in scientific forums. The historic ban on the use of oral hypoglycemic agents in pregnancy have been based on scant evidence of case reports[23,24] and one study in particular on fetal anomalies in 50 poorly controlled diabetics prior to pregnancy,[25] begging the question: is it the drug or is it the glucose?

The controversy surrounding the management of GDM with oral hypoglycemic agents stems from the lack of data from well-designed studies. The new term for emphasizing outcome-based approaches is 'evidence-based medicine'. When doctors continue to question established practices, and base decision-making on research evidence rather than on anecdotes and opinions of 'experts', they can perform at their best. The purpose of this review is to provide the reader with the evidence and the foundation for understanding the use of oral hypoglycemic drugs in pregnancy as an effective alternative to insulin therapy in achieving glycemic control. The concerns of teratogenicity due to possible placental transfer, neonatal and maternal outcome, and basic pharmacological benefits will be addressed.

Oral hypoglycemic agents: classification and characteristics

In contrast to systematic studies that led to the isolation of insulin, **sulfonylureas** were discovered accidentally. Additional clinical trials led to the discovery of tolbutamide in the 1950s and since that time many agents in this class of drugs have been developed, e.g.

chlorpropamide. Second-generation sulfonylureas were subsequently developed that today include drugs such as glyburide and glipizide. In 1997, the first drug in a new class of oral insulin secretagogues called meglitinides (benzoic acid derivatives) was approved for clinical use. The agent, repaglinide, has gained acceptance as a fast-acting, premeal therapy to limit postprandial hyperglycemia.[26]

Biguanides were recognized as early as 1920 but received clinical recognition in the US only in the past decade. Phenformin, the primary drug in this group, was withdrawn from American and European markets because of the side effects of lactic acidosis. Its replacement, metformin, although used extensively in Europe, has only been recognized for use in the US since 1995.[26]

Thiazolidinediones were introduced in 1997. The first agent, troglitazone, was reported to have a high rate of hepatic toxicity, and as a result was withdrawn from the market in 2000. However, newer agents in this class such as rosiglitazone and pioglitazone are widely used in clinical practice without reported hepatic toxicity. **Alpha-glucosidase inhibitors**, which reduce intestinal absorption of starch and glucose (acarbose), have now been introduced into clinical practice.[26]

The oral hypoglycemic agents act, depending upon the specific group, directly upon the beta cells to increase insulin secretion and/or to decrease hepatic glucose production, and to increase peripheral insulin sensitivity. The advantage of using these agents rather than administering exogenous insulin is because of their ability to have an impact by nutrient availability, extra pancreatic effect and/or to increase insulin availability through the physiological route.

The prevalence of Type 2 diabetes and GDM has increased by 33% in the past decade in the US.[6] This may be attributed to the increased rate of obesity in the general population in all ethnic groups and the trend towards advanced maternal age in pregnancy. Because of the relative ease of administration and the low cost involved in overall therapy with oral hypoglycemic agents, they have become the drug of choice in the treatment of Type 2 diabetes. One can assume that their popularity will only increase in the future, especially after confirmation from the large prospective study by the United Kingdom Prospective Diabetes Study (UKPDS) group. The results of the study demonstrated that Type 2 diabetic patients can maintain their desired level of control, thereby lowering their risk for microvascular complications.[27] The present author's group's randomized study of the use of oral hypoglycemic agents demonstrated that glyburide is an efficacious alternative to insulin in the treatment of diabetes in the pregnant subject.[28]

The reader should consider the following 'drug compass' when contemplating the use of an insulin secretagogue in pregnancy:

(1) will the drug–drug interactions complicate its use with the necessary and commonly administered drugs?
(2) can glycemic control be achieved by using the optimal dose?
(3) after nutrient ingestion, can the drug reduce the time lag between the plasma glucose rise and insulin secretion?
(4) can serious postprandial and fasting hypoglycemia be minimized because the drug duration of action is short enough or its dependence on plasma glucose levels sufficient?
(5) are there any side effects that can reduce the long-term beneficial effects?[29]

A major consideration in the efficacy of the drug will be its ability to cross the placenta and, if this is so, what toxicity, if at all, can it cause to the developing fetus. Often, the fear of drug-induced adverse outcome, especially after the thalidomide era in the 1960s, paralyzes the physician's ability to judge the scientific rationale for using a drug and evaluating it using evidence-based data instead of dogma. Very few medications have been shown not to cross the placental barrier. In fact, a pregnant woman is often exposed to four or five prescription drugs during pregnancy for a variety of complaints. Similar to other epithelial barriers, transfer of drugs across the placenta is affected by several factors: molecular weight; pK_a; lipophilicity; placental blood flow; blood protein binding; elimination half-life; and the specific placental transport system that affects the ability of drugs to enter the fetal compartment.[26,30,31]

Sulfonylureas

Sulfonylureas have been used in the treatment of Type 2 diabetes since 1942 because of their capacity to cause hypoglycemia by stimulating insulin release from pancreatic beta cells. Sulfonylureas bind to specific receptors on beta cells, forcing closure of potassium adenosine triphosphate (ATP) channels and opening of calcium channels that cause an increase in cytoplastic calcium that stimulates insulin release. The major effect of these drugs is to enhance insulin secretion.[32–36] Sulfonylureas may also further increase insulin levels by reducing hepatic clearance of the hormone, the main contributor to fasting hyperglycemia. Enhanced insulin secretion diminishes glucose toxicity and improves insulin secretion after meals, thus reducing postprandial hyperglycemia. These drugs can also enhance peripheral tissue sensitivity to insulin.[32,33] The sulfonylureas influence insulin secretion in direct proportion to plasma glucose levels from 60 to 180 mg/dl: they do not stimulate insulin secretion when the plasma glucose is < 60 mg/dl.[37,38] The mechanism of action of sulfonyureas is to facilitate insulin secretion rapidly in response to nutritional intake, which will result in a minimal to no lag time between the changes in plasma glucose and modification of the insulin secretory rate.[39,40]

Chlorpropamide has been available for > 30 years and is a highly effective oral hypoglycemic agent with a very long duration of action. The main side effect for Type 2 non-pregnant patients is a significantly high rate of severe and protracted hypoglycemia. This complication has not been reported to be a major concern for pregnant patients in previous studies.[11–22] The drug stimulates the antidiuretic hormone secretion, potentiating its effect at the renal tubular level, resulting in water retention and hyponatremia. With the development of second-generation sulfonylurea drugs that do not cross the placenta (glyburide), and with the high rate of hypoglycemia, chlorpropamide should not be recommended for use in pregnancy.[26]

Glyburide (also known as glibenclamide and glybenzcyclamide) is one of the second generation of hypoglycemic sulfonylureas; this group also includes glipizide, gliclazide and glimepiridel. These sulfonylureas are considerably more potent than the earlier agents. When given as a single agent, the peak plasma level of glyburide occurs within 4 hours; the absorption of the drug is not affected by food digestion. Metabolism of glyburide occurs in the liver and its metabolites are extracted in bile and urine in equal proportions. Ten hours is the approximate elimination half-life of glyburide. Adverse effects of the drug are infrequent, occurring in < 4% of patients receiving second-generation agents.[26] However, in c. 11–38% of Type 2 non-pregnant patients, the main side effect of glyburide is hypoglycemia, with symptoms being dose related: the older patient is at greater risk of a hypoglycemic episode.

The patient most receptive to glyburide therapy is one who has been hyperglycemic for < 5 years, is willing to follow a dietary protocol

and is either of normal weight or obese. Characteristic features of both Type 2 diabetes and GDM are beta-cell exhaustion and insulin resistance. Most often, patients of both diabetic types are comparable in obesity, are asymptomatic in the early stages of the disease and have similar prevalence in the same ethnic group. Given the similarity of the phenotypic features of these complications, it is safe to assume that the use of glyburide may be beneficial in the prevention of maternal–fetal GDM complications.

Glimeperide is a new sulfonylurea drug. Both this drug and glyburide displace one another from their respective binding sites. Glimeperide has a 2.5–3-fold faster rate of association and an 8–9-fold faster rate of dissociation from the beta-cells SUR binding site than glyburide. This results in a more rapid release of insulin and a shorter duration of insulin secretion. Glimeperide significantly increases second-phase insulin secretion, whole-body glucose uptake and insulin sensitivity.[29,41,42] The increase in insulin sensitivity may be explained by studies demonstrating lower fasting plasma insulin and C-peptide levels in patients using this drug compared to glyburide-treated patients with comparable levels of glycemic control. It should be noted that, to date, glimeperide has not yet been tested for use in pregnancy.[29,41,42]

Biguanides

Metformin is an oral antihyperglycemic agent that is chemically and pharmacologically unrelated to the sulfonylureas. Metformin is a second-generation biguanide that was reintroduced and distributed in the US after biguanide phenformin was withdrawn from the market in the 1970s: both were introduced in 1957. Metformin has universally been shown to be effective in improving the glycemic profile in diabetic patients. Its mechanism of action is thought to include decreased hepatic glucose production and intestinal absorption of glucose, and increased peripheral uptake of glucose and utilization. The two latter mechanisms result in improved insulin sensitivity, i.e. decreased insulin requirements.[43,44] Importantly, metformin does not stimulate insulin secretion and, therefore, does not cause hypoglycemia either in diabetic or control patients. The drug acts by causing the translocation of glucose transporters from the miscrosomal fraction to the plasma membrane of hepatic and muscle cells.[45]

Metformin has no significant effects on the secretion of glucagons, cortisol, growth hormone or somatostatin. The mechanism by which metformin reduces hepatic glucose production is controversial, but the preponderance of data indicates an effect on reducing gluconeogenesis.[45] It has a strong safety and efficacy record, with a frequency of lactic acidosis one-tenth that of the parent drug. The incidence of lactic acidosis with metformin is c. 0.03 cases/1000 patients annually. The elimination of plasma half-life time is c. 6 hours. Therefore, patients with renal compromise should not receive metformin, since the risk of lactic acidosis increases with the degree of renal impairment and patient age. Metformin should be introduced gradually in 500 or 850 mg increments to a maximum of 2000 mg daily.[43,44]

The peak plasma level when the drug is given as a single agent occurs within 4 hours. The extent of absorption is reduced with food intake, although it should be administered with meals to minimize gastrointestinal intolerance. Metformin is not metabolized and is eliminated unchanged in the urine. It has been effective in reducing plasma triglyceride and cholesterol levels, as well as in promoting weight loss in obese diabetic patients. Hypoglycemia is not an overt side effect of its use. Metformin does not stimulate the fetal pancreas to oversecrete insulin. The efficacy of the drug to reverse

known defects responsible for insulin resistance in Type 2 diabetes and its safety with regard to hypoglycemia suggests that it may be an ideal drug for a primary prevention study in GDM.

Thiazolidenediones

Thiazolidenediones are a class of drugs which may provide still another pharmacological alternative to insulin therapy, although to date there are no reported data on its use in pregnancy. **Troglitazone**, the first of these agents to be introduced, has been withdrawn from use because it was associated with severe hepatic toxicity, followed by a number of deaths. These oral hypoglycemic agents exert their principal effects by lowering insulin resistance in peripheral tissue. A decrease in systemic and local tissue lipid availability may also contribute to its positive effects in controlling the effects of diabetes. **Rosiglitazone**, another oral agent in this group, is more potent than troglitazone and claims to offer a lower risk of hepatotoxicity. It is absorbed within c. 2 hours but the maximum clinical effect is not observed for 6–12 weeks. It is recommended that liver function be measured before the start of therapy and monitored once initiated. Studies also report considerable weight gain with these drugs.[46,47]

Similarities exist between rosiglitazone and glyburide in their pharmacological characteristics, which may suggest that there is a possibility that they do not cross the placenta. If this proves to be the case, rosiglitazone, just like metformin, may be an ideal agent for the management of GDM and Type 2 diabetes in pregnancy, as a single therapy or in combination with glyburide.

Alpha-glucosidase inhibitors

Alpha-glucosidase inhibitors act by slowing the absorption of carbohydrates from the intestine, thereby reducing the postprandial rise in blood glucose. The postprandial rise is blunted in both normal and diabetic patients. Gastrointestinal side effects require gradual dosage increments over time after initiation of therapy. This group of drugs may be considered a monotherapy in elderly patients but are typically used in combination with other oral antidiabetic agents and/or insulin. **Acarbose**, the oral agent in this group currently in use, may be added to most other available therapies.[48,49]

Rationale for the use of oral hypoglycemic agents in the management of gestational diabetes mellitus

The intensified insulin approach in the management of GDM has been shown to result in perinatal outcomes comparable to those in the general population; thus, it has become the method of choice for control of glycemia.[1] A less invasive, efficacious alternative that would achieve similar perinatal outcome while enhancing patient compliance has been a major diabetes research goal for the past 20 years.

The underlying principle for the use of oral hypoglycemic agents in pregnancy has been motivated by three factors. Firstly, the similarity between Type 2 diabetes and GDM. In addition to the insulin secretion and resistance abnormalities found in both conditions, there is a loss of the first-phase insulin secretion with a striking lag time between the postprandial rise in glucose and the presence of significant insulin at the peripheral sites,[38,39] this results in an early increase in postprandial glucose values. As discussed before, second-generation sulfonylurea agents are rapid in onset and have a short duration of action, which makes them ideal agents for treatment in the very early

stages of Type 2 diabetes and possibly GDM patients.

Secondly, GDM and patients with impaired glucose tolerance (IGT) are characterized by a mild hyperglycemia in comparison to Type 2 diabetics. However, this mild hyperglycemia is significantly elevated in comparison to non-diabetic women. As the disease progresses to Type 2 diabetes, there is progressive loss of beta-cell function.[50,51] In the presence of insulin resistance with obesity, pregnancy and, especially, GDM, insulin secretion will initially increase to compensate for the impairment in insulin action. The ensuing decrease in secretion over time will, in turn, result in the progression from normal glucose tolerance to GDM, from there to IGT and to Type 2 diabetes.[51] Oral hypoglycemic agents have been successfully used to decrease glycemic levels in Type 2 diabetic patients. Since GDM subjects have the mildest form of the glucose tolerance abnormality, it is reasonable to assume that the use of oral hypoglycemic agents in the treatment of GDM should be even more effective than its current use with Type 2 diabetic patients.

Thirdly, the UKPDS of Type 2 diabetes supported the efficacy of these drugs and in particular the use of glyburide.[27] The study demonstrated that with the use of glyburide, 70% of the patients achieved a desirable level of glucose control with the most favorable effect achieved within the first 5 years of therapy.[27] The study also reported a decrease in microvascular and macrovascular complications. Rather than credit a specific therapy as the factor responsible for reduced risk of complications, the authors concluded that improvement in glycemic control was the crucial factor in treating the disease.

The UKPDS[27] and the Diabetes Control and Complications Trial (DCCT)[52] groups suggest that intensive therapy in patients with Types 1 and 2 diabetes will result in improved glycemic control and a decrease in the complication rate. Thus, intensified therapy can, by itself, provide the primary prevention for diabetic complications. Studies of pregnant diabetic women, including a study of > 2000 GDM,[1] demonstrated that intensified therapy results in improvement in glycemic control and in perinatal outcomes similar to those in the non-diabetic population.

Since GDM is characterized by a milder glycemic profile and occurs 2–10 years earlier than in Type 2 diabetics, the use of oral hypoglycemic agents to treat GDM patients should prove to be even more efficacious. In addition, it is reasonable to expect that the success rate for therapy with GDM patients should be ≥ 70%, as achieved with Type 2 diabetics. In evaluating the use of glyburide in comparison to insulin,[28] it was found that glyburide in GDM patients was as effective as the use of insulin, with 82% of the glyburide patients and 88% of the insulin patients achieving their targeted levels of control. In another randomized study,[19] 80% of subjects treated with oral agents or diet alone maintained targeted blood glucose levels of < 150 mg/dl. In contrast, only 38% of the insulin patients were able to achieve this level, probably due to poor compliance.

In two recent studies of the use of glyburide in pregnancy, the level of compliance in women using glyburide therapy to achieve glycemic control was re-examined. In both studies, the sample sizes were relatively small and the authors reached contradictory conclusions. In the first study of 42 women with GDM, success of glyburide therapy was defined as maintaining a fasting plasma level of < 90 mg/dl and a 1-hour postprandial level of < 130 mg/dl. Approximately 83% of the women achieved these goals with universal satisfaction with the mode of therapy.[53] In the other study, 73 women who had refused insulin therapy were assigned to glyburide therapy. In this study,

success of therapy was defined as achieving ≥ 80% of capillary blood values within normal glycemic levels. Approximately 47% of the subjects failed to achieve the targeted glycemic goals after 1–9 weeks of treatment.[54]

Analysis of the latter study revealed several confounding design flaws. The authors used a non-traditional method of glyburide administration. The initial dose was too large, the increments too rapid (in some cases every 3 days) and the maximal dose too small (17.5 mg). Finally, the duration of glyburide treatment was too short (1–9 weeks). The above factors suggest that a large number of patients did not receive a sufficient glyburide dose and/or insufficient time had been allocated so that subjects could achieve targeted goals. It is interesting to note, however, that none of the newborns demonstrated signs of hypoglycemia after delivery.[54]

Success in achieving targeted levels of glycemia will vary from study to study because of different doses, administration algorithms, length of therapy, type of patient (severity and ethnicity), and non-comparable groups (compliant versus non-compliant subjects). Finally, to date, there is no evidence that a diabetic medication will be able to maintain targeted levels of glycemic control in all patients. For example, in the present author's group's study,[28] only 88% of the insulin-treated patients achieved targeted levels of control. In the present author's unpublished data, analyzing 3000 GDM patients treated with intensified insulin therapy, it was found that 44% of subjects achieved targeted control within the first 3 weeks of treatment.

Basic science studies

The incidence of congenital anomalies in non-diabetic women is 2–3%: this rate increases to

7–9% overall in pregnant diabetic patients, and will be even higher in poorly controlled diabetics and as the severity of the disease increases. An unanswered question remains: what is the toxic agent that triggers the development of malformations – is it the glucose or is it the oral hypoglycemic agent? This dilemma has led to several investigations of animal species or tissue cultures as a source for answers. These types of studies provide the conditions with which to test separately and together the effect of different drug doses in conjunction with varying levels of glucose. However, a major difference exists between laboratory mice and the human embryo.

Smithberg and Runner[55] studied different hypoglycemia-inducing treatments, including insulin, tolbutamide and fasting of prepuberal mice, as well as combination treatments involving nicotinamide plus insulin or tolbutamide. They were all found to be potent teratogens in one or more inbred strains of mice. Teratogenic treatments, with the exception of fasting, also cause a variable proportion of deaths. The response of different strains of mice to individual treatments relevant to teratogenicity or lethality was highly variable. It is the variability of response elicited from each strain of mouse as a group which may be the most pertinent finding in these experiments. Most noteworthy is the 3% mortality produced by insulin treatment in strain BALB/c as compared to 17% in 129. This example demonstrates the variability in study results reported in the literature. It also makes one realize that it was the strain of mouse that was the determining factor in recommending or failing to recommend a particular drug.

However, first-generation sulfonylureas, such as tolbutamide and chlorpropamide, were found to be associated with congenital malformations in the majority of animal studies. Adverse effects appear to be caused by the drugs and not by the hypoglycemia they produce. Chlorpropamide appeared to be embryotoxic in mouse embryos in culture.[56–58] To date, no animal studies have been performed to evaluate second- and third-generation sulfonylureas and their associations with malformations.

Denno and Sadler[59] evaluated the effect of biguanides, using metformin and phenformin as embryotoxic agents at concentrations equal to serum levels obtained in patients treated with the agent clinically. They found that phenformin is embryotoxic, whereas metformin is not, suggesting that metformin is also the safer drug during pregnancy in patients with non-insulin-dependent diabetes mellitus (NIDDM). However, it should be noted that in the present study, metformin was not without adverse effects since it produced a delay in neural tube closure and also reduced yolk sac protein values at two different concentrations. While delayed closure of the neural tube may not have resulted in gross morphological abnormalities, it was not possible to assess subtler alterations that might result from such a delay using the culture system.

Shephard[60] and Schardein[61] reported that metformin did not appear to be a major teratogen because < 0.5% of the rat fetuses in mothers administered 500–1000 mg/kg developed anophthalmia and anencephaly. However, evidence of embryo toxicity was evident with higher doses of the drug. Since animal studies are not conclusive about the safety of the fetus regarding the association between drugs and malformations, additional research approaches are needed to determine drug transfer across the placenta and/or tests of fetal blood for evidence of the drug.

Unlike other species, the human placental barrier is composed of a single rate-limiting layer of multinucleated cells, the syncytiotrophoblasts. During the formation of the placenta, fetal tissues erode the maternal blood vessels to attain a closer proximity to the maternal circulation. Chorionic villi that contain fetal blood vessels infiltrate the maternal vessels and establish a sinusoid in which the villi are suffused by maternal blood.[62–65] The rate-limiting barrier for penetration across the human placenta is the syncytiotrophoblast layer. Therefore, animal studies addressing placental transfer (e.g. mice) will not necessarily be applicable in humans.[66]

The characteristics of individual drugs will determine their placental transfer capability. These factors will include: molecular weight, pK_a, lipophilicity, placental blood flow, blood protein binding and elimination half-life.[65] Although the cut-off for actual molecular weight passage across the placental barrier has not yet been accurately defined, it is generally agreed that molecular weights ≤ 1000 Da passively permeate across the placental barrier with sustained maternal blood concentrations.[67,68]

The recirculating single-cotyledon human placental model is widely used to characterize the transport and metabolism of numerous drugs and nutrients. It is a reliable *in vitro* model for human placental transfer since it facilitates the study of intact human placenta independent of fetal metabolism. Experiments can be validated against known substances that freely cross the placenta.[69–71]

The present author's group's studies evaluated whether or not first- and second-generation sulfonylureas will cross the placenta.[30,72,73] Glyburide's molecular weight is 494 units (U); it is one of the largest oral hypoglycemic or antihyperglycemic agents. First, transport and metabolism of glyburide across the human placenta was investigated, when the following were found. (1) There was virtually no significant transport of glyburide in either the maternal-to-fetal or fetal-to-maternal

directions, with an average transport of 0.26% at 2 hours. These levels are 3–8-fold higher than the therapeutic peak levels after a 5 mg oral dose in humans. In fact, when cord blood samples were tested using high-performance liquid chromatography (HPLC), glyburide was undetectable in these samples despite maternal plasma levels of 50–150 ng/ml. (2) Increasing the glyburide concentration to 100 times therapeutic levels did not alter transport appreciably. Equilibrium dialysis demonstrated that at least 98% of the glyburide was protein bound. (3) Glyburide is neither metabolized nor sequestered by the placenta. (4) The results of the study suggest passive transfer of the drug.

In the second studies in 1994[72] and 1997[73] it was demonstrated that second-generation oral hypoglycemic agents, especially glyburide, do not significantly cross the diabetic or non-diabetic placenta. Fetal concentrations reached no more than 1–2% of maternal concentrations. Although glipizide crossed the placenta in small amounts, this was significantly higher than glyburide. In contrast, tolbutamide diffused across the placenta most freely. Glyburide has not been demonstrated to be teratogenic in animal studies and is thus classified as a category B agent.

Clinical studies

The use of oral hypoglycemic agents is contraindicated in the US. This recommendation stems from the potential adverse effect on the developing fetus with the assumption that significant transfer occurs across the placenta. Three issues of concern have been raised: (1) the increased rate of congenital anomalies; (2) the possible induction of fetal macrosomia due to direct stimulation of the fetal pancreas resulting in hyperinsulinemia; and (3) the increased rate of hypoglycemia due to fetal hyperinsulinemia. The sources for the above concerns were based on clinical observations of case reports or small retrospective studies, the majority published in the 1960s and 1970s. The patient populations were mainly Type 2 diabetics and the drugs used were mainly first-generation sulfonylureas.[23–25]

An example of a study used to generate the recommendation that there is an increased risk for neonatal hypoglycemia with the use of these drugs was a case report of three infants whose mothers received chlorpropamide and another mother of an infant given acetohexamide; another case report reported prolonged symptomatic neonatal hypoglycemia.[23,24]

The recommendation not to use oral hypoglycemic or antihyperglycemic agents because of an increased rate of anomalies was based on a retrospective study involving 20 Type 2 diabetic patients, all with hyperglycemia prior to conception [glycosylated hemoglobin (HbA1c) levels > 8%].[25] The fact that maternal hyperglycemia existed preconception makes it impossible to determine if the increased rate of anomalies found in these study subjects was a result of the medication or of the elevated glucose level. In contrast, three studies in the past decade have suggested that there is no association between oral hypoglycemic agents and congenital malformations. Towner et al[74] treated 332 Type 2 diabetic patients with oral hypoglycemic agents or insulin prior to pregnancy. The authors demonstrated, using a stepwise logistic regression, that the mode of therapy did not have an adverse significant effect, while the level of glycemia and maternal age were significant factors contributing to the rate of anomalies. The present author's group demonstrated similar findings in a retrospective analysis of 850 Type 2 diabetic women exposed to different oral hypoglycemic agents, insulin and diet therapy prior to and during the

first trimester of pregnancy.[75] Again, it was the blood glucose and not the mode of therapy that had the net effect on the rate of anomalies. Finally, Koren,[76] at an National Institute Health (NIH) Food and Drug Administration (FDA) conference presented the results of eight studies and concluded that the use of oral hypoglycemic agents have no effect on the rate of fetal anomalies due to a very narrow confidence interval (CI) [odds ratio (OR) 1.0; 95% CI 1.05–1.85].

To date, no randomized study addressing the use of oral hypoglycemic agents during organogenesis has been performed. The results of early small-scale studies suggest that an association exists. However, these studies were not controlled for the level of glycemia. The above large-scale studies, although retrospective, demonstrated that the cause of anomalies is the level of glycemia and not the use of oral hypoglycemic drugs.

It remains unresolved if the treatment of Type 2 diabetes with oral hypoglycemic agents will accelerate the rate of anomalies. On the other hand, is it an overreaction to condemn these medications? With existing data, care providers need to objectively present information to patients so that issues are addressed and informed decisions are made. Moreover, there should be diligence in separating data from Type 2 diabetic studies when considering GDM.

In the case of GDM, the issue of anomalies is simpler. GDM patients are diagnosed and enter therapy after the first trimester (after the organogenesis period). There then remains concern about potential fetal hypoglycemia and stimulation for macrosomia if the drug crosses the placenta. However, as previously discussed, glyburide does not cross the placenta and therefore cannot stimulate adverse effects in the fetus. Finally, the present author's group's recent study[28] provides clinical support for this concern. It was demonstrated that in patients entering therapy after the first trimester, the rate of anomalies was comparable for insulin- and glyburide-treated patients, and similar to the rate reported in the non-diabetic general population.

There are several retrospective and two randomized studies in the literature that have evaluated the use of first- and second-generation sulfonylurea drugs and metformin in pregnancy.[11-22] Notolovitz[19] studied the utility of tolbutamide, chlorpropamine, diet and insulin in a randomized study with a small sample size with relatively low power (each of the four arms of the study contained c. 50 patients). There was no significant difference for perinatal mortality and congenital anomalies. Good glycemic control was defined as a blood glucose level < 150 mg/dl. Eighty percent of the subjects using oral hypoglycemic agents or diet and 36% of the insulin-treated patients achieved the targeted glycemic category (i.e. < 150 mg/dl).

In the present author's group's study,[29] 440 women between 11 and 33 weeks gestation, with a singleton pregnancy, having GDM requiring treatment (a failed oral glucose tolerance test and a fasting plasma glucose level of 95–140 mg/dl) were enrolled. The blood glucose profile characteristics prior to initiation of therapy were comparable for the glyburide and the insulin–treated groups (114±9 versus 116±22 mg/dl, respectively). Patients were randomly assigned to receive either glyburide (n = 201; initial dose 2.5 mg orally, increasing by 5 mg/week up to a total of 20 mg) or insulin (n = 203; initial dose 0.7 U/kg subcutaneously three times daily, increasing each week as necessary) for glycemic control. Patients were required to measure their glucose values seven times daily. The targets for glycemic control were a mean blood glucose level of 90–105 mg/dl, a fasting blood glucose level of 60–90 mg/dl, a preprandial blood glucose level of 80–95 mg/dl and a postprandial blood glucose level of <120 mg/dl.

Both treatments caused significant reductions in blood glucose levels compared with levels measured at home for 1 week prior to initiation of treatment. Mean blood glucose levels in the glyburide group decreased from 114 to 105 mg/dl, whereas those in the insulin group decreased from 116 to 105 mg/dl. Eighty-two percent of the glyburide- and 88% of the insulin-treated subjects were able to achieve targeted levels of glycemia. However, eight glyburide-treated women (4%) failed to achieve the desired level of control early in the third trimester and were transferred to insulin therapy. None of the patients developed severe symptoms of hypoglycemia. However, in the insulin-treated group a significantly higher rate of subjects had 1–6% of their self-monitoring blood glucose determinations values < 40 mg/dl compared to the glyburide subjects. The glyburide and insulin groups had similar rates of pre-eclampsia (6%) and Cesarean sections (23–24%). Neonatal outcomes did not differ significantly between the two groups. The glyburide and insulin groups had a similar incidence of large-for-gestational-age (LGA) infants (12 versus 13%) macrosomia (7 versus 4%) lung complications (8 versus 6%), hypoglycemia (9 versus 6%), admission to a neonatal intensive care unit (6 versus 7%) and fetal anomalies (2 versus 2%).

A clinical study confirmed basic science studies[30,72,73] that glyburide does not cross the placenta in significant amounts. Glyburide was undetectable in cord serum to the level of sensitivity of the test. As a quality control, simultaneous samples of maternal serum were obtained from 12 women at the time of delivery to determine whether sufficient gradient levels for glyburide exist. Maternal levels ranged from 50 to 150 ng/ml. To ascertain any potential effect of glyburide on fetal pancreas, insulin umbilical cord levels between the two groups were compared. The mean cord serum insulin concentrations were similar for both groups.

Three clinical trials studied the effect of metformin as a single or combination therapy in pregnancy. The results of the studies indicated a significant mean decline in plasma glucose concentrations.[16,21,22]

In one study,[22] the failure of metformin to achieve targeted levels of glycemic control was 53.8% for established diabetics and 28.6% in the GDM patients. Apart from a high incidence of neonatal jaundice requiring phototherapy, the infant morbidity in the metformin group was low. The rate of LGA infants was double the rate found in the authors' general population. However, the LGA rate was comparable in the metformin- and insulin-treated patients, approaching 20%. Finally, in this study,[22] the mothers of the three infants with congenital malformations in the metformin group initiated therapy in the third trimester. In another study by the same authors,[16] they compared patients treated with metformin and glibenclamide alone, and the combination of diet, metformin and glibenclamide. Patients who failed the oral hypoglycemic agent therapy were transferred to insulin therapy. The incidences of LGA neonates (> 90th percentile) were 15% (metformin), 27% (glibenclamide), 33% (combined therapy group) and 41% (failed oral insulin-treated group). The relative increase in the rate of LGA infants must be explained by the severity of the disease and the higher rate of poorly controlled subjects in the combination- and insulin-treated groups. Neonatal hypoglycemia is defined as <25 mg/dl: the overall rate of neonatal hypoglycemia was 11.5%, with the highest rates for the patients treated with glibenclamide (27%) and combination therapy (glibenclamide and metformin) (18%), and the lowest rate in metformin-treated patients (5%). The high rate of neonatal hypoglycemia corresponds with a rate of LGA infants reported in the present author's study, suggesting that a significant number of their patients were in suboptimal glucose control.

Conclusions

Different oral hypoglycemic and antihyperglycemic agents act via diverse mechanisms of action. These drug characteristics provide a more physiological approach to the treatment of Type 2 diabetes and GDM. Furthermore, combination therapies will enhance the effect of these drugs on glucose metabolism.

Insulin therapy involves daily injections which do not always result in optimal compliance by many women, and women in many developing countries cannot afford insulin therapy. Studies have demonstrated that both diet- and insulin-treated women have comparable psychological profiles in different ethnic groups.[77–79] However, given the choice of insulin injections versus tablets, almost all women will opt for the latter.

Although sulfonylureas are the only oral agents that have been studied in GDM women in randomized controlled trials, other oral hypoglycemic agents may have an even greater therapeutic effect in controlling glycemic levels. Evidence suggests that glyburide is as effective as insulin in maintaining desired glycemic levels and results in comparable outcomes. However, regardless of the mode of therapy, whole-patient care (glucose monitoring, education, diet adherence, etc.) will determine the overall success in managing this disease and maximizing the quality of perinatal outcome.[80–82]

References

1. Langer O, Rodriguez DA, Xenakis EMJ et al. Intensfied vs. conventional management of gestational diabetes. *Am J Obstet Gynecol* 1994; **170**:1036–47.

2. Bauman WA, Yallow RS. Transplacental passage of insulin complexed to antibody. *Proc Natl Acad Sci USA* 1981; **78**:4588–90.

3. Menon RK, Cohen RM, Sperling MA et al. Transplacental passage of insulin in pregnant women with insulin-dependent diabetes mellitus. *N Engl J Med* 1990; **323**:309–15.

4. Turner RC, Cull CA, Fright V et al. Glycemic control with diet, sulfonylurea, metformin, or insulin inpatients with type 2 diabetes mellitus: progressive requirement for multiple therapies. *J Am Med Assoc* 1999; **281**: 2005–12.

5. Lebovitz HE. Insulin secretagogues: old and new. *Diabetes Rev* 1999; **7**:139–53.

6. Coustan DR. Gestational diabetes. In: *National Institutes of Diabetes and Digestive and Kidney Diseases. Diabetes in America*, 2nd edn. (NIDDK: 1995) Bethesda, Maryland, NIH Publication No. 95–1468:703–17.

7. Coustan DR, Carpenter MW, O'Sullivan PS, Carr SR. Gestational diabetes: predictors of subsequent disordered glucose metabolism. *Am J Obstet Gynecol* 1993; **168**: 1139–45.

8. Freinkel N, Metzger BE, Phelps RL et al. Gestational diabetes mellitus: heterogeneity of maternal age, weight, insulin secretion, HLA antigens, and islet cell antibodies and the impact of maternal metabolism on pancreatic B-cell function and somatic growth in the offspring. *Diabetes* 1995; **34 (Suppl 2)**:1–7.

9. Catalano PM, Virgo KM, Bernstein IM, Amine SB. Incidence and risk factors associated with abnormal glucose tolerance in women with gestational diabetes. *Am J Obstet Gynecol* 1991; **165**:914–19.

10. Catalano PM, Tyzbir ED, Wolfe RR et al. Carbohydrate metabolism during pregnancy in control subjects and women with gestational diabetes. *Am J Physiol* 1993; **264**:E60–E67.

11. Douglas CP, Richards R. Use of chlorpropamide in the treatment of diabetes in pregnancy. *Diabetes* 1967; **16**:60–1.

12. Jackson WPU, Campbell GD, Notelovitz M, Blumson D. Tolbutamide and chlorpropamide during pregnancy in human diabetics. *Diabetes* 1963; **(Suppl)**:98–101.

13. Sutherland HW, Bewsher PD, Cormack JD et al. Effect of moderate dosage of chlorpropamide in pregnancy on fetal outcome. *Arch Dis Child* 1974; **49**:283–91.

14. Stowers JM, Sutherland HW. The use of sulphonylureas bigunides and insulin in pregnancy. In: (Stowers, Sutherland, eds) *Carbohydrate Metabolism in Pregnancy and the Newborn.* (Churchill Livingstone: Edinburgh, 1975) 205–20.

15. Coetzee EJ, Jackson WPU. Oral hypoglycemics in the first trimester and fetal outcome. *South Afr Med J* 1984; **65**:635–637.

16. Coetzee EJ, Jackson WPU. Pregnancy in established non-insulin-dependent diabetics. *S Afr Med J* 1980; **61**: 795–802.

17. Notelovitz M. Oral hypoglycemic therapy in diabetic pregnancies. *Lancet* 1974; **ii**:902–3.

18. Malins JM, Cooke AM, Pyke DA, Fitzgerald MG. Sulfonylurea drugs in pregnancy. *Br Med J* 1964; **ii**:187 (letter).

19. Notelowitz M. Sulfonylurea therapy in the treatment of the pregnant diabetic. *S Afr Med J* 1971; **45**:226–9.

20. Coetzee EJ, Jackson WPU. The management of non-insulin-dependent diabetes during pregnancy. *Diabetes Res Clin Pract* 1986; **1**:281–7.

21. Coetzee EJ, Jackson WPU. Diabetes newly diagnosed in pregnancy: a 4-year study at Groote Schuur Hospital. *SA Mediese Tydskrif* 1979; 467–75.

22. Coetzee EJ, Jackson WPU. Metformin in management of pregnant insulin-independent diabetics. *Diabetologia* 1979; **16**:241–5.

23. Kemball ML, McIvert C, Milner RDG et al. Neonatal hypoglycemia in infants of diabetic mothers given sulphonylurea drugs in pregnancy. *Arch Dis Child* 1970; **45**:696–701.

24. Zucker P, Simon G. Prolonged symptomatic neonatal hypoglycemia associated with maternal chlorpropamide therapy. *Pediatrics* 1968; **42**:824–5.

25. Piacquadio K, Hollingsworth DR, Murphy H. Effects of in-utero exposure to oral hypoglycemic drugs. *Lancet* 1991; **338**:866–9.

26. In: (Hardmons J, Limbird, editors-in-chief) *Goodman and Gillman's. The Pharmacologic Basis of Therapeutics*, 9th edn. (McGraw Hill: New York, 1996) 1712–92.

27. American Diabetes Association. Implications of the United Kingdom Prospective Diabetes Study. *Diabetes Care* 2000; **23 (Suppl 2)**:S27–S31.

28. Langer O, Conway DL, Berkus MD et al. A comparison of glyburide vs. insulin in women with gestational diabetes mellitus. *N Engl J Med* 2000; **343**:1134–8.

29. Lebovitz HE. Insulin secretagogues: old and new. *Diabetes Rev* 1999; **7**:139–53.

30. Elliot B, Langer O, Schenker S, Jonhson RF. Insignificant transfer of glyburide occurs across the human placenta. *Am J Obstet Gynecol* 1991; **165**:807–12.

31. Koren G. Glyburide and fetal safety; transplacental pharmacokinetic considerations. *Reprod Toxicol* 2001; **15**:225–9.

32. Rossetti L, Giaaccari A, DeFronzo RA. Glucose toxicity. *Diabetes Care* 1990; **13**:610–30.

33. Simonson DC, Farrannini E, Bevilacqua S et al. Mechanism of improvement in glucose metabolism after chronic glyburide therapy. *Diabetes Care* 1984; **33**: 838–45.

34. Groop L, Luzi L, Melanger A et al. Different effects of glyburide and glipizide on insulin secretion and hepatic glucose production in normal and NIDDM subjects. *Diabetes* 1987; **36**:1320–8.

35. Groop LC, Barzilai N, Ratheiser K et al. Dose-dependent effects of glyburide on insulin secretion and glucose uptake in humans. *Diabetes Care* 1991; **14**:724–7.

36. DeFronzo RA, Simonson DC. Oral sulfonylurea agents suppress hepatic glucose production in non-insulin-dependent diabetic individuals. *Diabetes Care* 1984; **7**:72–80.

37. Kahn SE, McCulloch DK, Porte Jr D. Insulin secretion in normal and diabetic humans. In: (Alberti KGMM, Zimmer P, DeFronzo RA, Keen H, eds) *International Textbook of Diabetes Mellitus*, 2nd edn. (Wiley: Chichester, 1997) 337–54.

38. Mitrakou A, Kelley D, Mokan M et al. Role of reduced suppression of glucose production and early insulin release in impaired glucose tolerance. *N Engl J Med* 1992; **326**:22–9.

39. Polansky KS, Given BD, Hirsch I et al. Abnormal patterns of insulin secretion in non-insulin dependent diabetes mellitus. *N Engl J Med* 1988; **318**:1231–9.

40. Leahy JL. Natural history of beta cell dysfunction in NIDDM. *Diabetes Care* 1990; **13**:992–1010.

41. Clark HE, Matthews DR. The effect of glimerpiride on pancreatic beta-cell function under hyperglycemic clamp and hyperinsulinaemic, euglycaemic clamp conditions in non-insulin dependent diabetes mellitus. *Horm Metab Res* 1996; **28**:445–50.

42. van der Wal PS, Draeger KE, van Iperen AM et al. Beta cell response to oral glimepiride administration during and following a hyperglycaemic clamp in NIDDM patients. *Diabet Med* 1997; **14**:556–63.

43. Product information. *Glucophage*. Bristol-Myers Squibb, 1997.

44. Klepser TB, Kelly MW. Metformin hydrochloride: an antihyperglycemic agent. *Am J Health-Syst Pharm* 1997; **54**:893–903.

45. Stumvoll M, Nurjhan N, Perriello G et al. Metabolic effects of metformin in non-insulin dependent diabetes mellitus. *N Engl J Med* 1995; **333**:550–4.

46. Buckingham RE, Al-Barazanji KA, Toseland N et al. Peroxisome proliferatated-activitated receptor-gamma agonist, rosiglitazone, protects against nephropathy and pancreatic islet abnormalities in Zucker fatty rats. *Diabetes* 1998; **47**:1326–34.

47. Lebovitz HE. Thiazolidinediones. In: (Lebovitz HE, ed) *Therapy for Diabetes Mellitus and Related Disorders*, 3rd edn. (American Diabetes Association: Alexandria, VA, 1998) 181–5.

48. Coniff RF, Seaton TB, Shjapiro JA et al. Reduction of glycosylated hemoglobin and postprandial hyperglycemia by acarbose in patients with NIDDM. *Diabetes Care* 1995; **18**:817–20.

49. Lebovitz HE. Alpha-glucosidase inhibitors. *Endocrinol Metab Clin N Am* 1997; **26**:539–51.

50. UK Prospective Diabetes Study Group V. Characteristics of newly presenting type 2 diabetic patients: estimates of insulin sensitivity and islet beta-cell function. *Diabet Med* 1988; **5**:444–8.

51. UK Prospective Diabetes Study Group 16. Overview of 6 years' therapy of type 2 diabetes: a progressive disease. *Diabetes* 1995; **44**:1249–58.

52. The Diabetes Control and Complications Trial Research Group. The effect of intensive treatment of diabetes on the development and progression of long-term complications in insulin-dependent diabetes mellitus. *N Engl J Med* 1993; **329**:977–86.

53. Chmait R, Dinise T, Daneshmand S et al. Prospective cohort study to establish predictors of glyburide success in gestational diabetes mellitus. *Am J Obstet Gynecol* 2001; **185** (abstract).

54. Kitzmiller J. Limited efficacy of glyburide for glycemic control. *Am J Obstet Gynecol* 2001; **185** (abstract).

55. Smithberg M, Runner MN. Teratogenic effects of hypoglycemic treatments in inbred strains of mice. *Am J Anat* 1963; **113**:479–89.

56. Sivan E, Feldman B, Dolitzki M et al. Glyburide crosses the placenta in vivo in pregnant rats. *Diabetologia* 1995; **38**:753–6.

57. Smoak IW. Teratogenic effects of chlorpropamide in mouse embryos in vitro. *Teratology* 1992; **45**:474.

58. Smoak IW, Sadler TW. Embryopathic effects of short-term exposure to hypoglycemia in the mouse. *Am J Obstet Gynecol* 1990; **163**:619–24.

59. Denno KM, Sadler TW. Effects of the biguanide class of oral hypoglycemic agents on mouse embryogenesis. *Teratology* 1994; **49**:260–6.

60. Shepard TH. *Catalog of Teratogenic Agents*, 8th edn. (John Hopkins University Press: Baltimore, 1995) 270.

61. Schardein JL. *Chemically Induced Birth Defects*, 2nd edn. (Marcel Dekker: New York, 1993) 417–18.

62. Audus KL. Controlling drug delivery across the placenta. *Eur J Pharmacol Sci* 1999; **8**:161–5.

63. Dancis J. Placental physiology. In: (Kretchmer N, Quilligan EJ, Johnson JD, eds *Prenatal and Perinatal Biology and Medicine, Physiology and Growth*, Volume 1. (Harwood Academic Publishers: Chur, Switzerland, 1987) 1–33.

64. Enders AC, Blakenship TN. Comparative placental structure. *Adv Drug Del Rev* 1999; **38**:3–16.

65. Ala-Kokko TL, Vahakangas K, Pelkonen O. Placental function and principles of drug transfer. *Acta Anaesth Scand* 1993; **37**:47–9.

66. Sibley CP. Mechanism of ion transfer by the rat placenta: a model for the human placenta? *Placenta* 1994; **15**:675–91. (review article).

67. Willis DM, O'Grady JP, Faber JJ, Thornburg KL. Diffusion permeability of cyanocobalamin in human placenta. *Am J Physiol* 1986; **250**:R459-R464.

68. Malek A, Blann E, Mattison DR. Human placental transport of oxytocin. *J Matern–Fetal Med* 1996; 5:245–55.

69. Brandes JM, Travoloni N, Potter JB et al. A new recycling technique for human placental cotyledon perfusion: application to studies of the fetomaternal transfer of glucose, insulin, and antipyrine. *Am J Obstet Gynecol* 1983; **146**:800–6.

70. Schenker S, Johnson R, Hays S et al. Effects of nicotine and nicotine/ethanol on human placental amino acid transfer. *Alcohol* 1989; **6**:289–96.

71. Schenker S, Dicke J, Johnson R et al. Human placental transport of cimetidine. *J Clin Invest* 1987; **80**:1428–34.

72. Elliot B, Schenker S, Langer O et al. Comparative placental transport of oral hypoglycemic agents. A model of human placental drug transfer. *Am J Obstet Gynecol* 1994; **171**:653–60.

73. Elliot B, Langer O, Schussling F. A model of human placental drug transfer. *Am J Obstet Gynecol* 1997; **176**: 527–30.

74. Towner D, Kjos SL, Montoro MM et al. Congenital malformations in pregnancies complicated by NIDDM. *Diabetes Care* 1995; **18**:1446–51.

75. Langer O, Conway D, Berkus M, Xenakis EMJ. There is no association between hypoglycemic use and fetal anomalies. *Am J Obstet Gynecol* 1999; **180**:S38 (abstract).

76. Koren G. *Proceedings of the NIH/FDA Toxicology in Pregnancy conference*, Toronto, 2000.

77. Langer N, Langer O. Emotional adjustment to diagnosis and intensified treatment of gestational diabetes. *Obstet Gynecol* 1994; **84**:329–34.

78. Langer O, Langer N, Piper JM et al. Is cultural diversity a factor in self-monitoring blood glucose in gestational diabetes? *J Assoc Acad Minor Phys* 1995; **6**:73–7.

79. Spirito A, Williams C, Ruggiero L et al. Psychological impact of the diagnosis of gestational diabetes. *Obstet Gynecol* 1989; **73**:562–6.

80. Langer O. The use of oral hypoglycemic agents in the pregnant diabetic woman. *Israel J Obstet Gynecol* 2001; **12**:179–84.

81. Langer O. When diet fails: insulin and oral hypoglycemic agents as alternatives for the management of gestational diabetes. *J Matern–Fetal Med* 2002; **11**:1–8.

82. Langer O. Insulin and other treatment alternatives in gestational diabetes mellitus. *Prenat Neonat Med* 1998; 542–9.

29

Continuous glucose monitoring during pregnancies complicated by diabetes mellitus

Lois Jovanovic, Yariv Yogev, Moshe Hod

Introduction

Gestational diabetes mellitus (GDM), defined as 'carbohydrate intolerance of variable severity with onset or first recognition during pregnancy',[1] occurs in nearly 4% of all pregnancies in the United States, but the actual prevalence may differ with ethnicity and maternal age.[2] Women with high blood glucose levels experience a greater risk of adverse maternal and fetal outcomes, including pre-eclampsia, Cesarean delivery, macrosomia, congenital anomalies and increased risk for future development of Type 2 diabetes.[3] The most common and significant neonatal complication clearly associated with GDM is macrosomia, an oversized infant with a birthweight > 90th percentile for gestational age and sex or a birthweight > two standard deviations (2 SD) above the mean of a normal population of neonates.[4] The greatest danger of macrosomia lies in its association with increased risk of birth injuries and asphyxia. In untreated GDM the risk of macrosomia is as high as 40% of neonates.[5] In addition, neonatal macrosomia is associated with the metabolic syndrome of hyperinsulinemia and deposition of fat in the visceral cavity.[6] Many feel that *in utero* hyperglycemia/hyperinsulinemia is the strongest predictor of Type 2 diabetes, overriding genetic predisposition.[3] The literature has documented that intensified management of GDM reduces the rate of neonatal complications and can normalize birthweight.[7] At the same time, others are concerned that attempts at tight control can increase the risk for severe hypoglycemia that may also compromise the well-being of both mother and fetus.[8] Therefore, the primary goal of treatment in GDM is to achieve and maintain as near normal glycemia as is feasible.

Importance of monitoring postprandial glucose levels in GDM

A review of the literature suggests that the risk of macrosomia rise as maternal glycemia increase.[9–11] Specifically, the risk of macrosomia appears to increase with increasing postprandial glucose levels.[12–14] In the present authors' experience,[12] the risk of macrosomia increases more rapidly when the peak postprandial glucose levels exceed 120 mg/dl (fingersitck capillary glucose). Others have confirmed this association and this has led the American Diabetes Association (ADA) to recommend postprandial glucose monitoring in pregnancies complicated by diabetes.[1] The controversy remains, however, as to the exclusive role of maternal glucose in the etiology of macrosomia. In fact, there are still reports that macrosomia can manifest 'despite normoglycemia'.[5,10] Also, there is no consensus as to the optimal timing of the postmeal test.[15] Traditionally, in the guidelines for the care of non-pregnant diabetic patients, a 2 hour after eating test has been recommended because of fear of hypoglycemia due to the peak action of human regular insulin. Now that more rapid-acting insulin analogues are available, it is possible to blunt the peak postprandial glucose response without fear of subsequent hypoglycemia.[16] The timing of the peak response is yet to be agreed upon. Once the timing of the highest blood glucose levels of the day in pregnant diabetic women are known, then treatment strategies to minimize this peak, and thus minimize the risk of macrosomia, can be developed.

Continuous glucose monitoring

One possibility that macrosomia has persisted despite intensified care protocols is that the times of the day that the glucose levels are elevated are being missed. The size of the meal dictates the number of hours that a patient will remain in the postprandial state.[17] Polonski et al[17] reported that a large dinner meal might be associated with sustaining the postprandial state for 4.7 hours. In addition, the most rigorous protocols only ask for postprandial glucose measurements three times a day. Many patients indulge in large between meal snacks that may be the cause of hidden hyperglycemia.

The current practice of glucose monitoring is by measuring glucose levels after each meal (postprandial) in addition to fasting by the self-blood glucose monitoring (SBGM)

method.[8,9] Optimal frequency of blood glucose testing in GDM patients has not been established. Using the SBGM method has the severe limitation of providing only a single value during the day, thus not allowing for continuous longitudinal monitoring. As such, it may be missing both hypoglycemic and hyperglycemic events.

Recently, the newly available technology of continuous glucose monitoring (CGM) was developed.[10] The MiniMed CGM system (Sylmar, CA, USA) is composed of a disposable subcutaneous glucose-sensing device and an electrode impregnated with glucose oxidase connected by a cable to a lightweight monitor, which is worn over clothing or a belt (Figs 29.1 and 29.2). The system takes a glucose measurement every 10 seconds, based on the electrochemical detection of glucose by its reaction with glucose oxidase, and stores an average value every 5 minutes, for a total of 288 measurements per day. The system measures, in subcutaneous tissue, interstitial glucose levels within a range of 40–400 mg/dl, every 5 minutes. The data are stored in the monitor for later downloading and reviewing on a personal computer. The patients are unaware of the results of the sensor measurements during the monitoring period. Glucose values obtained with CGM have been shown to correlate with laboratory measurements of plasma glucose levels[11] and with home glucose meter values.[10] CGM may facilitate the detection of all postprandial peaks, including those due to unscheduled meals and hypoglycemic events (Figs 29.3 and 29.4). CGM may provide an opportunity for better intervention, by providing the complete glucose profile. Over the past couple of years, systems that measure glucose continuously have helped in understanding the glycemia excursions possible in a daily profile in both diabetic and non-diabetic persons.[18–24] Reports using devices that measure interstitial fluid have shown that

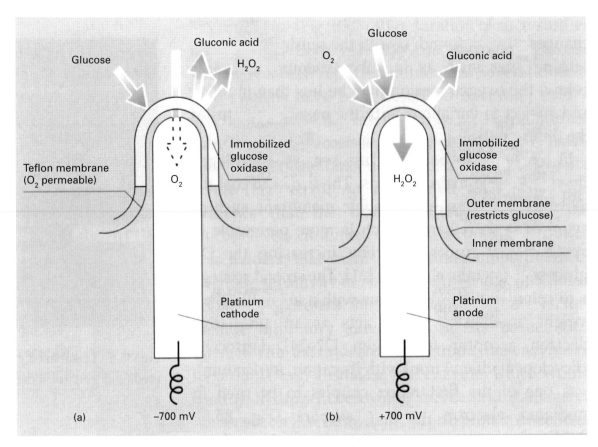

Figure 29.1. *The physics behind the MiniMed CGM system (Sylmar, CA, USA).*

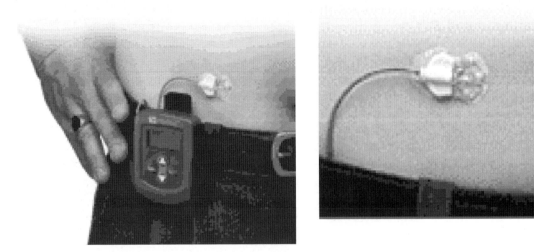

Figure 29.2. *Demonstration of how the MiniMed CGM system is worn (Sylmar, CA, USA).*

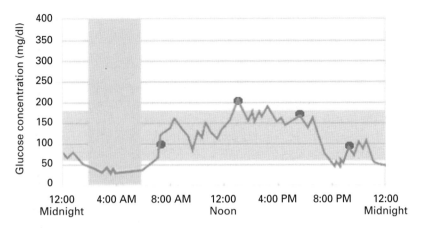

Figure 29.3. *Example of how intermittent blood glucose determinations (•) miss the glucose extremes of both hypoglycemia and postprandial hyperglycemia evident from the continuous glucose profile.*

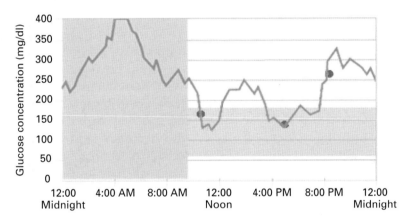

Figure 29.4. *Nocturnal hyperglycemia as documented by the continuous glucose profile missed by intermittent blood glucose monitoring (•).*

frequently monitored glucose levels can be used to adjust diabetes therapy and improve glucose control. Bode et al[20] reported on a pilot study in which hemoglobin A1c (HbA1c) values improved using the feedback of the continuously monitored interstitial fluid glucose levels calibrated to plasma glucose levels. A total of nine subjects with Type 1 diabetes and HbA1c values > 8.5% completed the study. Subjects wore a continuous glucose monitor for two 1 week periods during the study. After each sensor use, changes to diet, insulin dosage and SMBG schedules were made. HbA1c values decreased from 9.9% (SD = 1.1%) at baseline to 8.8%

(SD = 1.0%) 5 weeks after baseline (P = 0.0006), but daily insulin usage was unchanged over the same period of time (P = 0.428). The glucose sensors performed accurately, with a median correlation of 0.92 and a mean absolute difference of 19.1% (SD = 9.0%). The continuous glucose profiles allowed identification of glucose patterns and excursions that helped direct changes in therapy. These treatment changes would not have been made on the basis of meter data alone and were effective in improving glucose control. This pilot study highlighted the potential for CGM to provide the valuable information necessary to make therapy adjustments that can dramatically improve a patient's glycemic control and reduce the risk of long-term complications. Others have reported that a continuous glucose sensor utilizing the technique of reverse iontophoresis also can improve diabetes care. Tamada et al[24] reported that when the patients can see their blood glucose levels in real time, they can change their behavior accordingly and thus limit the rising or falling glucose levels before the extremes of glycemia occur. In addition, other techniques are on the horizon to improve the collection of interstitial fluid by non-invasive techniques.[22,23]

Continuous glucose monitoring in pregnancy

Almost 20 years ago, there were reports of continuous glucose profiles in patients who were studied using the Biostator glucose-controlled insulin infusion device (Bayer Pharmaceuticals Inc, Elkhart, Indiana).[25,26] The two reports of the use of this devise in pregnancy focused on the insulin and glucose requirements of labor,[25] and the 24 hour glucose profiles of non-diabetic and diabetic pregnant women.[26] The latter report confirmed the observation that non-diabetic pregnant women had fasting and postprandial glucose levels $\leq 20\%$ below non-pregnant ranges.[27] Because the Biostator weighted 250 pounds and required two indwelling intravenous catheters, ambient glucose levels could not be measured in the home setting. Unfortunately, there have not been any other reports of CGM in pregnancy since these publications. The only recent reports of CGM during pregnancy are limited to fetal heart rate testing and to maternal blood pressure levels. In these studies, using telemetry, the monitoring of uterine activity and fetal heart

rate responses have advanced the field of obstetrics and have allowed more targeted used of tocolytic agents.[28] Studies using a 'Holter' monitor to assess blood-pressure profiles during pregnancy have shown that loss of the nocturnal dip in blood pressure is associated with an increased risk of pre-ecalmpsia and that the mean arterial pressure is related to the mean insulin level. In fact, women with the insulin resistance of Type 2 diabetes and the insulin resistance of pregnancy have the highest mean arterial blood pressure, and there- fore are at the highest risk of pregnancy-induced hypertension.[29]

Using a continuous monitor to measure glucose in the home setting has been impeded by the ability to accurately measure glucose continuously without using an IV catheter. A major breakthrough was made when researchers found that measuring interstitial fluid glucose is a reflection of the blood glucose and is a way to continuously assess glucose with accuracy sufficient to make treatment decisions. Application of CGM may be the means whereby answers to the questions as to timing of the postprandial peak, the relationship between glucose and macrosomia, and the utility of monitoring all meal plans, not just the three prescribed meals, are obtained. Although maternal postprandial glucose (1 hour after the beginning of a meal) has been shown to be positively related to neonatal birthweight $(r = -0.72, P < 0.05)$ in pregnancies complicated by diabetes, many have reported that the infants may be large despite 'normoglycemia'. Numerous theories have been suggested that there may be other variables that negate or minimize the impact of maternal glucose. It is possible that fetal utilization of glucose compensates for the maternal hyperglycemia. The present authors have studied the relationship between fetal movement and birthweight, and found that the significance between birthweight and postprandial glucose could be increased if the maternal glucose was adjusted by the number of fetal movements in a 20 minute observation period ($r = 0.83$, $P < 0.02$).[30] However, there still remains a population of infants whose birthweight seems to be independent of maternal glycemia.[31]

Rather than assuming that there may be another variable, a CGM system (MiniMed) was utilized in 10 GDM women for a total of 30 days of continuous monitoring: it was observed that the total minutes/day of previously unknown hyperglycemia was a mean of 82.4 ± 18 (SD).[32] These events were discovered to be unscheduled meals not detected by conventional SBGM protocols. Furthermore, these elevations of blood glucose often occurred shortly after patients took fasting and postprandial fingerstick glucose determinations that indicated that their glucose levels were in the target ranges.[33] In another work by Yogev et al[34] a comparison of the daily glycemic profile reflected by continuous and intermittent blood glucose monitoring in pregnant women with Type 1 diabetes was evaluated. The study sample consisted of 34 gravid patients at gestational weeks 16–32 with Type 1 diabetes, being treated by multiple insulin injections. Data derived by the CGM System (MiniMed) for 72 hours were compared to fingerstick glucose measurements performed 6–8 times a day. An average of 780 ± 54 glucose measurements was recorded for each patient with continuous glucose monitoring. The mean total time of hyperglycemia (glucose level > 140 mg/dl) undetected by the fingerstick method was 192 ± 28 minutes/day. Nocturnal hypoglycemic events (glucose level < 50 mg/dl) were recorded in 26 patients; in all cases, there was an interval of 1–4 hours before clinical manifestations appeared or the event was revealed by random blood glucose examination. Based

on the additional information obtained by continuous monitoring, the insulin therapeutic regimen was adjusted in 24 patients (70%). Another recent work by Chen and Yogev et al (submitted for publication) the daily glycemic profile reflected by CGM versus SBGM in women with GDM was evaluated. This study sample consisted of 57 women with gestational diabetes; 47 in Israel and 10 in California, USA. Gestational age ranged from 24–32 weeks in the Israeli women, and 32–36 weeks in the American women. In the Israeli group, 23 women were being treated by diet alone, and 24 by diet plus insulin. An average of 763 ± 62 glucose measurements was recorded for each patient with continuous glucose monitoring. The mean total time of hyperglycemia (glucose level > 140 mg/dl) undetected by the fingerstick method was 132 ± 31 minutes/day in the insulin treated group and 94 ± 23 minutes/day in the diet treated group. Nocturnal hypoglycemic events (glucose levels < 50 mg/dl) were recorded in 14 patients, all insulin-treated. On the basis of the additional information provided by continuous monitoring, the therapeutic regimen (insulin therapy, diet adjustment, or both) was changed in 36 of the 47 patients. All of the 10 American women were being treated with insulin. The mean time of undetected hyperglycemia for the total group monitoring time of 30 days was 78 ± 13 minutes per day. Eight women had nocturnal hypoglycemia on at least one of the three nights of monitoring for a total of 12 nights. A change in insulin dosage was made in all women on the basis of the data provided by continuous glucose monitoring

Examining the sensor profile with each patient revealed important information about eating habits. In one patient, for example, the patient's CGM sensor profile showed glucose peaks of as much as 250 mg/dl occurring after the fingersitck reading of 120 mg/dl. Upon questioning, this patient indicated that she was measuring her blood glucose as instructed – before and after a low-carbohydrate meal – and then she would eat a high-carbohydrate snack. To patients such as this, the CGM sensor profiles demonstrated graphically the damaging effects of these high-carbohydrate between-meal snacks and led them to be more compliant with their prescribed diet. Instructions for fingerstick glucose monitoring were clarified to direct patients to check their blood glucose levels after each time they ate rather than just after formal meals. It is hypothesized that when real-time continuous glucose monitors become available, patients will be able to modify their behavior immediately. Thus, they can participate actively in normalizing their blood glucose levels, so preventing macrosomia and, perhaps, congenital anomalies, providing that this protocol is instituted in the first trimester.[35]

Algorithms for management using CGM

Over 20 years ago, SBGM performed eight to 10 times a day by Type 1 diabetic women resulted in normalization by outcome including normal birthweight and no increased risk of spontaneous abortion or neonatal malformation,[26,27] and no untoward outcomes.[26] The systems used in those days had > 20% coefficient of variation, but did detect hypoglycemia and hyperglycemia suffiently accurately to achieve and maintain normoglycemia.[33,35–37] The standard for SBGM systems today are to achieve < 15%, and many can achieve < 5%, variation. The CGM systems today have 94% of the values in the clinically significant A and B range on the Clack error grid.[38] Thus, when frequently measured glucose levels are available, the accuracy of each

determination can be less than optimal but improvements in outcome can still be achieved.

As recently described by Kaufman et al,[39] CGM could serve as a clinical tool for clinical decision-making and glycemic control in children with Type 1 diabetes. In another recent work, Hershkovitz et al[40] demonstrated the clinical implications of CGM use to assess and manage asymptomatic hypoglycemic events in children with glycogen storage disease.

In the present authors' work, CGM profiles allowed the physician to identify glucose patterns and to better target diabetic treatment. The treatment changes would not have been made on the basis of meter data alone.[32] A large prospective study on maternal and neonatal outcome is needed to evaluate the clinical implications of this new monitoring technique.

Detection of hypoglycemia

Despite years of meticulous study, there is still a paucity of information regarding the optimal level of glycemia in diabetic pregnancy that clinicians should target to safely reduce maternal and perinatal morbidity. Strict metabolic control in this patient population has been associated with an increased risk of maternal hypoglycemia. In the present authors' study, continuous monitoring of blood glucose in women with diabetic pregnancies confirmed the high occurrence rate of nocturnal hypoglycemia suspected in earlier studies. Rosenn and Midovnik[8] reported significant hypoglycemia, defined as hypoglycemia requiring assistance from another person, in 71% of gravid patients with Type 1 diabetes, with a peak incidence in the first trimester. The impact of maternal hypoglycemia on human fetal development and neonatal outcome has not been extensively studied. Although concern about the hazards of hypoglycemia are related primarily to the pregnant mother, the potential effects on the developing fetus need to be considered as well.

These findings were not apparent with intermittent blood glucose levels measured by fingerstick capillary glucose concentrations. Data derived from CGM[19,20,22,38,40] led the evaluating physician to change the insulin regimen by decreasing the night-time dose of intermediate-acting insulin. In over half of the patients, the hypoglycemic events were subclinical, diagnosed only by CGM, and in one quarter of the patients, more than one hypoglycemic event occurred during the night.

Use of CGM to prevent adverse fetal outcome

It seems clear that CGM is a superior tool over SBGM in detecting hypoglycemic events, as most of them are asymptomatic, occurring during the night. The clinical effect of these events is currently unknown.

On the other side of glycemic control, the most common and significant perinatal complication clearly associated with diabetic pregnancy is macrosomia, which poses an increased risk of birth injuries and asphyxia. The risk of macrosomia rises as maternal glycemia increases. Intensified management of GDM reduces the rate of perinatal complications, normalizes birthweight[7,12] and has a positive influence on the congenital malformation rate. Most likely, the high rates of macrosomia and perinatal morbidity persist despite intensified treatment protocols owing to the imperfect evaluation of the daily glucose profile, because intermittent blood glucose monitoring underestimates the hyperglycemic events. In addition, the most rigorous monitoring protocols only require postprandial

glucose measurements three times a day. Many patients indulge in large between-meal snacks, and these may be the cause of the hidden hyperglycemia.

The lack of a strong correlation between HbA1c and glucose levels by CGM may indicate that plasma blood glucose levels vary significantly day by day, and although CGM is more informative than sporadic non-longitudinal glucose monitoring, it cannot adequately describe daily glucose profiles over an 8–10 week period. It might that HbA1c is a better predictor of preprandial rather than postprandial glucose levels, as more hours are spent in the interprandial and nocturnal periods than in the postprandial phases.[12] CGM profiles allow the physician to identify glucose patterns and to better target insulin treatment; the treatment changes would not have been made on the basis of meter data alone. A large prospective study on maternal and neonatal outcome is needed to evaluate the clinical implications of this new monitoring technique.

Conclusions

Many physicians have had the experience of managing women with GDM who appeared to have good glycemic control based on their SBGM diaries and HbA1c; nonetheless, these women still delivered a macrosomic infant.[41] The present authors' experience has shown that CGM in GDM women can reveal high postprandial blood glucose levels unrecognized by intermittent blood glucose determinations. CGM shows where and how hyperglycemia that might contribute to neonatal complications is occurring, and provides a useful tool to help educate patients in behavior modifications that can improve compliance with the management regimen.

References

1. Jovanovic L. (editor-in chief). *Medical Management of Pregnancy Complicated by Diabetes*. (American Diabetes Association, Inc: Alexandria, 2000.)

2. Engelgau M, German R, Herman W, Aubert R, Smith J. The epidemiology of diabetes and pregnancy in the US, 1988. *Diabetes Care* 1995; **18**:1029–33.

3. McCance DR, Pettitt DJ, Hanson RL et al. Birth weight and non-insulin-dependent diabetes: thrifty genotype, thrifty phenotype, or surviving small baby genotype? *Br Med J* 1994; **398**:942–5.

4. Langer O, Mazze R. The relationship between large-for-gestational-age infants and glycemic control in women with gestational diabetes. *Am J Obstet Gynecol* 1988; **159**:1478–83.

5. Persson B, Hanson U. Neonatal morbidities in gestational diabetes mellitus. *Diabetes Care* 1998; **21 (Suppl 2)**:B79–B84.

6. Jovanovic L, Crues J, Durak E, Peterson CM. Magnetic resonance imaging in pregnancies complicated by diabetes predicts infant birthweight ratio and neonatal morbidity. *Am J Perinatol* 1993; **10**:432–7.

7. Jovanovic L, Bevier W, Peterson CM. The Santa Barbara County Health Care Services Program: birth weight change concomitant with screening for and treatment of glucose-intolerance of pregnancy: a potential cost-effective intervention. *Am J Perinatol* 1997; **14**:221–8.

8. Rosenn BM, Miodovnik M. Glycemic control in the diabetic pregnancy: is tighter always better? *J Maternal–Fetal Med* 2000; **9**:29–34.

9. Hod M, Rabinerson D, Peled Y. Gestational diabetes mellitus: is it a clinical entity? *Diabetes Rev* 1995; **3**:603–13.

10. Ogata ES. Perinatal morbidity in offspring of diabetic mothers. *Diabetes Rev* 1995; **3**:652–7.

11. Langer O. Is normoglycemia the correct threshold to prevent complications in the pregnant diabetic patient? *Diabetes Rev* 1995; **4**:2–10.

12. Jovanovic L, Reed GF, Metzger BE et al. Maternal postprandial glucose levels and infant birth weight: the Diabetes in Early Pregnancy Study. The National Institute of Child Health and Human Development – Diabetes in Early Pregnancy Study. *Am J Obstet Gynecol* 1991; **164**:103–11.

13. Combs CA, Gunderson E, Kitzmiller JL, Gavin LA, Main EK. Relationship of fetal macrosomia to maternal postprandial glucose control during pregnancy. *Diabetes Care* 1992; **15**:1251–7.

14. deVeciana M, Major CA, Morgan MA. Postprandial versus pre-prandial blood glucose monitoring in women with gestational diabetes mellitus requiring insulin therapy. *N Engl J Med* 1995; **333**:1237–41.

15. Moses RG, Lucas EM, Knights S. Gestational diabetes mellitus. At what time should the postprandial glucose level be monitored? *Aust NZ J Obstet Gynecol* 1999; **39**:457–60.

16. Jovanovic L, Ilic S, Pettitt DJ et al. Metabolic and immunologic effects of insulin lispro in gestational diabetes. *Diabetes Care* 1999; **22**:1422–7.

17. Polansky KS, Given BD, Hirsch LJ et al. Abnormal patterns of insulin secretion in non-insulin-dependent diabetes mellitus. *N Engl J Med* 1988; **318**:1231–9.

18. Aussedat B, Dupire-Angel M, Gifford R et al. Interstitial glucose concentration and glycemia: implications for continuous subcutaneous glucose monitoring. *Am J Physiol Endocr Metab* 2000; **278**:E716–E728.

19. Mastrototaro J. The MiniMed Continuous Glucose Monitoring System (CGMS). *J Pediatr Endocrinol Metab* 1999; **12 (Suppl 3)**:751–8.

20. Bode BW, Gross TM, Thornton KR, Mastrototaro JJ. Continuous glucose monitoring used to adjust diabetes therapy improves glycosylated hemoglobin: a pilot study. *Diabetes Res Clin Pract* 1999; **46**:183–90.

21. Haak T. New developments in the treatment of type 1 diabetes mellitus. *Exp Clin Endocrinol Diabetes* 1999; **107 (Suppl 3)**:S108–13.

22. Rebrin K, Steil GM, van Antwerp WP, Mastrototaro JJ. Subcutaneous glucose predicts plasma glucose independent of insulin: implications for continuous monitoring. *Am J Physiol* 1999; **277**:E561–E571.

23. Gerritsen M, Jansen JA, Lutterman JA. Performance of subcutaneously implanted glucose sensors for continuous monitoring. *Neth J Med* 1999; **54**:167–79.

24. Tamada JA, Garg S, Jovanovic L et al and the Cygnus Research Team. Noninvasive glucose monitoring comprehensive clinical results. *J Am Med Assoc* 1999; **282**:1839–44.

25. Jovanovic L, Peterson CM. Insulin and glucose requirements during the first stage of labor in insulin-dependent diabetic women. *Am J Med* 1983; **75**:607–12.

26. Jovanovic L, Druzin M, Peterson CM. Effect of euglycemia on the outcome of pregnancy in insulin dependent diabetic women as compared to normal controls. *Am J Med* 1981; **71**:921–7.

27. Jovanovic L, Peterson CM, Saxena BB, Dawood MY, Saudek CD. Feasibility of maintaining euglycemia in insulin-dependent diabetic women. *Am J Med* 1980; **68**:105–12.

28. Durak EP, Jovanovic L, Peterson CM. Comparative evaluation of five aerobic machines and their effect on uterine activity during pregnancy. *Am J Obstet Gynecol* 1990; **162**:754–6.

29. Jovanovic L, Meisel B, Bevier W, Peterson CM. The Rubenesque pregnancy: a progression towards higher blood pressure correlates with a measure of endogenous and exogenous insulin levels. *Am J Perinatol* 1997; **14**:181–6.

30. Jovanovic L, Jovanovic LL. Increased fetal movement negates postprandial glucose-mediated macrosomia.

American Diabetes Association's Fourth International Workshop – Conference on Gestational Diabetes Mellitus. *Diabetes Care* 1998; **21**:B131–B137.

31. Karlsson K, Kjellmer I. The outcome of diabetic pregnancies in relation to the mothers blood sugar level. *Am J Obstet Gynecol* 1972; **112**:213–20.

32. Jovanovic L. The role of continuous glucose monitoring in gestational diabetes mellitus. *Diabetes Tech Therapeut* 2000; **2 (Suppl 1)**:S67–S71.

33. Landon MB, Gabbe SG, Piana R, Menutti MT, Main EK. Neonatal morbidity in pregnancy complicated by diabetes mellitus: predictive value of maternal glycemic profiles. *Am J Obstet Gynecol* 1987; **156**:1089–95.

34. Yogev Y, Chen R, Ben-Haroush A et al. Continuous glucose monitoring for the evaluation of gravid women with type 1 diabetes mellitus. *Obstet Gynecol* 2003; **101**:633–38.

35. Damm P, Molsted-Pedersen L. Significant decrease in congenital malformations in newborn infants of an unselected population of diabetic women. *Am J Obstet Gynecol* 1989; **161**:1163–7.

36. Cryer PE. Iatrogenic hypoglycemia as a cause of hypoglycemia-associated autonomic failure in IDDM: a vicious cycle. *Diabetes* 1992; **41**:255–60.

37. Rosenn BM, Miodovnik M, Holcberg G, Khoury JC, Siddiqi TA. Hypoglycemia: the price of intensive insulin therapy for pregnant women with insulin-dependent diabetes mellitus. *Obstet Gynecol* 1995; **85**:417–22.

38. Mastortotoro J, Levy R, Georges LP, White N, Mestman J. Clinical results from a continuous glucose sensor multi-center study. *Diabetes* 1998; **47**:A61.

39. Kaufman FR, Gibson LC, Halvorson M et al. A pilot study of the continuous glucose monitoring system: clinical decisions and glycemic control after its use in pediatric type 1 diabetic subjects. *Diabetes Care* 2001; **24**:2030–4.

40. Hershkovitz E, Rachmel A, Ben-Zaken H, Phillip M. Continuous glucose monitoring in children with glycogen storage disease type-1. *J Inherit Metab Dis* 2001; **24**:863–9.

41. Kjos SL, Buchanan TA. Gestational diabetes mellitus. *N Engl J Med* 1999; **341**:1749–56.

30

Prenatal ultrasound assessment of the diabetic patient

Israel Meizner, Reuven Mashiach

Introduction

Diabetes is the most common medical complication of pregnancy. Patients can be separated into those who were known to have diabetes before pregnancy (overt) and those diagnosed during pregnancy [gestational diabetes mellitus (GDM)]. GDM is associated with 3–5% of all live births,[1] though the rate may be even higher in selected populations (e.g. Mexican-Americans, Asians, Indians).[2,3] The significant improvement in outcome of diabetic pregnancies since the advent of insulin therapy at the start of the twentieth century is attributable to improved perinatal maternal glycemic control, close antepartum surveillance and advances in neonatal care. With appropriately treated gestational diabetes, the likelihood of fetal death is no different from that in the general population.[4] Nevertheless, diabetic gravidas are still at high risk of adverse perinatal outcome. Ultrasonography is important for monitoring diabetic pregnancies, and potentially improving both perinatal management and fetal outcome. It is used to assess four major factors:

- Gestational age
- Congenital anomalies
- Growth abnormalities
    Macrosomia
    Intrauterine growth restriction
- Fetal well-being (dynamic assessment).

The evaluation should take the differences between gestational and pregestational diabetes into account and be tailored accordingly.

Gestational age

The evaluation of gestational age is vital to the management of diabetic gravidas because of the increased possibility of growth abnormalities and the importance of delivery at term. The clinical estimation of gestational age has been found to be unsatisfactory in a significantly large number of cases, even when the menstrual history is reliable, and it may therefore be inadequate for critical management decisions.[5] The two most widely used ultrasound measurements for determining gestational age are the crown–rump length (CRL) in the first trimester (up to 12 weeks gestation) and the biparietal diameter (BPD) in the second trimester (before 32 weeks gestation).[6,7] The CRL, assessed with transvaginal sonography, can predict the delivery date to within 5 days.[8] The BPD, assessed by serial ultrasound examinations, is used for confirmation. Femur length is also a valuable predictor of gestational age, especially when it is technically impossible to measure the BPD.[9] The first sonographic examination to determine dates should be performed in the first trimester, prior to 12 weeks gestation whenever possible. These data can assist in the interpretation of gestational-age-correlated biochemical data, such as alpha-fetoprotein and glycosylated hemoglobin levels, as well as in the early detection of fetal malformations. If the findings in the first ultrasound examination differ significantly from clinical dating, the ultrasound examination usually needs to be repeated after at least a 3-week interval. Gestational age can then be determined by the methods of mean projected gestational age or growth-adjusted sonographic age.[10] After 32 weeks gestation, ultrasound can estimate age only to within ±3 weeks. Clinicians should be aware that CRL measurements of fetuses of diabetic gravidas may lag behind those of normal fetuses at the same gestational age.[11] These fetuses also have a higher risk of being malformed.[12–14] Steel et al[15] reported that early growth delay is probably an artifact of an incorrectly estimated ovulation date. These observations can be confirmed only by the study of many diabetic women with conceptually timed pregnancies.

Congenital anomalies

An association between maternal diabetes mellitus and congenital malformations has been suspected since the nineteenth century.[16,17] Despite the considerable advances in the management of the pregnancy complicated by diabetes, the rate of congenital malformations has not changed dramatically. Congenital malformations and their sequelae have replaced intrauterine fetal death and respiratory distress syndrome as the major causes of morbidity and mortality in infants of diabetic mothers.[16] Their estimated frequency is 6–10%, or three- to fivefold higher than the rate in the general population.[18] Most researchers believe that high rates of severe malformations are the consequence of poorly controlled diabetes, both periconceptionally as

well as early in pregnancy,[19,20] though others have failed to totally corroborate these findings.[21–23] The precise mechanism underlying the abnormal development of fetuses of hyperglycemic mothers has not been completely elucidated. The pathogenesis may also involve factors other than hyperglycemia, such as free oxygen radical scavenging enzymes.[24] Diabetes in pregnancy is not associated with a specific fetal phenotype or syndrome, but rather affects multiple organ systems.[25]

The sonographic detection of recognizable congenital anomalies is an important aspect of the management of diabetic pregnancy. Diabetes-associated malformations occur very early in pregnancy, usually before the eighth week of gestation. Therefore, the evaluation should be done in the first trimester of pregnancy and repeated in the second. Cardiovascular anomalies are the most common, especially conotruncal and ventricular septal defects.[26–28] Indeed, maternal diabetes mellitus has been accepted as one of the indications for fetal echocardiography because congenital heart disease occurs four to five times more frequently in the offspring of women with diabetes than in the general population.[29–31] Antenatal identification is important because some defects are ductal-dependent and require immediate therapy after birth.[32] Second in frequency are neural tube defects (NTD) (Figs 30.1–30.3). The skeletal, genitourinary and gastrointestinal systems may also be affected. Maternal serum alpha-fetoprotein (MSAFP) testing is an important indicator of NTD: second-trimester values in women with pregestational diabetes are, on average, 20% lower than in the general population. In these cases, MSAFP levels are corrected without regard to diabetic control. The sensitivity of ultrasound for the detection of NTD associated with increased MSAFP values is reported as being as high as 94%.[33] Be that as it may, all diabetic

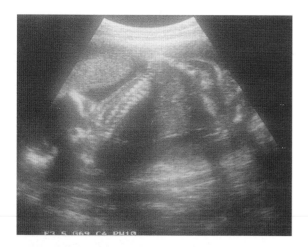

Figure 30.1. *Spina bifida – longitudinal scan of the fetal spine. Note the distortion of the spine due to spinal defects.*

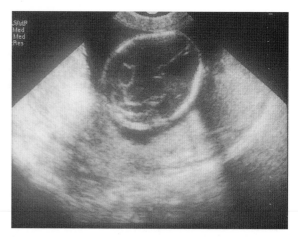

Figure 30.3. *Spina bifida – ultrasound picture of fetal head having the typical lemon-shape configuration.*

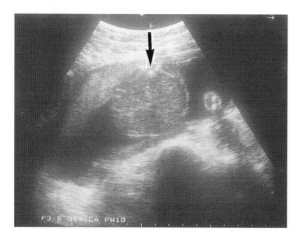

Figure 30.2. *Spina bifida – transverse scan of a fetus at 22 weeks gestation. Note the opening of the spinal canal (U-shaped vertebra) (arrow).*

of the prosencephalon. Interestingly, the lesion most associated with diabetic embryopathy, namely caudal regression syndrome (caudal dysplasia sequence)[35] is actually less common than cardiovascular malformations (Figs 30.4–30.8). However, it is difficult to estimate its incidence

pregnancies should be sonographically evaluated for NTD regardless of the MSAFP level. Anencephaly is the most common anomaly affecting the central nervous system, with an incidence of 0.57% in fetuses of diabetic pregnancies – threefold higher than in the normal population (0.19%).[34] Maternal diabetes is also thought to increase the risk of holoprosencephaly, which results from failure of cleavage

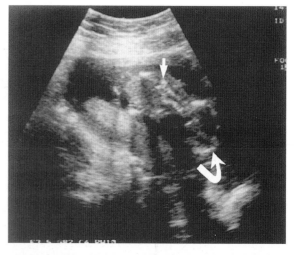

Figure 30.4. *Caudal regression syndrome – longitudinal scan of the fetus. Note the complete absence of the lumbosacral spine. The twelfth thoracic vertebra is prominent (arrow); the fetal head is marked by the curved arrow.*

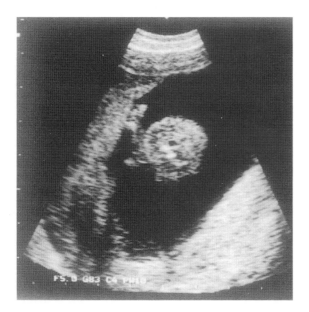

Figure 30.5. *Caudal regression syndrome – transverse scan through the fetal abdomen. Spinal vertebrae are absent; both approximated iliac crests are seen (transvaginal scan).*

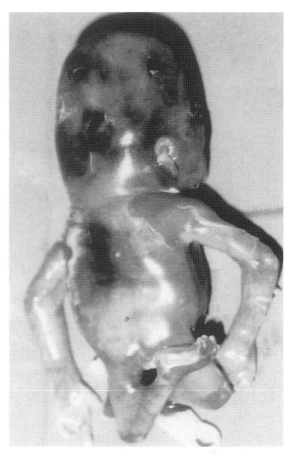

Figure 30.7. *Caudal regression syndrome – Picture of the abortus from the back. Note the short stature with reduced distance between chest and pelvis. The characteristic Buddha (frog-leg) position of the legs is evident.*

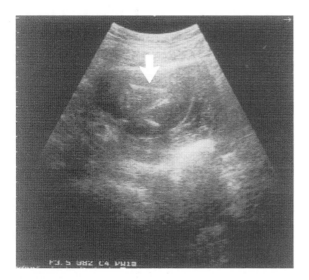

Figure 30.6. *Caudal regression syndrome – ultrasound picture of a fetal flexed leg; the arrow marks the femur.*

because it is often reported together with cases of sirenomelia. The pathogenesis is currently thought to be heterogeneous. The primary defect is in the midposterior axis mesoderm. All degrees of severity may occur, depending primarily on the relative length and width of the early caudal deficit.[35] The most severe form is presumably the consequence of a wedge-shaped early deficit of the caudal blastema.[36] Associated anomalies, in accordance with the severity of the syndrome, may include imperforate anus,

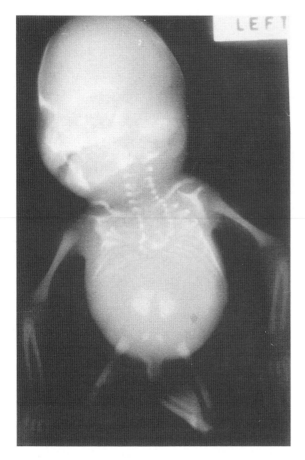

Figure 30.8. *Caudal regression syndrome – anteroposterior X-ray of the abortus. Complete absence of the lumbosacral spine is evident. Touching iliac bones and frog-leg position of the lower limbs are present.*

absence of external genitalia, renal agenesis, absence of internal genitalia except gonads, a single umbilical artery, absence of a bladder and fusion of the lower limbs. The principal findings of caudal regression syndrome on sonographic radiology are as follows: various types of lower limb anomalies ranging from hip dislocation to frog-leg deformity and equinovarus, hydrocephalus and Dandy-Walker malformation; complete absence of the spine below L1, partial or complete absence of the caudal part of the sacrum; intraspinal anomalies in the form of

meningomyelocele and sacral lipoma; the pelvis is small owing to the absence of a sacrum, and the iliac bones touch or even fuse.[37] Up to 16% of cases are associated with diabetes mellitus.[38,39] Although the disorder occurs 200 times more often in infants of diabetic mothers, only 1.3 per 1000 diabetic pregnancies are affected. Defects involving the genitourinary system that show preponderance in infants of diabetic mothers include ureteral duplication, renal agenesis and hydronephrosis.

Growth abnormalities

Monitoring fetal growth is a challenging and highly inexact process. Today's tools, which involve serial plotting of fetal growth parameters, are superior to earlier clinical estimations, but accuracy is still only *c.* 15%, even with the most sophisticated ultrasound equipment. Particular effort should be directed towards the diagnosis of fetal macrosomia, the most frequent fetal complication (up to 50%) of the diabetic pregnancy.[40–44] Macrosomia is a term used rather imprecisely to describe a very large fetus/neonate: there is no universally accepted definition. Macrosomia has been variously defined as a birth weight > 4000–4500 gram, a birth weight > two standard deviations (2 SD) above the mean for gestational age or above the 90th percentile for population-specific and sex-specific growth curves. Macrosomia is not only a result of maternal hyperglycemia, and elevated levels of lipids and amino acids, but are also characteristic of pregnancies complicated by GDM, also resulting in fetal overgrowth. Fetal organomegaly is also common, affecting the fetal liver, pancreas, heart and adrenal glands.[45] Fetal overgrowth or macrosomia can lead to some of the most common morbidities seen in infants of women with GDM. For example, the incidence of shoulder dystocia, which ranges from 0.2 to 2.8% in the general population,[46,47] can be as high as 3–9% in infants of women with GDM.[48] In addition, the growth of these infants tends to be asymmetric, with larger chest/head and shoulder/head ratios than those of infants born to women with normal glucose tolerance.[49] Shoulder dystocia may be associated with other birth trauma, such as Erb's palsy, clavicular fracture, fetal distress, low Apgar scores and birth asphyxia,[50] although 25–75% of brachial plexus injuries are unrelated to antecedent shoulder dystocia.[51] The management of fetal macrosomia has been the subject of much clinical concern and scientific investigation. Over the past 30 years, several investigators have attempted to derive formulas using sonographic measurements of fetal organs to estimate fetal weight. The older formulas used measures of the fetal head, abdomen and femur, either alone[52] or in combination.[53,54] Some authors demonstrated differences in accuracy and precision among these formulas.[55,56] Although most reported that, regardless of the formula used, the accuracy of the fetal weight estimation decreased with increasing birth weight.[57–59] Consequently, alternative sonographic markers for fetal macrosomia have been proposed that take advantage of the presumed correlation between subcutaneous fat deposition and fetal weight. Three-dimensional ultrasound measurements of fetal upper arm volume,[60,61] fetal chest,[62] abdominal[63] and humeral[64] soft tissue thickness, and cheek-to-cheek diameter,[65] as well as of the subcutaneous tissue/femur length ratio,[66,67] have yielded varying screening efficacies for macrosomia. Table 30.1 lists a number of population-based studies that have assessed the clinical performance of ultrasound in predicting macrosomia. The data in the last two columns suggest that 15–81% of babies (median 67%) predicted to be macrosomic are indeed macrosomic at birth,

and that 50–100% (median 62%) of all cases of macrosomia are successfully predicted by sonographic measurements.

Currently, no single sonographic measurement is capable of distinguishing between large for gestational age (LGA) and appropriate for gestational age (AGA) infants of diabetic mothers. The finding of an abdominal circumference above the 90th percentile during the second or third trimester is associated positively with fetal macrosomia, but actual birth weights of the babies predicted to be macrosomic on this basis overlap with those of AGA babies in a substantial proportion of cases.[68]

Other techniques for estimating fetal weight have been reported as well. In one study, magnetic resonance imaging (MRI) yielded estimates within 3% of the actual birth weight in 11 patients whose babies weighed between 1.6 and 3.3 kg. This compared favorably with the 6.5% error by sonographic examination of the same patients.[69]

The estimation of weight of fetuses of diabetic mothers involves special considerations. Because of the disproportionate contribution of fat to fetal body weight and because fat is less dense than lean body tissue, equations used derived from cross-sectional data may theoretically overestimate fetal weight when applied to the GDM population. Furthermore, the time from examination to delivery may influence the accuracy and precision of the sonographic estimates.[71–73]

Clinically, studies have found no significant differences in absolute percentage error of birthweight between infants of women with diabetes and those born to women without diabetes.[74] The accuracy of birthweight prediction by ultrasound and by clinical estimates has been analyzed in a number of studies.[75–80] When the sample was limited to babies with an actual birth weight of > 4 kg, no significant differences were found between the clinical and ultrasound estimates at or near the onset of labor.

Sonographic criteria* (reference)	No. scanned	Inclusion criteria	PPV[†] (%)	Sens[‡] (%)
AC, FL (55)	3512	Non-diabetic	15	94
AC, FL (59)	150	37+ weeks	52	54
AC, FL (56)	223	35–42 weeks	67	62
AC, FL, BPD (71)	479	40 weeks, non-diabetic	67	56
BPD, OFD, ALD, ASD, FL (72)	498	22–50 weeks	67	67
Abdominal subcutaneous tissue (63)	133	37–42 weeks	59	70
Humeral soft tissue (64)	95	Term, prior macrosomia: diabetic ≥ 41 weeks	81	88
AC, FL (95)	519	≥ 41 weeks,	64	56
AC, FL (96)	472	Non-diabetic, 36+ weeks	70	61
AC, FL, BPD, HC (97[§])	406	36+ weeks	51	50
AC, FL, HC (98)	86	Non-diabetic	67	100

* AC, abdominal circumference; FL, femur length; BPD, biparietal diameter; OFD, occipitofrontal diameter; ALD, abdominal longest diameter; ASD, abdominal shortest diameter; HC, head circumference.
[†] PPV, Positive predictive value.
[‡] Sens, Sensitivity.
[§] Macrosomia defined as birth weight ≥ 90th percentile for gestational age.

Table 30.1. Sonographic criteria for macrosomia in the general population and in diabetic mothers.

Intrauterine growth restriction (IUGR), broadly defined as a birthweight lower than the 10th percentile for a given gestational age or an infant with evidence of tissue wasting and malnutrition, is not common in diabetic pregnancies. Because IUGR is associated with conditions that predispose the fetus to utero-placental insufficiency, it is more likely to occur in diabetic pregnancies complicated by severe vasculopathy. The resultant decrease in placental nutrient transfer is thought to be responsible for the IUGR in these infants. Unlike macrosomic fetuses, fetuses with IUGR associated with pancreatic agenesis apparently stop growing at 28–30 weeks gestation.[81] The relative inaccuracy of clinical means for detecting IUGR may result in misdiagnosis in 50–70% of cases. Serial ultrasonography may be beneficial, as it is offered as a routine antenatal procedure.

Fetal well-being (dynamic assessment)

Assessment of fetal well-being

Dynamic assessment of diabetic pregnancies implies two types of investigations: the biophysical score (BPS) and Doppler ultrasound studies. The fetal BPS is often applied to evaluate the significance of a non-reactive NST (non-stress test). It may serve as an important tool for fetal surveillance, especially in order to prevent unnecessary early interventions, thereby allowing prolongation of pregnancy beyond 37 weeks.

Sonography has become one of the most common techniques for non-invasive evaluation of the body. It has taken on a major role in obstetrics largely because of its minimal bioeffects, flexibility and low cost. Sonography also offers several distinct diagnostic tools in one instrument, including imaging and Doppler, enabling both anatomic and dynamic information to be obtained in real time. More complicated instrumentation places additional demands on the clinician, who has to be able to appreciate the operational principles and inherent limitations of the apparatus, and accurately analyze the array of data available. Within the past few years, the application of Doppler ultrasound has allowed the examination of the following characteristics of blood flow: direction, velocity and volume. The sonographer, using principles that have been applied to the pediatric and adult patient, can therefore obtain valuable information concerning fetal cardiovascular flow dynamics.

The assessment of maternal and fetal placental circulation has been of special interest to the obstetrician for a long time. Normal fetal growth and oxygenation in diabetic patients is dependent on adequate perfusion of the placental bed. A better understanding of this circulation is essential in the management of the pregnant woman and her unborn child. After the introduction of Doppler ultrasound in the investigation of blood flow velocities in adults, the human maternal and fetal circulation has become accessible for this new non-invasive evaluation.

Placental vessels in diabetic pregnancy

The placenta in diabetic pregnancies is not closely related to the severity of the disease or the tightness of control.[82,83] Unlike maternal vessels exposed to many years of altered glycemic metabolism, placental vessels do not exhibit the changes characteristic of diabetic angiopathy. However, specific structural changes have been described in the diabetic placenta consisting of immature larger villi, relatively fewer capillaries and decidual microvascular pathology. Abnormal distributions and calibers of placental stem arteries have been reported,[84] probably reflecting the villous immaturity or the obliterative endarteritis that appear in diabetes mellitus. An abnormal cardiac flow has been described in fetuses of Type 1 diabetics, starting from early gestation.[84] All of these changes in placental anatomy have raised the expectations that Doppler ultrasound studies may depict specific findings in diabetic pregnancies. In addition, glucose levels could have an acute and chronic effect on placental and fetal blood flow, as has been shown by laboratory experiments.[85]

Clinical studies in diabetic patients

The effect of glucose on both fetal and maternal flow velocity waveforms (FVW) is controversial. Several large studies have shown that umbilical artery FVW indices are no different in a diabetic population without pregnancy complications than in normal controls.[86,87] No association has been observed when duration of diabetes and Doppler indices have been compared.[88] Mean umbilical artery systolic/diastolic (S/D) ratios were similar in patients with good and poor glycemic control, and there was only a weak correlation between hemoglobin A1c and umbilical artery S/D.[89]

On the other hand, a significant correlation between Doppler indices and serum glucose levels has been found. An elevated S/D ratio was associated with an increased incidence of stillbirths as well as neonatal morbidity.[90] Forty-three patients were enrolled into the study and the S/D ratio was serially examined with continuous wave Doppler from 30 to 40 weeks gestation. Simple regression analysis showed a positive correlation between mean third trimester S/D ratios and serum glucose measurements averaged over the last 2 weeks of pregnancy (resistance index = 0.52, $P < 0.001$). However, assessment of the glycemic control in this study was based only on small numbers of random blood glucose.

Well-designed studies have not been able to demonstrate any correlation between long-term glucose regulation and chronic changes in placental regulation. However, one should raise the question of whether acute or extreme changes in blood glucose levels may affect the placental vasculature in a manner that might be detected by Doppler ultrasound. Ishimatsu et al[91] studied 16 patients with insulin-dependent diabetes without vascular disease. The authors found two patients with mean daily serum glucose levels > 300 mg% at the time of enrollment: both of these patients demonstrated elevated umbilical artery resistance indices when Doppler velocimetry studies were undertaken. After a few weeks, when better control was achieved (mean glucose levels < 200 mg%), the resistance index in each patient returned to the normal range. In animal models (sheep), Crandell et al[92] induced maternal and fetal hyperglycemia by glucose infusion. When the glucose levels were elevated to two to three times normal

range, fetal hypoxemia and mixed metabolic and respiratory acidosis developed. Umbilical artery blood flow was significantly decreased. The same group of investigators has also shown, on an isolated placental cotyledon model, that high glucose levels cause a local decrease in prostacycline production, promoting vasoconstriction.[85] It is therefore possible that severe hyperglycemia can cause transient, humorally-mediated changes in placental blood flow that could be depicted by simultaneous Doppler studies, even though average glycemic control does not correlate with umbilical artery resistance.

The present authors have studied a group of 30 healthy pregnant women at 24–28 weeks gestation undergoing an oral glucose tolerance test (OGTT). Umbilical and uterine artery flow was assessed using Doppler apparatus and the following studies were made: prior to an oral 100 g glucose load; 1-hour intervals thereafter. All OGTT tests results were normal and Doppler signals were obtained in all patients. No abnormal flow ratios were detected in any of the tests. There were no significant differences in waveforms between either the right and left uterine arteries resistance indices during the various stages of testing (Table 30.2, and Figs 30.9 and 30.10).

Uterine artery FVW in diabetic patients has been examined only in few studies.[89,93] The limited data available suggest that it is appropriate to use uterine artery reference ranges

Time (minutes)	Umbilical artery	Right uterine artery	Left uterine artery
0	2.87±0.77	0.49±0.09	0.53±0.1
60	2.86±0.83	0.53±0.08	0.52±0.1
120	2.95±0.83	0.51±0.08	0.50±0.09
180	2.87±1.1	0.53±0.09	0.52±0.1

Table 30.2. Blood flow velocimetry during oral glucose tolerance test.

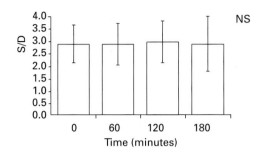

Figure 30.9. *Systolic/diastolic (S/D) ratio in the umbilical cord during oral glucose tolerance test.*

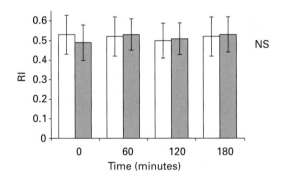

Figure 30.10. *Resistance index (RI) in right (■) and left (□) uterine arteries during oral glucose tolerance test.*

from the non-diabetic population. In the study by Johnstone and Steel,[94] the third trimester mean value for the uterine artery resistance index was 0.4 + 0.06 for both insulin-dependent diabetics and non-diabetic controls.

Conclusions

Antenatal ultrasound plays an important role in monitoring diabetic pregnancies. The main issues associated with sonographic assessment of these pregnancies include the following:

* Assessment of gestational age
* Detection of congenital anomalies
* Surveillance of growth

* Dynamic assessment of fetal status (BPS, Doppler).

The ultrasound evaluation should take into consideration the differences between GDM and preGDM and, therefore, the sonographic approach must be tailored accordingly.

Proposed ultrasound work-up in diabetes mellitus complicating pregnancy

GDM *patients*

Ultrasound evaluation should start immediately following diagnosis and continue as follows:

* Fetal growth and weight estimations starting at diagnosis and continuing at 3–4 weeks intervals
* Fetal weight estimation at 37–38 weeks gestation
* BPS at weekly intervals starting at 34 weeks gestation, only for insulin-treated patients and/or those with poor compliance and control
* Fetal echocardiography if fasting glucose values > 120 mg/dl.

PreGDM *patients*

First trimester:
* 8–10 weeks gestation – transvaginal sonography dating of pregnancy (CRL)
* 12 weeks gestation – nuchal translucency (optional).

Second trimester:
* 15 weeks gestation – transvaginal first detailed anatomical survey of the fetus (optional)
* 22 weeks gestation – second detailed anatomical survey of the fetus (abdominal)
* 20–24 weeks gestation – fetal echocardiography.

Third trimester:

- Fetal growth and weight estimations starting at 20 weeks gestation and at 3–4-week intervals
- Fetal weight estimation at 37–38 weeks gestation
- BPS at weekly intervals starting at 32–34 weeks gestation.

In all examinations a thorough assessment of all fetal growth parameters is mandatory (i.e. BPD, occipitofrontal diameter, head circumference, abdominal circumference and femur length).

References

1. Ventura SJ, Martin JA, Curtin SC et al. Births: final data for 1998. *Natl Vital Stat Rep* 2000; **48**.
2. King H. Epidemiology of glucose intolerance and gestational diabetes in women of childbearing age. *Diabetes* 1998; **2 (Suppl 2)**:9–13.
3. Engelgau NM, Herman WH, Smith PI et al. The epidemiology of diabetes and pregnancy in the US. *Diabetes Care* 1998; **18**:1029–33.
4. Metzger BE, Coustan DR. Summary and recommendations of the Fourth International Workshop–Conference on Gestational Diabetes Mellitus. *Diabetes Care* 1998; **21**:B161–B175.
5. Callen PW. *Ultrasonography in Obstetrics and Gynecology.* (Philadelphia: WB Saunders, 2000) 146–70.
6. Robinson HP. Sonar measurements of the fetal crown–rump length as a means of assessing maturity in first trimester pregnancy. *Br Med J* 1973; **4**:28–31.
7. Campbell S, Newman GB. Growth of the fetal biparietal diameter during pregnancy. *J Obstet Gynecol Br Commonwealth* 1971; **78**:513–16.
8. Robinson HP, Fleming JEE. A critical evaluation of sonar crown–rump length measurements. *Br J Obstet Gynecol* 1975; **82**:702–6.
9. O'Brien GD, Queenan JT, Campbell S. Assessment of gestational age in the second trimester by real-time ultrasound measurement of the femur length. *Am J Obstet Gynecol* 1981; **139**:540–4.
10. Kopta MM, Tomich PG, Crane JP. Ultrasound methods of predicting the estimated date of confinement. *Obstet Gynecol* 1981; **57**:657–60.
11. Pedersen JF, Molsted-Pedersen L. Early growth retardation in diabetic pregnancy. *Br Med J* 1979; **1**:18–19.
12. Pedersen JF, Molsted-Pedersen L. Early fetal growth delay detected by ultrasound marks increased risk of congenital malformation in diabetic pregnancy. *Br Med J* 1981; **283**:80–4.
13. Pedersen JF, Molsted-Pedersen L, Mortensen HB. Fetal growth delay and maternal hemoglobin A1c in early diabetic pregnancy. *Obstet Gynecol* 1984; **64**:351–61.
14. Pedersen JF, Molsted-Pedersen L. The possibility of an early growth delay in White's class A diabetic pregnancy. *Diabetes* 1985; **34 (Supp 2)**:47–50.
15. Steel JM, Wu PS, Johnstone DF et al. Does early growth delay occur in diabetic pregnancy? *Br J Obstet Gynaecol* 1995; **102**:224–7.
16. Mills JL. Malformations in infants of diabetic mothers. *Teratology* 1982; **25**:385–9.
17. Mills JL, Baker L, Goldman AS. Malformations in infants of diabetic mothers occur before the seventh gestational week: implications for treatment. *Diabetes* 1979; **28**:292–6.
18. Hanson U, Persson B. Outcome of pregnancy complicated by Type 1 insulin dependent diabetes in Sweden: acute pregnancy complications, neonatal mortality, and morbidity. *Am J Perinatol* 1993; **10**:330–3.
19. Miller E, Hare JW, Cloherty JP et al. Elevated maternal hemoglobin A_{1c} in early pregnancy and major congenital anomalies in infants of diabetic mothers. *N Engl J Med* 1981; **304**:1331–9.
20. Lucas MJ, Leveno KL, Williams ML et al. Early pregnancy glycosylated hemoglobin, severity of diabetes, and fetal malformations. *Am J Obstet Gynecol* 1989; **161**:426–30.
21. Mills JL, Knopp RH, Simpson JL et al. National Institute of Child Health and Human Development Diabetes in Early Pregnancy Study: incidence of spontaneous abortion among normal women and insulin-dependent diabetic women whose pregnancies were identified within 21 days of conception. *N Engl J Med* 1988; **318**:671–81.
22. Schaefer-Graf UM, Buchanan TA, Xiang A et al. Patterns of congenital anomalies and relationship to initial maternal fasting glucose levels in pregnancies complicated by type 2 and gestational diabetes. *Am J Obstet Gynecol* 2000; **182**:313–24.
23. Rose BJ, Graff S, Spencer R. Major congenital anomalies in infants and glycosylated hemoglobin levels in insulin-requiring diabetic mothers. *J Perinatol* 1988; **8**:309–11.
24. Reece EA, Homko CJ, Wu YK. Multifactorial basis of the syndrome of diabetic embryopathy. *Teratology* 1997; **54**:171–82.
25. Mills JL. Congenital malformations in diabetes. In: (Gabbe SG, Oh W, eds) *Infant of the Diabetic Mother. Report of the 93rd Ross Conference on Pediatric Research.* (Ross Laboratories: Columbus, OH, 1987) 12–19.
26. Adams MM, Mulinare J, Dooley K. Risk factors for conotruncal cardiac defects in Atlanta. *J Am Coll Cardiol* 1989; **14**:432–42.

27. Ferencz C, Rubin JD, McCarter RJ. Maternal diabetes and cardiovascular malformations: predominance of double outlet right ventricle and truncus arteriosus. *Teratology* 1990; 41:319–26.

28. Lowy C, Beard RW, Goldschmidt J. Congenital malformations in babies of diabetic mothers. *Diabet Med* 1986; 3:458–62.

29. Rowland TW, Hubbell JP, Nadas AS. Congenital heart disease in infants of diabetic mothers. *J Pediatr* 1973; 83:815–20.

30. Ramos-Arroyo MA, Rodriguez-Pinilla E, Cordero JF. Maternal diabetes: the risk for specific birth defects. *Eur J Epidemiol* 1992; 8:503–8.

31. Fraser R. Diabetes in pregnancy. *Arch Dis Child* 1994; 71:224–38.

32. Ramada SS, Christine HC, Robert PL et al. Maternal diabetes mellitus: which views are essential for fetal echocardiography. *Obstet Gynecol* 1997; 90:575–9.

33. Watson WJ, Chescheir NC, Katz VL. The role of ultrasound in evaluation of patients with elevated maternal serum alpha-fetoprotein: a review. *Obstet Gynecol* 1991; 78:123–8.

34. Soler NG, Walsh CH, Malins JM. Congenital malformations in infants of diabetic mothers. *J Med* 1976; 178:303–7.

35. Lenz W, Maier W. Congenital malformations and maternal diabetes. *Lancet* 1964; 2:1124–8.

36. Smith DW, Jones KL. *Recognizable Pattern of Human Malformation.* (WB Saunders: Philadelphia, 1982) 486–7.

37. Meizner I, Bar-Ziv J. *In Utero Diagnosis of Skeletal Disorders. An Atlas of Prenatal Sonographic and Postnatal Radiologic Correlation.* (CRC Press: FL, 1993) 72–7.

38. Rusnak SL, Driscoll SG. Congenital spinal anomalies in infants of diabetic mothers. *Teratology* 1965; 25:385–9.

39. Mills JL. Malformations in infants of diabetic mothers. *Teratology* 1982; 25:385–8.

40. Boyd ME, Usher RH, McLean FH. Fetal macrosomia: prediction, risks, proposed management. *Obstet Gynecol* 1983; 61:715–22.

41. Lubchenco LO, Hansman C, Dressler M, Boyd E. Intrauterine growth as estimated from liveborn birthweight data at 24 to 42 weeks of gestation. *Pediatrics* 1963; 32:793–800.

42. Spellacy WN, Miller S, Winegar A, Peterson PQ. Macrosomia – maternal characteristics and infant complications. *Obstet Gynecol* 1985; 66:185–90.

43. Langer O. Is normoglycemia the correct threshold to prevent complications in the pregnant diabetic patient? *Diabetes Rev* 1996; 4:2–10.

44. American College of Obstetricians and Gynecologists (ACOG). *Fetal Macrosomia. ACOG Technical Bulletin No. 159.* (ACOG: Washington, DC, 1991).

45. Persson B, Hanson U. Neonatal morbidities in gestational diabetes mellitus. *Diabetes* 1998; 21(Suppl 2): 79–84.

46. Acker DB, Sachs BP, Friedman EA. Risk factors for shoulder dystocia. *Obstet Gynecol* 1985; 66:762–7.

47. Langer O, Berkus HD, Huff RW, Sameloff A. Shoulder dystocia: should the fetus weighing ≥ 4000 g be delivered by cesarean section? *Am J Obstet Gynecol* 1991; 165:831–7.

48. Elliot JP, Garite TJ, Freedman RK et al. Ultrasonic prediction of fetal macrosomia in diabetic patients. *Obstet Gynecol Clin N Am* 1999; 26:445–58.

49. Ballard JL, Rosenn B, Khoury JC, Miodovnik M. Diabetic fetal macrosomia: significance of disproportionate fetal growth. *J Pediatr* 1993; 122:445–58.

50. Levine MG, Holroyde S, Woods JR et al. Birth trauma: incidence and predisposing factors. *Obstet Gynecol* 1984; 63:792–5.

51. Gherman RB, Goodwin TM, Ouzounian JG. Brachial plexus palsy associated with cesarean section: an in utero injury? *Am J Obstet Gynecol* 1997; 177:1162–4.

52. Campbell S, Wilkin D. Ultrasonic measurements of fetal abdomen circumference in the estimation of fetal weight. *Br J Obstet Gynaecol* 1975; 82:689–97.

53. Hadlock FP, Harrist RB, Carpenter RJ et al. Sonographic estimation of fetal weight: the value of femur length in addition to head and abdomen measurements. *Radiology* 1984; 150:535–40.

54. Shepard MJ, Richards VA, Berkowitz RL et al. An evaluation of two equations for predicting fetal weight by ultrasound. *Am J Obstet Gynecol* 1982; 142:47–4.

55. Smith GCB, Smith MFS, McNay MB, Fleming JEE. The relation between fetal abdominal circumference and birthweight: findings in 3512 pregnancies. *Br J Obstet Gynaecol* 1997; 104:186–90.

56. Shamley KT, Landon MB. Accuracy and modifying factors for ultrasonographic determination of fetal weight at term. *Obstet Gynecol* 1994; 84:926–30.

57. Dudley NJ. Selection of appropriate ultrasound methods for the estimation of fetal weight. *Br J Radiol* 1995; 68:385–8.

58. Hirata GI, Medearis AL, Horenstein J. Ultrasonographic estimation of fetal weight in the clinically macrosomic fetus. *Am J Obstet Gynecol* 1990; 162:238–42.

59. Miller JM, Korndorffer FA, Gabert HA. Fetal weight estimates in late pregnancy with emphasis on macrosomia. *J Clin Ultrasound* 1986; 14:437–42.

60. Favre R, Bader A-M, Nisand G. Prospective study on fetal weight estimation using limb circumferences obtained by three-dimensional ultrasound. *Ultrasound Obstet Gynecol* 1995; 6:140–4.

61. Liang R-I, Chang F-M, Yao B-L. Predicting birth weight by fetal upper-arm volume with use of three-dimensional ultrasonography. *Am J Obstet Gynecol* 1997; 177:632–8.

62. Winn NH, Rauk PN, Petrie RH. Use of the fetal chest in estimating fetal weight. *Am J Obstet Gynecol* 1992; 167:448–50.

63. Petrikovsky BM, Oleschuk C, Lesser M. Prediction of fetal macrosomia using sonographically measured

abdominal subcutaneous tissue thickness. *J Clin Ultrasound* 1997; **25**:378–82.

64. Sood AK, Yancey M, Richards D. Prediction of fetal macrosomia using humeral soft tissue thickness. *Obstet Gynecol* 1995; **85**:937–40.

65. Abramovicz JS, Sherer DM, Woods JR. Ultra-sonographic measurements of cheek-to-cheek diameter in fetal growth disturbances. *Am J Obstet Gynecol* 1993; **169**:405–8.

66. Santolaya-Forgas J, Meyer WJ, Gautier DW. Intrapartum fetal subcutaneous tissue/femur length ratio: an ultra-sonographic clue to fetal macrosomia. *Am J Obstet Gynecol* 1994; **171**:1072–5.

67. Rotmensch S, Celentano C, Liberati M et al. Screening efficacy of the subcutaneous tissue width/femur length ratio for fetal macrosomia in the non-diabetic pregnancy. *Ultrasound Obstet Gynecol* 1999; **13**:340–4.

68. Keller JD, Metzger BE, Doodly SL. Infants of diabetic mothers with accelerated fetal growth by ultrasonography: are they all alike? *Am J Obstet Gynecol* 1990; **163**:893–7.

69. Baker PN, Johnson IR, Gowland PA. Fetal weight estimation by echo-planar magnetic resonance imaging. *Lancet* 1994; **343**:644–5.

70. Crane SS, Avallone DA, Thomas AJ. Sonographic estimation of fetal body composition with gestational diabetes mellitus at term. *Obstet Gynecol* 1996; **88**:849–54.

71. O'Reilly-Green CP, Divon MY. Receiver operating characteristics curves of sonographic estimated fetal weight for prediction of macrosomia in prolonged pregnancies. *Ultrasound Obstet Gynecol* 1997; **9**:403–8.

72. Rossavik IK, Joslin GL. Macrosomatia and ultrasonography: what is the problem? *South Med J* 1993:86:1129–32.

73. Spinnato JA, Allen RD, Mendenhall HW. Birth weight prediction from remote ultrasonographic examination. *Am J Obstet Gynecol* 1989; **161**:742–7.

74. Alsulyman OM, Ouzounian JG, Kjos SL. The accuracy of intrapartum ultrasonographic fetal weight estimation in diabetic pregnancies. *Am J Obstet Gynecol* 1997; **177**:503–6.

75. Raman S, Urquhart R, Yusof M. Clinical versus ultra-sound estimation of fetal weight. *Aust NZ Obstet Gynaecol* 1992; **32**:196–9.

76. Chauhan SP, Cowan BD, Magann EF. Intrapartum detection of a macrosomic fetus: clinical versus 8 sonographic models. *Aust NZ J Obstet Gynaecol* 1995; **35**:266–70.

77. Watson WJ, Soisson AP, Harlass FE. Estimated weight of the term fetus. Accuracy of ultrasound vs clinical examination. *J Reprod Med* 1998; **33**:369–71.

78. Sherman DJ, Arieli S, Tovbin J. A comparison of clinical and ultrasonic estimation of fetal weight. *Obstet Gynecol* 1998; **91**:212–17.

79. Chauhan SP, Hendrix NW, Magann EF. Limitation of clinical and sonographic estimates of birth weight: expe-

rience with 1034 parturients. *Obstet Gynecol* 1998; **91**:72–7.

80. Johnstone FD, Prescott RJ, Steel JM. Clinical and ultra-sound prediction of macrosomia in diabetic pregnancy. *Br J Obstet Gynaecol* 1996; **103**:747–54.

81. Dourow N, Buyl-Strouvens ML. Agenesis du pancreas. *Arch Fr Pediatr* 1969; **26**:641–50.

82. Fox H. The placenta in diabetes mellitus. In: (Sutherland HW, Stowers JM, Pearson DWM eds) *Carbohydrate Metabolism in Pregnancy and the Newborn*. (Springer-Verlag: London, 1989) 109–17.

83. Bjork O, Persson B. Placental changes in relation to the degree of metabolic control in diabetes mellitus. *Placenta* 1982; **3**:367–78.

84. Rizzo G, Arduini D, Capponi A, Romanini C. Cardiac and venous blood flow in fetuses of insulin-dependant diabetic mothers: evidence of abnormal hemodynamics in early gestation. *Am J Obstet Gynecol* 1992; **173**: 1775–81.

85. Roth JB, Thorp JA, Palmer SM et al. Response of placental vasculature to high glucose levels in the isolated human placental cotyledon. *Am J Obstet Gynecol* 1990; **163**:1828–30.

86. Dicker D, Goldman JA, Yeshaya A, Peleg D. Umbilical artery velocimetry in insulin dependent diabetes mellitus pregnancies. *J Perinat Med* 1990; **18**:391–5.

87. Johnstone FD, Steel JM, Haddad NG et al. Doppler umbilical artery flow velocity waveforms in diabetic pregnancy. *Br J Obstet Gynecol* 1992; **99**:135–40.

88. Zimmerman P, Kujansuu E, Tuimala R. Doppler velocimetry of the umbilical artery in pregnancies complicated by insulin dependent diabetes mellitus. *Eur J Obstet Gynecol Reprod Biol* 1992; **47**:85–93.

89. Kofinas A, Penry M, Swain M. Uteroplacental Doppler flow velocity waveform analysis correlates poorly with glycemic control in diabetic pregnant women. *Am J Perinatol* 1991; **8**:273–7.

90. Bracero L, Schulman H, Fleisher A et al. Umbilical artery velocimetry in diabetes and pregnancy. *Obstet Gynecol* 1986; **68**:654–8.

91. Ishimatsu J, Yoshimura O, Manabe A. Umbilical artery blood flow velocity waveforms in pregnancy complicated by diabetes mellitus. *Arch Gynecol Obstet* 1991; **248**: 123–7.

92. Crandell SS, Fisher DJ, Morris FH. Effects of ovine maternal hyperglycemia on fetal regional blood flows and metabolism. *Am J Physiol* 1985; **249**:E454–E460.

93. Bracero LA, Jovanovic L, Rochelson B et al. Significance of umbilical and uterine artery velocimetry in the well-controlled pregnant diabetic. *J Reprod Med* 1989; **34**:273–6.

94. Johnstone F, Steel JM. Use of Doppler ultrasound in the management of diabetic pregnancy. In: (Pearce JM, ed). *Doppler Ultrasound in Perinatal Medicine*. (Oxford University Press: Oxford, 1992) 178–88.

95. Pollack RN, Hauer-Pollack G, Divon MY. Macrosomia in postdates pregnancies: the accuracy of routine ultra-

sonographic screening. *Am J Obstet Gynecol* 1992; **167**:7–11.

96. Chervenack JL, Divon MY, Hirsch J. Macrosomia in the postdate pregnancies: is routine ultrasonographic screening indicated? *Am J Obstet Gynecol* 1989; **161**:753–6.

97. Levine AB, Lockwood CJ, Brown B. Sonographic diagnosis of the large for gestational age fetus at term: does it make a difference? *Obstet Gynecol* 1992; **79**:55–8.

98. Delpapa EH, Muller-Heubach E. Pregnancy outcome following ultrasound diagnosis of macrosomia. *Obstet Gynecol* 1991; **78**:340–3.

31

Monitoring in labor

Roberto Luzietti, Karl G Rosén

Introduction

Alteration of fetal carbohydrate metabolism may contribute to intrauterine asphyxia. There is considerable evidence linking hyperinsulinemia and fetal hypoxemia. Hyperinsulinemia induced in fetal lambs by an infusion of exogenous insulin produces an increase in oxygen consumption and a decrease in arterial oxygen content. The fetus of the diabetic mother is also at increased risk of asphyxia because of other factors such as increased fetal metabolic rate and oxygen requirement, ketoacidosis and the increased incidence of certain pathological conditions in the diabetic pregnancy, e.g. preeclampsia and vasculopathy, that can result in a reduction in placental blood flow and fetal oxygenation.

All these factors make intrapartum fetal surveillance in pregnancies complicated by maternal diabetes of fundamental importance. In this chapter the basis and current development of intrapartum fetal monitoring, with particular reference to ST waveform analysis of the fetal electrocardiogram (ECG), will be reviewed.

The twentieth century saw dramatic developments in medical care as technological advances were applied to both diagnosis and treatment. However, some areas of obstetrics have been slow to benefit from these advances – and none more so than the care of the fetus in labor. Fetal surveillance during labor constitutes a challenge in information management. To give birth is a natural process for women. For the child it may constitute a threat for intact survival and ominous changes may appear within minutes, putting labor-ward management in the forefront of medical high-risk management. The nurse/ midwife/obstetrician manages this complex situation by visual analysis of a host of information, both clinical and that directly recorded, from the fetus in particular. The current situation is far from satisfactory and a new strategy has to be developed and implemented to take obstetric management further into this century.

What information is required?

The capacity of fetuses to handle hypoxemia may differ greatly, depending not only on the condition prior to labor but also due to events during labor which may affect the ability to mobilize these defence systems. Therefore, it may be difficult to rely only on the actual level of oxygenation. Instead, it may be more rewarding to try to interpret the reactions taking place in a high-priority organ like the heart or the brain.

Much would be gained if there were continuous information available providing direct measure on the ability of the fetus to respond to the stress of labor. The fetal ability to adapt to hypoxemia, hypoxia and asphyxia involves multiple defence mechanisms. These consist primarily of behavioral changes, i.e. reduced active sleep with fewer fetal movements and enhanced extraction of available oxygen. Cardiovascular compensation that increases blood flow to the most important organs, i.e. the brain, the heart and the adrenals, is of importance during hypoxia, as is the metabolic defence of anaerobic metabolism. It is only when these compensatory mechanisms are insufficient that asphyxia will develop and along with it the possibility of central nervous system damage and handicap (for review see Greene and Rosén).[1]

Available techniques

To achieve a change, we need to analyze what were the shortcomings when electronic fetal monitoring (EFM) was introduced some 30 years ago. With EFM obstetricians hoped to prevent the delivery of dead or impaired babies who had suffered from birth asphyxia. It is now realized that cardiotocography (CTG) does not provide all the information required to do this.[2,3] Misinterpretation of the CTG not only causes an increase in unnecessary intervention but is also implicated in a large proportion of patients with birth asphyxia and avoidable perinatal morbidity.[4] Misinterpretation could be corrected with improved understanding and enhanced identification of specific events in fetal heart rate (FHR) patterns. The automatic assessment of FHR variability and reactivity antenatally provides a good example of the latter. Physiologically, there are a multitude of factors influencing FHR in the term fetus and it should not be anticipated that there are FHR features that are specific enough to discriminate between different levels of hypoxia. However,

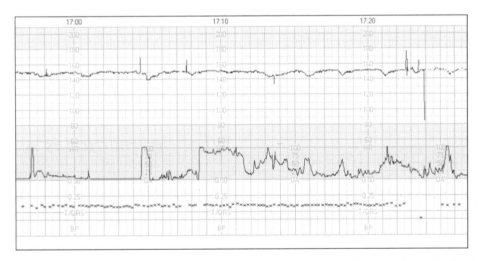

Figure 31.1. *Para 1, normal pregnancy, spontaneous onset at 39 weeks gestation, oligohydramnios plus decreased fetal movements noted by the mother. Emergency Cesarean section for fetal distress at 17:43. Female 2900 grams, Apgar score 1-3-5, cord artery data not obtained, cord vein data – pH 7.29, pCO$_2$ 6.5 kPa, BDecf (base deficit in the extra cellular fluid) 2.5 mmol/l. Initial ventilation by mask followed by intubation, meconium in upper airways. Adequate breathing at 25 minutes of age. Marked hypoglycemia (0.5 mmol/l) initially. No sign of meconium aspiration or RDS (respiratory distress syndrome). Increased neuromuscular tone but normal electroencephalogram. No suctioning reflex initially. Normal behavior after 4 days. Discharged home after 15 days.*

at the same time, EFM provides relevant information of fetal reactiveness, i.e. a fetus showing a completely normal CTG should have matters under control. At the same time, a CTG pattern with complete lack of FHR variability and reactivity (Fig. 31.1) should serve as the best indicator of a fetus that has lost its ability to respond and is in a preterminal situation.

Fetal blood sampling

Fetal blood sampling (FBS) can be used along with CTG monitoring to assess the fetal acid–base status during labor and can reduce operative intervention,[5] but it requires additional expertise, is time consuming and gives only intermittent information; therefore, it is not widely used.[3]

Considering the need to improve understanding of the process of intrapartum hypoxia, very little new information has emerged with regard to the analysis of scalp pH since the early work by Rosén et al.[6] At the same time as EFM and FBS have been shown to improve outcome, the use of FBS has also been questioned by analyzing outcome measures in a large clinical service where the rate of FBS decreased from 1.76 to 0.03% without any change in the Cesarean section rate or an increase in indicators of perinatal asphyxia.[7] Thus, the attitude towards the clinical usefulness of FBS and scalp pH is, after 30 years, still unclear.

To what extent should a scalp pH add to our ability to identify fetuses at risk of intrapartum hypoxia? The limitation of a scalp pH is that it will always reflect the status of the peripheral blood where an acidosis is inherent due to the accumulation of CO_2. Respiratory acidemia is generated in the blood, whereas metabolic acidemia is generated in the tissues. This means that a scalp sample *per se* will not always reflect the state of the tissues. If the aim is to identify those fetuses suffering from metabolic

acidosis, a scalp blood pH may be a poor predictor. Furthermore, the effectiveness of FBS in clinical practice is another problem. In the Plymouth trial, despite the use of a strict protocol, 39% of cases had FBS performed unnecessarily and 33% of cases did not have it performed when it was indicated.[5] The decision to perform FBS depends on the interpretation of the CTG: if the level of CTG interpretation is suboptimal, the value of monitoring by FBS is limited.[8]

Pulse oximetry

Pulse oximetry is focused on recording the actual level of fetal hypoxemia and relates the level of oxygenation of organ function as indicated by FHR.[9] A US multicentre randomized trial of 1010 laboring women with a non-reassuring FHR tracing showed a reduction in emergency Cesarean sections from 10 to 5%. However, unexpectedly, the study also showed an increase in the Cesarean section rate for failure to progress in the test group, 19 versus 9%, and the overall Cesarean section rates were not different between the test and control groups.

The current literature holds somewhat diverging views on the information available from fetal pulse oximetry during labor. The issue still to be resolved is the ability of CTG + pulse oximetry to provide diagnostic capacity on fetal metabolic acidosis.[10,11] Thus, the situation may arise where the two parameters in combination may not be specific enough to enable the obstetrician to grade the impact of hypoxemia on fetal organ function.

A different approach to assess fetal condition during labor is that based on evaluation of high-priority organ function. ST analysis of the ECG during exercise testing is well proven in assessing myocardial function in the adult.[10]

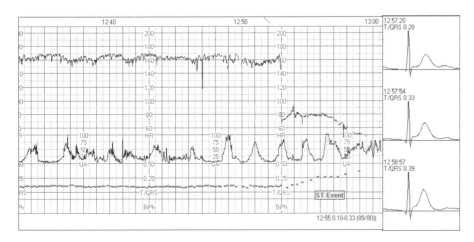

Figure 31.2. *STAN recording during the second stage of labor. Uneventful pregnancy at term. At 12:53 the midwife, who was a trained STAN user, noted as abrupt shift in the fetal heart rate (FHR) recording. She immediately informed the clinician about the situation of an emerging acute asphyxia. The clinician, who had **not** been trained, choose to verify that the FHR was recorded by applying an external sensor. The baby was delivered 14 minutes after the end of the recording, with Apgar scores of 3 at 1 minute and of 5 at 5 minutes, and developed signs of neonatal encephalopathy with seizures. Acute placental abruption with an immediate stop in cord vein blood flow was the cause of this acutely emerging intrapartum asphyxia.*

Fetal ECG

Similar to the adult stress test, ST waveform analysis of the fetal ECG, affected by the stress of labor, should provide key information about the ability of the high-priority organ, i.e. the fetal heart, to respond. This assumption seems to hold true and ST analysis has emerged not as an alternative to CTG but as a support tool, allowing more accurate interpretation of intrapartum events along the lines depicted in Fig. 31.2. Furthermore, the fetal ECG is readily obtainable during labor from the same scalp electrode used to obtain the FHR and no alterations are required in the patient handling routines.

Figure 31.3 indicates those parts of the ECG that provide specific information on the fetal response to hypoxia. The waveform marked P corresponds to the contraction of the atrium; the next sequence is the contraction of the ventricles, illustrated by the waveforms Q, R and S.

Physiology

The ST segment and the T wave relate to the repolarization of myocardial cells in preparation for the next contraction, a process that is energy consuming. An *increase* in T-wave height, quantified by the ratio between T and QRS amplitudes (the T/QRS ratio) (Fig. 31.2), occurs when the energy balance within the myocardial cells threatens to become negative.[1,8,12] A

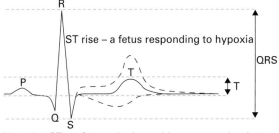

Negative ST – a fetus who is unable to respond or has not had time to react

Figure 31.3. *The ECG, with a schematic presentation of hypoxia-related changes; the T/QRS ratio measurement is also indicated.*

negative energy balance means a situation where the amount of oxygen supplied to the cells no longer covers the energy required for metabolic activity. During hypoxia this balance becomes negative and the cells produce energy by the beta-adrenoceptor-mediated anaerobic breakdown of glycogen reserves.[6] The ability of these cells to produce energy in this manner, and thereby maintain myocardial function, is a vital compensatory defence mechanism.[13] This process not only produces lactic acid but also potassium ions (K^+), which affects myocardial cell membrane potential and causes a rise in the ST waveform (Fig. 31.3).[12] Thus, the rise in T-wave amplitude and the increase in the T/QRS ratio reflect the rate of myocardial glycogenolysis and the utilization of a key fetal defence to hypoxia.

Hypoxemia is just one way in which this myocardial energy balance changes, so producing ST waveform changes. Another mechanism by which these ST changes may occur is the general surge of stress hormones (adrenaline) occurring in response to the squeezing and squashing of labor. This will stimulate the heart to increase its pumping activity, and at the same time induce glycogenolysis and high T waves. This general arousal is part of normal labor and in these cases the healthy fetus will display a reactive CTG, ensuring normality.[14]

Biphasic ST events

ST depression with negative T waves has been observed during hypoxia experiments in experimentally growth-retarded guinea pigs.[7] Clinically, these changes have emerged as a specific sign of myocardial hypoxic stress, reflecting a myocardium either unable or with insufficient time to mobilize its defence to hypoxemia. The result is a decrease in myocardial activity and a risk of cardiovascular failure.

The physiology behind biphasic ST events is related to the mechanical performance of the myocardium, and the relationship between the inner (endocardium) and outer (epicardium) layers of the walls of the ventricles in particular. As we know it, biphasic ST illustrates an imbalance between these two layers, the reason being that the perfusion pressure of the endocardium is always lower when the mechanical strain is greater. This means that unless the myocardium is generally activated (beta-receptor activation and enhanced Frank–Starling relationship, i.e. the ability of the myocardium to respond to volume load), any decrease in performance will cause biphasic ST. Thus, not only may hypoxia *per se* cause biphasic ST as a sign of maladaptation, but so will all factors substantially altering the balance and performance characteristics within the myocardial wall. Basically, biphasic ST is the pattern to be expected whenever the myocardium is exposed to factors that may decrease its ability to respond.

Probably the most clinically important aspect of biphasic ST is that once it has been identified, then a situation of potentially reduced myocardial performance has also been identified and 'classical' signs of fetal reactions to an emerging hypoxia should not be expected. From what is stated above, it should be noted that a fetus displaying biphasic ST events is not usually in a situation of immediate hypoxia and metabolic acidosis. However, with further progress of labor, especially during the second stage, these fetuses will suffer.

Recently, Westgate et al[15] reported on ST-waveform changes during repeated umbilical cord occlusions in near-term fetal sheep. As expected, they found an increase in the T/QRS ratio with cord occlusions that became more marked when the level of hypoxia was increased by reducing the time between occlusions from 5 to 2.5 minutes. Fetuses no longer capable of maintaining their cardiovascular response reacted with negative ST changes in between occlusions. The authors concluded that an increase in the T/QRS ratio indicated hypoxic stress, and that the appearance of biphasic and negative waveforms between contractions may be a useful marker for the development of severe fetal decompensation.

Clinical research

The concept of ST analysis has been developed through a continuous validation process, starting with experimental research followed by bioengineering developments and the generation of a dedicated medical device.

Plymouth randomized controlled trial

This was the first randomized controlled trial (RCT) where 2400 high-risk term deliveries were studied, comparing CTG monitoring plus ST-waveform analysis (CTG + ST) with standard CTG monitoring.[14] Strict clinical guidelines were developed and initially tested in the Plymouth RCT of CTG + ST versus CTG, which showed a safe reduction in operative deliveries for fetal distress (ODFD) by 46%, with fewer babies born with signs of intrapartum hypoxia. The trial also showed the need to improve data presentation, as three cases in the CTG + ST arm had clinical signs of asphyxia in spite of ST events which were missed. To improve the detection of ST events, a new STAN recorder was developed utilizing modern software to improve signal quality and allow for automatic identification of significant ST events. This work required extensive signal processing and not until fast-processing capacity became available (at reasonable costs) in the 1990s was the next step taken – the introduction of the event log.

This approach was tested in a European multicenter prospective trial of 320 high-risk pregnancies. The cases were managed according to the routine CTG with blinded ST information (data stored on a PC connected to a STAN prototype unit). There were six cases of marked hypoxia, all of which showed ST-waveform changes of a magnitude to signify immediate delivery.[16]

This ST log function in combination with the CTG + ST clinical guidelines was recently shown to accurately identify all 15 babies with marked oxygen deficiency among a group of 574 Swedish and Norwegian babies. Although conventional CTG monitoring was used to assess the condition of the babies these cases were still missed and, as a consequence, three of them are likely to suffer permanent brain damage.[9] These results have recently been verified in a second large randomized trial.

Swedish multicenter RCT

The aim of this large trial was to test the hypothesis that intrapartum monitoring of term fetuses with CTG + ST results in a reduced rate of both ODFD and of newborns with metabolic acidosis, as compared with CTG alone.[10,17]

The primary outcome of this RCT was published recently.[17] It showed a significant reduction in ODFD from 8.0 to 5.9%, at the same time as the risk of being born with cord artery metabolic acidosis, defined as cord artery pH < 7.05 and BDecf (base deficit in extracellular fluid) > 12 mmol/l, was reduced from 1.44 to 0.57%.

The Swedish RCT was designed with a power to assess potential improvements in neonatal outcome. The trial design also allowed testing of the effects of growing, with the new STAN technology in the three busy labor ward units with cases managed by > 300 midwives and physicians. The current analysis summarizes the findings associated with the 351 babies that were admitted to the Special Care Baby Unit (SCBU).

	CTG		CTG + ST	
	Before (n = 1250)	After retraining (n = 1197)	Before (n = 1333)	After retraining (n = 1186)
Perinatal death	1 (Asphyxia)	0	1 (Sepsis)	1 (Asphyxia)
Outcome of SCBU visit				
Neuromuscular symptoms				
Seizures	1	2	0	0
Increased neuromuscular tone	1	3	0	0
Irritability only	1	0	3	0
Met acid + other symptoms	3	7	4	1
Total	**7**	**12**	**8**	**2**

OR 0.17, 95% CI 0.03–0.78, P 0.01.

Table 31.1. *Distribution of cases with adverse/complicated neonatal outcome, related to the method of intrapartum fetal surveillance and their occurrence in relationship to retraining. (met acid, metabolic acidosis).*

Results

Table 31.1 gives neonatal outcome according to intention to treat. The case of intrapartum death after retraining in the CTG + ST arm had second-stage CTG and ST changes that were not recognized; the scalp electrode was disconnected due to ventouse extraction for failure to progress and a severely asphyxiated baby was delivered after 23 minutes. The other case had 10 minutes of a T/QRS ratio rise before a normal delivery, the Apgar score was normal and the baby was observed for 3 hours in the SCBU due to cord metabolic acidosis. All cases except for the one in the CTG + ST arm had intrapartum events detected as abnormal by the STAN clinical guidelines: this case had had the STAN recorder disconnected 3.5 hours before delivery.

Fetal scalp pH (i.e. FBS) has hitherto been regarded as the method of reference for detection of intrapartum hypoxia – 495 cases from both arms had fetal scalp pH samples. Of a total of 46 cases with metabolic acidosis at delivery, only six had FBS data. The ST waveform could be assessed in five of these six babies, showing abnormalities lasting from 25 to 276 (median 119) minutes before delivery. In only one case was an abnormal FBS obtained (pH 7.13), at which point ST events had been recorded for 80 minutes. In the other five cases, the scalp pH was normal (> 7.20) and not repeated as labor progressed.

A 1600 cases interim analysis revealed six cases where ST events had been ignored and the fetus exposed to hypoxia. This observation showed that ST analysis improved the sensitivity of detecting adverse events in labor and it was decided to continue with the trial, with the

	CTG		CTG + ST		OR, 95% CI, P
	n	%	n	%	
Total	1049		1054		
Apgar score 1 minute < 4	23	2.19	8	0.76	0.34, 0.14–0.80, 0.011
Apgar score 5 minutes > 7	13	1.24	8	0.76	0.61, 0.23–1.58, 0.37
Apgar score 5 minutes < 4	5	0.48	0	0.00	P = 0.031
Admissions to SCBU	78	7.44	54	5.12	0.67, 0.46–0.98, 0.036
Cord artery metabolic acidosis	14	1.54	4	0.44	0.28, 0.08–0.92, 0.032

Table 31.2. *Neonatal outcome among adequately recorded cases during the second phase of the Swedish RCT.*

addition of regular staff meetings to discuss cases.

According to the protocol, a secondary analysis was made, with the exclusion of neonates with severe malformations and inadequately monitored cases (those monitored for < 20 minutes and cases where the monitoring was interrupted > 20 minutes before delivery). Table 31.2 shows the outcomes among adequately monitored neonates during the second phase of the trial.

Thus, irrespective of what outcome measure was applied, the Swedish RCT documented marked improvements in neonatal outcome after retraining with enhanced experience of ST analysis. The improvements in the diagnosis of intrapartum hypoxia during the second phase of the trial also enabled a 44% reduction in ODFD, from 8.7 to 5.0% ($P = 0.001$).

The data from these two large RCTs, including 6826 cases, have shown that, with the support of fetal ECG ST-waveform analysis, the number of babies born with cord metabolic acidosis could be reduced from 1.43 to 0.57% [odds ratio (OR) 0.39, 95% confidence interval (CI) 0.21–0.72, $P = 0.0017$] whilst at the same time ODFD were reduced from 8.4 to 5.6% (OR 0.65, 95% CI 0.53–0.78, $P < 0.001$).

EU project

The expectation of society is that the application of the results of health technology assessment will improve the quality of care and ensure that available resources are used effectively. The objective of the EU project is to develop and validate a model whereby the user aspects are put to the fore to stimulate postgraduate training and an appropriate management structure.

Today, there are no specific requirements regarding the implementation of a medical device knowledge transfer process. Action according to regulatory requirements is only required when things go wrong – obviously too late in a situation, such as labor, when oxygen deficiency may institute a threat to life and intact survival. The prime objective of the EU-supported FECG project is to develop a model whereby 10 academic centers across Europe, as a joint effort, are made active partners of this knowledge-transfer process. These centers of excellence then become their regions' hub of experience.

Methodology

The aim of the STAN concept is to provide a more thorough understanding of fetal reactions to the stress and strain of labor. The EU-supported FECG (fetal ECG) project includes the development and testing of educational material, such as a trainer/simulator that allows midwives and doctors to gain experience from displaying real cases virtually from a database. This enables exposure to rare but important cases, not otherwise easily experienced. Multimedia-based teaching, together with conventional written material, is also used. In parallel to the educational efforts, STAN S21 fetal heart recorders are used clinically.

Results and discussion

Table 31.3 gives the initial data from the 10 obstetric units participating in the project.

One neonate developed increased neuromuscular tone during the first 24 hours, with signs of metabolic acidosis at 1 hour of age (no cord data available). The STAN recording showed an abnormal CTG + baseline rise in the T/QRS ratio that was missed for 60 minutes. The material includes another 13 cases with cord artery metabolic acidosis (pH < 7.05 and BDecf > 12 mmol/l), corresponding to 0.66%. Four of those required special neonatal care but no

neuromuscular abnormalities were noted. All but one of these five cases with signs of complicated neonatal outcome had ST events lasting ≥ 20 minutes. Only two of the 13 cases with cord metabolic acidosis did not show ST events, nor were the CTG abnormal. These data are comparable to those noted in the Swedish RCT. Thus, standard CTG recording would cause a metabolic acidosis incidence of 1.4%. The results achieved in the FECG project clearly indicate that the 0.6% incidence may be achieved even from the first day of STAN usage.

Conclusions

The primary aim of intrapartum fetal monitoring is to reduce the risk of babies being affected by oxygen deficiency during labor. The appropriate clinical use of combined CTG + ST of fetal ECG allow this to be achieved by improving the detection and prevention of intrapartum hypoxia, with consequent improvements in perinatal outcomes.

	EU project incidence (%) n = 2181	Swedish RCT incidence (%)	
		CTG + ST n = 2228	CTG n = 2164
ODFD, STAN indication	7.2		
ODFD, CTG indication	9.1		
ODFD, fetal scalp pH	1.3		
ODFD, total	17.6	5.9	8.0
Cord artery metabolic acidosis (pH < 7.05 and BDecf > 12 mmol/l)	0.66 (1921 cases with cord data available)	0.57	1.44
Neuromuscular symptoms, metabolic acidosis plus neonatal care	0.23	0.13	0.74

Table 31.3. *The FECG project: outcome of intrapartum fetal monitoring to April 01 2001 (corresponding data from the Swedish RCT are also given).*

Appendix

Case report

Para 0, complicated pregnancy with maternal diabetes and pre-eclampsia.

Induction after 35 + 6 weeks gestation.
The recording starts during the first stage of labor.

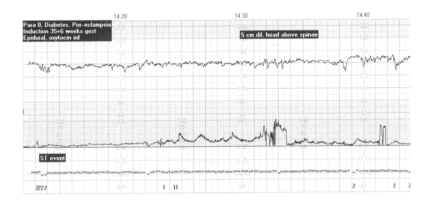

Already, at the onset of recording, a biphasic ST event is noted. The FHR is normal and

there was no need for intervention according to STAN clinical guidelines.

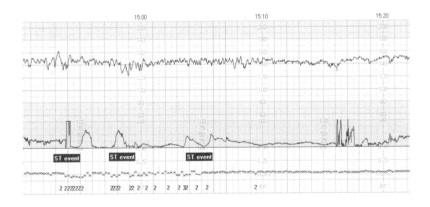

However, the biphasic pattern was repeating itself at 15:00, indicating that the fetal myocardium is operating under stress. A reason would be the early gestational age or cardiac

malformation/dystrostophy and the lessened ability of the fetal heart to manage the strain of labor.

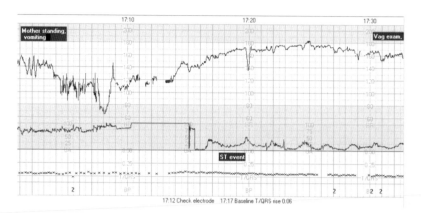

The recording continued and another ST event, consisting of a baseline rise in the T/QRS ratio, was noted at 17:17. At this point CTG abnormalities were noted and intervention was required according to CTG + ST guidelines. This pattern is often the initial sign of impending hypoxia and indicates of the inability of the placenta to meet the demands of the fetus. The fetus is not acidotic but the resources are inadequate to meet the further stress of active pushing in particular.

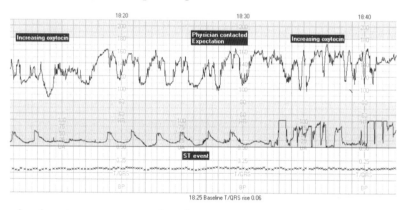

At 17:38, late decelerations commenced and another ST rise was indicated at 18:25. When the physician was informed by the midwife at 18:25, it was decided to continue with further augmentation of labor.

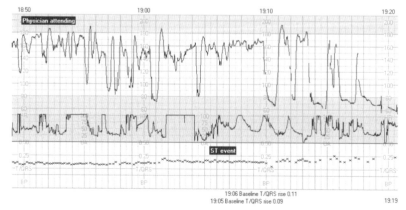

The last 30 minutes of the recording illustrate the occurrence of progressive hypoxia with a continuing rise in the T/QRS ratio. At 19:21, the head was delivered but shoulder dystocia occurred: the baby was delivered at 19:26. Apgar score 0–0–0; birthweight 4650 grams; cord artery data, pH 6.90, pCO_2 11.6 kPa, BDecf 14.1 mmol/l. The baby responded to resuscitation with heart activity at 12 minutes of age but died within the first 24 hours, no autopsy was performed.

Comments

This case illustrates the main problems of an uncontrolled diabetic pregnancy with a large-for-date fetus developing intrapartum hypoxia and shoulder dystocia. Furthermore, data are now available to continuously assess the condition of a fetus at risk to allow for a safe delivery, provided that STAN clinical guidelines are followed.

References

1. Greene KR, Rosén KG. Intrapartum asphyxia. In: (Levene MI, Bennett MJ, Punt J eds) *Fetal and Neonatal Neurology and Neurosurgery*. (Churchill Livingstone: Edinburgh, 1995) 265–72.
2. Larsen JF. Why has conventional intrapartum cardiotocography not given the expected results? *J Perinat Med* 1996; **24**:15–23.
3. Nelson KB, Dambrosia JM, Ting TY, Grether JK. Uncertain value of electronic fetal monitoring in predicting cerebral palsy. *N Engl J Med* 1996; **334**:613–18.
4. Greene KR. Intelligent fetal heart rate computer systems in intrapartum surveillance. *Curr Opin Obstet Gynaecol* 1996; **8**:123–7.
5. Murphy KW, Johnson P, Moorcraft J et al. Birth asphyxia and the intrapartum cardiotocograph. *Br J Obstet Gynaecol* 1990; **97**:470–9.
6. Rosén KG, Dagbjartsson A, Henriksson BA et al. The relationship between circulating catecholamines and ST waveform in the fetal lamb electrocardiogram during hypoxia. *Am J Obstet Gynaecol* 1984; **149**:190–5.
7. Rosén KG, Isaksson O. Alterations in fetal heart rate and ECG correlated to glycogen, creatine phosphate and ATP levels during graded hypoxia. *Biol Neonate* 1976; **30**: 17–24.
8. Rosén KG, Kjellmer I. Changes in the fetal heart rate and ECG during hypoxia. *Acta Physiol Scand* 1975; **93**:59–66.
9. Rosén KG, Luzietti R. Intrapartum fetal monitoring – its basis and current developments. *Prenat Neonat Med* 2000; **5**:155–68.
10. Sokolow M, McIlroy MB. In *Clinical Cardiology*. (Lange Medical Publications: Los Altos, CA, 1981) 97–112.
11. Sundström A-K for the Swedish STAN study group. Randomised controlled trial of CTG versus CTG+ST analysis of the fetal ECG. *J Obstet Gynaecol* 2001; **21**:18–19.
12. Hökegård KH, Eriksson BO, Kjellmer I et al. Myocardial metabolism in relation to electrocardiographic changes and cardiac function during graded hypoxia in the fetal lamb. *Acta Physiol Scand* 1981; **113**:1–7.
13. Dawes GS, Mott JC, Shelley HJ. The importance of cardiac glycogen for the maintenance of life in fetal lambs and newborn animals during anoxia. *J Physiol* 1959; **146**:516–38.
14. Westgate J, Harris M, Curnow JSH, Greene KR. Plymouth randomised trial of cardiotocogram only versus ST waveform plus cardiotocogram for intrapartum monitoring: 2,400 cases. *Am J Obstet Gynecol* 1993; **169**:1151–60.
15. Westgate JA, Bennet L, Brabyn C et al. ST waveform changes during repeated umbilical cord occlusions in near-term fetal sheep. *Am J Obstet Gynecol* 2001; **184**:743–51.
16. Luzietti R, Erkkola R, Hasbargen U et al. European community multi-center trial 'Fetal ECG analysis during labor': ST plus CTG analysis. *J Perinat Med* 1999; **27**:431–40.
17. Amer-Wåhlin I, Hellsten C, Norén H et al. Intrapartum fetal monitoring: cardiotocography versus cardiotocography plus ST Analysis of the Fetal ECG. A Swedish randomized controlled trial. *Lancet* 2001; **358**:534–8.

32

Timing and mode of delivery
Jeremy JN Oats, Oded Langer

Introduction

The decision about the optimum time to deliver the baby in the pregnancy complicated by diabetes has to consider the balance between the perceived risk of late intrauterine death and shoulder dystocia and the consequences of unnecessary prematurity and Cesarean section delivery.

It is important to emphasize the issue of fetal demise in pregnancy. Fetal death, excluding congenital anomalies, has been found to be associated with the level of glycemic control in the pregnant diabetic. The level of glycemia will be one of the factors that will mandate timing of delivery in these patients. A brief review of the existing literature reveals that the majority of studies in obstetrics are observational studies (approximately 80%),[1] while randomized studies account for about 11%. Since studies evaluating perinatal mortality of diabetes in pregnancy are under the constraints of strict ethical standards that prevent randomized trials, it is necessary that the basic characteristics of both the study and control populations be comparable, e.g. incidence of prolapse of cord, medical complications, parity, ethnicity and prenatal care. Only then does the disease in question, diabetes, become the main cause for the difference in rates between the groups for perinatal outcome.

Fetal demise in the pregnant diabetic is often defined as 'unexplained fetal death'. The demise is the result of the metabolic acidosis developed in the fetal compartment in the presence of an abnormal glucose level rather than the traditional explanation of fetal hypoxia. The second and up to the middle of the third trimesters of pregnancy are times of minimal rates of fetal demise; the majority of fetal deaths occur late in the third trimester. This mortality pattern is associated with fetal development and increase in insulin sensitivity during pregnancy. Although insulin can be detected as early as the latter part of the first trimester, the affinity to insulin action becomes significant around the 28th week of gestation, resulting in fetal hyperinsulinemia that leads to fetal acidemia and hyperlacticemia without evidence of fetal hypoxia. Supporting this concept, Pettitt et al's[2] study found that, of 236/1000 fetal deaths, the majority occurred in large-for-gestational age (LGA) infants of gestational diabetes mellitus (GDM) mothers. Needless to say, fetal hypoxemia can occur in all types of diabetes, especially pregnancies associated with hypertensive disorder and microvascular complications (Types 1 and 2). Maternal insulinemia alone can be a cause for vasoconstriction and fetal hypoxia.[1,2]

The association between level of glycemia and fetal demise during the antepartum period was demonstrated by O'Sullivan et al.[3] They found that GDM compared to non-diabetic pregnancies had a fourfold higher perinatal mortality. Pettitt et al[2] found similar mortality rates for GDM and pre-existing diabetic subjects (59/1000 versus 43–125/1000, respectively). Karlsson and Kjellmer[4] evaluated relationships between the degree of glycemic control and perinatal mortality and found a 3.8% perinatal mortality rate for the blood group < 100 mg/dl, 16% in the group of 100–150 mg/dl, and 24% in the group with > 150 mg/dl. Finally, keeping a mean blood glucose threshold of < 100 mg/dl during the prenatal period will result in the lowest rate of fetal demise and provides the opportunity to avoid unnecessary early deliveries.

Historically, it was believed that the fetus of the mother with diabetes matured early and reached the equivalent of term by 36 weeks gestation.[5] This view was championed by Peel and Oakley[6] from King's College Hospital, London, in the late 1940s. The reasoning behind this tenet was a classic example of the wrong conclusion being drawn from a study that had two major changes in management. On the one hand, they delivered all babies at 36 weeks but this was part of a regimen that paid much closer attention to the control of the mother's diabetes during pregnancy. The perinatal outcomes from their study showed that in comparison with other units in Great Britain, there was a halving of the fetal death rate from 29.4 to 11.3%. The overall perinatal mortality in comparison with the other units decreased from 40.1 to 25.5% and in their own unit from 37%. The key outcome parameter that was not given due importance was the rise in neonatal death from 10.7 to 14.2%. They were not alone in their teaching. White et al,[7] in Boston, were also recommending that women with Class D, E, and F should be delivered by 36 weeks, although they did allow those with Class B and C to reach 38 weeks and those with Class A to go to term.

In 1979, Roversi et al,[8] in Italy, challenged this now 30-year-old regimen demonstrating that it was meticulous attention to blood glucose control that was the key factor in reducing perinatal mortality and, in particular, late intrauterine fetal death. Using the maximum dose of insulin that could be tolerated by the mother, they carried 94% of the pregnancies to 38 weeks or more, 19% not being delivered until after 40 weeks. The only late fetal death occurred at 37 weeks in a woman with diabetic nephropathy. At the same time, Drury et al,[9] at the National Maternity Hospital in Dublin, reported their experience of the first 141 diabetic pregnancies managed using a regimen of tight control and not delivering the baby before full term irrespective of the severity of the diabetes unless obstetric complications necessitated intervention. This was done without the use of either cardiographic surveillance or ultrasonic assessment of fetal well-being. Spontaneous labor ensued in 57% of cases, the Cesarean section rate was 20% and perinatal mortality was 31/1000. A subsequent analysis of this management policy and outcome by Rasmussen et al[10] showed that the only deaths in normally formed infants occurred in those in whom there was poor metabolic control, clinical macrosomia or polyhydramnios.

Furthermore, the report from Murphy et al,[11] from Cardiff, showed that the additional benefit in allowing the pregnancies of women with diabetes to go to full term was that there was a fourfold increase in the spontaneous vaginal delivery rate. This came without a significant increase in the emergency Cesarean section rate and a modest fall in elective Cesarean section rate (Figs 32.1 and 32.2). A later update from the Dublin group[12] showed that between 1981 and 1994 their conservative

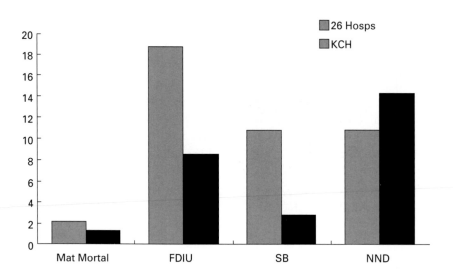

Figure 32.1 *Comparison of the outcome of diabetic pregnancies managed at King's College Hospital, London and at 26 other UK hospitals.*[1]

policy maintained a high vaginal delivery rate of 93% (90.5% of these being normal deliveries), with a Cesarean section rate of 7% compared with the non-diabetic population rate of 3.4%. The perinatal mortality rate had fallen to 13.5/1000. In Australia, in 1999, fetal demise not associated with congenital anomalies accounted for 15% of the total.[13] The cause of death in most diabetic pregnancies is not known (except for those associated with diabetic ketoacidosis) and it is possible that they are in fact unrelated to maternal diabetes *per se*. Consequently, it is not realistic to expect that all deaths can be prevented with the currently available tools for fetal surveillance.

Further reassurance for taking the pregnancy to term comes from the study of Sheiner et al.[14] In a multiple logistic regression analysis of 72,875 singleton deliveries, no association was found between intrapartum fetal death and maternal diabetes. The significant factors were maternal age > 35 years, polyhydramnios, congenital malformations, pathologic presentation, abruptio placentae and cord prolapse.

Lung maturation and iatrogenic prematurity

As mentioned above, the fear of stillbirths in the past, and even in current practice in several maternity units in the United States and Europe, encouraged the policy of planned delivery of these patients at approximately 34–37 weeks gestation. Indeed, this policy significantly decreased the stillbirth rate but, in contrast, resulted in iatrogenic prematurity with the accompanying neonatal

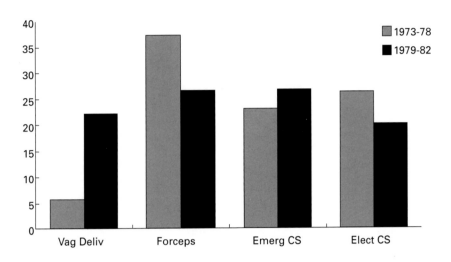

Figure 32.2 *The effect of change of management on mode of delivery.[7]*

complications, especially respiratory distress syndrome (RDS) (formerly known as hyaline membranous disease). The policy decreased stillbirths but created a higher rate of neonatal morbidity and mortality. All this led to the development of fetal maturity lung testing, which is addressed at length in Chapter 21. However, in the past two to three decades, lung maturity testing has enabled us to significantly decrease iatrogenic prematurity and to comprehend the impact of the level of glycemic control and the delay in lung maturation.

We now have the technology to synchronize planned deliveries and lung maturity in a relatively safe mode. In addition, the modern approach to fetal surveillance testing and the recognition of the importance of glucose control presented an opportunity to avoid planned deliveries due to fear of fetal demise.

On the other hand, perhaps there is now an opportunity to consider planned delivery for the oversized fetus (macrosomia) in order to prevent shoulder dystocia and its accompanying complications.[15–17]

Fetal overgrowth in the diabetic pregnancy

The other major factor that influences the decision on the timing of delivery is the likelihood of shoulder dystocia and particularly permanent brachial plexus nerve palsy. Shoulder dystocia has been aptly described as 'the infrequent, unanticipated, unpredictable nightmare of the obstetrician'.[18] The major dilemma for the obstetrician is the poor predictive power of methods of fetal weight assessment and particularly shoulder width in the fetus. Coupled with this is the dynamic interaction between the maternal pelvic girdle, the power of the uterine contractions, maternal expulsive efforts and the fetal diameters that will ultimately determine whether the shoulders pass easily through the outlet of the maternal pelvis. Fetal weight alone is a poor predictor. From cases with shoulder dystocia, approximately 40–50% will occur within the infant group weighing < 4000 grams.[19] However, it should be noted that pregnancies with infants weighing < 4000 grams are the majority, while the total number of infants weighing > 4000 grams is about 8–10%. Furthermore, although macrosomia is one of the classic markers of diabetes in pregnancy, a larger number of macrosomic babies will be identified in the general population while the prevalence of diabetes is 3–5%. Thus, policies for timing and method of delivery should consider the total population that may be affected by them.[18,19]

The overgrown fetus of a diabetic mother is at an increased risk for serious adverse outcomes due to shoulder dystocia during vaginal delivery. Traditionally, authors have emphasized Erb's palsy as the single most significant complication when shoulder dystocia occurs. However, the prevalence of Erb's palsy is relatively low. Shoulder dystocia without Erb's palsy remains a serious complication involving bone fractures, asphyxia and even fetal death. Cesarean delivery greatly reduces the likelihood of such outcomes and may, therefore, be used as the primary prevention approach. However, it should be noted that Cesarean delivery itself is not free from fetal and/or maternal complications, which may include increased maternal blood loss, traumatic organ injury (ureters), infection, as well as other long-term complications. Therefore, in light of the fact that Cesarean section rates are increasing univer-

sally, the benefit–risk ratio should be assessed for any given complication before surgery.

In diabetic patients, the majority of shoulder dystocia cases occur among macrosomic infants born vaginally. In a cohort study of nearly 75,000 non-diabetic women, it was found that the rate of macrosomic infants was 7.6% compared to 20.6% in the 1500 diabetic women.[18] Non-diabetic women had an overall shoulder dystocia rate of 0.5%, compared to 3.2% in diabetic women. The shoulder dystocia rate was 0.3% when birthweight was < 4000 grams and 4.9% when it was > 4000 grams in diabetic patients. Macrosomic infants of diabetic mothers had a more than threefold higher risk of shoulder dystocia than macrosomic infants of non-diabetic pregnancies (14.7 versus 4.4%). However, within each 250 gram birthweight category over 4000 grams, diabetics had significantly more shoulder dystocia than non-diabetics.

Anthropometric differences explain the discrepancy in the risk for shoulder dystocia between diabetic and non-diabetic women. In non-diabetic women, macrosomia is constitutional in origin, thus resulting in a proportionally larger infant. In contrast, for the diabetic macrosomic infant, its overgrowth is due to continuous fetal hyperinsulinemia resulting in disproportional growth and organomegaly in the majority of organs with the exception of the brain. It has been found that there is a significant difference in several anthropomorphic measures, such as abdominal and shoulder circumference, as well as an increase in fetal fat mass distribution. Organ overgrowth is used as the marker to identify the fetus compromised by diabetic macrosomia.[18,20,21] As compared to a macrosomic fetus of a non-diabetic woman, the macrosomic fetus in a diabetic pregnancy is disproportionately large, with much of the excess weight distributed in the trunk and shoulders.

This increased chest–head and shoulder–head size discrepancy results in a higher risk for shoulder dystocia.[22,23]

Just as the shoulder dystocia rate goes up with increasing birthweight, so too does the risk of injury when shoulder dystocia occurs. Ecker et al[24] found a relative risk for brachial plexus injury of 9.6 for infants weighing > 4000 grams versus < 4000 grams; the relative risk increased to 17.9 and 45.2 at birthweight thresholds > 4500 and 5000 grams, respectively. Increasing birthweight, maternal diabetes and vaginal delivery were all independently associated with an increased risk for brachial plexus injury.

Using ultrasonography to detect fetal overgrowth

The accurate prediction of fetal weight in intrauterine life is an attractive approach to identify the fetus at risk. Unfortunately, it has been demonstrated that the error in weight estimation is relatively high (10–20%), thus mothers are being subjected to often unnecessary interventions. Nevertheless, ultrasonographic estimation of fetal weight is commonly employed in clinical practice. In a survey of practitioners, approximately 75% of maternal–fetal specialists and almost 66% of general obstetricians utilized ultrasound to estimate fetal size prior to the delivery of the diabetic woman.[25]

Recently, it was demonstrated that 31 different sonographic estimations of fetal weight formulae had comparably poor accuracy for prediction of macrosomia. The 1986 formula devised by Ott had the lowest total score. Using Ott's formula, an estimated fetal weight (EFW) of > 4000 grams had a sensitivity of 45% to predict macrosomia and a positive predictive value (PPV) of 81%. In order to achieve 90% sensitivity using this formula, it would have required a diagnosis of macrosomia with an EFW > 3535 grams, but this would have comprised 46% of the population with a 42% false-positive rate.[26]

When EFW was predicted by ultrasound to be > 4000 grams, 75–85% of infants were macrosomic at birth.[27,28] In the present authors' experience, ultrasonic EFW by the Shepard formula correctly predicted presence or absence of macrosomia in 87% of diabetic pregnancies.[29] Maternal obesity, a common co-morbidity in a diabetic population, does not appear to diminish the accuracy of fetal weight estimation by ultrasound.[30] In general, over-estimation of fetal weight would seem to make the practice less beneficial.

Using a combination of approaches to detect fetal macrosomia in a population of both diabetic and non-diabetic women, Chauhan et al[31] compared the performance of various methods, including a standard formula for calculating fetal weight, clinical estimation and measures of fetal subcutaneous tissue by ultrasound. Using receiver operating characteristic curves to assess these diagnostic modalities, they found traditional fetal weight estimation by ultrasound to perform the best, and shoulder soft tissue width to perform the worst. Therefore, although formulae for fetal weight estimation used in daily clinical practice lack the level of accuracy in predicting fetal overgrowth that we would like to achieve, they appear to be the best tool available, and they do not require special expertise or equipment to obtain them.

Cohen et al[32] proposed the abdominal diameter (AD) minus the biparietal diameter (BPD) as a predictor of whether a fetus will be compromised by shoulder dystocia at delivery. The authors used severe shoulder dystocia as their end point, retrospectively examining the AD – BPD values obtained from infants of diabetic mothers with EFW of 3800–4200 grams within 2 weeks of delivery. Infants with shoulder dystocia had significantly larger AD – BPD measurements despite finding no difference in birthweight between the shoulder dystocia and normal delivery groups. No infant with an antenatal AD – BPD value < 2.6 cm suffered shoulder dystocia. However, the PPV for this cut-off was only 30%. Prospective studies using comparable models may provide improved predictors of shoulder dystocia.[33]

Benefits of Cesarean delivery in preventing shoulder dystocia and fetal injury

Avoidance of vaginal delivery for the large fetus of a diabetic mother eliminates the possibility of shoulder dystocia and should, therefore, eliminate the risk of nerve and bone injury, as well as the more serious outcomes of birth asphyxia and intrapartum death resulting from shoulder dystocia. Although it is recognized that brachial plexus injury can occur in the setting of Cesarean delivery,[34,35] the risk associated with vaginal birth is much greater.[36] Indeed, a population-based study of births in Washington State, USA, revealed no reported cases of brachial or Erb's palsy out of over 13,000 consecutive Cesarean deliveries.[37] Therefore, it is reasonable to conclude that performance of a Cesarean section will prevent Erb's–Duchenne palsy in the vast majority of cases. It is for this reason that Cesarean delivery has been proposed as the preferred route of delivery for the large fetus.

Among diabetic women, 84% of shoulder dystocia cases occur in infants with birthweights > 4000 grams. Among non-diabetic women, only 60% of deliveries complicated by shoulder dystocia involve a macrosomic fetus.[18] Thus, avoidance of vaginal delivery of macrosomic fetuses of diabetic mothers would eliminate most cases of shoulder dystocia, while the same practice in non-diabetic mothers would eliminate just over half of cases. The practicality of this plan in the clinical setting is hampered by two factors: first, accurate antenatal identification of macrosomia is difficult to accomplish; and second, most cases of shoulder dystocia do not result in permanent damage to the infant. We are currently unable to select those cases in which the fetus is excessively large, much less detect which overgrown fetus is at risk for handicap or death due to shoulder dystocia. This fact has diminished the enthusiasm of some authors for Cesarean delivery for suspected macrosomia.[38]

Rouse et al,[38] using a decision analysis methodology abstracting information available in the literature, calculated the probability of shoulder dystocia according to birthweight in both diabetic and non-diabetic pregnancies (Table 32.1). It is noteworthy that for

Birthweight (grams)	Diabetic pregnancy	Non-diabetic pregnancy
< 4000	0.022	0.007
4000–4499	0.139	0.067
≥ 4500	0.525	0.145

Table 32.1 Probability of shoulder dystocia by birthweight in diabetic and non-diabetic pregnancies (from Rouse et al[38]).

birthweights ≥ 4500 grams, the probability is 52% in diabetic pregnancies compared with 14% in non-diabetic pregnancies. The mean probability that a neonatal brachial plexus injury will persist was 6.7% (range 0–19%).[29] Rouse et al[38] calculated that to prevent one case of permanent brachial plexus injury in babies weighing ≥ 4500 grams would necessitate performing 153 Cesarean deliveries in diabetic mothers and 419 in non-diabetics. If a cut-off of 4000 grams is used, then 169 Cesarean sections would be required in diabetics and 654 in non-diabetics.

Rouse and Owen[39] have updated their initial analysis by factoring in information from recent population-based studies on the frequency of brachial plexus injury, both transient and persistent. These calculations suggest that an even greater number of Cesarean sections need to be performed to prevent permanent palsies. However, Erb's palsy should not be the only consideration in evaluation of morbidity prevention by Cesarean section. Although Erb's palsy is a severe complication, bone fractures, asphyxia, respiratory complications requiring neonatal intensive care admission, and neonatal and fetal demise should be considered when calculating the cost of Cesarean sections performed to prevent shoulder dystocia and adverse outcomes. In fact, when the composite outcome approach is used, 81% of shoulder dystocia cases of the infants of diabetic mothers will be identified compared to 34% for infants of non-diabetic mothers.[18]

Applying the same types of calculations to an actual obstetric population, Mullin et al[40] examined the results of their policy of offering Cesarean deliveries to all diabetic women with EFW > 4250 grams (by sonographic or clinical means). Of 72 women meeting this fetal weight threshold, during a 3 year period, 61% elected for Cesarean delivery. Seventeen of the remaining women delivered vaginally (39% Cesarean

section rate in women who labored), and four of these deliveries were complicated by shoulder dystocia (24%). Based on previously reported rates of brachial plexus injuries, the investigators then calculated the number of Cesarean sections needed to prevent one case of permanent Erb's palsy. In diabetic women, approximately 100–400 Cesarean sections would result in avoidance of one case of permanent palsy. This number is somewhat more favorable toward a policy of prophylactic Cesarean section than that estimated by Rouse and colleagues.[38,39] This highlights the fact that cost–benefit ratios of prophylactic Cesarean sections for suspected macrosomia in diabetic women may be most meaningful when calculated for, and applied to, an individual population taking into account overall morbidity rather than a single outcome parameter. Moreover, different diabetic programs report different rates of macrosomia (poor glycemic control) which affects the rate of shoulder dystocia. Probably, achievement of adequate glycemic control will be a major factor in decreasing the rate of this complication in diabetic mothers.

Theoretical models provide a foundation for clinical studies. However, paucity of information exists on the actual clinical impact of a policy of prophylactic Cesarean sections in reducing the frequency of shoulder dystocia events. If there is no significant decrease in shoulder dystocia rate, there cannot be an accompanying decrease in brachial plexus injury and other adverse outcomes. In one of the few published reports, Conway and Langer,[29] in a prospective study, addressed this issue. Diabetic women underwent Cesarean delivery when EFW by ultrasound was > 4250 grams, a threshold chosen to reduce unnecessary intervention due to sonographic error. Labor inductions of LGA fetuses with birthweights < 4250 grams were also performed. Although only 11% of the diabetic population underwent Cesarean section or inductions for macrosomia, the shoulder dystocia rate among diabetic women dropped significantly on implementing this procedure compared to the previous 3 year period [1.5 versus 2.8%; odds ratio (OR) 0.5, range 0.3–1.0]. Among macrosomic infants, the shoulder dystocia rate dropped from 19 to 7% (OR 0.3, range 0.1–1.0). The Cesarean delivery rate among diabetics rose from 21.7 to 25.1%. Conway and Langer's[29] study demonstrated the possibility of reducing the rate of shoulder dystocia in diabetic women using prophylactic Cesarean delivery for the macrosomic fetus.

Ultrasonic estimation of fetal weight needs to take into account whether or not the mother has diabetes. Otherwise, there is a significant underestimation of fetal weight of > 10% using conventional weight prediction tables.[41] Diabetic pregnancies, because of the larger fetal weight, are five times more likely to be complicated by shoulder dystocia than non-diabetic pregnancies (5 versus 1.1% for birthweights ≥ 4000 grams). Brachial plexus injuries are four times more likely in diabetic pregnancies, although due to the paucity of long-term follow-up the prevalence of the permanency of the injury is not yet well established.[39,42]

The concern that delaying delivery until full-term results in a greater morbidity rate led Kjos et al[43] to conduct an randomized controlled trial (RCT) of 200 pregnancies complicated by GDM. Patients were assigned either to elective delivery at 38 weeks or to expectant management, which included twice weekly cardiotocography and amniotic fluid volume evaluation. The Cochrane review[44] of this trial found that the risk of having a Cesarean section was similar for both groups [relative risk (RR) 0.81, 95% confidence interval (CI) 0.52–1.26]. The risk of macrosomia was reduced in the elective delivery group (RR

0.56, 95% CI 0.32–0.98) and there were three cases of mild shoulder dystocia in the expectant management group. They concluded that due to the limited number of studies, there is little evidence to support either elective delivery at 38 weeks or expectant management.

Cesarean section rates for women with diabetes are significantly greater than for their non-diabetic counterparts in most series. Remsberg et al[45] conducted a detailed analysis of 42,071 singleton births in South Carolina, USA. Diabetic mothers compromised 3.6% of the series, 80% of which had GDM. Of the pre-existing diabetic patients, 51.3% underwent a Cesarean section, as did 34.4% of those with GDM. For non-diabetic women, 22.9% of births were by Cesarean section. Regression analysis showed an association between diabetes and Cesarean section and showed that it was not mediated through infant size alone. The strongest reported associations were with disproportion, previous Cesarean delivery, failed induction and malpresentation. These results and those from other studies[12,46] suggest that the practice patterns of the clinicians and not macrosomia itself are the major factors in high Cesarean section rates.

One of the major contributors to the Cesarean section rate is the presence of a previous Cesarean section scar. Two studies have examined the outcome of vaginal birth after Cesarean (VBAC) in women with diabetes. In Coleman et al's[47] study, VBAC was offered if the sonographically EFW was < 4000 grams. Overall, the successful VBAC rate was lower in women with diabetes (64.1 versus 73.2%; OR 1.90, range 1.20–2.99). This was not due to the higher induction rate in women with diabetes (OR 2.16, range 1.37–3.40). Women with diabetes who delivered vaginally were more likely to have an operative vaginal delivery: forceps (OR 2.71, range 1.15–6.45); vacuum (OR 2.59, range 0.89–7.73). Most importantly, there were no significant differences between the two groups in the incidence of shoulder dystocia, pre-eclampsia, pelvic lacerations or prolonged hospitalization, and the only two ruptured uteri occurred in the control group. In the other study, Blackwell et al[48] compared diabetic women with and without a previous Cesarean section delivery. In the previous Cesarean section group, the rate of repeat Cesarean section was doubled (56.3 versus 26.3%) with a successful VBAC rate of 43.7%. From these two studies it can be concluded that for women with diabetes who have had a previous Cesarean delivery it is reasonable and safe to offer both a VBAC and induction of labor.

Returning to the debate about mode of delivery and EFW, the use of elective Cesarean section to prevent shoulder dystocia remains controversial. As discussed above, the dilemma is that current methods of determining the EFW have inherent inaccuracies. Furthermore, 50% of brachial plexus injuries occur in the absence of shoulder dystocia and can occur with a Cesarean delivery, which suggest that ante- and intrapartum factors are at least as important etiologically as shoulder dystocia.[49]

It is not possible to offer advice to the clinician with any degree of certainty on what should be the threshold for performing an elective Cesarean delivery in women with diabetes with the currently available evidence. Certainly, a past history of shoulder dystocia should influence the decision on the mode of delivery unless the EFW is significantly less than the previous birthweight. Unless obstetric complications dictate otherwise, the uncomplicated (normal estimated birthweight, amniotic fluid volume and metabolic control) diabetic pregnancy, both pregestational and gestational, can be left to go into spontaneous delivery at full term. Induction of labor and planned VBAC carry no greater risks than for the non-diabetic pregnancy. Elective Cesarean section for the pregnant diabetic patient should be actively considered if the EFW is ≥ 4250 grams,[18,28] although some authors recommend an EFW of 4000 grams.[50]

References

1. Gerstein HC, Haynes RB. *Evidence-based Diabetes Care.* (BC Decker, Inc: London, 2001) 1–48.
2. Pettitt DJ, Knowler WC, Baird HR et al. Gestational diabetes: infant and maternal complications of pregnancy in relation to third-trimester glucose tolerance in the Pima Indians. *Diabetes Care* 1980; 3:458–64.
3. O'Sullivan JB, Charles D, Mahan CM et al. Gestational diabetes and perinatal mortality rate. *Am J Obstet Gynecol* 1973; 1:901–4.
4. Karlsson K, Kjellmer I. The outcome of diabetic pregnancies in relation to the mother's blood sugar level. *Am J Obstet Gynecol* 1972; 112:213–20.
5. Peel J. A historical review of diabetes and pregnancy. *J Obstet Gynaecol Br Commonw* 1972; 79:385–95.
6. Peel J, Oakley WG. *Transactions of the 12th British Congress of Obstetrics and Gynaecology* 1949; 161.
7. White P, Koshy P, Duckers J. The management of pregnancy complicated by diabetes and of children of diabetic mothers. *Med Clin N Am* 1953; 37:1481–96.
8. Roversi GD, Gargulio M, Nicolini U et al. A new approach to the treatment of diabetic pregnant women. *Am J Obstet Gynecol* 1979; 135:567–76.
9. Drury MI, Stronge JM, Foley ME, MacDonald DW. Pregnancy in the diabetic patient: timing and mode of delivery. *Obstet Gynecol* 1983; 62:279–82.
10. Rasmussen MJ, Firth R, Foley M, Stronge JM. The timing of delivery in diabetic pregnancy: a 10-year review. *Aust NZ J Obstet Gynaecol* 1992; 32:313–17.
11. Murphy J, Peters J, Morris P et al. Conservative management of pregnancy in diabetic women. *Br Med J* 1984; 288:1203–5.
12. McAuliffe FM, Foley M, Firth R et al. Outcome of diabetic pregnancy with spontaneous labour after 38 weeks. *Irish J Med Sci* 1999; 168:160–3.
13. Nassar N, Sullivan EA 2001. Australia's mothers and babies 1999. AIHW Cat No. PER 19, Perinatal Statistics Series no. 11. (AIHW National Perinatal Statistics Unit: Sydney, 2001).
14. Sheiner E, Hallak M, Shomam-Vardi I et al. Determining risks for intrapartum fetal death. *J Reprod Med* 2000; 45:419–24.
15. Langer O, Conway, D. Level of glycemia and perinatal outcome in pregestational diabetes. *J Matern-Fetal Med* 2000; 9:35–41.

16. Langer O. A spectrum of glucose thresholds may effectively prevent complications in the pregnant diabetic patient. *Semin Perinatol* 2002; **26**:196–205.

17. Piper JM. Lung maturation in diabetes in pregnancy: if and when to test. *Semin Per* 2002; **26**:206–9.

18. Langer O, Berkus MD, Huff RW, Samueloff A. Shoulder dystocia: should the fetus weighing ≥4,000g be delivered by cesarean section? *Am J Obstet Gynecol* 1991; **165**: 831–7.

19. Keller JD, Lopez-Zeno JA, Dooley SL, Socol ML. Shoulder dystocia and birth trauma in gestational diabetes: a five-year experience. *Am J Obstet Gynecol* 1991; **165**:928–30.

20. Langer O. Macrosomia in the fetus of the diabetic mother. *In*: (Divon M, ed.) *Abnormal Fetal Growth*. (Elsevier Science Publishers: NY, 1991) 99–110.

21. Susa JB, McCormick KL, Widness JA et al. Chronic hyperinsulinemia in the fetal rhesus monkey: effects on fetal growth and composition. *Diabetes* 1979; **28**: 1058–63.

22. McFarland MB, Trylovich CG, Langer O. Anthropometric differences in macrosomic infants of diabetic and non-diabetic mothers. *J Matern-Fetal Med* 1998; **7**:292–5.

23. Modanlou HD, Komatsu G, Dorchester W et al. Large-for-gestational-age neonates: anthropometric reasons for shoulder dystocia. *Obstet Gynecol* 1982; **60**:417–23.

24. Ecker JL, Greenberg JA, Norwitz ER et al. Birth weight as a predictor of brachial plexus injury. *Obstet Gynecol* 1997; **89**:643–7.

25. Landon MB. Prenatal diagnosis of macrosomia in pregnancy complicated by diabetes mellitus. *J Matern-Fetal Med* 2000; **9**:52–4.

26. Combs CA, Rosenn B, Miodovnik Siddiqi TA. Sonographic EFW and macrosomia: is there an optimum formula to predict diabetic fetal macrosomia? *J Matern-Fetal Med* 2000; **9**:55–61.

27. Tamura RK, Sabbagha RE, Dooley SL et al. Real-time ultrasound estimations of weight in fetuses of diabetic gravid women. *Am J Obstet Gynecol* 1985; **153**:57–60.

28. Benson CB, Doubilet PM, Saltzman DH. Sonographic determination of fetal weights in diabetic pregnancies. *Am J Obstet Gynecol* 1987; **156**:441–4.

29. Conway DL, Langer O. Elective delivery of infants with macrosomia in diabetic women: reduced shoulder dystocia versus increased cesarean deliveries. *Am J Obstet Gynecol* 1998; **178**:922–5.

30. Field NT, Piper JM, Langer O. The effect of maternal obesity on the accuracy of fetal weight estimation. *Obstet Gynecol* 1995; **86**:102–7.

31. Chauhan SP, West DJ, Scardo JA et al. Antepartum detection of macrosomic fetus: clinical versus sonographic, including soft-tissue measurements. *Obstet Gynecol* 2000; **95**:639–42.

32. Cohen B, Penning S, Major C et al. Sonographic prediction of shoulder dystocia in infants of diabetic mothers. *Obstet Gynecol* 1996; **88**:10–13.

33. Jaffe R. Identification of fetal growth abnormalities in diabetes mellitus. *Semin Perinatal* 2002; **26**:190–5.

34. Morrison JC, Sanders JR, Magann EF et al. The diagnosis and management of dystocia of the shoulder. *Surg Gynecol Obstet* 1992; **175**:515–22.

35. Bar J, Dvir A, Hod M et al. Brachial plexus injury and obstetrical risk factors. *Int J Gynecol Obstet* 2001; **73**:21–5.

36. Gregory KD, Henry OA, Ramicone E et al. Maternal and infant complications in high and normal weight infants by method of delivery. *Obstet Gynecol* 1998; **92**:507–13.

37. Mocanu EV, Greene RA, Byrne BM et al. Obstetric and neonatal outcome of babies weighing more than 4.5 kg: an analysis by parity. *Eur J Obstet Gynecol Reprod Biol* 2000; **92**:229–33.

38. Rouse DJ, Owen J, Goldenberg RL et al. The effectiveness and costs of elective cesarean delivery for fetal macrosomia diagnosed by ultrasound. *J Am Med Assoc* 1996; **276**:1480–6.

39. Rouse DJ, Owen J. Prophylactic cesarean delivery for fetal macrosomia diagnosed by means of ultrasonography – a Faustian bargain? *Am J Obstet Gynecol* 1999; **181**:332–8.

40. Mullin P, Gherman R, Melkumian A et al. The relationship of shoulder dystocia to estimated fetal weight. Presented at the 68th Annual Meeting of the Pacific Coast Obstetrical and Gynecological Society, Ashland, OR, 2001.

41. Wong SF, Chan FY, Cincotta RB et al. Sonographic estimation of fetal weight in macrosomic fetuses: diabetic versus non-diabetic pregnancies. *Aust NZ J Obstet Gynaecol* 2001; **41**:429–32.

42. American College of Obstetricians and Gynecologists: Task Force on Cesarean Delivery Rates: Evaluation of cesarean delivery. (American College of Obstetricians and Gynecologists: Washington, DC, 2000).

43. Kjos SL, Henry OA, Montoro M et al. Insulin requiring diabetes in pregnancy: a randomised trial of active inductioin of labor and expectant management. *Am J Obstet Gynecol* 1993; **169**:611–15.

44. Boulvain M, Stan C, Irion O. Elective delivery in diabetic pregnant women. Cochrane Database of Systematic Reviews [computer file] (2): CD 001997, 2000.

45. Remsberg KE, McKeown RE, McFarland KF, Irwin LS. Diabetes in pregnancy and cesarean delivery. *Diabetes Care* 1999; **22**:1561–7.

46. Blackwell SC, Hassan SS, Wolfe HW et al. Why are cesarean delivery rates so high in diabetic pregnancies? *J Perinat Med* 2000; **28**:316–20.

47. Coleman TL, Randall H, Graves W, Lindsay M. Vaginal birth after cesarean among women with gestational diabetes. *Am J Obstet Gynecol* 2001; **184**:1104–7.

48. Blackwell SC, Hassan SS, Wolfe HM et al. Vaginal birth after cesarean in the diabetic gravida. *J Reprod Med* 2000; **45**:987–90.

49. Gherman EM, Forouzan I, Morgan MA. A retrospective analysis of Erb's palsy cases and their relationship to birth weight and trauma at delivery. *Am J Obstet Gynecol* 1998; **178**:423–7.

50. Hod M, Bar J, Peled Y et al. Antepartum management protocol. Timing and mode of delivery in gestational diabetes. *Diabetes Care* 1998; **21 (Suppl 2)**:B113–B117.

33

Prevention of fetal macrosomia

Giorgio Mello, Elena Parretti, Federico Mecacci, Moshe Hod

Introduction

Fetal growth and development are primarily determined by the fetal genome, but there are other factors which influence this genetic regulation and which can either increase or reduce its effects.[1] The capacity of the placenta to transport nutrients to the fetus has an important role in fetal growth determination, but the fetal growth factors also have an influence, particularly with regard to differentiation.[2] Normal growth demands an equilibrium in the interaction between these different compartments and between the stimulatory and inhibitory factors affecting each of these steps.[1] Disturbance of this equilibrium at any stage can result in abnormal fetal growth. The fetus receives the main growth substance, glucose, which it cannot synthesize for itself, from the maternal circulation by means of facilitated diffusion through the placenta.[2] This diffusion is regulated principally through maternal plasma glucose levels. The maternal metabolic condition is the first determinant of fetal growth. Maternal metabolic disorders of glucohomeostasis, ranging from slightly impaired glucose tolerance to overt diabetes, since they provide an excess of substrates, are able to provoke an increased stimulation of the fetal beta cell with consequent hyperinsulinemia, which is in turn responsible for fetal hyper-

somatism as seen clinically at birth as a higher incidence of macrosomia.[3]

The term macrosomia is often used to describe a birthweight > 4000 grams or ≥ 90th percentile for gestational age;[4–6] a birthweight > 4000 grams is found in *c*. 5.5–10% of all infants,[7] although the incidence is much higher in newborns of diabetic women (10–33%).[5–8]

There are two types of macrosomia: the first type is constitutional, or symmetric, macrosomia, that accounts for 70% of cases, in which overgrowth is genetically directed and does not imply an abnormal supply of nutrients *in utero*.[9,10] The fetus is big but normal and the only potential problem is to avoid trauma during delivery. In contrast, the second type of macrosomia (asymmetric) (30%) is typically related to maternal diabetes and is characterized by organomegaly, and should be considered a pathological entity.[9,10] This type of macrosomia is associated with an abnormal thoracic and abdominal circumference, which is relatively larger than the head circumference.[11] These infants also differ in terms of their body proportions when compared with neonates of mothers with normal glucose metabolism.[12] As a result, disproportion between the head and shoulder girdle of the fetus, causing difficulty in delivery of the shoulders, predisposes to birth trauma (shoulder dystocia, clavicular fracture and brachial palsy) and, as a consequence, an increased rate of Cesarean sections. In addition, it is has been postulated that asymmetric macrosomia could have long-term consequences, including obesity, coronary heart disease, hypertension and Type 2 diabetes.[1,13,14]

For these reasons the classical definition of macrosomia based on birthweight and gestational age is not perhaps appropriate to identify features of disproportionate growth in the fetuses of mothers with abnormal glucose metabolism.[15] In this respect, the use of weight-to-length ratios, such as the ponderal index[15] and the birth symmetric index,[16] should give a more accurate description of fetal overgrowth. In addition, recent advances in ultrasound techniques have made possible the precise measurement of fetal insulin-sensitive tissue growth, and therefore an accurate analysis of fetal body composition in terms of lean body mass and fat body mass.[16–18] The human body is classically divided into fat and lean body mass components; it is the fat content that most accurately reflects energy stores and thus substrate supply.[19] The use of an index of fat mass as a predictor of morbidity has been widely used in neonates.[19] These findings suggest the potential

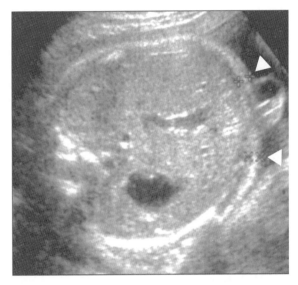

Figure 33.1. *Anterior abdominal wall thickness (arrowheads).*

usefulness of ultrasound measurements of fetal fat such as the anterior abdominal wall thickness (Fig. 33.1) and the mid-thigh subcutaneous (Fig. 33.2) areas for the determination and evaluation of fetal growth abnormalities. The distinction between fat and lean body mass seems to be relevant and efforts should be directed to the asymmetric overgrown fetus,

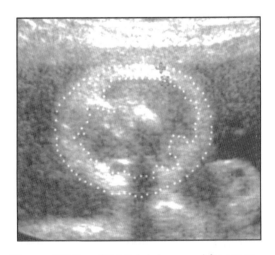

Figure 33.2. *Mid-thigh lean and fat areas.*

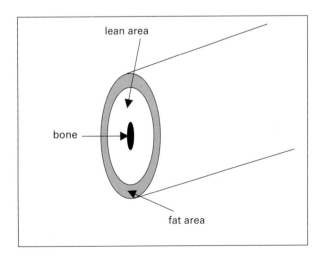

and to methods of primary prevention of this abnormality, by appropriate management approaches for both the mother and the fetus.[9]

The issue of preventing fetal macrosomia is somewhat puzzling; it would seem that, for some obstetricians, identification of the oversized fetus is aimed at reducing both the risk of shoulder dystocia and the rate of Cesarean sections. In fact, this goal is better described as preventing intrapartum complications associated with fetal macrosomia by appropriate management of the macrosomic fetus, rather than preventing the development of a macrosomic fetus. Although sonographic estimation of fetal weight is an important tool for the identification of fetal macrosomia, the sonographic fetal weight evaluation is less accurate the heavier the fetus is, reaching a mean error of ±20% for fetuses close to 4000 grams, thus increasing diagnostic uncertainty where accuracy is most needed. On the other hand, when the obstetrician delivers the infant early to stop the accelerated *in utero* growth, complications related to prematurity, such as hyperbilirubinemia, hypocalcemia and respiratory distress, may result.[20] In addition, this clinical approach is secondary, at the moment, to the lack of accurate diagnostic tools to identify all pregnant women at risk of macrosomia and of effective measures to control intrauterine fetal growth.

In the prevention of asymmetric fetal overgrowth in mothers with abnormal glucose metabolism, treatment strategies must be targeted to preventing overnutrition of the fetus,[21] even if to date there is no evidence-based study indicating that prevention and rigorous treatment of this metabolic condition can minimize fetal complications.[20]

If fetal macrosomia associated with maternal diabetes is related to maternal glucose levels,[22-25] then strategies to prevent hyperglycemia must be devised to treat the diabetic pregnant woman.[26] Indeed, glycemia is the single maternal metabolic parameter routinely assessed in diabetic pregnancies, and the criteria for metabolic control and therapeutic strategies of diabetes in pregnancy are based on maternal glucose levels,[27] since normoglycemia in pregnancy is associated with normal levels of other nutrients such as amino acids and lipids.[28] Overall, good perinatal outcomes have been achieved in diabetic pregnancies by aiming at normalization of maternal glucose values.[29-31] In many studies, however, the rate of macrosomia was still high, despite apparent rectification of glycemia. Therefore, it would appear that there are different thresholds of glycemic control for different known complications of diabetes,[31] and that tighter metabolic control needs to be achieved in order to prevent macrosomia.

Recently, a study has provided the true definition of normoglycemia during the third trimester in normal non-diabetic pregnancies (Table 33.1).[32] Overall, daily mean glucose levels showed a slight but progressive increase from 28 (71.9±5.7) to 38 (78.3±5.4) weeks. In addition, 1 hour postprandial glucose values were found to positively correlate with fetal abdominal growth as early as 28 weeks gestation, and this correlation was maintained throughout the third trimester. These findings are in agreement with those of diabetic pregnancies where 1 hour postprandial maternal blood glucose concentrations in the third trimester are considered a strong predictor of infant birthweight and fetal macrosomia.[22] Also in diabetic pregnancies, fetal hyperinsulinism and birthweight have been found to correlate best with 1 hour postprandial glucose values, as the postprandial glucose peak would breach the placental barrier.[33] In this context, the results from normoglycemic pregnancies seem to suggest that the fetal abdominal circumference – a parameter of growth of insulin-sensitive

Time	Gestational age (weeks)					
	28	30	32	34	36	38
08.00	54.8±6.2	55.9±4.9	53.7±4.2	56.3±4.7	57.2±3.9	59.0±4.1
09.00	92.0±7.5	94.2±5.9	95.2±4.3	96.5±5.1	101.2±4.9	104.2±5.1
10.00	78.2±5.8	80.5±6.7	82.9±6.5	83.7±9.8	90.1±4.9	89.2±9.5
12.00	67.1±5.5	66.2±5.5	63.4±4.8	66.3±5.9	68.1±6.7	64.2±6.2
13.00	92.9±7.1	94.9±4.8	95.9±6.8	98.8±4.5	101.9±3.4	105.2±4.9
14.00	85.2±4.9	82.5±4.7	87.4±6.6	87.9±3.9	94.2±4.1	95.0±6.2
16.00	70.1±5.8	66.1±4.0	68.1±5.7	66.1±7.0	69.8±5.6	68.2±6.1
18.00	63.0±6.5	61.9±5.1	63.4±3.6	65.9±3.9	65.1±5.0	66.2±5.0
20.00	62.4±4.1	62.9±4.8	63.3±2.8	64.0±3.1	64.9±4.1	65.1±7.7
21.00	91.1±7.8	92.5±7.5	94.9±4.7	99.0±4.5	102.2±3.2	105.2±4.0
22.00	79.5±6.3	81.1±5.7	85.2±3.6	89.5±8.4	93.5±5.1	95.2±4.2
00.00	64.5±5.1	62.1±7.6	64.5±4.4	60.8±7.7	64.9±5.9	69.2±7.0
02.00	60.5±3.9	64.0±4.4	64.0±5.2	66.3±3.4	67.1±4.1	66.2±4.6
04.00	59.8±3.4	60.8±3.7	61.2±5.6	64.2±4.1	61.5±5.8	63.1±3.8
06.00	58.7±6.0	59.7±4.2	58.8±5.1	60.3±5.9	59.8±4.1	60.1±3.2
Overall	**71.9±5.7**	**72.3±5.3**	**73.4±4.9**	**75.0±5.4**	**77.4±4.7**	**78.3±5.4**

Table 33.1. Diurnal glucose profiles at different gestational ages.

tissues – is influenced by postprandial glucose peaks even in glucose-tolerant women. This observation confirms that glycemia in pregnancy can be regarded as a 'continuum', ranging from normal glucose metabolism to overt diabetes, and that the consequences of hyperglycemia in terms of clinical outcome can be understood as an exaggeration of a mechanism that also occurs in normoglycemic pregnancies.[32] In the study by Parretti et al,[32] mean postprandial glucose levels never exceeded 105.2 mg/dl, a value well below the currently accepted thresholds for a good metabolic control in diabetic pregnancies, thus suggesting that simply blunting the peak postprandial response to such an extent can result in a decreased rate of macrosomia and lead to the absolute normalization of fetal growth. Nonetheless, the American Diabetes Association guidelines for pregnant diabetic women suggest that glucose levels can be as high as 140 mg/dl at the 1 hour and 120 mg/dl at the 2 hour postprandial time point, clearly recommending action only when glucose is in the hyperglycemic range. According to Jovanovic,[34] maintaining such a high threshold for action in the treatment of diabetic pregnant women may have contributed to sustained increased prevalence of macrosomia in infants of diabetic mothers despite good glucose control. In this respect, macrosomia despite normoglycemia would be better described as macrosomia because of undetected, and therefore undertreated, hyperglycemia.[35,36]

References

1. Van Assche FA, Holemens K, Aerts L. Fetal growth and consequences for later life. J Perinatol Med 1998; 26:337–46.
2. Aerts L, Pijnenborg R, Verhaeghe J et al. Fetal growth and development. In: (Dornhorst A, Hadden DR, eds) Diabetes and Pregnancy: An International Approach to

Diagnosis and Management. (Wiley & Sons: Chichester, 1996) 77–97.

3. Kalkhoff RK. Impact of maternal fuels and nutritional status on fetal growth. *Diabetes* 1991; **40 (Suppl 2):** 61–5.

4. Langer O, Michael D, Berkus MD et al. Shoulder dystocia: should the fetus weighing > 4000 grams be delivered by cesarean section? *Am J Obstet Gynecol* 1991; 165:831–7.

5. Keller DJ, Lopez-Zeno JA, Dooley SL et al. Shoulder dystocia and birth trauma in gestational diabetes: a five-year experience. *Am J Obstet Gynecol* 1991; 165:928–30.

6. Combs AC, Navkaran BS, Khoury J. Elective induction versus spotaneous labor after sonographic diagnosis of fetal macrosomia. *Obstet Gynecol* 1993; 81:492–6.

7. Macdonald PC, Gant NF, Leveno KJ, Gilstrap LC III (eds). *William Obstetrics,* 19th edn. (Appleton & Lange: New York, 1993); 493–520.

8. Kaufmann RC, McBride P, Amankwah KS, Huffman DG. The effect of minor degrees of glucose intolerance on the incidence of neonatal macrosomia. *Obstet Gynecol* 1992; 80:97–101.

9. Langer O. Fetal macrosomia: etiologic factors. *Clin Obstet Gynecol* 2000; 43:283–97.

10. Aschkenazi S, Chen R, Perri T et al. Size matters: management of the macrosomic infants. *Israel J Obstet Gynecol* 2001; 12:159–64.

11. Schwartz R. Hyperinsulinemia and macrosomia. *N Engl J Med* 1990; 323:340–2.

12. Mello G, Parretti E, Mecacci F et al. Anthropometric characteristics of full-term infants: effects of varying degrees of 'normal' glucose metabolism. *J Perinatol Med* 1997; 25:197–204.

13. Godfrey KM, Barker DJ. Fetal nutrition and adult diseases. *Am J Clin Nutr* 2000; **71 (Suppl 5):** S1344–S1352.

14. Van Assche EA. Symmetric and asymmetric fetal macrosomia in relation to long-term consequences. *Am J Obstet Gynecol* 1997; 177:563.

15. Lepercq J, Lahlou N, Timsit J et al. Macrosomia revisited: ponderal index and leptin delineate subtypes of fetal overgrowth. *Am J Obstet Gynecol* 1999; **181:** 621–5.

16. Landon MB, Sonek J, Foy P et al. Sonographic measurement of fetal humeral soft tissue thickness in pregnancy complicated by GDM. *Diabetes* 1991; **40 (Suppl 2):** 66–70.

17. Bernstein IM, Catalano PM. Ultrasonographic estimation of fetal body composition for children of diabetic mothers. *Invest Radiol* 1991; 26:722–6.

18. Winn HN, Holcomb NL. Fetal nonmuscular soft tissue: a prenatal assessment. *J Ultrasound Med* 1993; 4:107–99.

19. Bernstein IM, Goran MI, Amini SB et al. Differential growth of fetal tissues during the second half of pregnancy. *Am J Obstet Gynecol* 1997; 176:28–32.

20. Jovanovic L, Pettitt DJ. Gestational diabetes mellitus. *J Am Med Assoc* 2001; **286.**

21. Jovanovic L. Optimization of insulin therapy in patients with gestational diabetes. *Endocr Pract* 2000; **6:**98–100.

22. Jovanovic L, Peterson CM, Reed GF et al. and the National Institute of Child Health and Human Development–Diabetes In Early Pregnancy Study. Maternal postprandial glucose levels and infant birth weight: the Diabetes In Early Pregnancy Study. *Am J Obstet Gynecol* 1991; **164:**103–11.

23. DeVeciana M, Major CA, Morgan MA et al. Postprandial versus preprandial blood glucose monitoring in women with gestational diabetes mellitus requiring insulin therapy. *N Engl J Med* 1995; **333:**1237–41.

24. Combs CA, Gunderson E, Kitzmiller JL et al. Relationship of fetal macrosomia to maternal postprandial glucose control during pregnancy. *Diabetes Care* 1992; **15:**1251–7.

25. Mello G, Parretti E, Mecacci F et al. What degree of maternal metabolic control in women with type 1 diabetes is associated with normal body size and proportions in full-term infants? *Diabetes Care* 2000; **23:**1494–8.

26. Jovanovic L (ed.) *Medical Management of Pregnancy Complicated by Diabetes,* 3rd edn. (American Diabetes Association: Alexandria, VA, 2000.)

27. Buchanan TA, Kitzmiller JL. Metabolic interactions of diabetes and pregnancy. *Annu Rev Med* 1994; **45:**245–60.

28. Reece EA, Coustan DR, Sherwin RS et al. Does intensive glycemic control in diabetic pregnancies result in normalization of other metabolic fuels? *Am J Obstet Gynecol* 1991; **165:**126–30.

29. Weiss PAM. Diabetes in Pregnancy: lessons from the fetus. In: (Dornhost A, Hadden DR, eds) *Diabetes and Pregnancy: An International Approach to Diagnosis and Management.* (Widley & Sons: Chichester, 1996) 221–40.

30. Mello G, Parretti E, Mecacci F et al. Excursion of daily glucose profiles in pregnant women with IDDM: relationship with perinatal outcome. *J Perinatol Med* 1997; **25:**488–97.

31. Langer O. Is normoglycemia the correct threshold to prevent complications in the pregnant diabetic patient? *Diabetes Rev* 1996; **4:**2–10.

32. Parretti E, Mecacci F, Papini M et al. Third-trimester maternal glucose levels from diurnal profiles in non diabetic pregnancies: correlation with sonographic parameters of fetal growth. *Diabetes Care* 2001; **24:**1319–23.

33. Weiss PAM, Haeusler M, Kainer F et al. Toward universal criteria for gestational diabetes: relationships between seventy-five and one hundred gram glucose loads and between capillary and venous glucose concentrations. *Am J Obstet Gynecol* 1998; **178:**830–5.

34. Jovanovic L. Response to Fraser. *Diabetes Care* 2002; **25:**1104–5 (letter).

35. Jovanovic L. What is so bad about a big baby? *Diabetes Care* 2001; **24:**1317–18.

36. Mello G, Parretti E, Cioni R. Responce to Fraser. *Diabetes Care* 2002; **25:**1105–6. (letter).

34

Timing and delivery of the macrosomic infant: induction versus conservative management

David A Sacks

Introduction

The title of this chapter may be somewhat ambiguous, as the interpretation of the term 'conservative' in the current context has broad latitude. For example, induction of labor may be considered a more radical procedure than Cesarean delivery for pregnant women who have diabetes. Furthermore, the term 'macrosomic infant' has a variety of definitions, some of which are mutually exclusive.[1] This chapter will employ the definitions of macrosomia used by the authors of the cited studies. For clarity, large for gestational age (LGA) refers to a baby whose birthweight is ≥ 90th percentile for gestational age for a given population. The interested reader is advised to consult the original journal articles for the details of these definitions, as well as for indepth details of methodology and data analysis.

Rationale for induction of labor in diabetes

Before considering the relative virtues of offering an induction of labor to a woman who has diabetes, it is relevant to question the potential benefits to be derived from such a procedure. Four rationales present: (1) prevention of fetal death; (2) prevention of fetal overgrowth; (3) avoidance of shoulder dystocia; and (4) avoidance of Cesarean delivery. While the last three are interrelated, the first bears separate analysis.

Prior to the implementation of contemporary management of diabetes in pregnancy, including normalization of maternal glycemia, frequent daily monitoring of glucose and antepartum fetal assessment, unexplained fetal demise toward term was a known, feared complication of maternal diabetes. For several years, some have suggested that fetal demise in cases unassociated with major congenital anomalies or poor maternal glycemic control is a thing of the past.[2] However, recent data suggest that this may not be the case. Studies of Type 1[3] and Type 2[4] pregnant diabetic women found a statistically significantly increased risk of fetal mortality among these women in comparison with their non-diabetic controls. Among gestational diabetics a trend toward an increase in fetal demise was found, but the difference with non-diabetic controls did not achieve statistical significance.[5] In all three studies only ≤ 10% of the stillborns had recognizable anomalies. Furthermore, in an analysis confined to gestationally diabetic women who were managed with diet alone, the adjusted relative risk of perinatal death was three times that of the non-diabetic controls.[5] Data such as these suggest that the risk of fetal and perinatal demise may be attributable to factors intrinsic to maternal diabetes other than congenital anomalies and maternal glycemic control. Thus, the rationale of prevention of fetal demise for induction of labor appears to be justified.

The prevention of excessive fetal growth has also been applied as a rationale for delivery prior to term in pregnancies complicated by diabetes. A large database demonstrates that the rate of fetal growth peaks at 33–34 weeks gestation. At 40 weeks gestation the average rate of growth is 100 grams/week (Fig. 34.1). These data were derived from an unselected cohort of births in one study in the United States.[6] Data from a later study performed at an institution in the same state and limited to women who had diabetes suggested that the rate of *in utero* fetal growth in the latter population was twice that in the general population.[7] Thus, employing prevention of excessive fetal growth as a rationale for induction of labor in pregnancies complicated by diabetes also seems justified.

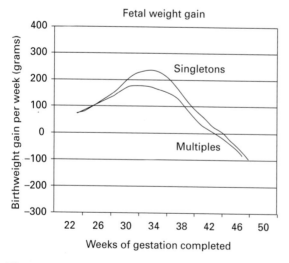

Figure 34.1. *Median growth curve for singleton and multiple births in California, 1970–1976 (from Williams et al[6]).*

Induction of labor: confounders

An analytical comparison of the risks and benefits of induction of labor for women who have diabetes is a very difficult undertaking. A major reason for this difficulty is that few publications deal with induction of labor exclusively in pregnant diabetic women. A second reason is that comparisons between induction of labor and elective Cesarean delivery involve comparisons of two very different procedures, each of which has a different set of risks and benefits. Finally, it is not possible to deal with the issue of induction of labor in isolation, as outcomes may be confounded by such factors as cervical ripeness, labor management, epidural anesthesia, fetal body composition and weight distribution, and the incorporation of estimates of fetal weight into the plan of management. Each of these factors will now be considered.

Cervical ripeness

On the basis of common sense alone, it may be intuited that the more effaced and/or dilated the cervix at the initiation of induction, the greater the likelihood that the woman will deliver vaginally. A large matched cohort study compared the outcomes of labor of uncomplicated women carrying singletons whose labor was induced with those who underwent spontaneous onset of labor. Matching was based on nulliparity, cephalic presentation, term gestational age and an actual birthweight of 3800–4000 grams. A higher incidence of Cesarean deliveries for dystocia and non-reassuring fetal heart rate tracings, as well as an increase in instrumented deliveries, in the induction group was reported.[8] Given the factors for which the subjects were matched, it is possible that the differences in outcomes may have been accounted for by differences in cervical status at the initiation of labor.

Another study which compared women undergoing induced labor with those who had spontaneous labor analyzed the influence of cervical status at the onset of induction. Women who had a Bishop score[9] ≤ 7 received vaginal prostaglandin as a cervical ripening agent. The authors found that regardless of the initial Bishop score, women undergoing labor induction had a higher cesarean rate than those whose labor was spontaneous in onset.[10] It therefore seems likely that, regardless of cervical status at the start of an induction and the use of cervical ripening agents, the fact that labor was induced rather than spontaneous predisposes a woman to have an operative delivery.

Available experience with cervical ripening limited to diabetic women is quite limited. One such study had as entry criteria a gestational age of at least 38.5 weeks, no vascular complications, and an estimated fetal weight of between 2000 and 4500 grams. In double-blind fashion, subjects and controls whose initial Bishop scores were ≤ 4 received either cervical misoprostil or placebo twice during the week following enrollment. Those not in labor within 1 week had their labors induced. There were no statistically significant differences between the misoprostil and the placebo groups with regard to the Bishop score on admission for either labor or induction. The incidence of spontaneous labor within 1 week of study (54 and 57%, respectively), was also not significantly different. The difference in Cesarean rates (25 and 17%, respectively) also did not achieve statistical significance.[11]

Labor management

The protocol for labor induction, the decision-making threshold for the diagnosis of an arrest disorder and the obstetrician's knowledge that his or her patient has diabetes may each influence the outcome of an induction of labor.

Differing regimens for labor induction have been proposed over the years. Active management of labor is one regimen that has received intensive scrutiny. Active management has four essential components. The first of these requires a strict definition of labor. Satisfaction of this criterion requires that the cervix be ≥ 80% effaced, that a bloody show be present and that there be spontaneous rupture of membranes, either alone or in combination. The second element is that amniotomy be performed early in labor. The third element is early use of oxytocin, utilized on indication of a cervix whose dilatation is progressing at a rate of < 1 cm/hour. The fourth requirement is the continuous personal support of the patient.[12] Four randomized controlled trials (RCT) limited to nulliparas comparing active with standard labor management reported similar findings. Active management did result in shortened labor by shortening the first stage of labor. Two of these studies additionally found a decreased incidence of maternal infection. Active management did not, however, effect a change in either the overall Cesarean rate or the rate of Cesarean deliveries for arrest disorders.[13–16] While none of these trials analyzed diabetic women as a separate subgroup, one may infer that, among nulliparous women in early labor, neither the timing of administration nor the dosage regimen of oxytocin appears to affect the Cesarean rate. Note must also be taken that entry into these studies required that the woman had a spontaneously initiated labor. Therefore, the relevance of these data to induction of labor may be at best tenuous.

One contentious issue in labor management is the functional definition of an arrest disorder. For several years, a standard definition of an arrest disorder included a cessation of dilatation for > 2 hours.[17] More recently, it was shown that by allowing labor augmentation to continue after 4 hours of dilatation at a rate of < 1 cm/hour, 56% of nulliparas and 88% of multiparas ultimately delivered vaginally; no severe complications of labor were noted.[18] Thus, the definition of arrest of labor is a parameter that requires scrutiny in the assessment of the rate of failed inductions.

A variable whose influence on the Cesarean rate has been demonstrated is the obstetrician's knowledge that the patient has diabetes. One study compared the labor outcomes of patients known to have gestational diabetes with those of women whose glucose intolerance was unknown to their obstetricians. The former group was treated with diet and insulin while the latter received no special care for diabetes. Babies in the former group weighed significantly less than those in the latter group. However, the Cesarean rate for both groups was not significantly different. In multivariate analysis, a significant independent relationship between the diagnosis of gestational diabetes and the Cesarean rate was demonstrated in the group in which the diagnosis of diabetes was known. However, the absence of such a relationship was found in the group in which the diagnosis of diabetes had been blinded.[19] From these data one may infer that the obstetrician knowing that his or her patient has diabetes may lower the threshold for finding an indication for Cesarean delivery, or for declaring an induction to have failed.

Epidural analgesia

Data and opinions have been published which suggest that the employment of epidural analgesia during labor may[20,21] or may not[22-25] prolong labor and/or predispose to Cesarean delivery. While a discussion of this debate, as well as an analysis of epidural technique, agents, risks and benefits, is beyond the scope of this chapter, it must be noted that there are no data available specific to the employment of this modality in the induction of labor for diabetic women.

Fetal body composition and weight distribution

Babies of diabetic women differ in body composition and weight distribution from those of non-diabetic women. A substantial portion of the variance in the birthweight of the former is accounted for by differences in the fat mass.[26] Merely calculating a ratio between weight and length (e.g. to determine if a baby is LGA) may not adequately reflect the differences in weight distribution. A study comparing LGA neonates of diabetic and non-diabetic mothers found no differences in birthweights, lengths and body mass indices (BMI) between both sets of infants. However, the sum of skinfold thicknesses (a surrogate measure for subcutaneous fat) was significantly greater for the infants of the diabetic mothers.[27] The differences in weight distribution may, in turn, be related to differences in average maternal glucose concentrations or related metabolic factors idiosyncratic to diabetic women. A comparison between two groups of LGA neonates of Type 1 diabetic mothers has been reported. The asymmetrically large group was defined by having abdominal circumferences > 90th percentile and biparietal diameters < 90th percentile, while the symmetrically large babies had both measures > 90th percentile.[28] The glycosylated hemoglobin (HbA1c) of the asymmetrical group was significantly greater than that of the symmetrical group, suggesting that differential distribution of truncal fat in infants of diabetic mothers may be more dependent on maternal glucose concentrations than is overall fetal growth.[28]

The distribution of larger amounts of body fat within the trunks of infants of diabetic mothers has some important clinical implications. When matched for birthweight, infants of diabetic mothers were found to have larger shoulder–head circumference differences than infants of non-diabetic mothers.[29] This observation may in part explain the finding that within 250 gram increments in birthweights > 3750 grams there is a significantly higher incidence of shoulder dystocia among infants of diabetic mothers compared with equivalent birthweight infants of non-diabetic mothers (Fig. 34.2).[30]

Incorporating estimates of fetal weight into the plan of management

Estimates of fetal weight have been incorporated into the plan of patient care in deciding whether to deliver by a trial of labor, labor induction or a primary Cesarean delivery.[1] The argument in support of using such estimates for women who have diabetes is that over three quarters of shoulder dystocias

occur among babies who weigh > 4250 grams.[30] Unfortunately, both two-[31–33] and three-dimensional[34,35] sonographic estimates of fetal weight have been found to have a wide margin of error. Of concern is the observation that the accuracy of sonographic estimates of fetal weight decreases with increasing birthweight.[36–38] Overall, sonographic estimates of fetal weight have been found to be no more accurate than clinical estimates of fetal weight by obstetricians.[39–40] Between 50 and 60% of both clinical and sonographic estimates of fetal weight come within 10% of the actual birthweights.[41] Furthermore, estimates of fetal weight made early in labor by parous women have been reported to be as accurate as those of their obstetricians.[42,43]

Induction of labor versus expectant management

The relative merits of induction of labor and expectant management have focused on three

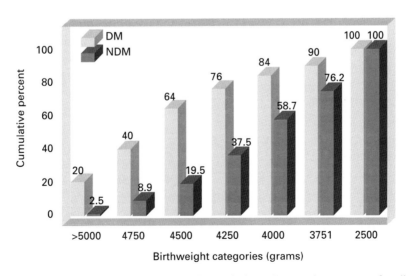

Figure 34.2. *Cumulative incidence of shoulder dystocia in 250 gram increments for diabetic (DM) and non-diabetic (NDM) women (from Langer et al[30]).*

Reference	Study type	Birthweight (grams)			Shoulder dystocia (%)			Cesarean delivery (%)		
		Induced	Exp*	P	Induced	Exp*	P	Induced	Exp*	P
Induction for estimated macrosomia at term in non-diabetic women										
44	RCT	4063	4133	0.024	4	4	NS	19	22	NS
45	RCT	4250	4253	NS	21	14	NS	32	38	NS
46	Case/ctl	4102	4355	< 0.05	6	11	NS	36	17	< 0.05
47	Cohort	4162	3887	< 0.01	5	3	NS	57	31	< 0.01
48	Cohort	4211	4180	NS	14	13	NS	24	10	< 0.03
Induction at term in diabetic women										
49	RCT	3446	3672	< 0.0001	0	3	NS	25	31	NS

* Expectant management.
RCT, Randomized controlled trial; case/ctl, case–control; NS, not significant.

Table 34.1. Clinical trials of induction of labor.

of the four rationales mentioned previously, namely prevention of excessive fetal growth, avoidance of shoulder dystocia and avoidance of Cesarean delivery. While several studies have examined induction of labor for the indication of estimated macrosomia in non-diabetic women,[44–48] little work limited to pregnancy complicated by diabetes has been reported.[49] Table 34.1 briefly summarizes some of the pertinent findings of these studies. All studies are limited by sample size, the largest consisting of 273 subjects.[44] Why continued fetal growth was not demonstrated in the expectantly managed group in one of the randomized controlled trials,[45] and why a decreased mean birthweight was found in the expectant group in one of the cohort studies[47] remains unexplained. Level II evidence, but not RCT suggested a higher Cesarean rate among those undergoing an induction of labor. Among the non-diabetics, the incidence of shoulder dystocia did not differ significantly by plan of management, and the direction of difference varied from study to study.

Only one trial comparing induction of labor with expectant management among diabetics has been published.[49] In this study, 200 insulin-requiring well-controlled Type 2 and gestationally diabetic women were randomized to either induction of labor or expectant management at 38 weeks. Although the mean gestational age difference between groups at delivery was only 1 week, the mean difference in birthweight was 226 grams. This weight difference stands in marked contrast with the average fetal weight gain of 100–150 grams/week at the same gestational age in the general obstetric population (Fig. 34.1). All three shoulder dystocias were found in the expectantly managed group. Although the Cesarean delivery rate was greater in the expectant group, this difference did not achieve statistical significance.

Conclusions

Insufficient data is available to justify recommending either for or against induction of labor at term in pregnancies complicated by diabetes. Considerations unique to pregnancies in diabetic mothers pertinent to deciding whether or not labor should be induced include the risk of fetal demise with continuation of pregnancy and that of accelerated *in utero* growth toward term. Of further concern is the differential distribution of subcutaneous fat to the fetal trunk in some infants of diabetic mothers. The latter likely predisposes toward shoulder dystocia and arrest disorders. Most published information about induction and cervical ripening is derived from either unselected or non-diabetic patient samples. These data suggest that, at least in nulliparas, active management shortens the first stage of labor.

While the ideal would be to await the publication of well-powered randomized clinical trials to assess the risks and benefits of induction of labor in diabetic women approaching term, such trials may never be performed. Thus, the practitioner who elects to induce labor for his or her patient whose pregnancy is complicated by diabetes is well-advised to observe the usual precautions attendant upon inductions for all pregnancies, while taking special care to follow maternal glucose during labor and to have the appropriate personnel and equipment available for the management of possible shoulder dystocia.

References

1. Sacks DA, Chen W. Estimating fetal weight in the management of macrosomia. *Obstet Gynecol Surv* 2000; 55:229–39.
2. Gabbe SG. Diabetes mellitus in pregnancy: have all the problems been solved? *Am J Med* 1981; 70:613–8.
3. Casson IF, Clarke CA, Howard CV et al. Outcomes of pregnancy in insulin dependent diabetic women: results of a five year population cohort study. *Br Med J* 1997; 315:275–8.
4. Cundy T, Gamble G, Townend K et al. Perinatal mortality in type 2 diabetes mellitus. *Diabet Med* 2000; 17:33–9.
5. Schmidt MI, Duncan BB, Reichelt AJ et al. Gestational diabetes mellitus diagnosed with a 2-h 75-g oral glucose tolerance test and adverse pregnancy outcomes. *Diabetes Care* 2001; 24:1151–5.
6. Williams RL, Creasy RK, Cunningham GC et al. Fetal growth and perinatal viability in California. *Obstet Gynecol* 1982; 59:624–32.
7. Kjos SL, Henry OA, Montoro M et al. Insulin-requiring diabetes in pregancy: a randomized trial of active induction of labor and expectant management. *Am J Obstet Gynecol* 1993; 169:611–15.
8. Cammu H, Martens G, Ruyssinck G, Amy JJ. Outcome after elective labor induction in nulliparous women: a matched cohort study. *Am J Obstet Gynecol* 2002; 186:240–4.
9. Bishop EH. Pelvic scoring for elective induction. *Obstet Gynecol* 1964; 24:266–8.
10. Xenakis EM-J, Piper JM, Conway DL, Langer O. Induction of labor in the nineties: conquering the unfavorable cervix. *Obstet Gynecol* 1997; 90:235–9.
11. Incerpi MH, Fassett MJ, Kjos SL et al. Vaginally administered misoprostol for outpatient cervical ripening in pregnancies complicated by diabetes mellitus. *Am J Obstet Gynecol* 2001; 185:916–19.
12. O'Driscoll K, Jackson JA, Gallagher JT. Prevention of prolonged labour. *Br Med J* 1969; 2:477–80.
13. Lopez-Zeno JA, Peaceman AM, Adashek JA, Socol ML. A controlled trial of a program for the active management of labor. *N Engl J Med* 1992; 326:450–4.
14. Frigoletto Jr FD, Lieberman E, Lang JM et al. A clinical trial of active management of labor. *N Engl J Med* 1995; 333:745–50.
15. Rogers R, Gilson GJ, Miller AC et al. Active management of labor: does it make a difference? *Am J Obstet Gynecol* 1997; 177:599–605.
16. Sadler LC, Davison T, McCowan LM. A randomised controlled trial and meta-analysis of active management of labour. *Br J Obstet Gynaecol* 2000; 107: 909–15.
17. Friedman EA (ed.). *Labor: Clinical Evaluation and Management*, 2nd edn. (Appleton-Century-Crofts: New York, 1978.)
18. Rouse DJ, Owen J, Hauth JC. Active-phase labor arrest: oxytocin augmentation for at least 4 hours. *Obstet Gynecol* 1999; 93:323–8.
19. Naylor CD, Sermer M, Chen E, Sykora K. Cesarean delivery in relation to birth weight and gestational glucose tolerance: pathophysiology or practice style? Toronto Trihospital Gestational Diabetes Investigators. *J Am Med Assoc* 1996; 275:1165–70.
20. Ramin SM, Gambling DR, Lucas MJ et al. Randomized trial of epidural versus intravenous analgesia during labor. *Obstet Gynecol* 1995; 86:783–9.
21. Lieberman E, Lang JM, Cohen A et al. Association of epidural analgesia with cesarean delivery in nulliparas. *Obstet Gynecol* 1996; 88:993–1000.
22. Sharma SK, Sidawi JE, Ramin SM et al. Cesarean delivery: a randomized trial of epidural versus patient-controlled meperidine analgesia during labor. *Anesthesiology* 1997; 87:487–94.

23. Gambling DR, Sharma SK, Ramin SM et al. A randomized study of combined spinal-epidural analgesia versus intravenous meperidine during labor: impact on cesarean delivery rate. *Anesthesiology* 1998; **89**:1336–44.

24. Chestnut DH, Vincent Jr RD, McGrath JM et al. Does early administration of epidural analgesia affect obstetric outcome in nulliparous women who are receiving intravenous oxytocin? *Anesthesiology* 1994; **80**:1193–200.

25. Chestnut DH, McGrath JM, Vincent Jr RD et al. Does early administration of epidural analgesia affect obstetric outcome in nulliparous women who are in spontaneous labor? *Anesthesiology* 1994; **80**:1201–8.

26. Kehl R, Krew M, Thomas A, Catalano P. Fetal growth and body composition in infants of women with diabetes mellitus during pregnancy. *Matern Fetal Med* 1996; **5**:273–80.

27. Vohr BR, McGarvey ST. Growth patterns of large-for-gestational-age and appropriate-for-gestational-age infants of gestational diabetic mothers and control mothers at age 1 year. *Diabetes Care* 1997; **20**:1066–72.

28. Keller JD, Metzger BE, Dooley SL et al. Infants of diabetic mothers with accelerated fetal growth by ultrasonography: are they all alike? *Am J Obstet Gynecol* 1990; **163**:893–7.

29. Modanlou HD, Komatsu G, Dorchester W et al. Large-for-gestational-age neonates: anthropometric reasons for shoulder dystocia. *Obstet Gynecol* 1982; **60**:417–23.

30. Langer O, Berkus MD, Huff RW, Samueloff A. Shoulder dystocia: should the fetus weighing greater than or equal to 4000 grams be delivered by cesarean section? *Am J Obstet Gynecol* 1991; **165**:831–7.

31. Ocer F, Kaleli S, Budak E, Oral E. Fetal weight estimation and prediction of fetal macrosomia in non-diabetic pregnant women. *Eur J Obstet Gynecol Reprod Biol* 1999; **83**:47–52.

32. Gilby JR, Williams MC, Spellacy WN. Fetal abdominal circumference measurements of 35 and 38 cm as predictors of macrosomia. A risk factor for shoulder dystocia. *J Reprod Med* 2000; **45**:936–8.

33. Smulian JC, Ranzini AC, Ananth CV et al. Comparison of three sonographic circumference measurement techniques to predict birth weight. *Obstet Gynecol* 1999; **93**:692–6.

34. Song TB, Moore TR, Lee JI et al. Fetal weight prediction by thigh volume measurement with three-dimensional ultrasonography. *Obstet Gynecol* 2000; **96**:157–61.

35. Schild RL, Fimmers R, Hansmann M. Fetal weight estimation by three-dimensional ultrasound. *Ultrasound Obstet Gynecol* 2000; **16**:445–52.

36. Dudley NJ. Selection of appropriate ultrasound methods for the estimation of fetal weight. *Br J Radiol* 1995; **68**:385–8.

37. Hirata GI, Medearis AL, Horenstein J et al. Ultrasonographic estimation of fetal weight in the clinically macrosomic fetus. *Am J Obstet Gynecol* 1990; **162**:238–42.

38. Miller Jr JM, Korndorffer 3rd FA, Gabert HA. Fetal weight estimates in late pregnancy with emphasis on macrosomia. *J Clin Ultrasound* 1986; **14**:437–42.

39. Sherman DJ, Arieli S, Tovbin J et al. A comparison of clinical and ultrasonic estimation of fetal weight. *Obstet Gynecol* 1998; **91**:212–17.

40. Johnstone FD, Prescott RJ, Steel JM et al. Clinical and ultrasound prediction of macrosomia in diabetic pregnancy. *Br J Obstet Gynaecol* 1996; **103**:747–54.

41. O'Reilly-Green C, Divon M. Sonographic and clinical methods in the diagnosis of macrosomia. *Clin Obstet Gynecol* 2000; **43**:309–20.

42. Chauhan SP, Sullivan CA, Lutton TC et al. Parous patients' estimate of birth weight in postterm pregnancy. *J Perinatol* 1995; **15**:192–4.

43. Chauhan SP, Lutton PM, Bailey KJ et al. Intrapartum clinical, sonographic, and parous patients' estimates of newborn birth weight. *Obstet Gynecol* 1992; **79**:956–8.

44. Gonen O, Rosen DJ, Dolfin Z et al. Induction of labor versus expectant management in macrosomia: a randomized study. *Obstet Gynecol* 1997; **89**:913–17.

45. Tey A, Eriksen NL, Blanco JD. A prospective randomized trial of induction versus expectant management in nondiabetic pregnancies with fetal macrosomia. *Am J Obstet Gynecol* 1995; **172**:293.

46. Leaphart WL, Meyer MC, Capeless EL. Labor induction with a prenatal diagnosis of fetal macrosomia. *J Matern Fetal Med* 1997; **6**:99–102.

47. Combs CA, Singh NB, Khoury JC. Elective induction versus spontaneous labor after sonographic diagnosis of fetal macrosomia. *Obstet Gynecol* 1993; **81**:492–6.

48. Friesen CD, Miller AM, Rayburn WF. Influence of spontaneous or induced labor on delivering the macrosomic fetus. *Am J Perinatol* 1995; **12**:63–6.

49. Kjos SL, Henry OA, Montoro M et al. Insulin-requiring diabetes in pregnancy: a randomized trial of active induction of labor and expectant management. *Am J Obstet Gynecol* 1993; **169**:611–15.

35

Management of the macrosomic fetus

Gerard HA Visser, Inge M Evers, Giorgio Mello

Introduction

Fetal macrosomia is a frequent complication in pregnancies of women with diabetes. Its incidence depends, among other things, on the definition of macrosomia. On the one hand, birthweight centiles (> 90th or > 97.7th centile) are used and, on the other, weight (i.e. > 4000 grams or > 4500 grams) are used. The use of centiles is preferable from an epidemiological point of view, since such a definition is independent of gestational age. However, weight is more directly related to complications during labor. National studies show an incidence of a birthweight > 90th centile in pregestational diabetic pregnancies of 20% (Sweden 1982–1985), 33.5% (Sweden 1991–1996) and 45% (The Netherlands, 1999–2000).[1-3] These data suggest that there might have been an increase of macrosomia during the past decade: regional and/or multicenter studies show an incidence of 19–43%.[4-10] A birthweight of > 4000 grams occurs in *c.* 20–25% of infants of women with insulin-dependent diabetes[3,11-13] and a weight > 4500 grams in 7–10%.[3,12,14]

Macrosomia is related to glucose control [glycosylated hemoglobin (HbA1c) levels] during pregnancy, but the percentage of variance in weight explained by HbA1c values is limited (i.e. < 10%).[3] Macrosomia in diabetic pregnancy is related to unexplained death *in utero*, prolonged labor, shoulder dystocia and, as a consequence, fetal asphyxia, clavicle fracture and/or Erb's palsy. Macrosomic newborns are at increased risk of hypoglycemia, hyperbilirubinemia and hypertrophic cardiomyopathy.[2,15-17] Prevention of macrosomia is therefore of great importance. This should be achieved by reducing weight (centiles); however, since this seems as yet impossible – at least at a nationwide level – a timed early delivery may be an option.

Obstetric management

Management of the macrosomic fetus depends on several factors, such as actual fetal weight (and/or centile) at which perinatal risks increase and the reliability of fetal weight estimations. Moreover, as to the timing of delivery, gestational age (and fetal maturity) and the cervix score are of importance.

Stillbirth is more frequent in macrosomic fetuses and data from the Swedish Medical Birth Register from 1991 to 1996 show an incidence of 2.4% in large-for-date infants as compared to 1.2% for appropriate-for-date infants of insulin-dependent diabetic women.[2] Prevention of stillbirth in the macrosomic fetus is, apart from improving maternal glucose control and intensified fetal monitoring, only

(in the non-diabetic population too).[26,27] Assessment of fetal lung maturation should therefore be made if a Cesarean section before that time is considered. It is not known if the same holds for a planned induction of labor, since labor itself might stimulate fetal lung maturation. However, it is the present authors' policy to perform lung maturity testing if labor is induced before 38 weeks of gestation.

Timing of delivery

There is no convincing data as to the optimal timing of delivery of the macrosomic fetus of the woman with diabetes. Gestational age, estimated fetal weight and the degree of glucose control all play a role.

The present authors start delivering infants with an estimated fetal weight > 97.7th centile from 36 weeks onwards, after determination of fetal lung maturation. Labor may be induced in the case of a favorable cervix. Poor glucose control and excessive fetal weight may result in an even earlier intervention; good glucose control may lead to a later intervention. If longitudinal ultrasound measurements of fetal weight indicate an estimated weight > 4250 grams, then a Cesarean section is considered.

Conclusions

- The problem of fetal macrosomia in maternal Type 1 diabetes is increasing rather than decreasing.
- Intrauterine death occurs more often of large-for-gestational-age fetuses than of appropriate-for-gestational-age fetuses. There is some evidence that the highest incidence of stillbirth occurs *c*. 37–39 weeks of gestation.
- Complicated vaginal delivery of infants with shoulder dystocia occurs more often in

diabetic women than in non-diabetic women when the infant weighs > 4250 grams.

- In Type 1 diabetes an elective Cesarean section is recommended in cases where the estimated fetal weight is > 4250 grams, despite limitations in fetal weight estimation.
- In cases where an elective delivery is considered before 38 weeks of gestation, then fetal lung maturity testing is recommended.

References

1. Hanson U, Persson B. Outcome of pregnancies complicated by type-1 insulin dependent diabetes in Sweden: acute pregnancy complications, neonatal mortality and morbidity. *Am J Perinatol* 1993; 4:330–3.
2. Djerf P, Hanson U. Perinatal complications in large-for-gestational age (LGA) infants compared to non LGA-infants of type-1-diabetic mothers. *Abstracts Diabetic Pregnancy Study Group of the EASD, 32nd meeting*, Galilee, Israel, 2000, 38.
3. Evers IM, De Valk HW, Visser GHA. Macrosomia despite good glycemic control in type-1 diabetic pregnancy; results of a nationwide prospective study. *Diabetologia* 2002; 45:1484–9.
4. Nordström L, Spetz E, Wallström K, Wålinder O. Metabolic control and pregnancy outcome among women with insulin-dependent diabetes mellitus. A twelve-year follow-up in the country of Jåmtland, Sweden. *Acta Obstet Gynecol Scand* 1998; 77:284–9.
5. GDF study group – France. Multicenter survey of diabetic pregnancy in France. Gestation and Diabetes in France Study Group. *Diabetes Care* 1991; 14:994–1000.
6. Vääräsmäki MS, Hartikainen A, Anttila M et al. Factors predicting peri- and neonatal outcome in diabetic pregnancy. *Early Hum Dev* 2000; 59:61–70.
7. Evers IM, Bos AME, Aalders AL et al. Pregnancy in women with type 1 diabetes mellitus; still maternal and perinatal complications in spite of good blood sugar control. *Ned T Geneesk* 2000; 144:804–9.
8. Leads from the MMWR. Diabetes in Pregnancy Project-Maine, 1986–1987. *J Am Med Assoc* 1987; 258:3495–6.
9. Casson IF, Clarke CA, Howard CV et al. Outcomes of pregnancy in insulin dependent diabetic women: results of a five year population cohort study. *Br Med J* 1997; 315:275–8.
10. Hawthorne G, Robson S, Ryall EA et al. Prospective population based survey of outcome of pregnancy in diabetic women: results of the Northern Diabetic Pregnancy Audit. *Br Med J* 1994; 315:279–81.

11. Jervell J, Bjerkedal T, Moe N. Outcome of pregnancies in diabetic mothers in Norway 1967–1976. *Diabetologia* 1980; **18**:131–4.

12. Langer O, Berkus MD, Huff RW, Samueloff A. Shoulder dystocia: should the fetus weighing ≥ 4000 grams be delivered by cesarean section? *Am J Obstet Gynecol* 1991; **165**:831–7.

13. Gabbe SG. Management of diabetes mellitus in pregnancy. *Am J Obstet Gynecol* 1985; **153**:824–8.

14. DCCT group. Pregnancy outcomes in the Diabetes Control and Complications Trial. The DCCT Research Group. *Am J Obstet Gynecol* 1996; **174**:1343–53.

15. Berk MA, Mimouni F, Miodovnik M et al. Macrosomia in infants of insulin–dependent diabetic mothers. *Pediatrics* 1989; **86**:1029–34.

16. Small M, Cameron A, Lunan CB, MacCuish AC. Macrosomia in pregnancy complicated by insulin-dependent diabetes mellitus. *Diabetes Care* 1987; **10**:594–9.

17. Gutgesell HP, Speer ME, Rosenberg HS. Characterization of the cardiomyopathy in infants of diabetic mothers. *Circulation* 1980; **61**:441–50.

18. Lowy C, Beard RW, Goldschmidt J. Congenital malformations in babies of diabetic mothers. *Diabet Med* 1986; **3**:458–62.

19. Lowy C. Type 1 diabetes and pregnancy. *Lancet* 1995; **346**:966–7.

20. Lipscomb KR, Gregory K, Shaw K. The outcome of macrosomic infants weighing at least 4500 grams: Los Angeles + University of Southern California experience. *Obstet Gynecol* 1995; **85**:558–64.

21. Modanloü HD, Komatsu G, Dorchester W et al. Large-for-gestational age neonates: anthropometric reasons for shoulder dystocia. *Obstet Gynecol* 1982; **60**:417–23.

22. Foran AM, Donnelly V, Eligott MMc et al. Erb's Palsy, prevalence, prediction and management. *J Matern Fetal Neonat Med* 2002; **11 (Suppl 1)**: 46 (abstract).

23. McLaren RA, Puckett JL, Chauhan SP. Estimations of birth weight in pregnant women requiring insulin: a comparison of seven sonographic models. *Obstet Gynecol* 1995; **85**:565–9.

24. Watson W, Seeds J. Sonographic diagnosis of macrosomia. In: (Divon MR, ed.) *Abnormal Fetal Growth*. (Elsevier: New York, 1991) 237–42.

25. Carrera JM, Mallafré J. Macrosomia: obstetric management. In: (Kurjak A, ed.) *Textbook of Perinatal Medicine*. (Parthenon Publishing Group: London, 1998) 1294–5.

26. Graziosi GC, Bakker CM, Brouwers HAA, Bruinse HW. Elective cesarean section is preferred after the completion of a minimum of 38 weeks of pregnancy. *Ned T Geneesk* 1998; **142**:2300–3.

27. Donaldsson S, Thorkelsson T, Bergsteinsson H et al. The effect of gestational age at the time of delivery on the incidence of respiratory dysfunction in neonates born by elective caesarean section without labour. *J Matern Fetal Neonat Med* 2002; **11 (Suppl 1)**:20.

28. Garner PR, D'Alton ME, Dudley DK et al. Preeclampsia in diabetic pregnancies. *Am J Obstet Gynecol* 1990; **163**:505–8.

29. Landon MB, Langer O, Gabbe SG et al. Fetal surveillance in pregnancies complicated by insulin dependent diabetes mellitus. *Am J Obstet Gynecol* 1992; **167**: 617–21.

30. Lagrew DC, Pircon RA, Towers MD et al. Antepartum fetal surveillance in patients with diabetes: when to start? *Am J Obstet Gynecol* 1993; **168**:1802–6.

31. Evers IM. *Pregnancy outcome in women with type-1 diabetes mellitus: a nationwide study in The Netherlands*. PhD Theses, University of Utrecht, 2002.

36

Hypertensive disorders and diabetic pregnancy

Jacob Bar, Michael Kupferminc, Moshe Hod

Fetal origin of adult disease

Barker[1] pioneered the idea that the epidemic of coronary heart disease in Western countries in the twentieth century, which paradoxically coincided with improved standards of living and nutrition, originated in fetal life. In the early 1900s, deprived areas had the highest rates of neonatal mortalities and low birthweights. Barker[1] postulated that the impaired fetal growth might have predisposed the survivors to heart disease in later life. This hypothesis was supported by studies conducted in Hertfordshire, UK, showing a higher rate of cardiovascular mortality in the men who had been small at birth and at 1 year of age.[1] Thereafter, at least seven retrospective cohort studies based on anthropometric measurements in infancy reported an association of a low birthweight with a high risk of later ischemic heart disease[2-7] and stroke,[8,9] or impaired glucose tolerance (IGT) and diabetes mellitus (DM).[10,11] Accordingly, low birthweight was also found to be associated with high blood pressure (BP) in childhood[12,13] and adult life.[14] The evidence was strongest with regard to blood pressure and IGT,[15] which could be measured earlier in life and for which more data, and sometimes also prospective data, were available.[14,16] Evidence was weaker, though still convincing, for heart disease, for which data

were sparse and often confined to men. The few studies on stroke, particularly the hemorrhagic type, suggest the same association.[9]

In another study, Barker et al[17] observed that the effects of impaired fetal growth are modified by subsequent growth. As such, individuals who were small at birth but became overweight in adulthood were at the highest risk of heart disease and Type 2 (non-insulin-dependent, NID) DM, a physiological resistance to insulin action. This finding led to the second part of the hypothesis, the thrifty phenotype (see Fig. 36.1). The authors proposed that the process of adaptation to undernutrition in fetal life leads to permanent metabolic and endocrine changes. These are beneficial if the undernutrition persists after birth, but may predispose the individual to obesity and IGT if it does not. The most unfavorable growth pattern is smallness and thinness at birth, continued slow growth in early childhood, followed by acceleration of growth so that height and weight approach the population means. A continuing rise in the body mass index (BMI) above the mean is associated with IGT. The growth pattern differs by sex[1,18] and ponderal index.[1] However, as birthweight and ponderal index, as well as BMI, are only crude measures of the manner in which fetal nutrition affects body composition and the balance of lean body mass to fat, the true impact of fetal growth on

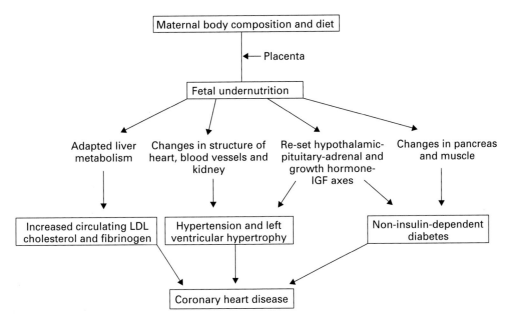

Figure 36.1. *Possible mechanisms linking fetal undernutrition and coronary artery disease. IGF, Insulin-like growth factor.*

later disease remains unclear. Be that as it may, there is no doubt that low birthweight and high BMI interact, and that their effects on BP and IGT are multiplicative.[1]

The thrifty phenotype paradigm has stimulated a wealth of animal and human research on fetal growth restriction and its sequelae. The hypothesis predicts that a population undergoing a transition from poor to better nutrition will be characterized by more heart disease and IGT. This is supported by the rapidly rising incidence of Type 2 DM, ischemic heart disease and obesity in increasingly urbanized India.[19–21] Indian infants are exceptionally small, with a mean birthweight of 2700 grams, and their mothers tend to be short and underweight. The infants also have low muscle mass, small viscera and a relative excess of fat – a body composition particularly likely to lead to insulin resistance.[22] In a cohort study in Indian children, Yajnik et al[23] showed that lower weight at birth and higher BMI in childhood are associated

with IGT. Although improving the growth and nutrition of the mother before pregnancy would seem to be the ideal strategy to improve fetal growth, animal studies have shown that more than one generation of improved maternal nutrition may be necessary for an optimal outcome.[24,25] Thus, in India, where women begin childbearing in their teens, before they are fully grown, postponing marriage might be a good first step.[26] There is only limited evidence that nutritional supplements in pregnancy improve fetal growth in undernourished mothers.[27] Furthermore, the effect of supplements varies according to the stage of pregnancy: giving supplements early in pregnancy may even worsen fetal growth.[1]

Recently, Stene et al,[28] in a large population-based cohort study, noted a relatively weak, but significant and nearly linear, association between birthweight and the risk of Type 1 (insulin-dependent, ID) DM. The rate ratio of children with a birthweight of ≥ 4500 grams to children with a birthweight of < 2000 grams was 2.21. This finding raises the possibility that perinatal factors influence the risk of Type 1 DM. The underlying mechanisms of this association are unknown, but they probably differ from those responsible for the association between low birthweight and later onset of Type 2 DM.

There may also be factors other than nutrition that play a role in the casual pathway leading to high BP, cardiovascular disease or Type 2 DM. The fetal origin hypothesis assumes that a poor nutrient supply during a critical period of *in utero* life may 'program' a permanent structural or functional change in the fetus, altering the distribution of cell types, gene expression, or both. Some authors have accused the original authors of the hypothesis of incorrect statistical interpretations, due to chance, artifact or confounding factors in later life, but these have recently been resolved.[29] Nevertheless, it should be emphasized that support for the hypotheses comes mainly from studies in rodents[30] and they cannot rule out environmental causes, particularly those associated with socioeconomic status,[31,32] genetic predisposition to low birthweight or hypertension and hypertension-related diseases, and postnatal factors.[33,34] Unfortunately, studies testing these parameters in humans are neither ethical nor practical.

In an attempt to separate genetic from extrauterine environmental influences, some researchers have studied multiple pregnancies. For example, the Tasmanian Infant Health Survey cohort of monozygotic, dizygotic and singleton pregnancies reported a stronger association between birthweight and BP in children from the multiple pregnancies. The association also held true within the monozygotic pairs, suggesting that a genetic predisposition may need to be combined with specific mechanisms within the feto-placental unit.[35] A recent study

of 492 pairs of female twins showing an inverse relationship of birthweight and adult BP[36] lent further support to the assumption that retarded intrauterine growth is due to placental dysfunction rather than inadequate maternal nutrition or genetic factors.

Two recent studies stress both the importance of primary prevention of high BP and cardiovascular disease, and the controversy still surrounding Barker's fetal origin hypothesis. In the first, school children with a history of low birthweight were found to have impaired endothelial function and a trend towards carotid stiffness, which may represent early expressions of vascular compromise.[37] However, another group of investigators showed no difference in flow-mediated endothelial-dependent vasodilatation (early stage in the development of atherosclerosis) between adolescents who had low birthweights and controls.[38]

Insulin resistance syndrome

The insulin resistance syndrome is characterized by a cluster of clinically recognizable physiological abnormalities, i.e., glucose intolerance, high BP and an unfavorable lipid profile, all alterations induced by the compensatory hyperinsulinemia. It also involves biochemical abnormalities. Insulin resistance now appears to be the epidemiological link between high BP and obesity, both risk factors for developing cardiovascular disease later in life. Insulin resistance can induce hypertension via mechanisms at the cellular, circulatory and neurological levels, as well as via possible polygenic factors. Acquired or transient insulin resistance is associated with certain physical conditions, such as pregnancy, obesity, oral contraceptive use and severe distress. Type 2 (NID) DM is a state of increased insulin secretion owing to the physiological resistance of insulin action and a lower than normal beta-cell reserve. Diabetes in pregnancy or gestational DM (GDM) may precede the clinical expression of Type 2 DM in the non-pregnant state, even by several years. Pre-eclampsia and other hypertensive disorders, which are known to have a higher incidence in GDM, can be linked to increased insulin resistance.

Essential hypertension

To understand the association between insulin resistance and hypertensive disorders in pregnancy, the role of insulin resistance in hypertensive disorders in the non-pregnant state first need to be elucidated. The pathogenesis of essential hypertension is multifactorial, involving complex interactions between endocrine, metabolic and genetic factors. Obesity, aging and diabetes can amplify genetic tendencies toward the clinical expression of the disorder

(see Fig. 36.2). Familial clustering of DM and hypertension has been reported by several investigators, who also observed a close association of insulin resistance with obesity-related hypertension.[39,40] Several other metabolic disturbances, such as elevated triglycerides, decreased high-density lipoproteins (HDL), cholesterolemia, glucose intolerance and hyperuricemia, have also been related to hyperinsulinemia.[41] The metabolic consequences of insulin resistance and subsequent hyperinsulinemia include changes in the lipid profile resulting in atherosclerosis, increased deposition of body fat and proliferation of vascular smooth muscle cells. Thus, the hypertensive, hyperinsulinemic individual is at increased risk of cardiac complications and stroke.[42] The study of the evolution of the clinical and biological disturbances in women with a polycystic ovary (PCO) supports the view that insulin resistance, dyslipidemia and hypertension are

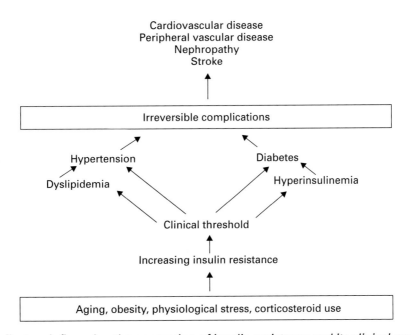

Figure 36.2. *Factors influencing the generation of insulin resistance and its clinical correlates in the non-pregnant state.*

all manifestations of a single syndrome. Often obese, these women have hyperinsulinemia that disrupts sex hormone production,[43] resulting in androgenization and certain clinical manifestations, such as hirsutism and infertility. During pregnancy, they have more glucose intolerance[44] and pregnancy-induced hypertension (PIH).[45] Later in their life, women with PCO will develop a male-pattern risk profile for coronary artery disease, including dyslipidemia and hypertension.[46]

Mechanisms of action

Physiologic studies suggest that insulin resistance occurs primarily in the peripheral muscle and is mediated through the non-oxidative intracellular pathways of glucose disposal.[47–49] Insulin modulates BP through several pathways, including stimulation of sympathetic neural activity, direct vasculopathic actions, changes in cellular ion flux and promotion of sodium (Na) retention.

Actions on the sympathetic nervous system

Insulin stimulates the release of plasma norepinephrine,[50] increases heart rate and systolic pressure, and stimulates vascular tone. In younger subjects, and in subjects with acute hyperinsulinemia,[51] these effects appear to override insulin's direct vasodilatory effect on the vascular beds. The observation that insulin administration sometimes leads to hypotensive episodes in diabetic patients with autonomic neuropathy is convincing proof of insulin's vasodilatory ability. The complexity of the situation is apparent from the finding that insulin therapy normalizes angiotensin responsiveness[52] and increases pressor responses.[53] Therefore, the possible attenuating effect of insulin on vasoconstrictor responses may be blunted in the presence of a pathological resistance to insulin action at the cellular level.[54]

Effect on vascular smooth muscle and epithelium

Hyperinsulinemia triggers hypertrophy of the vascular smooth muscle cells, leading to vasoconstriction and stiffening of the blood vessels and also the development of left ventricular hypertrophy.[55] The additional hyperinsulinemia-induced lipid changes also promote atherosclerosis with further stiffening and narrowing of the arteries. Evidence regarding the role of insulin resistance and hyperinsulinemia in the pathogenesis of endothelial dysfunction is less clear. McCarthy[56] presumed that the dysregulation of the transmembranous electrolyte pumps, which causes increased basal vascular tone, is a result of relative lack of insulin rather than hyperinsulinemia at the smooth muscle level.

Effect on the transmembranous electrolyte pump

In acute hyperinsulinemic states, transmembranous calcium (Ca) influx is usually lowered and vascular tone is decreased. However, the effect of chronic hyperinsulinemia on Ca^{2+}-adenosine triphosphatase, Na^+K^+-adenosine triphosphate (ATP) and the Na^+–H^+ countertransport mechanism may actually raise intercellular Ca^{2+} levels and increase vascular tone.[57,58] Erythrocyte Na^+–Li^+ countertransport is elevated in hypertensive patients with insulin resistance and hyperinsulinemia. At the cellular level, a rise in cytosolic Ca is promoted along with smooth muscle proliferation.[59]

Genetic components in insulin resistance

Type 2 DM has a strong genetic component. The genetic contribution varies from population group to population group, suggesting that more than one gene is involved and that more than one gene defect may cause similar phenotypic clinical syndromes.[60,61] Research in this area has concentrated on the steps in the insulin-signaling cascade between receptor and transport protein, but a lack of information about specific postreceptor signaling currently hampers these efforts.

Clinical consequences of insulin resistance

Insulin resistance impairs glucose tolerance while promoting dyslipidemia, obesity, hypertension and atherosclerosis. Its effects on salt handling by the kidneys predisposes the individual to renal dysfunction. Obesity, glucose intolerance, hyperinsulinemia, hypertension and dyslipidemia represent cumulative risk factors that generate an escalating cycle of vascular compromise and collapse. Patients with three or more of these risk factors have an increased incidence of stroke, nephropathy, ischemic heart disease and peripheral vascular disease.[62] Long-term diabetic complications are currently the most common cause of blindness, renal failure and limb amputation in the USA. Meticulous glycemic control has been shown to decrease the incidence of eye disease among diabetic patients. Antihypertensive therapy, specifically angiotensin-converting enzyme (ACE) inhibitors, is effective in reducing the rate of progression of diabetic kidney disease. To prevent the peripheral vascular remodeling that results in stroke, limb loss and heart disease, the underlying pathophysiologic mechanism needs to be reversed. This has become possible with the introduction of metformin[63] and troglitazone,[64] which are prototypes of the new classes of insulin-sensitivity-enhancing agents. These drugs are an important addition to the weight loss, exercise and diet modification programs used to date; lifestyle changes can be very effective but are rarely adhered to for more than a few years.

Insulin resistance and pregnancy

In normal pregnancy, insulin resistance results in a metabolic advantage for the fetus. The mother enters a state of accelerated starvation in which she increases her reliance on lipolysis and protein catabolism as a source of energy. Thus, glucose is reserved for the fetus, which uses it as its primary fuel.[65] A steady supply of glucose is essential for the growing feto-maternal unit; normally, pregnant women are able to increase their insulin secretion to three times that of non-pregnant women.[66] In GDM, however, there is no increase in maternal insulin secretion in reaction to the increasing insulin resistance.[67] Some investigators believe that this effect is due to a metabolically limited beta-cell reserve.[68,69] In most women with GDM, insulin sensitivity is restored after pregnancy; however, some may later develop Type 2 DM. The reported cumulative incidence rate of Type 2 DM after GDM is c. 50% after 5 years.[70,71] This rate is higher in women with excessive weight gain, or in those with repeated pregnancies who continue to experience insulin resistance.[72] Thus, the strong association between insulin resistance, hypertension, obesity and dyslipidemia as part of the insulin resistance syndrome, or sharing a common pathway in intrauterine life, may explain the higher incidence of hypertensive complications in diabetic pregnancy. Recently, researchers reported that the insulin resistance syndrome may also involve other metabolic abnormalities besides hyperglycemia, hyperinsulinemia and dyslipidemia, namely, increased concentrations of plasminogen activator inhibitor (PAI)-1,[73] leptin[74] and tumor necrosis factor-alpha (TNF-α).[75] Although these markers are surrogate measures of insulin sensitivity, they have been associated with a risk of hypertension in pregnancy.

GDM *and hypertensive disorders*

The study of both GDM and PIH has suffered from the lack of international consensus about classification, definitions and nomenclature, leading to difficulties in comparing studies that used different diagnostic criteria. Nevertheless, epidemiological and physiological evidence suggests that GDM and PIH are etiologically distinct entities, and that GDM is strongly associated with insulin resistance and glucose intolerance, whereas pre-eclampsia is probably not.

Epidemiological studies

Diabetic pregnancy is associated with a higher rate of hypertensive complications than normal pregnancy,[76,77] and a slightly increased risk of pre-eclampsia (15–20 versus 5–7%).[78–80] The latter is maintained even when the diagnosis of GDM is based on the 2 hour 75 gram oral glucose tolerance test (OGTT).[81] Mean arterial pressure is further increased in the presence of early diagnosis of GDM and the need for insulin therapy.[82]

The increased risk of hypertensive disorders in GDM is probably a result of the combination of insulin resistance and a genetic predisposition (Fig. 36.3). A genetic predisposition to PIH was described in southwestern Navajo Indians who, like other Native Americans, are also at increased risk of hypertension, obesity and DM.[83] Pre-eclampsia was also found to be associated with increased fasting plasma insulin levels in African-American women.[84] However, these findings have not been confirmed in more heterogeneous populations.[85]

Physiological studies

Patients with the severest form of glucose intolerance are more likely to exhibit pre-eclampsia[86] than those with milder forms.[85] Controlled studies of the association between insulin resistance and pre-eclampsia have been performed in several populations. Martinez et al[87] found that among women with normal glucose tolerance in the third trimester, those who subsequently developed severe pre-eclampsia had similar fasting and postprandial glucose levels to normotensive controls, but their fasting plasma insulin levels were twofold higher and their post-load insulin concentrations fourfold higher. Moreover, Joffe et al[88] recently reported that the level of plasma glucose at 1 hour after a 50 gram oral glucose challenge was an important predictor of pre-eclampsia, even if it was within the normal range. This also suggests that

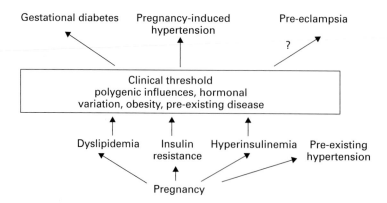

Figure 36.3. *Factors influencing the generation of insulin resistance and its clinical correlates during pregnancy.*

there is a continuum of insulin resistance in women with normal glucose tolerance that may predispose them to hypertensive disease. This assumption was supported by a similar study in China wherein higher serum insulin concentrations were detected in women with pre-eclampsia.[89] Besides insulin resistance, women with GDM and women with pre-eclampsia have similar hemodynamic profiles, namely, similar significant left ventricular hypertrophy and a reduction in diastolic function.[90] The mechanism by which insulin resistance may link these physiological findings is still unknown. One possibility is an interference of insulin resistance with the function of an endogenous sodium- pump inhibitor or digitalis-like factor. Graves et al[91] demonstrated that levels of serum digoxin-like immunoreactive factor are higher in women with pre-existing diabetes and pre-eclampsia than in normotensive diabetic women.

In hypertensive diabetic patients, some of the physiological changes that occur during pregnancy may persist after pregnancy. In one study, women with a pre-eclamptic pregnancy showed greater plasma insulin responses and steady-state plasma glucose levels 2 months after delivery than women with uncomplicated pregnancies.[92] A longer term study reported persistent mild hyperinsulinemia in women 17 years after a pre-eclamptic pregnancy, despite their current normoglycemic state.[93] Other investigators, however, failed to detect these changes at 3–6 months after delivery.[94]

Pregestational diabetes and hypertensive complications

In most cases, pregestational diabetes refers to Type 1 DM; the incidence of Type 1 DM in pregnancy ranges from 0.2 to 0.5%.[95,96] These women make up a heterogeneous group in terms of duration of diabetes (White's Classification), presence of hypertension and end-organ damage, especially damage to the eye (retinopathy) and kidney (nephropathy). Pregnancy in women with Type 1 diabetes is associated with increased risks of pre-eclampsia, intrauterine growth restriction (IUGR), neonatal morbidity and perinatal mortality.[95–103] The diagnosis of pre-eclampsia is difficult in women with pre-existing hypertension and proteinuria,[96] and women with chronic hypertension are at increased risk of superimposed pre-eclampsia independent of the presence of diabetes.[104] The rate of hypertensive disorders (PIH and

Author (reference)	No. of women	White's Class	Pre-eclampsia (%)	
			*	
Garner et al (108)	107	B, C	13	12.2
Greene et al (97)	361	B-R	86	23.8*
Hanson and Persson (95)	463	B-R	53	11.5
Miodovnik et al (105)	136	B-R	12	9.0
Kovilam et al (106)	238	B-D	36	15
Sibai et al (107)	462	B-D	92	20
Total	**1767**		**293**	**16.4**

* Includes women with pregnancy-induced hypertension.

Table 36.1. Rates of pre-eclampsia in women with Type 1 diabetes (excluding nephropathy).

Author (reference)	No. of women	Pre-eclampsia (%)	
Hanson and Persson (95)	31	18	58
Greene et al (97)	59	39	66
Reece et al (101)	31	11	35
Gordon et al (100)	45	24	53
Miodovnik et al (105)	46	30	65
Kovilam et al (106)	73*	32	44
Sibai et al (107)	58	21	36
Bar et al (111)	24	11	46
Total	**367**	**186**	**52**

* Includes women with R/F.

Table 36.2. Rates of pre-eclampsia in women with diabetic nephropathy.

pre-eclampsia) in the various studies ranged from 9 to 66%. The lowest rate occurred in women with milder forms of DM (Class B), and the highest rate in women with diabetic nephropathy. Table 36.1 summarizes the reported rates of pre-eclampsia in women with Type 1 DM (White's Classification Class B-R).[95,97,105–108] Four of the six studies reported increased rates of pre-eclampsia with increased severity of diabetes, with a mean of 16% (range 9–24%); however, rates were higher in patients with diabetic nephropathy (mean 52%, range 35–66%) (Table 36.2). Box 36.1 summarizes the risk factors for pre-eclampsia in women with Type 1 DM.[95,98,99,109–111] Siddiqi et al[98]

listed nulliparity, duration of diabetes and poor glycemic control, and Caritis et al[109] listed nulliparity and mean arterial pressure. Combs et al[99] added a glycohemoglobin (HbA1c) level > 9% at 12–16 weeks of gestation and proteinuria > 190 mg/dl. Accordingly, Hanson and Persson[95] noted a pre-eclampsia rate of 31% when HbA1c levels were > 10.1%, and a rate of 10.2% when HbA1c levels were < 10.1%. These findings indicate that PIH/pre-eclampsia might be preventable by aggressive control of maternal BP before and during pregnancy, and prevention of microalbuminuria or reduction of proteinuria levels in women with diabetic nephropathy: ACE inhibitors seem to be the

Duration of diabetes
Pre-existing hypertension
Microalbuminuria prior to pregnancy
Glycemic control prior to 20 weeks gestation
Nulliparity
Minimal proteinuria (190–499 mg/dl) before 20 weeks gestation
Nephropathy
Pre-pregnancy angiotensin-converting enzyme (ACE) inhibitor treatment

Box 36.1. Risk factors for pre-eclampsia in women with Type 1 diabetes.

ideal agents for this purpose.[111,112] Women with Type 1 DM and pre-existing hypertension and proteinuria need to be strictly controlled starting at least 6 months before conception.[111] According to recent evidence, ACE inhibitors do not pose an increased teratogenic risk with first-trimester exposure.[113,114] Nevertheless, most physicians advise stopping them before pregnancy, or at least immediately at diagnosis of pregnancy if they were continued inadvertently as part of the preconception program. Preconception medication should be accompanied by strict glycemic control.[111] Some authors have suggested the use of low-dose aspirin to prevent pre-eclampsia, since alterations in the metabolism of prostacyclin and thromboxane A2 have been reported in DM.[96,115] However, Caritis et al,[115] in a study of 462 women with Type 1 DM, found no significant differences in the rate of pre-eclampsia between the aspirin and placebo groups, although there was a non-significant trend toward a lower rate of pre-eclampsia in the aspirin group (19 versus 32%, respectively). It is possible that larger studies in patients with diabetic nephropathy might show a benefit of aspirin in preventing pre-eclampsia.

Microalbuminuria, diabetes and hypertension in pregnancy

The role of microalbuminuria in DM has been established over the past 10 years. At the early stage of DM, when glucose metabolism is not controlled, the increase in glomerular plasma flow and intraglomerular pressure is probably responsible for the increased protein excretion.[116] Some authors consider these hemodynamic alterations as major determinants of both the initiation and progression of diabetic nephropathy.[117] Several studies have reported that patients with Type 1[118] and/or Type 2 DM[119] who have above-normal urinary albumin excretion rates are more likely to

develop diabetic nephropathy, eventually progressing to renal failure.[120] Microalbuminuria is also associated with an excess of known and potential cardiovascular risk factors, and is a marker of established cardiovascular disease in both hypertensive[121] and non-hypertensive[122] individuals. While microalbuminuria serves as an important marker for an underlying vascular disease in the general population, its role in diabetic and hypertensive pregnancy is less clear,[123] but is becoming increasingly recognized. One study found that the presence of microalbuminuria in the early third trimester was predictive of pre-eclampsia in pregnant women at risk.[124] Furthermore, among women whose pregnancy was complicated by pre-eclampsia, 40% had microalbuminuria 5 years later – a significantly higher rate than in women with uncomplicated pregnancies.[125] The presence of microalbuminuria was also demonstrated in 30% of 72 women who had not conceived since a previous GDM pregnancy 5–8 years previously, again, a significantly higher rate than in women who did not have a history of GDM.[126] Recently, Ekbom et al[110] evaluated the role of microalbuminuria as a risk factor for pre-eclampsia in 68 women with Type 1 DM. They found that pre-eclampsia developed in 60% of those who had microalbuminuria before pregnancy. When the data were fitted to a logistic regression model, a significant association was revealed between microalbuminuria and duration of diabetes and pre-eclampsia. As in patients with hypertension, the progression to diabetic nephropathy in patients with Type 1 DM and microalbuminuria can be slowed by blockage of the renin–angiotensin system. Angiotensin II receptor antagonists were also recently found to be renoprotective in patients with Type 2 DM and microalbuminuria.[127] This evidence and other preliminary results[111,112] suggest that pregnancy outcome may be improved after pre-pregnancy ACE inhibitor treatment (discontinued at conception) in diabetic patients with overt proteinuria or microalbuminuria.

References

1. Barker DJP. *Mothers, Babies and Health in Later Life.* (Churchill Livingstone: London, 1998.)

2. Leon DA, Lithell HO, Vagero D et al. Reduced fetal growth rate and increased risk of death from ischaemic heart disease: cohort study of 15,000 Swedish men and women born 1915–29. *Br Med J* 1998; 317:241–5.

3. Rich-Edwards JW, Stampfer MJ, Manson JE et al. Birth weight and risk of cardiovascular disease in a cohort of women followed up since 1976. *Br Med J* 1997; 315:396–400.

4. Stein CE, Fall CHD, Kumaran K et al. Fetal growth and coronary heart disease in south India. *Lancet* 1996; 348:1269–73.

5. Eriksson JB, Forsen T, Tuomilehto J et al. Catch-up growth in childhood and death from coronary heart disease: longitudinal study. *Br Med J* 1999; 318: 427–31.

6. Forsen T, Eriksson JG, Tuomilehto J et al. Growth in utero and during childhood among women who develop coronary heart disease: longitudinal study. *Br Med J* 1999; 319:1403–7.

7. Frankel S, Elwood P, Sweetnam P et al. Birth weight, adult risk factors and incident coronary heart disease: the Caerphilly study. *Public Health* 1996; 110:139–43.

8. Eriksson JG, Forsén T, Tuomilehto J et al. Early growth and coronary heart disease in later life: longitudinal study. *Br Med J* 2001; 322:949–53.

9. Martyn CN, Barker DJP, Osmond C. Mothers' pelvic size, fetal growth, and death from stroke and coronary heart disease in men in the UK. *Lancet* 1996; 348:1264–8.

10. Barker DJP, Hales CN, Fall CHD et al. Type 2 (non-insulin-dependent) diabetes mellitus, hypertension and hyperlipidaemia (syndrome X): relation to reduced fetal growth. *Diabetologia* 1993; 36:62–7.

11. Bavdekar A, Chittaranjan S, Fall CHD et al. Insulin resistance syndrome in 8-year-old Indian children. Small at birth, big at 8 years, or both? *Diabetes* 1999; 48:2422–9.

12. Law CM, de Swiet M, Osmond C et al. Initiation of hypertension in utero and amplification throughout life. *Br Med J* 1993; 306:21–7.

13. Moore WM, Miller AG, Boulton TJ et al. Placental weight, birth measurements, and blood pressure at age 8 years. *Arch Dis Child* 1996; 74:538–41.

14. Barker DJ, Osmond C, Golding J et al. Growth in utero, blood pressure in childhood and adult life, and mortality from cardiovascular disease. *Br Med J* 1989; 298:564–7.

15. Hales CN. Non-insulin-dependent diabetes mellitus. *Br Med Bull* 1997; 53:109–22.

16. Whincup P, Cook D, Papacosta O et al. Birth weight and blood pressure: cross-sectional and longitudinal relations in childhood. *Br Med J* 1995; 311:773–6.

17. Barker DJP, Martyn CN, Osmond C et al. Abnormal liver growth in utero and death from coronary heart disease. *Br Med J* 1995; 310:703–4.

18. Taylor SJ, Whincup PH, Cook DG et al. Size at birth and blood pressure: cross-sectional study in 8–11 year old children. *Br Med J* 1997; 311:475–80.

19. Gupta R, Gupta VP, Ahluwalia NS. Educational status, coronary heart disease, and coronary risk factor prevalence in a rural population of India. *Br Med J* 1994; 309:1332–6.

20. McKeigue PM, Shah B, Marmot MG. Relation of central obesity and insulin resistance with high diabetes prevalence and cardiovascular risk in South Asians. *Lancet* 1991; 337:382–6.

21. Pais P, Pogue J, Gerstein H et al. Risk factors for acute myocardial infarction in Indians: a case–control study. *Lancet* 1995; 346:778–9.

22. Hales CN, Barker DJP, Clark PMS et al. Fetal and infant growth and impaired glucose tolerance at age 64. *Br Med J* 1991; 303:1019–22.

23. Yajnik CS, Fall CHD, Vaidya U et al. Fetal growth and glucose and insulin metabolism in four-year-old Indian children. *Diabet Med* 1995; 12:330–6.

24. McLeod KJ, Goldrick RB, Whyte HM. The effect of maternal malnutrition on the progeny in the rat: studies on growth, body composition and organ cellularity in first and second generation progeny. *Aust J Exp Biol Med Sci* 1972; 50:435–46.

25. Lemonnier D, Suquet J, Aubert R, Rosselin G. Long term effect of mouse neonate food intake on adult body composition, insulin and glucose serum levels. *Horm Metab Res* 1973; 5:223–4.

26. Philip W, James T, Wallace JM. The role of the mother's body composition in programming. *Pediatr Res* 2001; 50:?

27. Moore SE, Prentice AM. Glucose, insulin and lipid metabolism in rural Gambians exposed to early malnutrition. *Pediatr Res* 2001; 50.

28. Stene LC, Magnus P, Lie RT et al. Birth weight and childhood onset type 1 diabetes: population based cohort study. *Br Med J* 2001; 322:889–92.

29. Leon D. Twins and fetal programming of blood pressure. *Br Med J* 1999; 319:1313–14 (editorial).

30. Langley-Evans SC, Gardner DS, Welham SJ. Intrauterine programming of cardiovascular disease by maternal nutritional status. *Nutrition* 1998; 11:39–47.

31. Kramer MS. Determinants of low birth weight: methodological assessment and meta-analysis. *Bull WHO* 1987; 65:663–737.

32. Gliksman MD, Kawachi I, Hunter D et al. Childhood socioeconomic status and risk of cardiovascular disease in middle aged US women: a prospective study. *J Epidemiol Commun Health* 1995; **19**:10–15.

33. Susser M, Levin B. Ordeals for the fetal programming hypothesis. *Br Med J* 1999; **318**:883–6.

34. Lucas A, Fewtrell MS, Cole TJ. Fetal origins of adult disease – the hypothesis revisited. *Br Med J* 1999; **319**:245–9.

35. Dwyer T, Blizzard L, Morley R et al. Within pair association between birth weight and blood pressure at age 8 in twins from a cohort study. *Br Med J* 1999; **219**:1325–9.

36. Poulter NR, Chang CL, MacGregor AJ et al. Association between birth weight and adult blood pressure in twins: historical cohort study. *Br Med J* 1999; **319**:1330–3.

37. Martin H. Hu I, Gennser G et al. Impaired endothelial function and increased carotid stiffness in 9-year-old children with low birth weight. *Circulation* 2000; **102**:2739–44.

38. Singhal A, Kattenhorn M, Cole TJ et al. Preterm birth, vascular function, and risk factors for atherosclerosis. *Lancet* 2001; **358**:1159–60.

39. Modan M, Halkin H, Almog S et al. Hyperinsulinemia: a link between hypertension, obesity and glucose intolerance. *J Clin Invest* 1985; **75**:809–17.

40. O'Hare JA. The enigma of insulin resistance and hypertension. *Am J Med* 1988; **84**:505–11.

41. Schmidt MI, Watson RL, Duncan BB et al. Clustering of dyslipidemia, hyperuricemia, diabetes and hypertension and its association with fasting insulin and central and overall obesity in a general population. Atherosclerosis Risk in Communities Study Investigators. *Metabolism* 1996; **45**:699–706.

42. Harano Y, Suzuki M, Shinozaki K et al. Clinical impact of insulin resistance syndrome in cardiovascular diseases and its therapeutic approach. *Hypertens Res* 1996; **19 (Suppl 1)**:S81–S85.

43. Crave J, Fimbal S, Lejeune H et al. Effects of diet and metformin administration on sex hormone binding globulin, androgens, and insulin in hirsute and obese women. *J Clin Endocrinol Metab* 1995; **80**:2057–62.

44. Lanzone A, Caruso A, Disimone N et al. Polycystic ovarian disease: a risk factor for gestational diabetes? *J Reprod Med* 1995; **40**:312–16.

45. Urman B, Sarac E, Dogan L et al. Pregnancy in infertile PCOD patients: complications and outcome. *J Reprod Med* 1997; **42**:501–5.

46. Talbott E, Guzick D, Cleria A et al. Coronary heart disease in women with polycystic ovarian syndrome. *Arteroscler Thrombovasc Biol* 1995; **15**:821–6.

47. Capaldo B, Lembo G, Napoli et al. Skeletal muscle is a primary site of insulin resistance in essential hypertension. *Metabolism* 1991; **40**:1320–2.

48. Levy J, Zemel MB, Sowers JR. Role of cellular calcium metabolism in abnormal glucose metabolism and diabetic hypertension. *Am J Med* 1989; **87 (Suppl 6A)**: 7S–16S.

49. Resnick LM. Cellular ions in hypertension, insulin resistance, obesity and diabetes: a unifying theme. *J Am Soc Nephrol* 1992; **3**:S78–S85.

50. O'Hare JA, Minaker K, Young JB et al. Insulin increases plasma norepinephrine (NE) and lowers plasma potassium equally in lean and obese men. *Clin Res* 1985; **33**:441A.

51. Rowe JW, Young JB, Minaker K et al. Effect of insulin and glucose infusions on sympathetic nervous system activity in normal man. *Diabetes* 1981; **30**:219–25.

52. Christlieg AR. Renin, angiotensin and norepinephrine in alloxan diabetes. *Diabetes* 1974; **23**:962–70.

53. Weidmann P, Beretta-Piccoli C, Trost BN. Pressor factors and responsiveness in hypertension accompanying diabetes mellitus. *Hypertension* 1985; **7 (Suppl II)**:II33–II42.

54. Zemel MB. Insulin resistance vs. hyperinsulinemia in hypertension: insulin regulation of Ca^{2+} transport and Ca^{2+} regulation of insulin sensitivity. *J Nutr* 1995; **125 (Suppl 6)**:1738S–1743S.

55. Weidmann P, Bohlen L, de Courten M. Insulin resistance and hyperinsulinemia in hypertension. *J Hypertens* 1995; **13 (Suppl 2)**:S65–S72.

56. McCarthy MF. Insulin resistance – not hyperinsulinemia – is pathogenic in essential hypertension. *Med Hypotheses* 1994; **42**:226–36.

57. Byyny RL, Lo Verde M, Lloyd S et al. Cytosolic calcium and insulin resistance in elderly patients with essential hypertension. *Am J Hypertens* 1992; **5**: 459–64.

58. Weidmann P, de Courten M, Boehlen L. Insulin resistance, hyperinsulinemia and hypertension. *J Hypertens* 1993; **11 (Suppl 5)**:S27–S38.

59. Canessa M. Erythrocyte sodium–lithium countertransport: another link between essential hypertension and diabetes. *Curr Opin Nephrol Hypertens* 1994; **3**: 511–17.

60. Olefsky JM. Pathogenesis of non-insulin dependent diabetes (type II). In: (DeGroot LJ, Besser GM, Cahill JC, eds) *Endocrinology*, 2nd edn. (WB Saunders: Philadelphia, 1989) 1369–88.

61. Rotter JL, Vadheim CM, Rimoin DL. Genetics of diabetes mellitus. In: (Rifkin H, Porte D JR, eds) *Diabetes Mellitus: Theory and Practice*. (Elsevier: New York, 1990) 378–413.

62. Gilbert RE, Jerums G, Cooper ME. Diabetes and hypertension: prognostic and therapeutic considerations. *Blood Press* 1995; **4**:329–38.

63. DeFronzo RA, Goodman AM et al. Efficacy of metformin in patients with non-insulin dependent diabetes mellitus. *N Engl J Med* 1995; **333**:541–9.

64. Nolan JJ, Ludvik MD, Beerdsen RN et al. Improvement in glucose tolerance and insulin resistance in obese subjects treated with troglitazone. *N Engl J Med* 1995; **331**:1188–93.

65. Kalkhoff RK, Kissebah AH, Kim HJ. Carbohydrate and lipid metabolism during normal pregnancy: relationship to gestational hormones. In: (Merkatz IR, Adam PAJ, eds) *The Diabetic Pregnancy: A Perinatal Perspective.* (Grune & Stratton: New York, 1979.)

66. Bergmann RN, Phillips LS, Cobelli C. Physiologic evaluation of factors controlling glucose tolerance in man. Measurement of insulin sensitivity and beta-cell sensitivity from the response to intravenous glucose. *J Clin Invest* 1981; **68**:1456–67.

67. Buchanon TA, Metzger BE, Freinkel N et al. Insulin sensitivity and B-cell responsiveness to glucose during late pregnancy in lean and moderately obese women with normal glucose tolerance or mild gestational diabetes. *Am J Obstet Gynecol* 1990; **162**:1008–14.

68. Freinkel N, Metzger BE, Phelps RL et al. Gestational diabetes mellitus: heterogeneity of maternal age, weight, insulin secretion, HLA, antigens, and islet cell antibodies and the impact of maternal metabolism on pancreatic B-cell function and somatic growth in the offspring. *Diabetes* 1985; **34 (Suppl 2)**:1–7.

69. Yen SCC, Tsai CC, Vela. Gestational diabetogenesis: quantitative analysis of glucose–insulin interrelationship between normal pregnancy and pregnancy with gestational diabetes. *Am J Obstet Gynecol* 1971; **111**:792–800.

70. Metzger BE, Cho NH, Roston SM et al. Prepregnancy weight and antepartum insulin secretion predict glucose tolerance five years after gestational diabetes mellitus. *Diabetes Care* 1995; **16**:1598–605.

71. O'Sullivan JB. The Boston gestational diabetes studies: review and perspectives. In: (Sutherland HW, Stowers JM, Pearson DWM, eds) *Carbohydrate Metabolism in Pregnancy and the Newborn.* (Springer-Verlag: London, 1989) 287–94.

72. Peters RK, Kjos SL, Xiang A et al. Long-term diabetogenic effect of a single pregnancy in women with prior gestational diabetes mellitus. *Lancet* 1996; **347**:227–30.

73. Abbasi F, McLaughlin T, Lamendola C et al. Comparison of plasminogen activator inhibitor-1 concentration in insulin-resistant versus insulin-sensitive healthy women. *Arterioscler Thromb Vasc Biol* 1999; **19**:2818–21.

74. Segal KR, Landt M, Klein S. Relationship between insulin sensitivity and plasma leptin concentration in lean and obese men. *Diabetes* 1996; **45**:988–91.

75. Fernandez-Real JM, Broch M, Ricart W et al. Plasma levels of the soluble fraction of tumor necrosis factor receptor 2 and insulin resistance. *Diabetes* 1998; **47**:1757–62.

76. Greco P, Loverro G, Selvaggi L. Does gestational diabetes represent an obstetric risk factor? *Gynecol Obstet Invest* 1994; **37**:242–5.

77. Rudge MV, Calderon IM, Ramos MD et al. Hypertension disorders in pregnant women with diabetes mellitus. *Am J Perinatol* 1997; **44**:11–15.

78. Sacks DA, Greenspoon JS, Abu-Fadil S et al. Toward universal criteria for gestational diabetes: the 75-gram glucose tolerance test in pregnancy. *Am J Obstet Gynecol* 1995; **172**:607–14.

79. Sermer M, Naylor CD, Gare DJ et al. Impact of increasing carbohydrate intolerance on maternal–fetal outcomes in 3637 women without gestational diabetes. *Am J Obstet Gynecol* 1995; **173**:146–56.

80. Pennison EH, Egerman RS. Perinatal outcomes in gestational diabetes: a comparison of criteria for diagnosis. *Am J Obstet Gynecol* 2001; **184**:1118–21.

81. Schmidt MI, Duncan BB, Reichelt AJ et al. Gestational diabetes mellitus diagnosed with a 2-h 75-g oral glucose tolerance test and adverse pregnancy outcomes. *Diabetes Care* 2001; **24**:1151–5.

82. Schaffir JA, Lockwood CJ, Lapinski R et al. Incidence of pregnancy-induced hypertension among gestational diabetics. *Am J Perinatol* 1995; **12**:252–4.

83. Levy MT, Jacoaber SJ, Sowers JR. Hypertensive disorders of pregnancy in southwestern Navajo Indians. *Arch Intern Med* 1994; **154**:2181–3.

84. Sowers JR, Saleh AA, Sokol RJ. Hyperinsulinemia and insulin resistance are associated with pre-eclampsia in African-American women. *Am J Hypertens* 1995; **8**:1–4.

85. Cioffi FJ, Amorosa LF, Vintzileos AM et al. Relationship of insulin resistance and hyperinsulinemia to blood pressure during pregnancy. *J Matern Fetal Med* 1997; **6**:174–9.

86. Solomon CG, Graves SW, Greene MF et al. Glucose intolerance as a predictor of hypertension of pregnancy. *Hypertension* 1994; **23**:717–21.

87. Martinez AE, Gonzales OM, Quninones GA et al. Hyperinsulinemia in glucose-tolerant women with pre-eclampsia: a controlled study. *Am J Hypertens* 1996; **9**:610–14.

88. Joffe GM, Esterlitz JR, Levine RJ et al. The relationship between abnormal glucose tolerance and hypertensive disorders of pregnancy in healthy nulliparous women. *Am J Obstet Gynecol* 1998; **179**:1032–7

89. Gu H, Rong L, Sai JY. Insulin resistance and pregnancy-induced hypertension. *Chung Hua Fu Chan Ko Tsa Chih* 1994; **29**:711–3.

90. Oren S, Golzman B, Reitblatt T et al. Gestational diabetes mellitus and hypertension in pregnancy: hemodynamics and diurnal arterial pressure profile. *J Hum Hypertens* 1996; **10**:505–9.

91. Graves SW, Lincoln K, Cook SL et al. Digitalis-like factor and digoxin-like immunoreactive factor in

diabetic women with pre-eclampsia, transient hypertension of pregnancy and normotensive pregnancy. *Am J Hypertens* 1995; 8:5–11.

92. Fuh MM, Yin CS, Pei D et al. Resistance to insulin-mediated glucose uptake and hyperinsulinemia in women who had pre-eclampsia in pregnancy. *Am J Hypertens* 1995; 8:768–71.

93. Laivuori II, Tikkanen MJ, Ylikorkala O. Hyperinsulinemia 17 years after pre-eclamptic first pregnancy. *J Clin Endocrinol Metab* 1996; 81:2908–11.

94. Jacober SJ, Morris DA, Sower JR. Postpartum blood pressure and insulin sensitivity in African-American women with recent pre-eclampsia. *Am J Hypertens* 1994; 7:933–6.

95. Hanson U, Persson B. Epidemiology of pregnancy-induced hypertension and preeclampsia in type 1 (insulin-dependent) diabetic pregnancies in Sweden. *Acta Obstet Gynecol Scand* 1998; 77:620–4.

96. Garner PR. Type 1 diabetes mellitus and pregnancy. *Lancet* 1995; 346:152–61.

97. Greene MF, Hare JW, Krache M et al. Prematurity among insulin-requiring diabetic gravid women. *Am J Obstet Gynecol* 1989; 161:106–11.

98. Siddiqi T, Rosenn B, Mimouni F et al. Hypertension during pregnancy in insulin-dependent diabetic women. *Obstet Gynecol* 1991; 77:514–19.

99. Combs CA, Rosenn B, Kitmiller JL et al. Early-pregnancy proteinuria in diabetes related to preeclampsia. *Obstet Gynecol* 1993; 82:802–7.

100. Gordon M, Landon MB, Samuels P et al. Perinatal outcome and long-term follow-up associated with modern management of diabetic nephropathy. *Obstet Gynecol* 1996; 87:401–9.

101. Reece EA, Coustan DR, Hayslett JP et al. Diabetic nephropathy: pregnancy performance and fetomaternal outcome. *Am J Obstet Gynecol* 1988; 59:56–66.

102. Hanson U, Persson B. Outcome of pregnancies complicated by type 1 insulin-dependent diabetes in Sweden: acute pregnancy complications, neonatal mortality and morbidity. *Am J Perinatol* 1993; 10:330–3.

103. Diamond MP, Shah DM, Hester RA et al. Complication of insulin-dependent diabetic pregnancies by preeclampsia and/or chronic hypertension: analysis of outcome. *Am J Perinatol* 1985; 2:263–7.

104. Sibai BM, Lindheimer ML, Hauth J et al. Risk factors for preeclampsia, abruptio placentae, and adverse neonatal outcomes among women with chronic hypertension. *N Engl J Med* 1998; 339:667–71.

105. Miodovnik M, Rosenn BM, Khoury JC et al. Does pregnancy increase the risk for development and progression of diabetic nephropathy? *Am J Obstet Gynecol* 1996; 174:1180–91.

106. Kovilam O, Rosenn B, Miodovnik M et al. Is proliferative retinopathy a risk factor for adverse pregnancy outcome in women with Type 1 diabetes? *J Soc Gynecol Invest* 1997; 4 (Suppl 1):152A.

107. Sibai BM, Caritis S, Hauth J et al. Risks of preeclampsia and adverse neonatal outcomes among women with pregestational diabetes mellitus. *Am J Obstet Gynecol* 2000; 182:364–9.

108. Garner PR, D'Alton ME, Dudley DK et al. Preeclampsia in diabetic pregnancies. *Am J Obstet Gynecol* 1990; 163:505–8.

109. Caritis S, Sibai B, Hauth J et al. Predictors of preeclampsia in women at high risk. National Institution of Child Health and Human Development Network of Maternal–Fetal Medicine Units. *Am J Obstet Gynecol* 1998; 179:949–51.

110. Ekbom P and the Copenhagen preeclampsia in Diabetic Pregnancy Study Group. Pre-pregnancy microalbuminuria predicts preeclampsia in insulin-dependent diabetes mellitus. *Lancet* 1999; 353:377.

111. Bar J, Chen R, Schoenfeld A et al. Pregnancy outcome in patients with insulin dependent diabetes mellitus and diabetic nephropathy treated with ACE inhibitors before pregnancy. *J Pediatr Endocrinol Metab* 1999; 12:659–65.

112. Hod M, van Dijk DJ, Karp M et al. Diabetic nephropathy and pregnancy: the effect of ACE inhibitors prior to pregnancy on fetomaternal outcome – preliminary report. *Nephrol Dialysis Transplant* 1995; 10:2328–33.

113. Bar J, Hod M, Merlob P. Angiotensin-converting enzyme inhibitors use in the first trimester of pregnancy. *Int J Risk Safety Med* 1997; 9:1–4.

114. Feldkamp M, Jones KL, Ornoy A et al. ACE inhibitors use in the first trimester of pregnancy. *MMWR* 1997; 46:240–2.

115. Caritis S, Sibai B, Hauth J et al. Low-dose aspirin to prevent preeclampsia in women at high risk. *N Engl J Med* 1998; 339:667–71.

116. Viberti CC, Mackintosh D, Keen H. Determinants of the penetration of proteins through the glomerular barrier in insulin-dependent diabetes mellitus. *Diabetes* 1983; 32 (Suppl 2):92–5.

117. Hostetter TH, Rennke HG, Brenner BM. The case for intrarenal hypertension in the initiation and progression of diabetic and other glomerulopathies. *Am J Med* 1982; 72:375–80.

118. Viberti GC. Prognostic significance of microalbuminuria in insulin dependent diabetes mellitus. *Kidney Int* 1992; 41:836–9.

119. Schmitz A, Vaeth M. Microalbuminuria: a major risk factor in non insulin dependent diabetes. A 10 year follow-up study of 503 patients. *Diabet Med* 1988; 5:126–34.

120. Viberti GC, Hill BD, Jarrett RJ et al. Microalbuminuria is a predictor of clinical nephropathy in insulin dependent diabetes mellitus. *Lancet* 1982; 2:1430–2.

121. Parving HH, Jensen H, Mogensen CE et al. Increased urinary albumin excretion rate in benign essential hypertension. *Lancet* 1974; 1:1190–2.

122. Yudkin JS, Forrest RD, Jackson CA. Microalbuminuria as a predictor of vascular disease in non diabetic subjects. Islington Diabetic Survey. *Lancet* 1988; **2**:530–3.

123. Bar J, Hod M, Erman A et al. Microalbuminuria: prognostic and therapeutic implications in diabetic and hypertensive pregnancy. *Diabet Med* 1995; **12**:649–56.

124. Bar J, Hod M, Erman A et al. Microalbuminuria as an early predictor of hypertensive complications in pregnant women at high risk. *Am J Kidney Dis* 1996; **28**:220–5.

125. Bar J, Kaplan B, Wittenberg C et al. Microalbuminuria after pregnancy complicated by pre-eclampsia. *Nephrol Dial Transplant* 1999; **14**:1129–32.

126. Friedman S, Rabinerson D, Bar J et al. Microalbuminuria following gestational diabetes. *Acta Obstet Gynecol Scand* 1995; **74**:176–81.

127. Parving HH, Lehnert H, Brochner-Mortensen J et al. The effect of irbesartan on the developement of diabetic nephropathy in patients with Type 2 diabetes. *N Engl J Med* 2001; **345**:870–8.

37

Diabetic retinopathy
Tamar Perri, Nino Loya, Moshe Hod

Introduction

Diabetic retinopathy is the most common chronic complication of diabetes mellitus.[1] The estimated incidence is up to 98% in patients with Type 1 (insulin-dependent) diabetes mellitus of > 15 years duration, and 100% in patients with Type 1 diabetes of 25 years duration.[2] It is the leading cause of blindness in patients between the ages of 24 and 64 in both the United States and the United Kingdom,[3,4] affecting 20–30% of all diabetic women in the reproductive age group. However, the mutual effects of pregnancy and retinopathy, though long a subject of research and debate, remain unclear, and data on methods of diagnosis and management in pregnancy are sparse. There is some evidence indicating that retinopathy may worsen during pregnancy, at least in some women.[5,6] Therefore, all pregnant women with diabetes should undergo ophthalmic evaluation and follow-up.

Classification of diabetic retinopathy

Diabetic retinopathy is graded according to the semiquantitative assessment of the morphological lesions on fundus photographs. The grading system considers mainly the type and number of retinopathy lesions, while the diagnostic value of the regional distribution of the lesions is largely unknown.[7]

Diabetic retinopathy has a wide spectrum of presentations, from early background or nonproliferative disease to preproliferative and proliferative disease. The retinal changes are a consequence of the systemic microangiopathy of diabetes, with modifications related to the intraocular environment. The underlying vascular disorders are arteriolar hyalinosis (which together with abnormalities in the circulating blood can give rise to focal capillary closure), venular dilatation, and capillaro-pathy in the form of pericyte degeneration, basement membrane thickening and microaneurysm formation.[8]

The earliest changes result from damage to the small blood vessels in the retina. Microaneurysm, or a protrusion of a retinal capillary, is the first lesion noted, appearing ophthalmoscopically as a red dot. It can be identified in 2% of patients with Type 1 diabetes within 2 years of onset of the disease, and in 98% of patients within 15 years.[9] In some cases, extravasation of blood from the retinal capillaries into the inner nuclear layer of the retina creates 'blots' of varying sizes with irregular margins and uneven densities. Yellow collections of lipoproteins, called hard exudates, that leak from the microaneurysms into the outer layer of the retina, may be seen, scattered or grouped

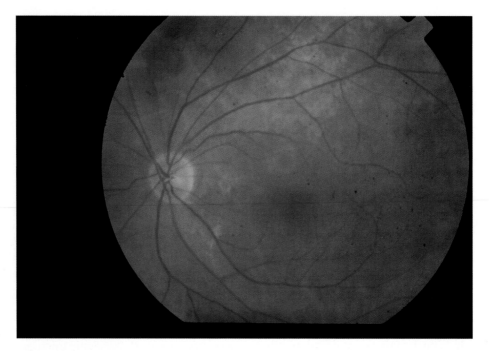

Figure 37.1. *Normal fundus.*

together, filling or partially filling the area surrounding the microaneurysm (Fig. 37.1 represents the normal fundus while background retinopathy is shown in Fig. 37.2).[5]

The preproliferative stage of diabetic retinopathy is characterized by ischemic lesions caused by the increasing closure of the capillaries. The ischemia-induced interruption of axoplasmic transport leads to the localized accumulation of axoplasmic debris resembling white or grayish-white cottonwool spots in the retinal nerve fiber layer.

The hallmark of proliferative retinopathy is retinal and preretinal neovascularization, which occurs in response to the increased ischemia (Fig. 37.3).[8] Presumably, the nutrient-starved retina sends out a chemical message to stimulate the growth of new blood vessels (neovascularization) in the eye. These vessels often grow on the surface of the retina, at the optic nerve, or on the iris, and may penetrate the outlining membrane of the retina. They are fragile and

prone to bleeding, placing the patient at significant risk of visual impairment due to vitreous hemorrhage, retinal detachment and uncontrolled glaucoma. The Diabetic Retinopathy Study Research Group[10] has identified four risk factors for severe visual loss in diabetic retinopathy (Box 37.1). When untreated, affected patients have a 30% risk of visual acuity deterioration to less than 5/200 within 3 years and a 50% risk within 5 years. In their series of patients with diabetic retinopathy, Fong et al[11] listed the following reasons for persistent visual loss: vitreous or preretinal hemorrhage; macular edema or macular pigmentary changes related to macular edema; macular or retinal detachment; neovascular glaucoma.

Pathogenesis

Chronic hyperglycemia is considered to be the primary cause of diabetic retinopathy and

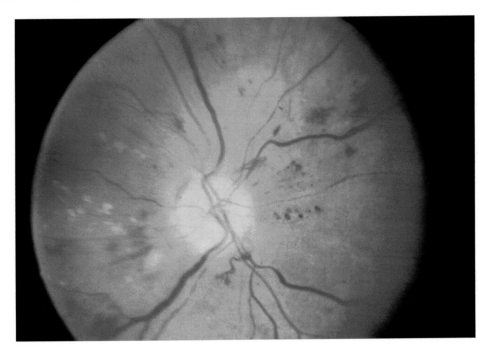

Figure 37.2.   *Background diabetic retinopathy.*

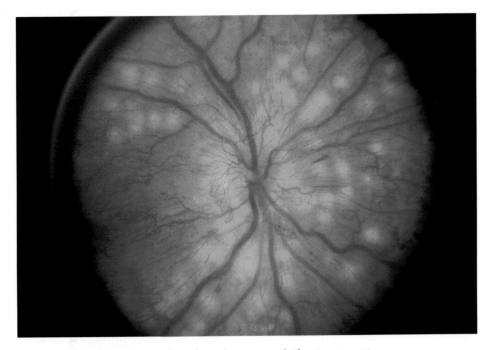

Figure 37.3.   *Proliferative retinopathy, after photocoagulation treatment.*

- New vessels on or within one disk diameter of the optic disk and at least one quarter of the disk area in extent, with or without preretinal or vitreous hemorrhage.
- Any new vessels on or within one disk diameter of the optic disk, with preretinal or vitreous hemorrhage.
- New vessels anywhere in the retina more than one disk diameter from the optic disk and at least one half of the disk area in extent (including the total area of all new vessels in the ocular fundus), with preretinal or vitreous hemorrhage.
- Extensive preretinal or vitreous hemorrhage that hides probable new vessels meeting the above criteria.

Box 37.1. High-risk characteristics for severe visual loss from proliferative retinopathy (from Van Dyk et al,[20] with permission).

other complications of diabetes, though this has not been proven definitively. It appears to act by different mechanisms in different tissues.[12] Genetic, environmental, immunologic and hormonal factors may also play a role.[12–18]

Hyperglycemia affects various biochemical pathways in the retinal microvasculature. The excess sorbitol and fructose may accumulate in the retinal capillary endothelial cells, with consequent osmotic damage to the cells and thickening of the basement membrane.[19] The basement membrane thickening is the earliest histologic abnormality seen in diabetic retinopathy, followed by loss of pericytes because of the interruption in their nutritional transport weakening of the capillary wall, and formation of microaneurysms.[20] The microaneurysms are permeable to water and large molecules, allowing the accumulation of fluid and lipids in the retina, and, consequently, further thickening and rupture of the capillary wall and intraretinal hemorrhage. The enzyme aldose reductase in the polyol pathway may play a major role in the development of diabetic retinopathy, though evidence remains contradictory.[21]

Proliferative diabetic retinopathy is apparently promoted by the hypoxic regulation of angiogenic growth factors, particularly the vascular endothelial growth factors (VEGF)

family. Boulton et al[22] reported that the intensity of immunostaining of VEGF in diabetic eyes was directly correlated with the severity of the retinopathy. Khaliq et al[23] found that placental growth factor (PGF) immunoreactivity was intensely localized to the endothelial and perivascular regions of the newly formed blood vessels in excised fibrovascular preretinal membranes, and also in the adjacent superficial retinal vessels. PGF localization was weak or absent in diabetic retinas with non-vascular proliferation, in normal retinas and in diabetic retinas treated extensively with scatter laser photocoagulation. These results imply that PGF plays a role in the pathogenesis of proliferative diabetic retinopathy.

Frank et al[24] reported that epiretinal and choroidal neovascular membranes contain both VEGF and basic fibroblast growth factor, possibly a critical mitogen for neovascularization. They suggested that since expression of some growth factors is stimulated by hypoxia, their localization within the choroidal neovascular membranes may indicate that hypoxia is an etiologic factor in both choroidal and retinal neovascularization. Furthermore, more than one growth factor may contribute to pathologic angiogenesis.

Katsura et al[25] found that levels of hepatocyte growth factor (HGF) are elevated in the active proliferative diabetic retinopathy stage, and two studies reported an upregulation of serum insulin-like growth factor (IGF) preceding retinal deterioration, indicating a possible cause–effect relationship.[26,27]

Impact of pregnancy on the progression of diabetic retinopathy

The question of whether pregnancy influences the development of retinopathy or the progression of established retinopathy is still unanswered.[28–36] Some investigators have reported that pregnancy is related to retinopathy exacerbation, with reported rates of progression from 17 to 70%,[28–34] whereas other, more recent, studies failed to support these findings.[6,35,36] Be that as it may, certain risk factors are apparently associated with poorer outcomes of retinopathy in pregnancy.

The effect of pregnancy on retinopathy might be explained by such normal pregnancy-associated changes such as the rise in growth hormone level, which in turn stimulates IGF-I production, a possible mechanism in the deterioration of retinopathy,[26,27] as mentioned above. Pregnancy is also associated with marked physiological changes, such as increased blood volume, heart rate and contractility, and, as a result, a marked increase in cardiac output. It may also induce an increase in retinal blood flow, which could damage diabetic vessels. Chen et al,[37] in a laser Doppler velocimetry study, found that in pregnant diabetic patients who showed retinal deteriorations, blood flow increased throughout pregnancy as compared with the postpartum period. However, as these patients also had worse glycemic control (higher HbA1c levels prior to and throughout pregnancy), it was not clear if the deterioration

was attributable to the increase in blood flow alone.

In a 12-year prospective study, Horvat et al[29] noted that proliferative retinopathy was present at the beginning of pregnancy or developed during or after pregnancy in 16% of women with Type 1 diabetes. The only known factor directly related to ocular complications was the duration of the diabetes. Thus, women with gestational or recent-onset diabetes are at minimal risk of acquiring diabetic retinopathy during pregnancy, whereas 97% of those who have had diabetes for 20 years or more will have retinopathy, including up to 50% with proliferative disease.[2] A similar correlation was also reported by Moloney and Drury[28] and Price et al.[38]

The severity of retinopathy prior to pregnancy may also be important: Serup[39] found that retinopathy worsened in pregnancy in 50% of the women in whom it was present at the onset of pregnancy, although postpartum regression was common as well. A third potential risk factor is poor glycemic control prior to pregnancy on the one hand, or too-tight glycemic control during pregnancy on the other. Lauszus et al[40] noted a relationship between changes in retinopathy and 24 hour blood pressure, blood glucose level, albuminuria and adverse perinatal outcome. Grade of retinopathy was also associated with HbA1c levels before and after pregnancy, but only when glycemia was not well controlled. However, in a systematic review, Walkinshaw[41] found no clear benefit for very tight glycemic control in pregnant diabetic women.

Chew et al[42] prospectively followed 155 diabetic women from the preconceptional period to 1 month postpartum. Proliferative retinopathy developed in 6.3% of the patients who had baseline retinopathy and in 29% of those with moderate to severe baseline retinopathy. The risk of progression of the retinopathy was increased when initial glycosylated hemoglobin levels increased, even by only 6 standard deviations (SD) above the control mean. The risk may have been related to the suboptimal control itself or to the rapid improvement in metabolic control that occurred in early pregnancy. They concluded that the abrupt institution of improved diabetic control during pregnancy could lead to a deterioration in background retinopathy. These findings were supported by other studies as well.[43]

To test the hypothesis that women with Type 1 (insulin-dependent) diabetes and chronic or pregnancy-induced hypertensive disorders are at risk of developing retinopathic complications during pregnancy, Rosenn et al[44] conducted ophthalmologic evaluations in 154 diabetic women throughout pregnancy and at 6–12 weeks postpartum. They found that retinopathy progressed in 51 patients. The factors significantly associated with the progression of retinopathy were changes in glycemic control early in pregnancy, chronic hypertension and pregnancy-induced hypertension. In a recent literature review by Aiello et al,[45] intensive blood glucose control and control of systemic hypertension were found to reduce the risk of new-onset diabetic retinopathy and to slow the progression of existing diabetic retinopathy. Both hypertension and retinopathy might be considered part of the spectrum of the systemic vasculopathy of diabetes that affects different organs.

In summary, the progression of retinopathy in pregnancy depends on a variety of factors, including the severity of retinopathy at conception, adequacy of treatment, duration of diabetes, metabolic control before and during pregnancy, and the presence of additional vascular damage (i.e. pre-existing or concomitant hypertensive disorder).

Rosenn et al,[44] in the same prospective study, also noted that the diabetic retinopathy regressed to the near-normal state in the postpartum period. Other authors have reported similar findings in women with mild diabetic retinopathy. Hellstedt et al,[46] in a follow-up study of 13 women during pregnancy and for 1 year afterwards, suggested that pregnancy is associated with a continuous microaneurysm turnover, with the count increasing continuously during pregnancy, peaking at 3 months postpartum and dropping thereafter. Once blood glucose levels are normalized, they suggested that mild retinopathy is temporarily aggravated. Thus, a long follow-up period after pregnancy is needed to assess the influence of pregnancy on diabetic retinopathy.

Several investigators have addressed the issue of a possible relationship between diabetic retinopathy and newborn outcome. Moloney and Drury[28] assessed 53 diabetic women by retinal photography every 6 weeks throughout pregnancy and for 6 months postpartum. They noted that maternal retinal hemorrhages or neovascularization was associated with increased infant morbidity. McElvy et al[47] performed ophthalmologic evaluations in 205 women with Type 1 diabetes before 14 weeks and 20 weeks gestation, and again in late gestation or postpartum. Fifty-nine showed progression of retinopathy (29%) and advanced White classification. There was a direct correlation between retinopathy and reduced fetal growth: affected women had infants of lower mean birthweights and more infants who were small for gestational age. There were no differences between the progression and non-progression groups in gestational age at delivery, macrosomia, preterm delivery, respiratory distress syndrome, neonatal hypoglycemia or neonatal death. Similar results were reported by Klein et al[48] in a logistic regression analysis of maternal age, duration of diabetes, glycosylated hemoglobin, proteinuria, cigarette smoking status and severity of diabetic retinopathy. Only the last variable significantly predicted an adverse neonatal outcome.

Lauszus et al[40] reviewed the ophthalmic, obstetric and pediatric records of 26 women with known proliferative retinopathy before pregnancy. The results yielded significant elevations in the preterm delivery rate and serious neonatal morbidity. However, low birth weight was more frequently associated with combined nephropathy and proliferative retinopathy than with retinopathy alone.

Treatment of diabetic retinopathy during pregnancy

The introduction of retinal laser photocoagulation was one of the greatest therapeutic advances in ophthalmology of the twentieth century.[5] Studies have shown that it can reduce the rate of progression to blindness in patients with severe proliferative retinopathy.[49,50] Argon laser photocoagulation therapy is equally effective in pregnant and non-pregnant diabetic patients;[51] however, Sinclair et al[52] claimed that proliferative lesions occurring early in pregnancy tended to be resistant to treatment. The current standard treatment for proliferative retinopathy consists of panretinal (scatter) placement of 1200–1800 closely spaced photocoagulation burns around the midperipheral retina, sparing the macula and the region immediately surrounding the optic nerve. Extensive photocoagulation leads to significant regression of the neovascular complexes in 63% of cases:[53] it has a protective effect when performed prior to or during pregnancy.[32]

Routine ophthalmologic examinations have little utility in class A (gestational) diabetes. In a chart study of 100 pregnant patients with diabetes, Puza and Malee[54] noted retinopathy rates of 19, 56 and 92% in patients with White classes B, C and D, respectively, with a

concomitant progression in background retinopathy of 0, 33 and 45%. In patients with classes F, R and RF, 100% demonstrated retinopathy and 46% progressed, 77% with proliferative disease; 15% required laser treatment during pregnancy. The authors proposed that subsequent ophthalmologic examinations be based on White's classification and the initial examination results. Rigorous follow-up is warranted for classes D–R. Since proliferative retinopathy rarely progresses after complete regression,[55] photocoagulation treatment should optimally be completed before conception.

According to the Early Treatment Diabetic Retinopathy Study Research Group[56] criteria, in patients with diabetic macular edema, photocoagulation should be performed during pregnancy, because spontaneous improvement rarely occurs after delivery. If the edema does not respond well to photocoagulation, hospitalization is required, with diuretic treatment and occasionally steroids.

Management recommendations

Pregnant patients with Type 1 diabetes need to be managed by a protocol based on early recognition, a rigid follow-up schedule and vision-sparing therapies when indicated to prevent visual loss. In general, patients are advised to plan pregnancy earlier in life. At the first preconception visit, metabolic control is initiated gradually, since rapid control to attain euglycemia may actually increase the risk of retinopathy progression, as discussed earlier. Complete eye evaluation should be performed before conception, every trimester, and at 3 and 6 months postpartum. Dilated fundus examination, 60° stereoscopic color fundus photography and laser treatment are all safe during pregnancy. If retinopathy is detected before or right after conception, fluorescein angiography is done; if retinopathy is detected during pregnancy, fluorescein angiography is usually avoided, though it has not been proven to have an adverse effect on the fetus.

Closer follow-up is warranted when moderate to severe proliferative retinopathy is noted at the beginning of pregnancy or when progression is noted. Panretinal photocoagulation is performed in the presence of proliferative or severe non-proliferative disease. Macular edema is treated by laser, diuretics and steroids. A schema of the recommended therapeutic approach is presented in Table 37.1. Although the earlier studies recommended early delivery, as soon as lung maturation was achieved, in pregnancies complicated by retinopathy and other vascular diseases, more recent research has shown that a well-controlled diabetic pregnancy can be allowed to continue to term in order to avoid iatrogenic prematurity, the risk of amniocentesis, failed induction of labor due to an unfavorable cervix and an unnecessary Cesarean section.[57] The obstetric protocol that best correlated with outcome was a combination of intensive diabetes control, self-monitoring of fetal movements, and regular fetal growth and cervical assessment.

The Valsalva maneuver during labor might induce vitreous hemorrhage from active neovascularization;[58,59] the role of an elective Cesarean section in these cases is controversial. The patient and the obstetrician should discuss the mode of delivery in advance.

Summary

Diabetes poses a considerable risk during pregnancy for both mother and fetus, especially if

Stage of diabetes	Therapeutic measures before conception	Therapeutic measures during pregnancy
No DR	–	Follow-up only
Mild NPDR	Inform patient about risk of aggravation	Follow-up each trimester
Moderate to severe NPDR		
PDR	PRP before conception; postpone conception until regression is observed	PRP; consider cesarean section

DR, diabetic retinopathy; NPDR, non-proliferative DR; PDR, proliferative DR; PRP, panretinal photocoagulation.

Table 37.1. *Schema of therapeutic approaches to pregnant diabetic women. (Copyright © 1995 American Diabetes Association. Reprinted with permission from American Diabetes Association, Diabet Rev 1995;**3**:632–40.)*

vascular disease such as retinopathy was present before conception. Not only may the pregnancy itself be complicated, but the retinopathy may also worsen. Nevertheless, it is now clear that White's[60] advice in 1971 to terminate pregnancies in diabetic patients with progressive proliferative retinopathy is no longer valid. Preconception preparation by a multidisciplinary team is required to achieve an optimal diabetic and ophthalmologic status, with strict follow-up during pregnancy. Each complication that arises during pregnancy should be treated promptly, and towards the end of pregnancy, the delivery route and date should be discussed between the patient and the treating physician(s). Follow-up should be continued after delivery to detect and treat late complications. Only on rare occasions should the patient with diabetic retinopathy be advised against pregnancy.[61] Nowadays, with careful professional care, a favorable pregnancy outcome can usually be expected with minimal or no deterioration in ophthalmologic status.

References

1. Reece EA, Homko CJ, Hagay Z. Diabetic retinopathy in pregnancy. *Obstet Gynecol Clin N Am* 1996; **23**: 161–71.
2. Klein R, Klein BE, Moss SE et al. The Wisconsin epidemiologic study of diabetic retinopathy. II. Prevalence and risk of diabetic retinopathy when age at diagnosis is less than 30 years. *Arch Ophthalmol* 1984; **102**:520–6.
3. Kahn HA, Moorehead HB. Statistics on blindness in the model reporting area, 1969–1970. Department of Health, Education and Welfare, Publication no. NIH 73-427. (US Government Printing Office: Washington, DC, 1973.)
4. Foulds WS, MacCuish A, Barrie T et al. Diabetic retinopathy in the west of Scotland: its detection and prevalence and the cost-effectiveness of a prospective screening program. *Health Bull (Edinburgh)* 1983; **41**:318–26.
5. Elman KD, Welch RA, Frank RN et al. Diabetic retinopathy in pregnancy: a review. *Obstet Gynecol* 1980; **75**:119–27.
6. Axer-Siegel R, Hod M, Fink-Cohen S et al. Diabetic retinopathy during pregnancy. *Ophthalmology* 1996; **103**:1815–19.
7. Bek T, Helgesen A. The regional distribution of diabetic retinopathy lesions may reflect risk factors for progression of the disease. *Acta Ophthalmol Scand* 2001; **79**:501–5.
8. Garner A. Histopathology of diabetic retinopathy in man. *Eye* 1993; **7**:250–3.
9. Klein R. The epidemiology of diabetic retinopathy: findings from the Wisconsin Epidemiologic Study of Diabetic Retinopathy. *Int Ophthalmol Clin* 1987; **27**:230–8.
10. The Diabetic Retinopathy Study Research Group. Four risk factors for severe visual loss in diabetic retinopathy. The third report from the Diabetic Retinopathy Study. *Arch Ophthalmol* 1979; **97**:654–5.
11. Fong DS, Ferris III FL, Davis MD et al. Causes of severe visual loss in the Early Treatment Diabetic Retinopathy Study: ETDRS report no. 24. Early Treatment Diabetic Retinopathy Study Research Group. *Am J Ophthalmol* 1999; **127**:137–41.
12. Frank RN, Hoffman WH, Podgor MJ et al. Retinopathy in juvenile-onset type I diabetes of short duration. *Diabetes* 1982; **31**:874–82.
13. Rand LI, Krolewski AS, Aiello LM et al. Multiple factors in the prediction of risk of proliferative diabetic retinopathy. *N Engl J Med* 1985; **313**:1433–8.
14. Baker RS, Rand LI, Krolewski AS et al. Influence of HLA-DR phenotype and myopia on the risk of nonproliferative and proliferative diabetic retinopathy. *Am J Ophthalmol* 1986; **102**:693–700.
15. Nguyen HT, Luzio SD, Dolben J et al. Dominant risk factors for retinopathy at clinical diagnosis in patients with type II diabetes mellitus. *J Diabetes Complicat* 1996; **10**:211–19.
16. Sone H, Okuda Y, Kawakami Y et al. Progesterone induces vascular endothelial growth factor on retinal pigment epithelial cells in culture. *Life Sci* 1996; **59**:21–5.
17. Siperstein MD. Diabetic microangiopathy, genetics, environment, and treatment. *Am J Med* 1988; **85**: 119–30.
18. Kawate R, Yamakido M, Nishimoto Y et al. Diabetes mellitus and its vascular complications in Japanese migrants on the Island of Hawaii. *Diabetes Care* 1979; **2**:161–70.
19. Frank RN. On the pathogenesis of diabetic retinopathy. A 1990 update. *Ophthalmology* 1991; **98**:586–93.
20. Van Dyk DJ, Axer-Siegel R, Erman A et al. Diabetic vascular complications and pregnancy. *Diabetes Rev* 1995; **3**:632–40.
21. Park HK, Ahn CW, Lee GT et al. Polymorphism of aldose reductase gene and diabetic microvascular complications in type 2 diabetes mellitus. *Diabetes Res Clin Pract* 2002; **55**:151–7.

22. Boulton M, Foreman D, Williams G et al. VEGF localisation in diabetic retinopathy. *Br J Ophthalmol* 1998; **82**:561–8.

23. Khaliq A, Foreman D, Ahmed A et al. Increased expression of placental growth factor in proliferative diabetic retinopathy. *Lab Invest* 1998; **78**:109–16.

24. Frank RN, Amin RH, Eliott D et al. Basic fibroblast growth factor and vascular endothelial growth factor are present in epiretinal and choroidal neovascular membranes. *Am J Ophthalmol* 1996; **122**:393–403.

25. Katsura Y, Okano T, Noritake M et al. Hepatocyte growth factor in vitreous fluid of patients with proliferative diabetic retinopathy and other retinal disorders. *Diabetes Care* 1998; **21**:1759–63.

26. Chantelau E. Evidence that upregulation of serum IGF-1 concentration can trigger acceleration of diabetic retinopathy. *Br J Ophthalmol* 1998; **82**:725–30.

27. Burgos R, Mateo C, Canton A et al. Vitreous levels of IGF-I, IGF binding protein 1, and IGF binding protein 3 in proliferative diabetic retinopathy: a case–control study. *Diabetes Care* 2000; **23**:80–3.

28. Moloney JB, Drury MI. The effect of pregnancy on the natural course of diabetic retinopathy. *Am J Ophthalmol* 1982; **93**:745–56.

29. Horvat M, Maclean H, Goldberg L et al. Diabetic retinopathy in pregnancy: a 12-year prospective survey. *Br J Ophthalmol* 1980; **64**:398–403.

30. McElvy SS, Demarini S, Miodovnik M et al. Fetal weight and progression of diabetic retinopathy. *Obstet Gynecol* 2001; **97**:587–92.

31. Klein BE, Moss SE, Klein R. Effect of pregnancy on progression of diabetic retinopathy. *Diabetes Care* 1990; **13**:34–40.

32. Dibble CM, Kochenour NK, Worley RJ et al. Effect of pregnancy on diabetic retinopathy. *Obstet Gynecol* 1982; **59**:699–704.

33. Soubrane G, Coscas G. Influence of pregnancy on the evolution of diabetic retinopathy. *Int Ophthalmol Clin* 1998; **38**:187–94.

34. The Diabetes Control and Complications Trial Research Group. Effect of pregnancy on microvascular complications in the Diabetes Control and Complications Trial. *Diabetes Care* 2000; **23**:1084–91.

35. Temple RC, Aldridge VA, Sampson MJ et al. Impact of pregnancy on the progression of diabetic retinopathy in Type 1 diabetes. *Diabet Med* 2001; **18**:573–7.

36. Lovestam-Adrian M, Agardh CD, Aberg A et al. Preeclampsia is a potent risk factor for deterioration of retinopathy during pregnancy in Type 1 diabetic patients. *Diabet Med* 1997; **14**:1059–65.

37. Chen HC, Newson RSB, Patel V et al. Retinal blood flow changes during pregnancy in women with diabetes. *Invest Ophthalmol Vis Sci* 1994; **35**:3199–208.

38. Price JH, Hadden DR, Archer DB et al. Diabetic retinopathy in pregnancy. *Br J Obstet Gynecol* 1984;**91**:11–17.

39. Serup L. Influence of pregnancy on diabetic retinopathy. *Acta Endocrinol Suppl (Copenhagen)* 1986; **277**:122–4.

40. Lauszus F, Klebe JG, Bek T. Diabetic retinopathy in pregnancy during tight metabolic control. *Acta Obstet Gynecol Scand* 2000; **79**:367–70.

41. Walkinshaw SA. Very tight versus tight control for diabetes in pregnancy. *Cochrane Database Syst Rev* 2000; 2:CD000226.

42. Chew EJ, Mills JL, Metzger BE et al. Metabolic control and progression of retinopathy. The Diabetes in Early Pregnancy Study. National Institute of Child Health and Human Development Diabetes in Early Pregnancy Study. *Diabetes Care* 1995; **18**:631–7.

43. Phelps RL, Sakol P, Metzger BE et al. Changes in diabetic retinopathy during pregnancy. Correlations with regulation of hyperglycemia. *Arch Ophthalmol* 1986; **104**:1806–10.

44. Rosenn B, Miodovnik M, Kranias G et al. Progression of diabetic retinopathy in pregnancy: association with hypertension in pregnancy. *Am J Obstet Gynecol* 1992; **166**:1214–18.

45. Aiello LP, Cahill MT, Wong JS. Systemic considerations in the management of diabetic retinopathy. *Am J Ophthalmol* 2001; **132**:760–76.

46. Hellstedt T, Kaaja R, Teramo K et al. The effect of pregnancy on mild diabetic retinopathy. *Graefes Arch Clin Exp Ophthalmol* 1997; **235**:437–41.

47. McElvy SS, Demarini S, Miodovnik M et al. Fetal weight and progression of diabetic retinopathy. *Obstet Gynecol* 2001; **97**:587–92.

48. Klein BE, Klein R, Meuer SM et al. Does the severity of diabetic retinopathy predict pregnancy outcome? *J Diabet Complicat* 1988; **2**:179–84.

49. The Diabetic Retinopathy Study Research Group. Photocoagulation treatment of proliferative diabetic retinopathy: clinical application of Diabetic Retinopathy Study (DRS) findings. DRS Report No. 8. *Ophthalmology* 1982; **88**:583–600.

50. British Multicentre Study Group. Proliferative diabetic retinopathy: treatment with xenon-arc photocoagulation. Interim report of multicentre randomised controlled trial. *Br Med J* 1977; **19**:739–41.

51. Frank RN. Diabetic retinopathy: current concepts of evaluation and treatment. *Clin Endocrinol Metab* 1986; **15**:933–69.

52. Sinclair SH, Nesler C, Foxman B et al. Macular edema and pregnancy in insulin-dependent diabetes. *Am J Ophthalmol* 1984;**97**:154–67.

53. Hercules BL, Wozencroft M, Gayed II et al. Peripheral retinal ablation in the treatment of proliferative diabetic retinopathy during pregnancy. *Br J Ophthalmol* 1980; **64**:87–93.

54. Puza SW, Malee MP. Utilization of routine ophthalmologic examinations in pregnant diabetic patients. *J Matern Fetal Med* 1996; **5**:7–10.

55. Cassar J, Kohner EM, Hamilton AM et al. Diabetic retinopathy and pregnancy. *Diabetologia* 1987; **15**: 105–11.

56. Early Treatment Diabetic Retinopathy Study Research Group. Treatment techniques and clinical guidelines for photocoagulation of diabetic macular edema. Early Treatment Diabetic Retinopathy Study Report No. 2. *Ophthalmology* 1987; **94**:761–74.

57. Jovanovic R, Jovanovic L. Obstetric management when normoglycemia is maintained in diabetic pregnant women with vascular compromise. *Am J Obstet Gynecol* 1984; **149**:617–23.

58. Kassoff A, Catalano RA, Mehu M. Vitreous hemorrhage and the Valsalva maneuver in proliferative diabetic retinopathy. *Retina* 1988; **8**:174–6.

59. Jones WL. Valsalva maneuver induced vitreous hemorrhage. *J Am Ophthalm Assoc* 1995; **6**:301–4.

60. White P. Pregnancy and diabetes. In: (Marble A, White P, Bradley RF, eds) *Joslin's Diabetes Mellitus*. (Lea & Febiger: Philadelphia, 1971) 581–98.

61. Rossen BM, Miodovnik M. Medical complications of diabetes mellitus in pregnancy. *Clin Obstet Gynecol* 2000; **43**:17–31.

38

Diabetic vascular complications in pregnancy: nephropathy
Barak M Rosenn, Menachem Miodovnik

Introduction

During the past few decades there has been a steady improvement in the perinatal outcome of pregnancies in women with diabetes. Several factors have contributed to these changes, including improved maternal glycemic control, advances in neonatal care and close antepartum surveillance. Even women with advanced diabetes can now gain access to specialized prenatal care and can often expect a successful pregnancy outcome. But even with the best of care, maternal and perinatal complications in women with diabetes are consistently more frequent than in the general population, particularly in those who have diabetic nephropathy, often coexisting with hypertension. Furthermore, questions regarding the possible short-term and long-term effects of pregnancy on maternal diabetic disease loom large in the minds of these women and their health care providers. Indeed, diabetes and pregnancy may mutually affect each other over a range of interactions from conception to delivery, and possibly even later.

Pathophysiology of diabetic nephropathy

Diabetic nephropathy is a progressive disease that affects 30–40% of patients with diabetes and is the most common cause of end-stage renal disease in the USA. Mogensen et al[1] described several distinct clinical and subclinical stages of the desease. Initially, renal hypertrophy and microscopic lesions appear in genetically susceptible individuals within a few years of the onset of diabetes. These lesions are characterized by scattered sclerosis of glomeruli that can be demonstrated on renal biopsy even in the absence of clinical findings. Within 5–10 years, minute amounts of albumin (30–300 mg 24 hours) and other anionic proteins appear in the urine, constituting the phase of incipient nephropathy with microalbuminuria. Within a few years, overt nephropathy develops (> 300 mg albumin 24 hours) characterized by progressive, widespread glomerular sclerosis resulting in excretion of progressively larger amounts of protein. Ultimately, progressive renal insufficiency and end-stage renal disease occur, manifest as decreasing creatinine clearance, increasing serum creatinine and uremia. The incidence of diabetic nephropathy is related to the duration of diabetes: *c.* 15% of people with diabetes have nephropathy within 15 years, 30% within 20 years and 40% within 30 years from the onset of diabetes.[2] Once nephropathy is established, renal function continues to deteriorate progressively, with the glomerular filtration rate declining at an average rate of 10 ml/minute each year.

Progression to end-stage renal disease occurs in at least 75% of patients within the following 10 years.[3]

Pregnancy and the pathophysiology of diabetic nephropathy

Several factors have been implicated in the development of diabetic nephropathy, many of which may be affected by pregnancy. These include glomerular filtration rate, hypertension, protein intake and excretion, and glycemic control.

The primary insult leading to diabetic nephropathy is most likely increased glomerular capillary pressure that leads to glomerular hyperfiltration that, in turn, results in structural damage and renal functional deterioration.[4] During normal pregnancy, there is a 40–60% increase in glomerular filtration rate that, theoretically, may accelerate the progression of nephropathy.[5]

Diets with a high-protein content can result in hyperaminoacidemia and consequently in increased glomerular filtration rates.[6] Several studies have shown that a low-protein diet has a beneficial effect on the course of incipient or overt diabetic nephropathy.[7,8] Conversely, increased dietary protein intake, such as recommended during pregnancy, may exacerbate glomerular hyperfiltration and accelerate the course of diabetic nephropathy.

Systemic arterial hypertension also appears to play a role in the rate of progression of nephropathy.[9] Hypertension is common in patients with overt diabetic nephropathy, as it is with many renal disorders. Strict control of blood pressure using angiotensin-converting enzyme (ACE) inhibitors or other antihypertensive agents appears to delay the progression

from incipient to overt nephropathy, and may also slow the progression from overt nephropathy to end-stage renal disease.[10] Because pregnancy-induced hypertension (PIH) affects 10–20% of all women with Type 1 diabetes, and an even greater proportion of those with nephropathy,[11] pregnancy may be expected to exert a detrimental effect on nephropathy in a considerable number of women with diabetes.

Poor glycemic control has consistently been found to increase the glomerular filtration rate, and recent studies have demonstrated that strict glycemic control results in improved renal function or a slower rate of progression of nephropathy.[12] Because pregnant women with diabetes are usually managed with intensive insulin therapy during pregnancy, this factor might actually be expected to have a beneficial effect on renal function.

Effects of pregnancy on diabetic nephropathy

Consideration of the factors described above suggests that pregnancy may have profound effects on the course of nephropathy. But how these different factors interact is essentially a matter of speculation, because only a few studies, involving relatively few pregnant women, have examined the short-term and long-term effects of pregnancy on renal function, and most have no non-pregnant controls.

Several studies have attempted to determine how pregnancy affects the course of diabetic nephropathy. Even though pregnancy in these women is often associated with a marked increase in proteinuria, this is generally an acute and transient phenomenon. In most cases, even when massive proteinuria develops during pregnancy, proteinuria subsides after delivery and returns to prepregnancy levels. It is much more difficult to determine the ultimate long-term effects of pregnancy on the course of diabetic nephropathy. Because it is impossible to conceive a prospective, randomized trial in which women with diabetic nephropathy would be randomized into either becoming pregnant or remaining childless, the answer to this question is far from definite. In general, studies on this issue fall into three groups.

(1) Longitudinal retrospective or prospective studies that examine the progression of nephropathy in women with diabetic nephropathy who have experienced one or more pregnancies. The actual average rate of progression in these women is compared to a control group or to the expected rate of progression in the general population of patients with diabetic nephropathy, as reported in the literature.

(2) Cross-sectional and case–control studies comparing the prevalence of diabetic nephropathy in women who have previously been pregnant to those who have never been pregnant.

(3) Longitudinal or cross-sectional studies examining the effect of parity on the incidence of nephropathy or the progression of nephropathy to end-stage renal disease.

Because of their design, none of these studies can account for all the possible confounding factors that might affect the outcome. Additionally, most studies include a relatively small number of subjects, explaining some of the conflicting conclusions.

A summary of the longitudinal studies on pregnant women with diabetic nephropathy is presented in Table 38.1.[13–23] Eight of these studies[13–17,19,22,23] determined that pregnancy did not alter the rate of decline in renal function, while one study[20] concluded that this is true only for women with early nephropathy who start their pregnancy with a creatinine clearance > 90 ml/minute and with < 1000 mg proteinuria per 24 hours; otherwise, the rate of decline was higher than expected. Of note, only one of these studies had non-pregnant controls,[23] while all the others compared the

Author (reference)	Year	No. of subjects	Follow-up (months)	Accelerated progression	Progressed to ESRD*
Kitzmiller et al (13)	1981	23	9–35	No	3
Dicker et al (14)	1986	5	6–12	No	0
Grenfell et al (15)	1986	20	6–120	No	2
Reece et al (16)	1988	31	1–86	No	6
Reece et al (17)	1990	11	10–45	No	0
Biesenbach et al (18)	1992	5†	13–42	Yes	5
Kimmerle et al (19)	1995	29	4–108	No	8
Gordon et al (20)	1996	34	34 (mean)	Yes	3
Purdy et al (21)	1996	11†	6–138	Yes	7
Mackie et al (22)	1996	6†	6–96	No	3
Rossing et al (23)	2002	26	36–164	No	5

* End-stage renal disease.
† Study subjects with moderate renal dysfunction at beginning of follow-up.

Table 38.1. Association of pregnancy with progression of diabetic nephropathy.

average rate of decline in renal function to the expected rate of decline in the general non-pregnant population of subjects with diabetic nephropathy.

At least two studies have suggested that pregnancy may accelerate the decline in renal function in women with advanced nephropathy, i.e. women who have not only proteinuria but also higher serum creatinine concentrations or decreased creatinine clearance. Biesenbach et al[18] studied five women with Type 1 diabetes who had diabetic nephropathy with compromised renal function (creatinine clearance < 75 ml/minute) and hypertension. The mean rate of decline in creatinine clearance was greater than expected both during pregnancy and during the postpartum follow-up period. Hypertension worsened in all five women during pregnancy, and all developed end-stage renal disease within 42 months postpartum (average 29 months). The authors suggested that the accelerated decline in renal function may be related to increasing hypertension during pregnancy. Similarly, Purdy et al[21] found that in patients with moderate to severe nephropathy (serum creatinine > 1.4 mg/dl), there is a 40% risk of accelerated, permanent decline in renal function during pregnancy, leading to accelerated progression to end-stage renal disease, compared to non-pregnant women with comparable severity of nephropathy. In contrast, Mackie et al[22] studied six women with moderate nephropathy (serum creatinine 1.4–2.8 mg/dl) who were followed up to 8 years after pregnancy and demonstrated that, although changes in renal function differed from patient to patient during pregnancy, pregnancy had no systematic adverse long-term effect on renal function.

At least four cross-sectional studies have examined the prevalence of diabetic nephropathy among parous women compared to nulliparous women. Kaaja et al[24] compared 28 parous women, 7 years after an index of pregnancy, to 17 nulliparous controls, and found no differences in the prevalence of nephropathy. Similarly, Carstensen et al[25] matched 22 pairs of parous and nulliparous women with Type 1 diabetes by age and duration of disease. They found no differences between the two groups with respect to the prevalence of microvascular complications up to 17.7 years after the birth of the oldest child and up to 24 years after the onset of diabetes. Hemachandra et al[26] matched 80 nulliparous women to 80 parous women by age, duration of diabetes, race and marital history, and found no differences between the groups regarding the prevalence of microvascular complications. Chaturvedi et al[27] determined the prevalence of microalbuminuria and macroalbuminuria in 776 nulliparous women compared to 582 parous women with Type 1 diabetes. After adjusting for age and duration of diabetes, there was no significant difference between groups with respect to the presence of microalbuminuria, while the prevalence of macroalbuminuria was lower in parous women (6%) compared to nulliparous women (10%). These findings suggest that pregnancy may actually have a protective effect on nephropathy, although explaining this phenomenon would necessarily be speculative.

Two small, prospective, controlled studies compared the incidence of diabetic nephropathy among parous women to that among nulliparous women over a short period of time. Hemachandra et al[26] followed a group of 30 primiparous women for a mean period of 11.8 months following their pregnancy, matched to a group of 30 nulliparous women followed for the same period, and found no difference in the incidence of diabetic nephropathy. Miodovnik et al[28] studied 23 pregnant women with Type 1 diabetes matched to 23 non-pregnant controls, all of whom had no evidence of microvascular disease at enrollment. Both groups were managed identically during the 9 month pregnancy period (sham 9 month pregnancy period for controls) and were then prospectively followed for an additional 14–43 months with regular evaluation of renal function. Neither the study patients nor the controls developed nephropathy during the follow-up period, suggesting that pregnancy is not associated with accelerated development of diabetic nephropathy.

To determine whether parity affects the course of diabetic nephropathy, Miodovnik et al[29] retrospectively studied 182 women with Type 1 diabetes, of whom 46 had overt diabetic nephropathy. These patients were followed for a period of 3–16 years (median 9.1 years) after delivery. Of the 136 women without nephropathy at the time of pregnancy, only 13 (10%) eventually developed nephropathy later in life, within a mean of 10.1 years following the pregnancy. Proteinuria appearing during pregnancy and poor glycemic control during pregnancy, but not parity *per se*, were significantly associated with the subsequent development of nephropathy. Of the 46 women who had overt nephropathy prior to pregnancy, 12 (26%) progressed to end-stage renal disease after a median period of 6 years, but again this was not associated with parity. Using life-table analysis, the investigators found that in this parous population, the overall risk of developing nephropathy was 44% after 27 years of diabetes, and the risk of progressing to end-stage renal disease was 30% after 10 years of overt diabetic nephropathy. Thus, the risk of developing nephropathy *de novo*, and the risk of progressing from nephropathy to end-stage renal disease, does not appear to be associated with pregnancy or with increasing parity.

Taken together, most of the aforementioned studies suggest that pregnancy is not associated with development of nephropathy or with

accelerated progression of pre-existing nephropathy, but some data suggest that in patients with moderate or advanced renal disease, pregnancy may accelerate progression to end-stage renal disease. This fact should be taken into account when counseling this selective group of high-risk patients.

Effects of diabetic nephropathy on pregnancy outcome

The presence of diabetic nephropathy significantly affects the outcome of pregnancy, primarily due to three reasons: (1) the increased risk of maternal hypertensive complications; (2) the increased risk of fetal prematurity due to deteriorating maternal hypertension and pre-eclampsia; and (3) the increased risk of fetal growth restriction and fetal distress. In general, the worst perinatal outcomes occur in women who have measurable impaired renal function, with decreased creatinine clearance and increased serum creatinine concentrations. A summary of selected perinatal complications from the literature is presented in Table 38.2.[13–16,19,20,30–34]

Many women with diabetic nephropathy have pre-existing chronic hypertension, and even in those that do not, perinatal complications are frequently associated with hypertension that develops during pregnancy, which can often be severe. Pre-eclampsia, or superimposed pre-eclampsia, are common complications of diabetic nephropathy, although the definition of these situations in women who have pre-existing proteinuria and hypertension is somewhat vague and arbitrary. This may explain some of the differences in the reported rates of pre-eclampsia depicted in Table 38.2.

Few studies have examined the association of microalbuminuria and perinatal outcome. Combs et al[35] found that even women with

					Author (reference)					
	Kitzmiller et al (13)	Grenfell et al (15)	Reece et al (16)	Pierce et al (30)	Gordon et al (20)	Kimmerle et al (19)	Rosenn et al (31)	Reece et al (32)	Khoury et al (33)	Ekbom et al (34)
No. of subjects	26	22	31	39	45	36	61	27	72	11
Chronic hypertension (%)	31	NA	23	NA	27	61	47	77	33	NA
Pre-eclampsia (%)	15	NA	35	NA	53	19	51	53	33	64
Cross-section (%)	NA	73	71	NA	80	86	82	63	68	NA
Perinatal survival (%)	89	100	94	97	100	100	94	96	96	100
Congenital malformations	3 (11%)	1 (4%)	3 (10%)	3 (8%)	2 (4%)	2 (6%)	4 (6%)	2 (9%)	4 (4%)	1 (9%)
IUGR (%)	21	14	16	10	11	22	11	9	10	45
Delivery < 34 weeks (%)	31	27	23	26	16	31	25	26 (≤ 36 weeks)	13 (< 32 weeks)	45
Delivery 34–36 weeks (%)	41	23	32	23	35	NA	28		NA	46
Delivery > 36 weeks (%)	28	50	45	51	49	NA	47	74	NA	9

IUGR, Intrauterine growth restriction; NA, not available.

Table 38.2. Outcome of pregnancy in women with diabetic nephropathy.

total protein excretion in the microalbuminuric range (< 500 mg total protein/24 hours) have an increased risk of developing pre-eclampsia. The cut-off for increased risk, determined by a characterstic receiver-operating curve (ROC) analysis was 190 mg protein/24 hours, above which the rate of pre-eclampsia rose dramatically to a level that remained essentially unchanged, even at higher levels of proteinuria. Similarly, Ekbom et al[34] found that the rate of prematurity among women with microalbuminura was significantly increased, primarily due to an increased incidence of pre-eclampsia in this subpopulation.

As mentioned above, in the patient with overt nephropathy (albuminuria > 300 mg/24 hours or > 500 mg total protein/24 hours), the actual amount of proteinuria as well as the increase in proteinuria during pregnancy appear to have no adverse effect on pregnancy outcome.[36] Not surprisingly, there are no studies examining the association of decreased creatinine clearance with adverse perinatal outcome, since most published studies include too few subjects to analyze this variable. However, Khoury et al[33] found that very low birthweight and neonatal hypoglycemia (in women with Type 1 diabetes) were significantly associated with a high serum creatinine concentration at the onset of pregnancy, independent of total proteinuria and glycemic control. There was also a trend of increased rates of perinatal death, growth restriction and respiratory distress syndrome in association with a high maternal serum creatinine level.

It appears that aggressive control of maternal hypertension is of utmost importance to optimize pregnancy outcome, but the choice of antihypertensive medications is somewhat limited. The ACE inhibitors are particularly useful in women with diabetic nephropathy, but their use is contraindicated in pregnancy due to their potential adverse effects on the fetus. The most widely used medications are methyldopa, nifedipine and alpha-adrenergic blockers, for a targeted blood pressure < 130/80.

Fetal outcome is often affected by prematurity as a result of deteriorating maternal status requiring early delivery, but also due to an increased risk of fetal growth restriction and fetal hypoxia. Worsening nephropathy and superimposed pre-eclampsia appear to be the most significant risk factors associated with fetal distress, while hypertension and decreased creatinine clearance are the strongest predictors of fetal growth restriction.[37]

As depicted in Table 38.2, perinatal survival of infants born to mothers with diabetic nephropathy has been consistently close to 100% during the past two decades. However, the increased rate of prematurity in this population is associated with an increased risk of long-term infant morbidity. Kimmerle et al[19] followed 36 infants of mothers with diabetic nephropathy for 0.5–11 years after delivery, and found that five had severe psychomotor retardation and three had mild developmental retardation, primarily associated with prematurity.

Thus, although women with diabetic nephropathy may usually expect to deliver a viable fetus and take home a reasonably healthy infant, this group of patients is the one most likely to have a complicated course of pregnancy, requiring expert care and intensive management.

References

1. Mogensen CE, Christensen CK, Vittinghus E. The stages in diabetic renal disease. With emphasis on the stage of incipient diabetic nephropathy. *Diabetes* 1983; **32 (Suppl 2)**: 64–78.
2. Andersen AR, Christiansen JS, Andersen JK et al. Diabetic nephropathy in Type 1 (insulin-dependent) diabetes: an epidemiological study. *Diabetologia* 1983; 25:459–501.

3. Krolewski AS, Warram JH, Christlieb AR et al. The changing natural history of nephropathy in Type I diabetes. *Am J Med* 1985; 78:785–94.

4. Hostetter TH. Pathogenesis of diabetic glomerulopathy: hemodynamic considerations. *Semin Nephrol* 1990; 10:219–27.

5. Sturgiss SN, Dunlop W, Davision JM. Renal haemodynamics and tubular function in human pregnancy. *Baillieres Clin Obstet Gynaecol* 1994; 8:209–34.

6. Bank N. Mechanisms of diabetic hyperfiltration. *Kidney Int* 1991; 40:792–807.

7. Zeller KR. Low-protein diets in renal disease. *Diabetes Care* 1991; 14:856–66.

8. Dodds RA, Keen H. Low protein diet and conservation of renal function in diabetic nephropathy. *Diabet Metab* 1990; 16:464–9.

9. Mauer SM, Sutherland DE, Steffes MW. Relationship of systemic blood pressure to nephropathology in insulin-dependent diabetes mellitus. *Kidney Int* 1992; 41: 736–40.

10. Parving HH. Impact of blood pressure and antihypertensive treatment on incipient and overt nephropathy, retinopathy, and endothelial permeability in diabetes mellitus. *Diabetes Care* 1991; 14:260–9.

11. Rosenn B, Miodovnik M, Combs CA et al. Poor glycemic control and antepartum obstetric complications in women with insulin-dependent diabetes. *Int J Gynaecol Obstet* 1993; 43:21–8.

12. The Diabetes Control and Complications Trial Research Group. The effect of intensive treatment of diabetes on the development and progression of long-term complications in insulin-dependent diabetes mellitus. *N Engl J Med* 1993; 329:977–86.

13. Kitzmiller JL, Brown ER, Phillippe M et al. Diabetic nephropathy and perinatal outcome. *Am J Obstet Gynecol* 1981; 141:741.

14. Dicker D, Feldberg D, Peleg D et al. Pregnancy complicated by diabetic nephropathy. *J Perinat Med* 1986; 14:299.

15. Grenfell A, Brudenell JM, Doddridge MC et al. Pregnancy in diabetic women who have proteinuria. *Q J Med* 1986; 59:379.

16. Reece EA, Coustan DR, Hayslett JP et al. Diabetic nephropathy: pregnancy performance and fetomaternal outcome. *Am J Obstet Gynecol* 1988; 159:56.

17. Reece EA, Winn HN, Hayslett JP et al. Does pregnancy alter the rate of progression of diabetic nephropathy? *Am J Perinatol* 1990; 7:193.

18. Biesenbach G, Stoger H, Zazgornik J. Influence of pregnancy on progression of diabetic nephropathy and subsequent requirement of renal replacement therapy in female type I diabetic patients with impaired renal function. *Nephrol Dial Transplant* 1992; 7:105.

19. Kimmerle R, Zass RP, Cupisti S et al. Pregnancies in women with diabetic nephropathy: long-term outcome for mother and child. *Diabetologia* 1995; 38:227.

20. Gordon M, Landon MB, Samuels P et al. Perinatal outcome and long-term follow-up associated with modern management of diabetic nephropathy. *Obstet Gynecol* 1996; 87:401.

21. Purdy LP, Hantsch CE, Molitch ME et al. Effect of pregnancy on renal function in patients with moderate-to-severe diabetic renal insufficiency. *Diabetes Care* 1996; 19:1067.

22. Mackie AD, Doddridge MC, Gamsu HR et al. Outcome of pregnancy in patients with insulin-dependent diabetes mellitus and nephropathy with moderate renal impairment. *Diabet Med* 1996; 13:90.

23. Rossing K, Jacobsen P, Hommel E et al. Pregnancy and progression of diabetic nephropathy. *Diabetologia* 2002; 45:36–41.

24. Kaaja R, Sjoberg L, Hellsted T et al. Long-term effects of pregnancy on diabetic complications. *Diabet Med* 1996; 13:165.

25. Carstensen LL, Frost-Larsen K, Fugleberg S et al. Does pregnancy influence the prognosis of uncomplicated insulin-dependent diabetes mellitus? *Diabetes Care* 1982; 5:1.

26. Hemachandra A, Ellis D, Lloyd CE et al. The influence of pregnancy on IDDM complications. *Diabetes Care* 1995; 18:950.

27. Chaturvedi N, Stephenson JM, Fuller JH. The relationship between pregnancy and long-term maternal complications in the EURODIAB IDDM Complications Study. *Diabet Med* 1995; 12:494.

28. Miodovnik M, Rosenn B, Berk M et al. The effect of pregnancy on microvascular complications of insulin-dependent diabetes (IDDM): a prospective study. *Am J Obstet Gynecol* 1998; 178:S53.

29. Miodovnik M, Rosenn BM, Khoury JC et al. Does pregnancy increase the risk for development and progression of diabetic nephropathy? *Am J Obstet Gynecol* 1996; 174:1180.

30. Pierce J. California Diabetes and Pregnancy Program data system report, 1992. *Clin Perinatol* 1993; 20:565–6.

31. Rosenn BM, Miodovnik M, Khoury JC et al. Outcome of pregnancy in women with diabetic nephropathy. *Am J Obstet Gynecol* 1997; 176:S179.

32. Reece EA, Leguizamon G, Homko C. Stringent control in diabetic nephropathy associated with optimization of pregnancy outcomes. *J Matern Fetal Med* 1998; 7: 213–6.

33. JC Khoury, Miodovnik M. LeMasters G et al. Pregnancy outcome and progression of diabetic nephropathy. What's next? *J Matern Fetal Neonatal Med* 2002; 11:238–44.

34. Ekbom P, Damm P, Feldt-Rasmussen B et al. Pregnancy outcome in type 1 diabetic women with microalbuminuria. *Diabetes Care* 2001; 24:1739–44.

35. Combs CA, Rosenn B, Kitzmiller JL et al. Early-pregnancy proteinuria in diabetes related to pre-eclampsia. *Obstet Gynecol* 1993; 82:802–7.

36. Kitzmiller JL, Combs CA. Diabetic nephropathy and pregnancy. *Obstet Gynecol Clin N Am* 1996; 23: 173–203.

37. Kitzmiller JL, Combs CA. Maternal and perinatal implications of diabetic nephropathy. *Clin Perinatol* 1993; 20:561–70.

39

Diabetic ketoacidosis in pregnancy

Yariv Yogev, Avi Ben-Haroush, Moshe Hod

Introduction

Diabetic ketoacidosis (DKA) is characterized by accelerated gluconeogenesis and ketogenesis. It occurs most often in the presence of predisposing factors such as insulin deficiency (absolute or relative), excess counter-regulatory hormones, fasting and dehydration; infection is a common catalyst.

The principles of management include rehydration, insulin therapy, electrolyte replacement, and identification and treatment of the underlying cause. DKA in pregnancy is an acute metabolic situation, jeopardizing both maternal and fetal well-being. DKA affects 1–3% of pregnancies complicated with diabetes, and is rare in women with previously undiagnosed diabetes.

DKA in pregnancy warrants assessment of fetal well-being during management of the mother. The pathophysiology, effect on the fetus and management of DKA in pregnancy are discussed in detail in this chapter.

Prevalance, precipitating factors and prognosis

DKA during pregnancy occurs more often in women with insulin-dependent diabetes mellitus (IDDM) than in women with Type 2 or gestational diabetes mellitus (GDM).[1] As the majority of studies on DKA during pregnancy have been done on samples of < 30 patients, the actual prevalence has to be extrapolated from that data. According to the National Diabetes Data Group, the incidence of DKA in non-pregnant diabetics indicates an annual incidence of 3–8 episodes/1000 diabetic patients.[2] However, pregnant diabetic women are at greater risk of DKA than non-pregnant diabetic women.[3] DKA usually appears in the second and third trimesters, when there is an increase in insulin resistance,[4] and it is more frequent in undiagnosed new-onset diabetic gravida. The rate of maternal mortality secondary to diabetes has fallen remarkably from 50 to 60% in the pre-insulin era to < 1% today.[4] The maternal mortality rate secondary to DKA is not well established, owing to the relatively low prevalence of DKA, but most likely ranges from 5 to 15%.[4,5] Gabbe et al[4] reported seven maternal deaths among 24 cases of metabolic complications during pregnancy, four of which were related to DKA. Fetal mortality has also decreased markedly since the introduction of the routine use of insulin, although it is still excessively high, ranging from 30 to 90%.[6,7]

Montoro et al[8] reported a fetal death rate of 35% in 20 pregnant women with IDDM and DKA on admission; however, once therapy was begun, none of the remaining 13 women sustained fetal loss. Kilvert et al[9] reported only one fetal loss in seven cases of DKA occurring after the first trimester. In a study of 26 pregnant women with brittle diabetes (i.e. recurrent DKA episodes and frequent hospitalizations) and 27 pregnant women with stable disease, Kent et al[10] noted 15 (54%) live births, 10 (48%) spontaneous abortions and one (5%) stillbirth in the first group, compared to 25 (95%) live births and no stillbirths in the second group.

Increased insulin requirements and accelerated ketosis imposed by pregnancy predisposes the pregnant diabetic patient to an increased risk of DKA. Several factors predispose pregnant diabetic women to ketoacidosis: accelerated starvation, dehydration secondary to emesis, lowered buffering capacity (respiratory alkalosis of pregnancy), increased insulin resistance and stress. Box 39.1 summarizes the precipitating factors for the development of DKA in diabetic pregnancies.

Rodgers and Rodgers[11] reviewed these clinical variables and found that emesis and the use of beta-sympathomimetic drugs were etiologic in 57% of cases, and patient non-compliance and physician management errors were etiologic in 24% of cases and contributory in 16% of cases. Thirty percent of the patients with emesis on admission had a prepregnancy history of diabetic gastroenteropathy, thus identifying this group as being at particularly high risk for DKA. This finding emphasizes the importance of patient education and early initiation of treatment in pregnant diabetic patients with emesis. Using tocolytic agents such as beta-adrenergic drugs and steroids for fetal lung maturation should be approached cautiously.

Smoking has been demonstrated to have ketogenic effect (increased production of 3-hydroxybutyric acid) in diabetic women that has not been reproducible in healthy pregnant controls.[12]

Pathogenesis

DKA can result from either a relative or an absolute lack of insulin in the presence of glucose counter-regulatory hormones, resulting in an overproduction of glucose and ketones in the liver, with release of free fatty acids from adipose tissue (Fig. 39.1). Glucagon seems to be the primary insulin antagonist in the development of DKA.

Gerich et al[13] demonstrated that in patients with IDDM, acute withdrawal of insulin and suppression of glucagon secretion by somatostatin prevented the development of ketoacidosis, whereas in the control group ketoacidosis occurred. These findings indicate that it is not

Infection
Acute illness
Endocrine disorders (hyperthyroidism, pheochromocytoma)
Failure to take insulin (non-compliance)
Insulin pump failure
Medications (steroids, adrenergic agonists)
Physician management errors
Smoking

Box 39.1. Precipitating factors for the development of DKA in diabetic pregnancies.

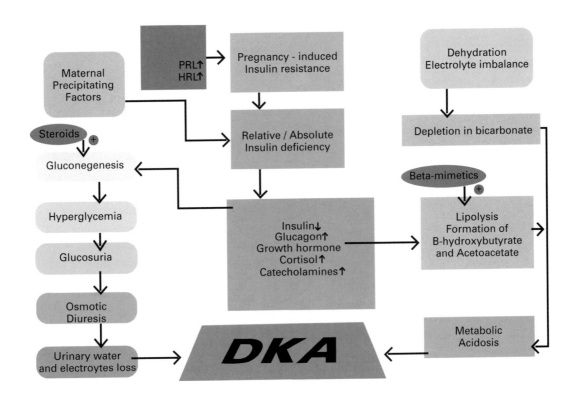

Figure 39.1. *Pathogenesis and biochemical changes of diabetic ketoacidosis (DKA). HPL, human placental lactogen; PRL, prolactin.*

only the lack of insulin that leads to fulminant diabetic ketoacidosis but that glucagon, by means of its gluconeogenic, ketogenic and lipolytic actions, is a prerequisite for its development. Support for this has been provided by studies in pancreatomized humans with low insulin levels, in whom glucose levels rise only slightly in direct correlation with blood glucose and glucagon levels.[14]

Other glucose counter-regulatory hormones include catecholamines, growth hormone and cortisol. In advancing gestation, human placental lactogen and prolactin also play a role, and have been incriminated in the pathogenesis of DKA. Owing the relative lack of insulin, increased levels of catecholamines and cortisol (due to stress and dehydration) result in significantly increased lipolysis in the adipose tissue and delivery of free fatty acids to the liver. Beta-oxidation of these fatty acids leads to the formation (up to 300%) of ketone bodies, namely β-hydroxybutyrate and acetoacetate, concomitant with a decrease in ketone used by muscle. As ketone bodies are acidic, ion concentrations in body fluids increases and so the pH decreases.

Acidosis is further exacerbated by the decrease in bicarbonate levels owing to bicarbonate neutralization of the ketone bodies prior to their excretion in urine.[5] As a result, a compensatory respiratory alkalosis is added to the baseline relative respiratory alkalosis and metabolic acidemia (renal excretion of bicarbonate) of pregnancy. Thus, the already diminished buffering capacity of pregnancy is compounded by the reduction in ketone use and severe impairment in bicarbonate regeneration. Acidosis, if untreated, leads to pronounced dehydration, oliguria and electrolyte imbalance. Hyperglycemia due to the accumulation of carbohydrates leads to an increase in serum osmolarity, profound osmotic diuresis (when glucose levels exceed those of the renal threshold), a decrease in cardiac output with a drop in blood pressure, and loss of sodium and potassium. Dehydration and severe hyperosmolarity may be further aggravated by the loss of water and electrolytes through acidosis-related vomiting. In advanced DKA, all body compartments become dehydrated, with a significant depletion in water, sodium, potassium, chloride, magnesium, phosphate and bicarbonate. Although the total body sodium deficit is high, the serum sodium level can be low, normal or high. The apparent hyponatremia ('pseudohyponatremia') is secondary to the hyperglycemic and hypertriglyceridemic state; this may be corrected by increasing measured sodium by 1.6 mEq/l for each 100 mg/dl of glucose above normal.[16] The drop in pH is compensated, in part, by the intracellular shift of hydrogen ions from the extracellular space in balance with the potassium flux from the intracellular space. Therefore, although the true serum potassium level is low, the measured serum potassium level will be at the upper end

of the normal range. Shock secondary to the depleted intravascular volume may ensue, with decreased tissue perfusion and increased lactic acid production.

Diagnosis

A high index of suspicion and prompt diagnosis is the key to improved outcome of both the fetus and the mother. The classic presentation of DKA in pregnancy consists of vomiting, thirst, polyuria, weakness, altered sensorium and air hunger. Malaise, headache, weight loss, nausea and abdominal pain occur less frequently. Importantly, symptoms can vary in severity. On examination, patients will have a characteristic fruity acetone breath odor with rapid and deep respiration (to release more carbon dioxide and prevent further pH deterioration). The diagnosis is confirmed by laboratory documentation of hyperglycemia, acidosis and ketonuria. Importantly, DKA in this patient population may be followed by euglycemia or mild hyperglycemia.[8,17] In a 10-year study of 11 cases of DKA in pregnancy, Cullen et al[18] noted symptoms of nausea, vomiting and decreased caloric intake in 10 patients (90%), and plasma glucose levels <200 mg/dl in four patients (36%). Ketonemia and prerenal azotemia with elevations in blood urea nitrogen and creatinine levels are also common findings. Arterial blood gas analysis revealed acidosis, with the pH usually <7.30, along with an anion gap of 12 mEq/l or greater; serum bicarbonate is often ≤15 mEq/l. As described earlier, sodium and potassium levels can vary significantly.

Fetal effects of diabetic ketoacidosis (DKA)

The greatest hazard facing the pregnant diabetic patient with DKA is fetal loss. The exact fetal loss rate is difficult to assess because of the small reported series in the literature. Historically, the reported fetal mortality ranged between 30 and 90%,[7] but remarkable progress has been made both in fetal assessment techniques and in the treatment of DKA, and mortality rates in more recent reviews are 10%.[18] Needless to say, fetal loss is primarily related to the severity of the maternal illness and the degree of metabolic decompensation. Most fetal losses occur prior to diagnosis and therefore to the onset of efficient treatment. As ketone bodies freely cross the placenta, maternal acidosis is assumed to cause fetal acidosis; however, the exact mechanism by which maternal DKA affects the fetus remains unclear. Suggestions include a decrease in uterine blood flow and fetal hypoxemia, maternal hyperketonemia inducing fetal hypoxemia, and fetal hyperglycemia causing an increased fetal oxidative mechanism and a decreased fetal myocardial contractility. Indeed, fetal potassium deficit has been found to lead to fetal cardiac arrest.[7] Fetal hypoxia may also be attributed to a DKA-associated phosphate deficit which leads to depletion of red cell 2,3-diphosphoglycerate and consequent impairment of oxygen delivery. The risk of fetal distress, and even death, during the maternal DKA state makes it mandatory to continuously monitor the fetal heart and to assess the biophysical score, and to evaluate the fetal acid–base balance by cordocentesis if necessary. In the few case reports of fetal monitoring during maternal DKA, a non-reassuring pattern with tachycardia, reduced variability and late decelerations was reported.[19,20] LoBue and Goodlin[21] found that the administration of just sodium bicarbonate for 2 hours led to the resolution of the late deceleration and decreased variability of uterine contractions. Hughes[20] reported the resolution of a similar fetal heart rate pattern 40 minutes after intravenous administration of insulin with no mention of maternal rehydration. Other researchers reported that a combination of massive intravenous hydration, insulin therapy and intensive care of the mother lead to resolution of fetal acidosis and on improvement in fetal heart rate monitoring.

The long-term effects of DKA episodes during pregnancy on the fetus remain unclear, but a relationship between plasma ketone levels in the pregnant diabetic women and a lower intelligence quotient in the child has been suggested.[22]

Treatment

Prompt and vigorous treatment in an obstetric intensive care unit is generally needed to decrease the high maternal and fetal mortalities accompanying DKA. All treatment protocols are based on correcting volume depletion, supplying insulin, correcting acidosis and electrolyte imbalance, and, most importantly, identifying and correcting any possible precipitating factor. Continuous fetal heart rate monitoring and biophysical assessment are mandatory to assess fetal well-being during the third trimester. Induction of labor or an emergency Cesarean section should be done only after maternal stabilization. In the event of preterm labor, magnesium sulfate is the tocolytic drug of choice, as beta-mimetic drugs only exacerbate the metabolic disorder. Major consideration should be given to the use of steroids for lung maturation, as they also worsen the metabolic consequences. A search for a source of infection or other severe illness must be undertaken concomitant with onset of treatment.

Several protocols have recently been suggested for the treatment of DKA. It should be borne in mind, however, that these protocols are only general guidelines and the therapeutic regimen must be tailored to the individual patient on the basis of her prominent clinical features. Only the therapeutic rationale and the physiological basis are outlined in this chapter.

An estimated 4–10l of deficit occurs in DKA;[23] therefore, fluid administration is considered the first priority of treatment in order to improve renal perfusion and thereby increase glucosuria. The initial therapy should be based on isotonic saline for effective restoration of the intravascular volume. In cases of hypernatremia, other isotonic solutions may be used. Importantly, it has been postulated that using hypotonic saline as initial treatment may cause a rapid drop in plasma osmolarity that can lead to fatal cerebral edema, which is a rare event among adults. Thus, when serum glucose falls to <250 mg/dl, the intravenous fluids can be changed to 5% dextrose solution.

There are many dosing regimens for insulin replacement in DKA, and each has its advantages and disadvantages. In recent years, the constant low-dose regimen rather than the high-dose bolus therapy has become popular,[3,24] owing both to its simplicity and to the lower rates of complications of hypoglycemia and hypokalemia. However, bolus or continuous infusion therapy also works well, and the clinician should choose the method with which they have the most experience.[3]

Acidemia in DKA takes longer to correct than the hyperglycemic state. Therefore, insulin therapy should be continued even when normal glucose levels have been achieved. When blood glucose reaches 150–200 mg/dl, a 5% dextrose solution should be used along with insulin.[25] Plasma electrolytes should be frequently evaluated, and once adequate renal function is established, potassium should be replaced, bearing in mind that the often normal or elevated serum potassium level may not reflect the true total deficit of 5–15 mEq/kg of body weight. Potassium is usually administered for 1–3 hours, when the level begins to normalize due to the intracellular shift. It is noteworthy that the serum potassium level can fall rapidly as a result of vigorous potassium loss in urine and correction of acidemia.[26]

If phosphorus is low, replacement of 10–20 mEq/l of potassium phosphate for each 10–20 mEq/l of potassium chloride should be used. The use of bicarbonate is the most controversial area in the treatment of DKA.[3,21,24] Routine bicarbonate therapy may be unnecessary, as the retained ketone bodies are metabolized and regenerated to bicarbonate. Overzealous replacement should be avoided in order to prevent rapid and complete maternal acidemia that may actually increase fetal pCO_2 levels and reduce oxygen delivery to maternal tissues.[7] Bicarbonate therapy should probably be used only in patients with severe acidosis (pH <7.1 or 7.0). There is currently no evidence to support a beneficial effect of bicarbonate in patients with a pH >6.9, though some authors recommend it only for such cases.[25]

Importantly, alkali therapy is associated with many side effects, e.g. hypokalemia, sodium overload, reduction in oxygen delivery capacity and a decrease in cerebrospinal fluid pH.

Conclusions

DKA is an extreme condition in the spectrum of decompensated diabetes mellitus. Its pathogenesis is related to an absolute or relative deficiency in insulin levels and elevations in insulin counter-regulatory hormones that lead to altered metabolism of carbohydrate, protein, and fat, and varying degrees of osmotic diuresis and dehydration, ketosis, and acidosis. Clinical presentation is characterized by insulin deficiency and ketoacidosis, and insulin therapy is the cornerstone of therapy. The therapeutic regimen is tailored to the prominent clinical features of the individual patient. In gravid patients, rapid correction of the metabolic abnormalities and, consequently, of hyperosmolarity by administration of hypotonic fluids and insulin should be avoided to decrease the risk for precipitating cerebral edema. Intensive care unit admission is indicated in the management of DKA, in the presence of cardiovascular instability, an inability to protect the airway, obtundation, the presence of blood pressure instability, or if there is not adequate capacity to provide the frequent and necessary monitoring that must accompany its use. Prompt diagnosis and early treatment, along with continuous monitoring of fetal well-being, is well correlated with favorable outcomes of both mother and infant.

Reference

1. Cousins L. Pregnancy complications among diabetic women. Review, 1965–1985. *Obstet Gynecol Surv* 1987; 42:140–9.
2. Fishbein HA. DKA, hyperosmolar coma, lactic acidosis and hypoglycemia. In: (Harris MI, Hammon RF, eds) *Diabetes in America*. (US Dept. of Health and Human Sciences: Washington, DC) 1985 XII.I–XII.19.
3. Hollingsworth DR. Medical and obstetrics complications of diabetic pregnancies: IDDM, NIDDM, and GDM. In: (Brown C-L, Mitchell, eds) *Pregnancy, Diabetes and Birth: A Management Guide*, 2nd edn. (Williams & Wilkins: Baltimore, 1992.)
4. Gabbe SG, Mestman HJ, Hibbard LT. Maternal mortality in diabetes mellitus: an 18 year survey. *Obstet Gynecol* 1976; 48:549–54.
5. Goto Y, Sato S, Masuda M. Causes of death in 3151 diabetic autopsy cases. *Tohoku J Exp Med* 1974; 112:3390–343.
6. Drury MI, Greene AT, Stronge JM. Pregnancy complicated by clinical diabetes mellitus: a study of 600 pregnancies. *Obstet Gynecol* 1977; 49:519–24.
7. Kitzmiller JL. Diabetic ketoacidosis and pregnancy. *Contemp Obstet Gynecol* 1982; 20:141–5.
8. Montoro MN, Myers VP, Mestman JH et al. Outcome of pregnancy in diabetic ketoacidosis. *Am J Perinatol* 1993; 10:17–21.
9. Kilvert JA, Nicholson HO, Wright AD. Ketoacidosis in diabetic pregnancy. *Diabet Med* 1993; 10:278–81.
10. Kent LA, Gill GV, Williams G. Mortality and outcome of patients with brittle diabetes and recurrent ketoacidosis. *Lancet* 1994; 17: 778–81.
11. Rodgers BD, Rodgers DE. Clinical variables associated with diabetic ketoacidosis during pregnancy. *J Reprod Med* 1991; 36:797–800.
12. Nylund L, Lunell NO, Persson B et al. Smoking exerts a ketogenic influence in diabetic pregnancy. *Gynecol Obstet Invest* 1988; 25:35–7.
13. Gerich JE, Lorenzi M, Bier DM et al. Prevention of human diabetic ketoacidosis by somatostatin. Evidence for an essential role of glucagon. *N Engl J Med* 1975; 8:985–9.
14. Machoff CD, Pohl SL, Kaiser DL et al. Determinants of glucose and ketoacid concentration in acutely hyperglycemic diabetic patients. *Am J Med* 1984; 77:275–85.
15. Riley Jr, LJ Cooper M, Narins RG. Alkali therapy of diabetic ketoacidosis: biochemical, physiologic, and clinical perspectives. *Diabetes Metab Rev* 1989; 5:627–36.
16. Katz MA. Hyperglycemia-induced hyponatremia – calculation of expected serum sodium depression. *N Engl J Med* 1973; 18: 843–4.
17. Clark JD, McConnell A, Hartog M. Normoglycaemic ketoacidosis in a woman with gestational diabetes. *Diabet Med* 1991; 8:388–9.
18. Cullen MT, Reece EA, Homko CJ, Sivan E. The changing presentations of diabetic ketoacidosis during pregnancy. *Am J Perinatol* 1996; 13:449–51.
19. Hagay ZJ, Weissman A, Lurie S, Insler V. Reversal of fetal distress following intensive treatment of maternal diabetic ketoacidosis. *Am J Perinatol* 1994; 11:430–2.
20. Hughes AB. Fetal heart rate changes during diabetic ketosis. *Acta Obstet Gynecol Scand* 1987; 66:71–3.
21. LoBue C, Goodlin RC. Treatment of fetal distress during diabetic keto-acidosis. *J Reprod Med* 1978; 20:101–4.
22. Stehbens JA, Baker GL, Kitchell M. Outcome at ages 1, 3, and 5 years of children born to diabetic women. *Am J Obstet Gynecol* 1977; 15:408–13.
23. Raskin P, Unger RH. Hyperglucagonemia and its suppression. Importance in the metabolic control of diabetes. *N Engl J Med* 1978; 31: 433–6.
24. Foster DW, McGarry JD. The metabolic derangement and treatment of diabetic ketoacidosis. *N Engl J Med* 1983; 21:159–69.
25. Walker M, Marshall SM, Alberti KG. Clinical aspects of diabetic ketoacidosis. *Diabetes Metab Rev* 1989; 5:651–63.
26. Owen OE, Licht JH, Sapir DG. Renal function and effects of partial rehydration during diabetic ketoacidosis. *Diabetes* 1981; 30:510–18.

40

Diabetes and multiple pregnancies
Yenon Hazan, Isaac Blickstein

Introduction

Multiple pregnancies have reached epidemic magnitudes in most developed countries. The various methods of infertility treatment – the major contributors to this epidemic – did not arise *ex vaccuo*. Over the past two decades women have relied on effective fertility treatment when deciding to postpone childbirth. It follows that when children are desired, usually when other phases in life are complete, women are at an advanced age, which by itself is a known risk factor for natural multiple pregnancies. The reduced fecundity of older age, on the other hand, significantly increases the need for infertility treatment. Thus, social trends and available effective therapy act in concert to increase the risk of multiple births.[1,2] According to the East Flanders Prospective Twin Survey, the ratio of induced to spontaneous twins has increased from 1:46 in the 1970s to 1:2 twins in the late 1990s.[3] This population-based trend is even more accentuated in centers with busy infertility clinics, where induced conceptions presently comprise the majority of multiple pregnancies. The rate of multiple births in most developed countries is currently as high as 2–4%, a figure that is two- to four times the rate of that in developing countries. Figs 40.1 and 40.2 show the rates of singleton and multiple births in women > 29 and > 39 years of age,

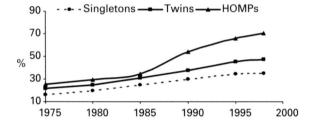

Figure 40.1. *Percentage of singleton and multiple births by maternal age of > 29 between 1975 and 2000 (adapted from Ventura et al[4]). HOMPs, High-order multiple pregnancy.*

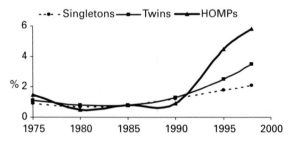

Figure 40.2. *Percentage of singleton and multiple births by maternal age of > 39 between 1975 and 2000 (adapted from Ventura et al HOMPs, High-order multiple pregnancy.*

respectively, during the last quarter of the twentieth century.[4] These figures demonstrate that one should expect higher ages among mothers of multiple pregnancies.

Based on the combined effect of hyperplacentosis and older maternal age during a multiple pregnancy, a corresponding increase in gestational diabetes mellitus (GDM) could be expected during these gestations. However, there is little to no information regarding the potential association between GDM and the epidemic of iatrogenic multiple pregnancies. This chapter offers a critical discussion that focuses on the available data related to GDM and multiple pregnancies, and possible lines of further investigation are proposed.

Supporting data

GDM is a relatively common perinatal complication of human pregnancies. This problem relates to other pregnancy complications such as premature delivery, fetal macrosomia, birth trauma, unexplained antepartum fetal demise, pregnancy-induced hypertension and placental abruption.

Pregnancy causes changes in carbohydrate metabolism and produces a pro-diabetic condition. One of the theories forwarded in the past to explain why multiple pregnancies were more prone to GDM was placental size – commonly referred to as hyperplacentosis. Hyperplacentosis in multiple pregnancies was alleged to increase hormonal levels and these, in turn, to increase the susceptibility to GDM.

In their study, Spellacy et al[5] compared levels of human placental lactogen (hPL) – a known pro-diabetic hormone – in singleton and twin pregnancies. Serum levels, established by radioimmunoassay, were evaluated in 75 singleton and 37 twin pregnancies. The results showed a significantly increased hPL level at 30 weeks (7.0 versus 6.0 µg/ml) as well as at 36 weeks (9.2 versus 7.4 µg/ml) in twins versus the singletons pregnancies, respectively. This study supported the theory that twin pregnancies are associated with an increased level of the principal diabetogenic hormone. Also in

support of the view that GDM is related to multiple pregnancies is the evaluation of carbohydrate metabolism by Spellacy et al.[6] They compared 24 cases of twin pregnancies with 24 control singleton pregnancies. Cases and controls were not different in age, parity, weight or gestational age. A 25 gram glucose tolerance test was done in the second half of gestation to measure blood glucose, hPL and plasma insulin levels. The hPL levels were significantly higher, and the fasting as well as the 5 and 15 minute insulin levels were significantly lower, in the women expecting twins. The effect of hPL in twin as compared with singleton pregnancies may also be indirectly appreciated by its augmentation of erythropoietin action as measured by the age-distribution shift of erythrocytes in women with twin gestations.[7]

The alteration in the response to eating and fasting may be exaggerated in twin gestations. Casele et al[8] conducted a 40 hour metabolic study in non-diabetic gestations and compared the metabolic response to normal meal eating and the vulnerability to starvation ketosis in 10 twin versus 10 matched-for-age and matched-for-prepregnancy-weight singleton pregnancies. The glucose, beta-hydroxybutyrate, and insulin excursions in response to meal eating from 8 a.m. to 12 noon on day 1 were similar in twin and singleton pregnancies. On day 2, when breakfast was delayed, a progressive but not significantly different decrement in glucose was observed in both twin and singleton pregnancies. Concurrently, there was a significantly greater progressive rise in beta-hydroxybutyrate in twins compared to singletons pregnancies. These observations may indicate that twin gestations are more vulnerable to the accelerated starvation of late normal pregnancy than singletons are.

If hyperplacentosis is indeed the link between a multiple gestation and GDM, it could be expected that the frequency of GDM will correlate with the number of fetuses (i.e. plurality).

Marconi et al[9] evaluated the glucose disposal rate in 11 singleton, five twin and one triplet pregnancies. Maternal fasting glucose concentration, and the total fetal and placental weight significantly correlated with an increased maternal glucose disposal rate, but glucose concentration and total pregnancy weight were interdependent variables. From the above mentioned studies it could be speculated that the difference between multiple and singleton pregnancies may be the result of a plurality-dependent increased metabolic demand of the multiple gestation.

The association between GDM and plurality was also examined by evaluating the effect of multifetal pregnancy reduction (MFPR) on the incidence of GDM. Sivan et al[10] studied 188 consecutive triplet pregnancies during the period of 1994–1998, of which 103 continued as triplets whereas 85 women underwent MFPR to twins. The frequency of GDM was significantly higher in the triplet group than in the (reduced) twin group (22.3 versus 5.8%), leading to the conclusion that plurality influences the frequency of GDM. It is interesting to note that Skupski et al[11] used the same methodology to compare the risk for pre-eclampsia in triplet and (reduced from triplets) twin gestations. As with GDM, the triplet group had a higher rate of severe pre-eclampsia (26.3%) than the twin group (7.9%); however, these authors did not find a difference in other maternal complications of pregnancy. In the two mentioned studies,[10,11] both cases and controls started as triplets and MFPR was performed during the early second trimester. This methodological construct excludes an early effect of the trophoblastic mass and may indirectly point to a later effect, whereby fetal number, placental mass or factors unrelated to the success of implantation are more important to the development of pre-eclampsia and GDM than is successful implantation alone.

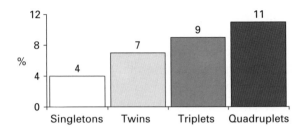

Figure 40.3. *Prevalence of gestational diabetes mellitus by plurality (adapted from Newan and Luke[12]).*

Finally, Newman and Luke[12] complied data from numerous reports on the frequency of GDM in multiple pregnancies. Fig. 40.3 shows that the frequency of GDM has a definite plurality-dependent trend.

Conflicting data

Over the years, relevant clinical data failed to support the high prevalence of GDM in multiple pregnancies. Naicker et al[13] compared 26 women carrying twins with 26 women carrying singletons matched for age, parity and gestational age. Each woman had an oral glucose tolerance test (OGTT); venous blood glucose levels and insulin responses were not significantly different between the two groups. The same researcher subsequently reported on 21 twin pregnancies and 21 matched-for-age, -weight, -parity and -gestational-age singleton pregnancies.[14] All 42 subjects had a 100 gram OGTT: the only difference was a lower plasma insulin level at 60 minutes in the twin pregnancy group, but again no significant differences in venous plasma glucose responses and insulin levels were found between singleton and twin pregnancies. It is unknown, however, if cases in the two studies[13,14] were the same.

Another approach to the debate was reported by Naidoo et al.[15] The authors compared 20 twin pregnancies with 20 matched-for-age, -weight, -parity, and -gestational-age singleton pregnancies. Intravenous glucose tolerance tests (IVGTT) (0.5 gram/kg bodyweight) were preformed on all women in the third trimester of pregnancy. No significant differences in mean venous insulin levels or glucose responses were found between singleton and twin pregnancies.

Spellacy et al[16] assessed the risk of GDM in a cohort of 101,506 pregnancies, including 1253 twin pregnancies. The twin pregnancy group was compared with a 5% random sample of singleton pregnancies (n = 5119). The data showed that women in the twin pregnancy group were slightly older, were of higher parity, gained more weight during gestation and had a higher body weight at delivery. Twin pregnancies were complicated with a higher rate of hypertension [odds ratio (OR) 2.5; 95% confidence interval (CI) 2.1–3.1], placental abruption (OR 3.0; 95% CI 1.9–4.7) and anemia (OR 2.4; 95% CI 1.9–3.0), but there was no increased risk for GDM.

Henderson et al[17] used the 50 gram 1 hour OGTT to screen 9185 pregnancies, including 138 (1.5%) twin gestations. GDM was diagnosed when abnormal screens (> 129 mg/dl) were followed by two or more abnormal values on the 3 hour, 100 gram glucose tolerance test (National Diabetes Data Group criteria). The incidence of GDM was similar for singleton and twin gestations – 5.8 and 5.4%, respectively.

Blickstein and Weissman[18] evaluated 56 twin pregnancies representing the tenth decile of the mean twin birthweight distribution to investigate whether 'macrosomic' twins face the same increased perinatal risk as do macrosomic singletons. In both study and control groups, GDM was infrequent and could not explain the increased birthweight among twins.

Multiple pregnancies with gestational diabetes mellitus

The control of GDM during twin pregnancies was evaluated by Schwartz et al,[19] who compared the frequency, maternal age, weight, 1 hour screen, OGTT results, post-treatment blood glucose values, insulin requirements and insulin dose in twin and singleton pregnancies associated with GDM and carbohydrate intolerance. They found an increased incoherence of GDM among twins (7.7 versus 4.1%) but insulin requirements were not different. This observation may suggest a mild disturbance of carbohydrate tolerance in twins, which may be effectively managed by similar strategies used to control blood glucose in singletons.

The data concerning the effect of GDM on perinatal outcome in multiple pregnancies is scant. Tchobroutsky et al[20] reported on a high frequency of fetal malformations in Type I diabetic women with twin pregnancies, however, the small number of cases precluded a final conclusion. Keller et al[21] compared 13 twin pregnancies complicated with GDM to matched-by-gestational-age twin pregnancies. There was a trend of greater likelihood of respiratory distress syndrome, hyperbilirubinemia and prolonged neonatal intensive care nursery admission in the diabetic group.

Conclusions

If both GDM and multiples pregnancy affect four out of every 100 pregnancies but are stochastically independent, their co-occurrence is expected to be as low as 16 out of every 10,000 (0.16%), a figure which is much lower that the observed figure in all studies. On the other hand, the data presented in this chapter, despite the inherent logical expectations, do

---

Reasons why multiple pregnancies are prone to GDM
Hyperplacentosis
Older women
Higher weight gain and body mass in twin gestations
Exaggerated response to fasting and food
Plurality-dependent frequency of GDM

Conflicting data concerning GDM and multiple pregnancies
Similar prevalence of GDM in twin and singleton pregnancies
No difference in glucose challenge and tolerance tests between twin and singleton pregnancies
Management of twin gestations complicated by GDM is similar to singleton pregnancies
Similar insulin requirements in twin and singleton pregnancies complicated by GDM

Box 40.1. Summery of clinical data related to gestational diabetes mellitus (GDM) and multiple pregnancies.

not support a clear-cut association between GDM and multiple pregnancies (Box 40.1). The question then arises if the data are appropriate to draw any conclusions. In fact, there are several reservations concerning the available data.

First, the few quasi-epidemiological studies performed are quite old and do not include multiple pregnancies resulting from the current epidemic of iatrogenic conceptions. The remarkable difference between mothers before and after the 1990s[1,2] cast serious doubts on whether the prevalence cited in older studies is still valid today. Second, most, if not all, information is hospital based and points to the serious flaw due to the lack of population-based data. As a result, prospective studies on maternal adaptation to carbohydrate metabolism during a multiple pregnancy are flawed because of a small sample size and the lack of sufficient statistical power. Moreover, time-lead bias, which overlooks changes in management over time, have not been considered. For example, it would be interesting to know how recommendations for excess weight gain during early stages of a multiple pregnancy[12] would influence carbohydrate metabolism.

Finally, there is a striking paucity of studies related to high-order multiple, especially triplet, pregnancies. Obviously, triplets were rare – and of negligible importance – before the current epidemic of iatrogenic pregnancies. However, this is no longer true in most developed countries.[1,2] It follows that, except for compiled data,[12] the reciprocal effect between GDM and triplet gestations are unknown.

The most pertinent question may be related to the most significant cause of morbidity of multiple gestations, i.e. low birthweight. In this respect, perinatal outcome related to the balance between the fetal growth-promoting effect of GDM and the inherent growth-restricting effect of the limited and overwhelmed uterine milieu is absolutely unknown.

Taken together, further study is needed to answer these and many other uncertainties related to the co-occurrence of GDM and multiple pregnancies.

References

1. Blickstein I, Keith LG. The spectrum of iatrogenic multiple pregnancy. In: (Blickstein I, Keith LG, eds.) *Iatrogenic Multiple Pregnancy: Clinical Implications.* (Parthenon Publishing: New York, 2001) 1–7.

2. Blickstein I, Keith LG. The epidemic of multiple pregnancies. *Postgrad Obstet Gynecol* 2001; **21**:1–7.

3. Loos R, Derom C, Vlietinck R, Derom R. The East Flanders Prospective Twin Survey (Belgium): a population-based register. *Twin Res* 1998; **1**:167–75.

4. Ventura SJ, Martin JA, Curtin SC et al. Births: final data for 1998. *Natl Vital Stat Rep* 2000; **28**:1–100.

5. Spellacy WN, Buhi WC, Birk SA. Human placental lactogen levels in multiple pregnancies. *Obstet Gynecol* 1978; **52**:210–12.

6. Spellacy WN, Buhi WC, Birk SA. Carbohydrate metabolism in women with a twin pregnancy. *Obstet Gynecol* 1980; **55**:688–9.

7. Lurie S, Blickstein I. Age distribution of erythrocyte population in women with twin pregnancy. *Gynecol Obstet Invest* 1993; **36**:163–5.

8. Casele HL, Dooley SL, Metzger BE. Metabolic response to meal eating and extended overnight fast in twin gestation. *Am J Obstet Gynecol* 1996; **175**:917–21.

9. Marconi AM, Davoli E, Cetin I et al. Impact of conceptus mass on glucose disposal rate in pregnant women. *Am J Physiol* 1993; **264**:514–18.

10. Sivan E, Maman E, Homko CJ et al. Impact of fetal reduction on the incidence of gestational diabetes. *Obstet Gynecol* 2002; **99**:91–4.

11. Skupski DW, Nelson S, Kowalik A et al. Multiple gestations from in vitro fertilization: successful implantation alone is not associated with subsequent preeclampsia. *Am J Obstet Gynecol* 1996; **175**:1029–32.

12. Newman RB, Luke B. *Multifetal Pregnancy.* (Lippincott, Williams & Wilkins: Philadelphia, 2000).

13. Naicker RS, Subrayen KT, Jialal I et al. Carbohydrate metabolism in twin pregnancy. *S Afr Med J* 1983; **63**:538–40.

14. Moodley SP, Jialal I, Moodley J et al. Carbohydrate metabolism in African women with twin pregnancy. *Diabetes Care* 1984; **7**:72–4.

15. Naidoo L, Jailal I, Moodley J, Desai R. Intravenous glucose tolerance tests in women with twin pregnancy. *Obstet Gynecol* 1985; **66**:500–2.

16. Spellacy WN, Handler A, Ferre CD. A case-control study of 1253 twin pregnancies from a 1982–1987 perinatal data base. *Obstet Gynecol* 1990; **75**:168–71.

17. Henderson CE, Scarpelli S, LaRosa D, Divon MY. Assessing the risk of gestational diabetes in twin gestation. *Natl Med Assoc* 1995; **87**:757–8.

18. Blickstein I, Weissman A. 'Macrosomic' twinning: a study of growth-promoted twins. *Obstet Gynecol* 1990; **76**:822–4.

19. Schwartz DB, Daoud Y, Zazula P et al. Gestational diabetes mellitus: metabolic and blood glucose parameters in singleton versus twin pregnancies. *Am J Obstet Gynecol* 1999; **181**:912–14.

20. Tchobroutsky C, Vray M, Papoz L. Fetal malformations in twin pregnancies of type I diabetic women. *Lancet* 1991; **337**:1358.

21. Keller JD, Utter GO, Dooley SL et al. Northwestern University Twin Study X: outcome of twin gestations complicated by gestational diabetes mellitus. *Acta Genet Med Gemellol* 1991; **40**:153–7.

41

Evidence-based medicine and diabetic pregnancy
Pauline Green, Zarko Alfirevic

Introduction

It seems that increasing number of clinicians are joining one of two very vocal camps. There are the 'evangelists' of evidence-based medicine, who believe that grading of evidence and guidelines based on clinical trials and meta-analyses are the panacea for all clinical mishaps, versus clinicians, who believe that medicine is an art and that so-called evidence has no meaning for doctors who want to provide holistic, individualized patient care. Of course, the truth is somewhere in between. The challenge for tomorrow's doctors is to combine the best of both worlds. It is important to be able to critically appraise the evidence quickly and accurately, and then to apply the knowledge at the bedside, taking into account both the individual needs of the patient and the population perspective.

Critical appraisal of the evidence is only the first step on this journey and not the end of it. Unfortunately, most attempts to start the journey of evidence-informed medicine have failed because the evidence is inadequate or non-existent. This has been a source of frustration for doctors from both camps and also for users of health care.

The public has been increasingly frustrated by the fact that most interventions currently used by health care professionals have not been evaluated according to standards demanded from the pharmaceutical industry. In principle, an evaluation of effectiveness and safety of a 'new' policy of elective Caesarean section to prevent birth trauma or a 'new' diet in diabetic pregnancy should not be less stringent than the evaluation of a new drug. The arguments that clinicians have used successfully to impose strict regulatory mechanisms on the pharmaceutical industry are also relevant when clinicians evaluate new ideas.

Rather than lament on the lack of evidence to guide the management of diabetes in pregnancy, this chapter will try to explain the reasons for it. It is suggested that most of the research related to the management of the diabetic pregnancy follows the pattern seen in other areas of medicine. Published research has concentrated on the clinical questions that have been possible to answer rather than the questions that need to be answered. In order to prove this 'hypothesis', in Table 41.1 the types of diabetic pregnant women and the interventions that may be offered to them in everyday clinical practice are summarized.

The contents of Table 41.1 are only the first part of the clinical question, for example is dietary advice of value for women with pre-existing insulin diabetes or should insulin be given to women with impaired glucose tolerance? The other important part of the

Pregnant women*	Interventions
Pregestational IDDM	Blood sugar control
Pregestational IDDM with complications	Dietary advice
Pregestational diet-controlled IDDM	Exercise
Pregestational drug-controlled IDDM	Insulin
Gestational diabetes requiring insulin	Oral hypoglycaemics
Gestational diabetes, diet controlled	Alternative medicine (e.g. herbs, acupuncture)
Impaired glucose tolerance test	Optimizing fetal and maternal outcome, prepregnancy counselling, vitamins/antioxidants, fetal assessment by ultrasound (e.g. fetal growth velocity, Doppler), cardiotocography, antenatal steroids, induction of labour before or at term, Caesarean section before labour, tight glycaemic control

* IDDM, Insulin-dependent diabetes mellitus.

Table 41.1. *Types of diabetic pregnant women and health care interventions suitable for inclusion in clinical trials.*

question is what is hoped to be achieved by the proposed interventions. Table 41.2 gives the clinical outcomes that should guide the choice of intervention(s) in the diabetic pregnancy. When reading clinical trial data, it is apparent that many different outcomes have been measured, e.g. fetal or neonatal macrosomia is often used as an outcome measure. This is not included in the present list of important clinical outcomes, as the macrosomia *per se* is not the end point one would wish to judge interventions by. The important end points are those subsequent upon the macrosomia, i.e. birth trauma, shoulder dystocia and Erb's palsy, cerebral haemorrhage due to difficult delivery, seizures due to birth asphyxia or metabolic disturbance in the newborn, and perinatal mortality. Macrosomia would not necessarily lead to any of these problems, therefore the measured outcome needs to be set at a clinically meaningful level. It must be asked whether an intervention being proposed to a patient is capable of reducing the adverse outcomes listed

in Table 41.2. The present authors suggest that if an intervention has no impact on these outcomes then it is unlikely to be of clinical value. So, what sort of impact is being sought? Often one finds that researchers are completely unrealistic in their expectations, anticipating reductions in adverse pregnancy outcomes of $\geq 50\%$. Very few interventions can achieve this. If they do, the impact is so obvious that clinical trials are at best unnecessary, if not unethical (e.g. Caesarean section for prolonged fetal bradycardia, glucagon for severe maternal hypoglycaemia). The vast majority of proposed interventions and management policies can only achieve modest benefits, e.g. $\leq 25\%$ reduction in important adverse outcomes. With this in mind, the number of women who would be needed to prove that an intervention is capable of achieving its intended aim has been calculated. (Table 40.2) As a rule, studies with < 1000 participants will not be able to give much information about the impact of an intervention on the outcomes that are important to pregnant women with diabetes. The studies will often claim that 'there is no difference in perinatal mortality or birth trauma', but this does not mean that an important clinical difference does not exist. 'No evidence of a difference', which is almost a rule in small studies, should not be confused with 'evidence of no difference'.

The aim of the next section of this chapter is to identify published clinical trials that have set out to answer the questions posed in Tables 41.1 and 41.2. For example, whether elective delivery of a pregnant diabetic woman is better than allowing her to await spontaneous labour or whether the elective use of insulin in mild glucose intolerance will have any advantages over diet alone.

Current evidence from clinical trials

One hundred and three publications of randomized trials from the Cochrane Register of Clinical Trials that may have contained relevant information for the management of diabetes in pregnancy were identified. Of these, 28 publications were excluded: one trial was still recruiting, there was insufficient data collected from a number of other trials, several trials were excluded as they did not contain information relevant to pregnancy and diabetes, and, finally, there were a number of publications which reported on the same randomized trial.

Clinically relevant adverse outcomes	How many participants are required in a two-arm trial to prove that an intervention can reduce an adverse outcome by 25%?*		
	Likely incidence in the control (untreated) group (%)	Anticipated 25% reduction (%)	Total sample size (both groups)
Fetal/neonatal			
Miscarriages/early pregnancy loss	17[80]	12.75	2292
Fetal anomalies	9.7[80]	7.3	8720
Perinatal mortality	3.6[80]	2.7	12,262
Shoulder dystocia	2.8[68]	2.1	15,878
Erb's palsy	1 (0.7 in neonates < 4.5 kg, 5 in neonates > 4.5 kg)[81]	0.75 3.75	45,157
Serious neonatal morbidity (seizures, intracranial haemorrhage, encephalopathy, cerebral palsy)	1	0.75	45,157
Maternal			
Maternal death	0.11[82]	0.08	344,284
Maternal ketoacidosis	1.73[83]	1.3	26,254
Maternal hypoglycaemic coma	36[84]	27	878

* Power 80%, alpha 0.05.

Table 41.2. Complications that should be used as main outcomes in clinical trials.

Fetal assessment by ultrasound

Two trials were identified which sought to answer the question as to whether ultrasound could help to identify pregnant women with diabetes who were likely to benefit from an intervention. Buchanon et al[1] used the third trimester ultrasound to measure the fetal abdominal circumference in women with mild gestational diabetes mellitus (GDM). If the fetal abdominal circumference was large ($\geq$ 75th centile), women were randomized either to continue with their diet or to start insulin in addition to their dietary therapy: 59 women completed the study but no serious clinically important adverse outcomes were reported (Table 41.2). Rossi et al[2] also started insulin therapy when ultrasound measurements of the fetal abdominal circumference exceeded the 75th centile in women with mild, diet-controlled GDM: 73 women had an ultrasound fetal abdominal circumference measurement at 28 and 32 weeks gestation, and 68 women had a single measurement at 32 weeks. There were no maternal hypoglycaemic episodes in 73 women who took part in the study, but other important adverse outcomes were not reported. For a clinically significant difference in the rate of serious maternal hypoglycaemia to be assessed, a sample size of over 800 women would have been required.

Intrapartum glucose control

One study from the USA[3] compared intravenous infusion of 10% invert sugar with lactated Ringer's solution and 5% dextrose in 32 insulin-requiring diabetics prior to labour induction or elective Caesarean section. No serious adverse outcomes were reported. This trial therefore failed to inform of a management strategy which would be of important clinical relevance.

Diet

A Cochrane review by Walkinshaw,[4] included four trials where GDM was managed either by dietary manipulation or with no specific treatment[5,6] (also Ford FA, unpublished work and Okum N, unpublished work). The reviewer concluded that the results were inconclusive, with only one trial of 158 women[6] reporting 'corrected' perinatal mortality of 0% (one baby died with multiple congenital malformations). In this same study there were no reported cases of birth trauma in either group and there were five babies with congenital abnormalities, three in the control group (including the baby with multiple abnormalities that died) and two in the treatment group. Okum reported the reduced incidence of birth trauma with diet [zero of 234 versus four of 223; odds ratio (OR) 0.13, 95% confidence interval (CI) 0.02–0.96].

A study by Bevier et al,[7] not included in the Cochrane review, also compared diet and home monitoring with routine care in 103 women with a positive glucose challenge test. There were two cases of shoulder dystocia in the control group and one case in the experimental group. However, only 83 of the 103 randomized women were reported on, 48 in the control group and 35 in the experimental group. These numbers are inadequate for assessing any clinically useful difference in the incidence of shoulder dystocia with the chosen intervention.

Seven small trials, with the number of participants ranging from five to 125, compared different types of diet.[8–14] Only trials by Ney et al[8] and Rae et al[10] reported substantive outcomes. Ney et al[8] reported no congenital malformations in 20 diabetic pregnancies, while Rae et al[10] reported three cases of shoulder dystocia in 124 women.

Insulin

A Cochrane review by Walkinshaw[15] included two trials[16,17] with 182 pre-existing insulin-dependent diabetics. He concluded that there was no clear evidence favouring very tight glycaemic control in these women. However, out of the nine clinically important outcomes (as listed in Table 41.2), only the perinatal mortality was reported by Farrag (0%).[17]

A preliminary report by Snyder et al[18] also described a trial of tight versus very tight diabetic control and reported no difference in the birth trauma between the two groups.

The present authors have identified a further 26 trials focusing on the use of insulin, either comparing its use with diet alone or with no treatment, or in trials comparing different types of insulin, different regimes of delivery of insulin or comparing insulin with oral hypoglycaemics.[5,19–43] The population of pregnant women in these studies were either gestational or pregestational diabetics.

Serious maternal morbidity was explicitly reported in nine trials.[27–36] Ketoacidosis was found in one of 10 women in Botta et al's[22] study, one of 89 women in Burkhart et al's[29] study, three of 23 women in Nosari et al's[31] study and no cases in 22 patients in Coustan et al's[35] study. The ketoacidosis rate reported in these trials was c. 3.5%, which is higher than in observational studies (Table 41.2). Nevertheless, thousands rather than tens of women are needed to show that an intervention does not affect the incidence of ketoacidosis. Seven studies have also reported severe maternal hypoglycaemia.[22,30–33,35,36] The incidence ranged from zero to a high rate of hypoglycaemia, with 0% in four studies,[22,30,32,36] 7% in Nachum et al's[33] study, 12.5% in Nosari et al's[31] study and the high rate of 36.4% in Coustan et al's[35] study. It is most likely that these large differences reflect the varying definitions of severe hypoglycaemia rather than any true differences in quality of care. This is the reason why severe hypoglycaemia is defined by the authors as one that causes unconciousness. In the three studies with cases of severe hypoglycaemia, Coustan et al[35] defined it as an episode of hypoglycaemia requiring hospital treatment with intravenous glucose or glucagon, Nosari et al[31] characterized it as coma, seizure or a situation requiring hospitalization, intravenous glucose or glucagon, and Nachum et al[33] defined it as an episode requiring the help of another person.

Perinatal deaths were reported in 14 of the trials.[28–33,36–43] The rates ranged from 0 to 14.5%,[42] but the majority of trials reported a perinatal death rate < 5%. Given the low number of patients in these studies and the relatively low perinatal mortality rates it is not surprising that no firm conclusions can be drawn regarding the safety of the various insulin regimens.

No trials reported serious neonatal morbidity as an outcome and only one trial reported Erb's palsy.[43]

Different screening practices

Bebbington et al's[44] randomized trial compared routine universal screening of low-risk pregnant women for GDM with selective screening when clinical indications (risk factors) were present: no clinically important outcomes were reported for the 2401 randomized women. A similar trial with 3152 women showed a higher rate of diagnosis of GDM in the universal screening group.[45] Two intrauterine deaths occurred in the routinely screened group after a positive glucose challenge test. Three further randomized trials were identified related to screening for GDM but none referred to clinically important outcomes.[46–48]

Induction versus expectant management

A Cochrane review by Boulvain et al[49] assessed the effectiveness and safety of elective delivery compared with expectant management in term diabetic pregnant women: only the trial by Kjos et al[50] was included in the review. This study randomized 200 insulin-requiring diabetic pregnant women to either active induction of labour or expectant management up to 42 weeks gestation. Spontaneous labour occurred in 44% of the expectant management group. Of the clinically significant outcomes that were detailed in the study, only shoulder dystocia actually occurred. All three documented cases occurred in the expectant management group and all were described as mild. There were no cases of birth trauma (including Erb's palsy), no perinatal deaths and no major congenital abnormalities. No maternal outcomes were reported. Again, one is unable to ascertain from this study whether elective delivery in the gestational diabetic confers any benefit as the numbers required to show a 25% improvement in the clinically important outcomes measured would require many more women (Table 41.2).

Vaginal delivery versus Caesarean section

Only one randomized trial compared vaginal delivery and Caesarean section as the mode of delivery at term in pregnant women diagnosed with GDM.[51] All women had been monitored during pregnancy and been given dietary advice, there was no indication that any women required insulin. Out of 84 randomized women with GDM, 44 were allocated to Caesarean section at term. It is reassuring that there were no reported cases of perinatal deaths or congenital malformations. However, > 10,000 women would have had be to randomized to exclude the possibility that one of these interventions increases perinatal mortality by 25%.

Exercise

Four studies were identified that assessed the effect of exercise on pregnant women with diabetes.[52-55] Only two of them reported on the present authors' pre-specified outcomes.[52,53] In the randomized trial comparing diet versus diet plus an exercise programme in the management of GDM, Jovanovic et al[52] reported that there were no cases of maternal hypoglycaemia and no neonatal morbidity in 19 gestational diabetics. The authors concluded that a cardiovascular-conditioning programme might obviate the need for insulin treatment in many women with GDM, but the observations in their study required further testing. Referring to Table 41.2, *c.* 900 women would be required to assess a difference of 25% in the rate of severe maternal hypoglycaemia. Similarly, in the trial by Bung et al,[53] 41 patients with failed diet therapy who would have been treated with insulin were randomized to either receive diet plus exercise or diet plus insulin. There were no reported episodes of hypoglycaemia in either group.

Glucose monitoring

Twelve clinical trials studying the various methods of monitoring glucose levels were identified.[56-67] Two studies based the clinical decision to commence insulin therapy on either amniotic fluid insulin levels or mean blood glucose monitoring.[57,67] In both of these studies the present authors' pre-specified outcomes were not reported, although Hopp et al[67] commented that there were no statistically significant differences in the rates of miscarriage, stillbirth or neonatal death in their two groups. Langer et al[62] randomized 2461 women with GDM into either conventional (weekly clinic visits) or intensified (home blood glucose monitoring) management groups. A threefold higher rate of shoulder dystocia was found in the conventional management group compared with the intensified management group (1.4 versus 0.4%, $P < 0.0001$). Langer et al[62] also reported on the percentages of other neonatal trauma events and the number of perinatal deaths. In the following list the conventional management group results come first and the intensified management group results second: seizures, 0.3 versus 0.2%; fracture, 0.7 versus 0.3%; Erb's palsy, 0.1 versus 0%; stillbirths, five versus one; neonatal deaths, three versus three. Langer et al[62] commented that two neonatal deaths were related to anomalies (anencephaly and holoprosencephaly) and one stillbirth had a cardiac anomaly, but they did not report whether other anomalies had occurred nor which group the anomalies occurred in.

Varner,[59] Rey[60] and Stubbs et al[63] all compared clinic visits with the more intensive home blood glucose monitoring in women with either GDM or insulin-dependent diabetes mellitus (IDDM). Varner[59] reported on miscarriage and perinatal death, but only 30 insulin-dependent diabetics were recruited. Rey[60] reported that a significant increase in shoulder dystocia occurred in the clinic visit group (one case in the home-monitoring group versus four cases in the clinic visits group), but on small numbers (347 randomized women). There was one fetal death in the home-monitoring group associated with a true knot of the cord. Stubbs et al[63] reported one perinatal loss (cot death) in 13 randomized women, but no other clinically important outcomes.

De Veciana et al[64] recruited 66 gestational diabetics on insulin to monitor blood glucose either pre- or postprandially. Shoulder dystocia (defined as requiring one or more manoeuvres) was reported to occur in 18% (six of 33) of the preprandial monitoring group and in 3% (one of 33) of the postprandial monitoring group. Overall, the rate of shoulder dystocia in the 66 gestational diabetics (10.6%) was much higher

than in observational studies (2.8%).[68] Such a high incidence of shoulder dystocia probably reflects the definition that was used. As expected, the incidence of Erb's palsy was lower (6 and 3%, respectively) but in all cases the palsy resolved before discharge. One infant in each group had a fracture (one of the clavicle and one of the humerus). There was one unexplained stillbirth in the preprandial monitoring group.

Reller et al[56] randomized 63 women to either early or late careful diabetic management, but the study design precluded any of the present authors' stated important outcomes. Di Biase et al[58] randomized 20 IDDM patients to either a telemedicine computerized device, enabling 24-hour communication of data, or conventional home blood glucose monitoring. Again, no significant outcome data was reported.

Two trials compared the effect of glycaemic control and routine antenatal care in GDM.[61,66] Both trials were in fact pilot studies and too small to draw any conclusions, but both authors concluded that a large randomized trial was feasible.

Hanson et al[65] studied the effect of hospitalization from 32 weeks gestation compared with a policy of home blood glucose monitoring in 100 pregnant diabetic women. Major congenital abnormalities were reported in three of 46 infants (hospital management) and one of 56 infants (home glucose monitoring). There was one perinatal death in each group. It must be emphasized again that the numbers were too small to draw any meaningful conclusions regarding effectiveness and safety of these interventions.

Diagnosis of gestational diabetes mellitus

Proving that a diagnostic test is reproducible and accurate is only the beginning, and not the end, of its evaluation. Introduction of an effective new screening policy, or a diagnostic test, into clinical practice should be expected to have a major impact on the outcome of diabetic pregnancies. One expects that a test with a better performance (sensitivity, specificity) would restrict interventions, such as blood glucose monitoring and treatment (diet, insulin), to those women who are likely to benefit from such interventions. However, an excellent diagnostic test may be followed by an ineffective or dangerous treatment package, or vice versa, with the net result of harm rather than benefit. At present, the randomized clinical trial is the only research method that allows an unbiased comparison of various management policies (diagnosis plus treatment) for diabetic pregnant women.

Ten studies were identified that sought to compare different diagnostic tests for GDM,[69–78] but only Court et al[70] reported the impact of these tests on clinically important outcomes, i.e. perinatal deaths. There were six perinatal deaths in the group of 230 women who used glucose polymer as the test beverage compared with zero deaths in the group of 48 women who were given glucose: two of six deaths were due to congenital abnormality. As far as the present authors could ascertain, no other important clinical outcomes were reported in any of the other studies of diagnostic tests in diabetic pregnancies.

Other

In 1955, Reid[79] evaluated the use of stilboestrol and progesterone in 147 pregnant women with either pre-existing diabetes or GDM. Women were randomized (after stratification by age and parity) to receive (76 women) or not to receive (71 women) hormones from 16 weeks to term. One mother died in each group after Caesarean section. There were four congenital abnormalities in the hormone-treated group and seven in the control group. There were six miscarriages in each group and 17 perinatal deaths in each group.

Summary

In this chapter, the present authors have deliberately set out to be controversial in their approach to evidence-based care of the diabetic pregnancy. It has been attempted to show, by using examples of published clinical trials in this field, that an enormous amount of research time and energy, and patient good will, has produced remarkably little evidence. It is suggested that the way forward is multicentre collaboration rather than intercentre competition. The research agenda should be driven by questions relevant to pregnant diabetic women and their families, rather than the present 'publish or perish' policy.

References

1. Buchanon TA, Kjos SL, Montoro MN et al. Use of fetal ultrasound to select metabolic therapy for pregnancies complicated by mild gestational diabetes. *Diabetes Care* 1994; **17**:275–83.
2. Rossi G, Somigliana E, Moschetta M et al. Adequate timing of fetal ultrasound to guide metabolic therapy in mild gestational diabetes mellitus. Results from a randomised study. *Acta Obstet Gynecol Scand* 2000; **79**:649–54.
3. Wright TE, Martin D, Qualls C, Curet LB. Effects of intrapartum administration of invert sugar and D5LR on neonatal blood glucose levels. *J Perinatol* 2000; **20**:217–18.
4. Walkinshaw SA. Dietary regulation for 'gestational diabetes' (Cochrane review). In: *The Cochrane Library, Issue 1.* (Oxford: Update Software, 2002).
5. Langer O, Anyaegbunam A, Brustman L, Divon M. Management of women with one abnormal oral glucose tolerance test value reduces adverse outcome in pregnancy. *Am J Obstet Gynecol* 1989; **161**:593–9.
6. Li DFH, Wong VCW, O'Hoy KMKY et al. Is treatment needed for mild impairment of glucose tolerance in pregnancy? A randomised controlled trial. *Br J Obstet Gynaecol* 1987; **94**:851–4.

7. Bevier WC, Fischer R, Jovanovic L. Treatment of women with an abnormal glucose challenge test (but a normal oral glucose tolerance test) decreases the prevalence of macrosomia. *Am J Perinatol* 1999; 16:269–75.

8. Ney D, Hollingsworth DR, Cousins L. Decreased insulin requirement and improved control of diabetes in pregnant women given a high-carbohydrate, high-fiber, low-fat diet. *Diabetes Care* 1982; 5:529–33.

9. Reece EA, Hagay Z, Gay LJ et al. A randomised clinical trial of a fiber-enriched diabetic diet vs. the standard American Diabetes Association recommended diet in the management of diabetes mellitus in pregnancy. *J Matern Fetal Invest* 1995; 5:8–12.

10. Rae A, Bond D, Evans S et al. A randomised controlled trial of dietary energy restriction in the management of obese women with gestational diabetes. *Aust NZ J Obstet Gynaecol* 2000; 40:416–22.

11. Nolan CJ. Improved glucose tolerance in gestational diabetic women on a low fat, high unrefined carbohydrate diet. *Aust NZ J Obstet Gynaecol* 1984; 24:174–7.

12. Magee MS, Knopp RH, Benedetti TJ. Metabolic effects of 1200-kcal diet in obese pregnant women with gestational diabetes. *Diabetes* 1990; 39:234–40.

13. Lauszus FF, Rasmussen OW, Henriksen JE et al. Effect of a high monounsaturated fatty acid diet on blood pressure and glucose metabolism in women with gestational diabetes mellitus. *Eur J Clin Nutr* 2001; 55:436–43.

14. Ilic S, Jovanovic L, Pettitt DJ. Comparison of the effect of saturated and monounsaturated fat on postprandial plasma glucose and insulin concentration in women with gestational diabetes mellitus. *Am J Perinatol* 1999; 16:489–95.

15. Walkinshaw SA. Very tight versus tight control for diabetes in pregnancy (Cochrane review). In: *The Cochrane Library, Issue 1*. (Oxford: Update Software, 2002).

16. Demarini S, Mimouni F, Tsang RC et al. Impact of metabolic control of diabetes during pregnancy on neonatal hypoglycemia: a randomised study. *Obstet Gynecol* 1994; 83:918–22.

17. Farrag OAM. Prospective study of 3 metabolic regimens in pregnant diabetics. *Aust NZ J Obstet Gynaecol* 1987; 27:6–9.

18. Snyder J, Morin L, Meltzer S, Nadeau J. Gestational diabetes and glycemic control: a randomised clinical trial. *Am J Obstet Gynecol* 1998; 178:55.

19. Pardi G, Buscaglia M, Kustermann A et al. Foetal pulmonary maturation in pregnancies complicated by diabetes and Rh immunization. *Eur Respir J* 1989; 2 (**Suppl** 3):50S–52S.

20. Gillmer MDG, Maresh M, Beard RW et al. Low energy diets in the treatment of gestational diabetes. *Acta Endocrinol* 1986; 277:44–9.

21. Schuster MW, Chauhan SP, McLaughlin BN et al. Comparison of insulin regimens and administration modalities in pregnancies complicated by diabetes. *J Mississippi State Med Assoc* 1998; 39:51–5.

22. Maresh M, Alderson C, Beard RW et al. Comparison of insulin against diet treatment in the management of abnormal carbohydrate tolerance in pregnancy. In: (Campbell DM, Gillmer MDG, eds) *Nutrition in Pregnancy, Proceedings of the 10th Study Group of the RCOG*. (London: RCOG, 1983) 255–67.

23. Li P, Yang H, Dong Y. Treating women with gestational impaired glucose tolerance reduces adverse outcome of pregnancy. *Chin J Obstet Gynecol* 1999; 34:462–4.

24. Laatikainen L, Teramo K, Hieta-Heikurainen H et al. A controlled study of the influence of continuous subcutaneous insulin infusion treatment on diabetic retinopathy during pregnancy. *Acta Med Scand* 1987; 221:367–76.

25. Jovanovic-Peterson L, Palmer JP, Sparks S, Peterson CM. Jet-injected insulin is associated with decreased antibody production and postprandial glucose variability when compared with needle-injected insulin in gestational diabetic women. *Diabetes Care* 1993; 16:1479–83.

26. Jovanovic-Peterson L, Kitzmiller JL, Peterson CM. Randomised trial of human versus animal species insulin in diabetic pregnant women: improved glycemic control, not fewer antibodies to insulin, influences birth weight. *Am J Obstet Gynecol* 1992; 167:1325–30.

27. Jovanovic L, Ilic S, Pettitt DJ et al. Metabolic and immunologic effects of insulin lispro in gestational diabetes. *Diabetes Care* 1999; 22:1422–7.

28. Botta RM, Sinagra D, Angelico MC, Bompiani GD. Intensified conventional insulin therapy as compared to micropump therapy in pregnant women affected by type 1 diabetes mellitus. *Minerva Medica* 1986; 77:657–61.

29. Burkart W, Hanker JP, Schneider HPG. Complications and fetal outcome in diabetic pregnancy. Intensified conventional versus insulin pump therapy. *Gynecol Obstet Invest* 1988; 26:104–12.

30. Langer O, Conway DL, Berkus MD et al. A comparison of glyburide and insulin in women with gestational diabetes mellitus. *N Engl J Med* 2000; 343:1134–8.

31. Nosari I, Maglio ML, Lepore G et al. Is continuous subcutaneous insulin infusion more effective than intensive conventional insulin therapy in the treatment of pregnant diabetic women? *Diabet Nutr Metab* 1993; 6:33–7.

32. Thompson DJ, Porter KB, Gunnells DJ et al. Prophylactic insulin in the management of gestational diabetes. *Obstet Gynecol* 1990; 75:960–4.

33. Nachum Z, Ben-Shlomo I, Weiner E, Shalev E. Twice daily versus four times daily insulin dose regimens for diabetes in pregnancy: randomised controlled trial. *Br Med J* 1999; 319:1223–7.

34. Maresh M, Gillmer MDG, Beard RW et al. The effect of diet and insulin on metabolic profiles of women with gestational diabetes mellitus. *Diabetes* 1985; 34 (**Suppl** 2):88–93.

35. Coustan DR, Reece EA, Sherwin RS et al. A randomised clinical trial of the insulin pump vs intensive conventional therapy in diabetic pregnancies. *J Am Med Assoc* 1986; 255:631–6.

36. Carta Q, Meriggi E, Trossarelli GF et al. Continuous subcutaneous insulin infusion versus intensive conventional insulin therapy in Type I and Type II diabetic pregnancy. *Diabete et Metabolisme (Paris)* 1986; **12**:121–9.

37. Persson B, Stangenberg M, Hansson, Nordlander E. Gestational diabetes mellitus (GDM): comparative evaluation of two treatment regimens, diet vs insulin and diet. *Diabetes* 1985; **34**:101–5.

38. O'Sullivan JB. Prospective study of gestational diabetes and its treatment. In: (Stowers JB, Sutherland HW, eds) *Carbohydrate Metabolism in Pregnancy and the Newborn.* (Churchill Livingstone: 1975) 195–204.

39. O'Sullivan JB, Charles D, Dandrow RV. Treatment of verified prediabetes in pregnancy. *J Reprod Med* 1971; **7**:21–4.

40. O'Sullivan JB, Gellis SS, Dandrow RV, Tenney BO. The potential diabetic and her treatment in pregnancy. *Obstet Gynecol* 1966; **27**:683–9.

41. O'Sullivan JB, Mahan CM, Charles D, Dandrow RV. Medical treatment of the gestational diabetic. *Obstet Gynecol* 1974; **43**:817–21.

42. Notelovitz M. Sulphonylurea therapy in the treatment of the pregnant diabetic. *S Afr Med J* 1971; **45**:226–9.

43. Coustan DR, Lewis SB. Insulin therapy for gestational diabetes. *Obstet Gynecol* 1978; **51**:306–10.

44. Bebbington M, Milner R, Wilson R, Harris S. A RCT comparing routine screening vs selected screening for GDM in low risk population. *Am J Obstet Gynecol* 1999; **180**:S36.

45. Griffin ME, Coffey M, Johnson H et al. Universal vs risk factor-based screening for gestational diabetes mellitus: detection rates, gestation at diagnosis and outcome. *Diabet Med* 2000; **17**:26–32.

46. Hidar S, Chaieb A, Baccouche S et al. Post-prandial plasma glucose test as screening tool for gestational diabetes: a prospective randomised trial. *J Gynecol Obstet Biol Reprod* 2001; **30**:344–7.

47. Murphy NJ, Meyer BA, O'Kell RT, Hogard ME. Carbohydrate sources for gestational diabetes mellitus screening. A comparison. *J Reprod Med* 1994; **39**: 977–81.

48. Lamar ME, Kuehl TJ, Cooney AT et al. Jelly beans as an alternative to a fifty-gram glucose beverage for gestational diabetes screening. *Am J Obstet Gynecol* 1999; **181**:1154–7.

49. Boulvain M, Stan C, Irion O. Elective delivery in diabetic pregnant women (Cochrane review). In: *The Cochrane Library, Issue 1.* (Oxford: Update Software, 2002).

50. Kjos SL, Henry OA, Montoro M et al. Insulin-requiring diabetes in pregnancy: a randomised trial of active induction of labor and expectant management. *Am J Obstet Gynecol* 1993; **169**:611–15.

51. Khojandi M, Tsai AY/M, Tyson JE. Gestational diabetes: the dilemma of delivery. *Obstet Gynecol* 1974; **43**:1–6.

52. Jovanovic-Peterson L, Durak EP, Peterson CM. Randomised trial of diet versus diet plus cardiovascular

53. conditioning on glucose levels in gestational diabetes. *Am J Obstet Gynecol* 1989; **161**:415–19.

53. Bung P, Artal R, Khodiguian N, Kjos S. Exercise in gestational diabetes. An optional therapeutic approach? *Diabetes* 1991; **40**:182–5.

54. Avery M, Leon AS, Kopher RA. Effects of a partially home-based exercise program for women with gestational diabetes. *Obstet Gynecol* 1997; **89**:10–15.

55. Lesser KB, Gruppuso PA, Terry RB, Carpenter MW. Exercise fails to improve postprandial glycemic excursion in women with gestational diabetes. *J Matern Fetal Med* 1996; **5**:211–17.

56. Reller MD, Tsang RC, Meyer RA, Braun CP. Relationship of prospective diabetes control in pregnancy to neonatal cardiorespiratory function. *J Pediatr* 1985; **106**:86–90.

57. Novak A, Hopp H, Vollert W et al. Fetal indication for insulin therapy in gestational diabetes. Proceedings of the 14th European Congress of Perinatal Medicine, Helsinki, Finland, 1994, 318.

58. Di Biase N, Napoli A, Sabbatini A et al. Telemedicine in the treatment of diabetic pregnancy. *Annali dell Istituto Superiore di Sanita* 1997; **33**:347–51.

59. Varner MW. Efficacy of home glucose monitoring in diabetic pregnancy. *Am J Med* 1983; **75**:592–6.

60. Rey E. Usefulness of a breakfast test in the management of women with gestational diabetes. *Obstet Gynecol* 1997; **89**:981–8.

61. Garner P, Okun N, Keely E et al. A randomised controlled trial of strict glycemic control and tertiary level obstetric care versus routine obstetric care in the management of gestational diabetes: a pilot study. *Am J Obstet Gynecol* 1997; **177**:190–5.

62. Langer O, Rodriguez DA, Xenakis EMJ et al. Intensified versus conventional management of gestational diabetes. *Am J Obstet Gynecol* 1994; **170**:1036–47.

63. Stubbs SM, Brudenell JM, Pyke DA et al. Management of the pregnant diabetic: home or hospital, with or without glucose meters? *Lancet* 1980; **1**:1122–4.

64. De Veciana M, Major CA, Morgan MA et al. Postprandial versus preprandial blood glucose monitoring in women with gestational diabetes mellitus requiring insulin therapy. *N Engl J Med* 1995; **333**:1237–41.

65. Hanson U, Persson B, Enochsson E et al. Self-monitoring of blood glucose by diabetic women during the third trimester of pregnancy. *Am J Obstet Gynecol* 1984; **150**:817–21.

66. Bancroft K, Tuffnell DJ, Mason GC et al. A randomised controlled pilot study of the management of gestational impaired glucose tolerance. *Br J Obstet Gynaecol* 2000; **107**:959–63.

67. Hopp H, Vollert W, Ragosch V et al. Indication and results of insulin therapy for gestational diabetes mellitus. *J Perinat Med* 1996; **24**:521–30.

68. Conway DL, Langer O. Elective delivery of infants with macrosomia in diabetic women: reduced shoulder dystocia

versus increased cesarean deliveries. *Am J Obstet Gynecol* 1998; **178**:922–5.

69. Sammarco MJ, Mundy DC, Riojas JE. Glucose tolerance in pregnancy. Proceedings of the 41st Annual Clinical Meeting Of The American College of Obstetricians and Gynecologists, USA, 1993, 10–11.

70. Court DJ, Mann SL, Stone PR et al. Comparison of glucose polymer and glucose for screening and tolerance tests in pregnancy. *Obstet Gynecol* 1985; **66**: 491–9.

71. Court DJ, Stone PR, Killip M. Comparison of glucose and glucose polymer for testing oral carbohydrate tolerance in pregnancy. *Obstet Gynecol* 1984; **64**: 251–5.

72. Cheng LC, Salmon YM, Chen C. A double-blind, randomised, cross-over study comparing the 50 g OGTT and the 75 g OGTT for pregnant women in the 3rd trimester. *Ann Acad Med* 1992; **21**:769–72.

73. Harlass FE, McClure GB, Read JA, Brady K. Use of a standard preparatory diet for the oral gl tol test. Is it necessary? *J Reprod Med* 1991; **36**:147–50.

74. Helton DG, Martin RW, Martin JN et al. Detection of glucose intolerance in pregnancy. *J Perinatol* 1989; **9**:259–61.

75. Berkus MD, Langer O. Glucose tolerance test periodicity: the effect of glucose loading. *Obstet Gynecol* 1995; **85**:423–7.

76. Bergus GR, Murphy NJ. Screening for gestational diabetes mellitus: comparison of a glucose polymer and a glucose monomer test beverage. *J Am Board Fam Plan* 1992; **5**:241–7.

77. Jones JS, Horger E. A comparative study of the standard oral and intravenous glucose tolerance tests in pregnancy. *Am J Obstet Gynecol* 1993; **168**:407.

78. Weiss PAM, Haeusler M, Kainer F et al. Toward universal criteria for gestational diabetes: relationships between seventy-five and one hundred gram glucose loads and capillary and venous glucose concentrations. *Am J Obstet Gynecol* 1998; **178**:830–5.

79. Reid DD. Report to the medical research council. The use of hormones in the management of pregnancy in diabetics. *Lancet* 1955; **2**:833–6.

80. Casson IF, Clarke CA, Howard CV et al. Outcomes of pregnancy in insulin dependent diabetic women: results of a five year population cohort study. *Br Med J* 1997; **315**:275–8.

81. Persson B, Hanson U. Neonatal morbidities in gestational diabetes mellitus. *Diabetes Care* 1998; **21** (**Suppl 2B**):79–84.

82. Reece EA, Hobbins JC, Mahony MJ, Petrie RH. *Handbook of Medicine of the Fetus and Mother*. (JB Lippincott Co: Philidelphia, 1995).

83. Kilvert JA, Nicholson HO, Wright AD. Ketoacidosis in diabetic pregnancy. *Diabet Med* 1993; **10**:278–81.

84. Rayburn W, Piehl E, Jacober S et al. Severe hypoglycaemia during pregnancy: its frequency and predisposing factors in diabetic women. *Int J Gynaecol Obstet* 1986; **24**:263–8.

42

Databases: a tool for quality management of diabetic pregnancies

Dina Pfeifer, Rony Chen, Moshe Hod

Introduction

Predicting the likelihood that databases will become an important instrument for medical quality improvement is at least as obvious as the prediction that a woman in labour will deliver. Databases are not a novelty. Although used by clinicians for only a century, there are earlier historical examples of simple types of database that served as a major engine of change and progress, displaying a convincing evidence of its usefulness over a respectable period of time.[1]

In most instances, the benefits of clinical databases have long been recognized. Formerly, data were stored in paper form, analysis meant calculation by hand or with a simple calculator, and statistical tables were used for accepting or rejecting hypothesis at defined levels of statistical significance.[2] In practice this has led to a restricted number of comparisons. Today we have databases, statistical and graphical packages, and comparisons between many variables and data sets are done with ease. Meta-analysis is becoming an increasingly popular method of comparing, combining and summarizing the outcomes of published studies, though provoking controversies at the same time. Some authors believe that meta-analysis may be as reliable as randomized controlled trials, whereas others believe that the technique should be used only to generate rather than test hypotheses.[3–5]

Database research is generally considered to be cheaper and faster than trials, but is weaker on research design. Such problems include incomplete data on the case mix, a lack of concurrent controls, and an inability to ascertain important outcomes or to identify the role of association among the multiple outcomes of interest.[6,7] While a lack of progress has partly been a consequence of a lack of interest on the part of clinicians, managers and researchers, it has also reflected the demanding requirements for creating high-quality databases.[8]

Database developments

Developments in computer technology and mass production of computer processors and other components have made computers and data-input devices affordable. The rapid development of newer and better equipment has made cutting-edge technology affordable even for low-income countries. In response to growing demand, the software market has become ultrasophisticated in addressing the vast range of user needs.

Various database architectures are in use. Database structures must be defined prior to data entry and are set as institutional administrative databases, clinical databases or national registries.[9] As a result, users of statistical techniques need no longer be concerned with the arithmetical and algebraic details of various statistical methods, and can concentrate instead on understanding the underlying ideas and basic principles of statistical analyses, and look into outcomes of the analysis.[10,11] The advantages of electronic databases include: minimal storage space, fast and accurate searches, ease of updating data, easy data management, merge of data from various sources, multiuser access, interactivity, networking, internet access, data presentation and reporting, and simple back-up.

When making a decision concerning which database software to use, care must be taken not to be unduly influenced by price and availability, but primarily by hardware capacity, software compatibility, programming requirements and technical expertise required. The analysis process frequently requires the simultaneous use of a number of complementary software packages. Therefore, the decision for software purchase should be established on the ability for the interface of various applications, the format in which the data are stored and simplicity of use.

Evidence-based medicine and databases

Evidence-based medicine integrates the best available data from clinical research into clinical practice to enhance the quality of decisions made, so achieving the best possible outcomes.[12-14] The precise role of evidence-based medicine is being widely debated in view of its applicability to individual patients. Continuous collation of data at the level of provision of medical services, though not being

pure clinical research, as an alternative approach is considered closer to reality.[8] The advantages include high generalizability through the participation of a wider scale of health care providers, the ability to rapidly generate large samples, and the opportunity to study conditions and interventions.[8,15] However, practitioners have difficulty in finding, assessing, interpreting and applying current best evidence.

The importance of data comparison of institutional data is invaluable for increasing excellence through the Hawthorne effect. An example of this approach is the Obstetrical Quality Indicators and Datacollection (OBSQID) database of the World Health Organization's (WHO) Regional Office for Europe, which includes aggregated data on more than 14 million births in 43 countries and offers a forum for comparing obstetrical quality data at its internet site for either aggregated or case-based data (Fig. 42.1).[16] In coordination with representatives of most participating institutions, the OBSQID project variables and coding were standardized, nevertheless mostly reflecting uniformity with clinical data already available. Thus, comparison of data was made possible and so increased the ability to effectively reuse data to produce further information of evidence-based medicine.

Despite of the wealth of available data, the issue of data quality should also be assessed. The incomplete data, limited detection of outcomes (e.g. maternal mortality 42 days after delivery, congenital malformations diagnosed after discharge), interrupted time series, coding accuracy and methods of data verification applied, are some of the problems encountered in the endeavour to maintain such regional databases. A substantial challenge of maintaining or improving obstetrical outcomes spins the process of comparing the data on more than initially agreed basic information. An increase

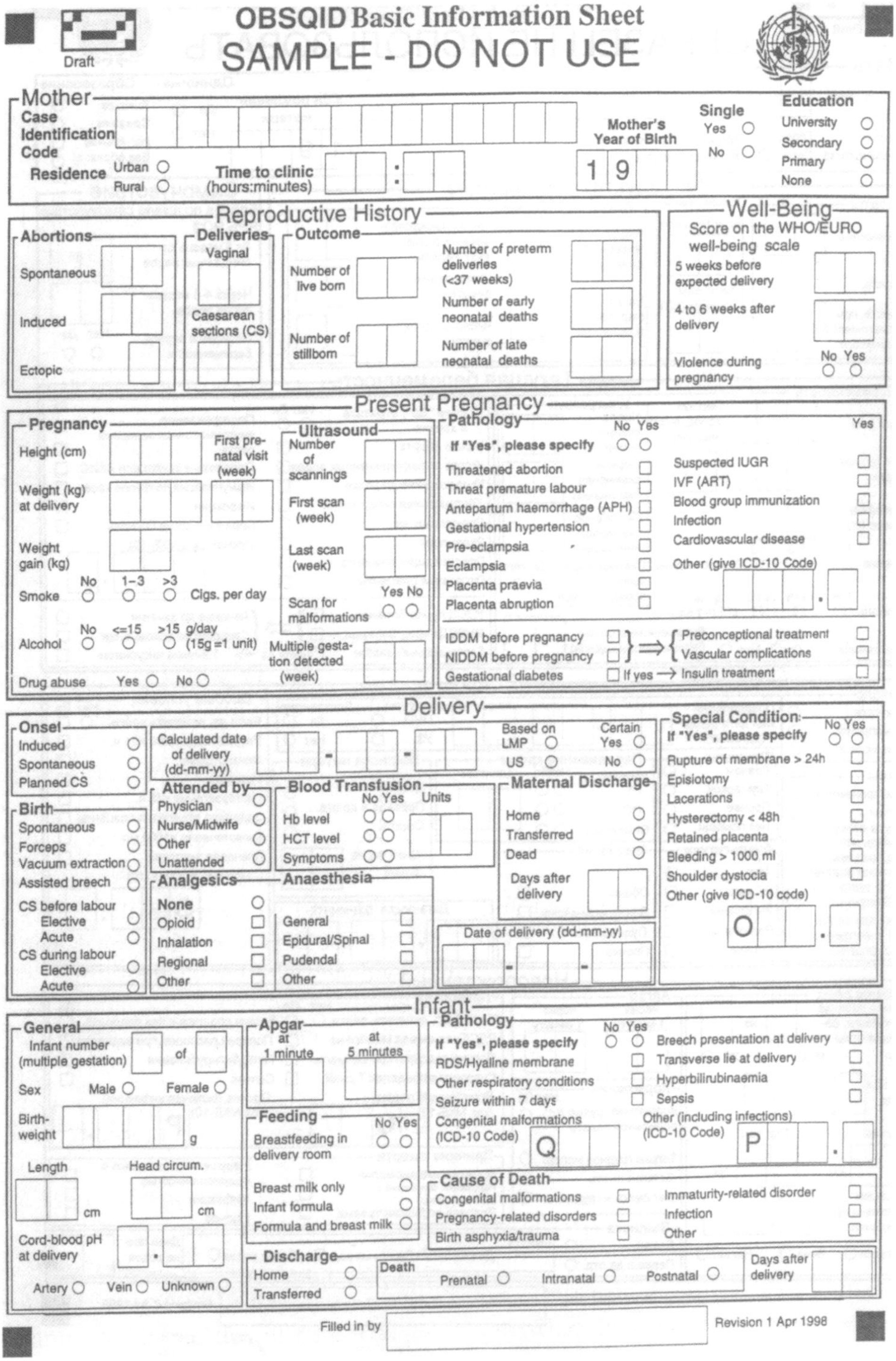

Draft

OBSQID Basic Information Sheet

SAMPLE - DO NOT USE

Mother

Case Identification Code

Residence: Urban ○ Rural ○

Time to clinic (hours:minutes)

Mother's Year of Birth: 1 9

Single: Yes ○ No ○

Education: University ○ Secondary ○ Primary ○ None ○

Reproductive History

Abortions: Spontaneous; Induced; Ectopic

Deliveries: Vaginal; Caesarean sections (CS)

Outcome: Number of live born; Number of stillborn; Number of preterm deliveries (<37 weeks); Number of early neonatal deaths; Number of late neonatal deaths

Well-Being

Score on the WHO/EURO well-being scale: 5 weeks before expected delivery; 4 to 6 weeks after delivery

Violence during pregnancy: No ○ Yes ○

Present Pregnancy

Pregnancy: Height (cm); Weight (kg) at delivery; First pre-natal visit (week); Weight gain (kg)

Smoke: No ○ 1–3 ○ >3 ○ Cigs. per day

Alcohol: No ○ <=15 ○ >15 ○ g/day (15g =1 unit)

Drug abuse: Yes ○ No ○

Ultrasound: Number of scannings; First scan (week); Last scan (week); Scan for malformations Yes ○ No ○; Multiple gestation detected (week)

Pathology (No ○ Yes ○) If "Yes", please specify:
Threatened abortion □; Threat premature labour □; Antepartum haemorrhage (APH) □; Gestational hypertension □; Pre-eclampsia □; Eclampsia □; Placenta praevia □; Placenta abruption □; Suspected IUGR □; IVF (ART) □; Blood group immunization □; Infection □; Cardiovascular disease □; Other (give ICD-10 Code)

IDDM before pregnancy □; NIDDM before pregnancy □ ⇒ Preconceptional treatment □; Vascular complications □

Gestational diabetes □ If yes → Insulin treatment □

Delivery

Onset: Induced ○; Spontaneous ○; Planned CS ○

Calculated date of delivery (dd-mm-yy) — Based on LMP ○ US ○; Certain Yes ○ No ○

Birth: Spontaneous ○; Forceps ○; Vacuum extraction ○; Assisted breech ○; CS before labour: Elective ○, Acute ○; CS during labour: Elective ○, Acute ○

Attended by: Physician ○; Nurse/Midwife ○; Other ○; Unattended ○

Blood Transfusion (No Yes, Units): Hb level ○ ○; HCT level ○ ○; Symptoms ○ ○

Maternal Discharge: Home ○; Transferred ○; Dead ○; Days after delivery

Analgesics: None ○; Opioid □; Inhalation □; Regional □; Other □

Anaesthesia: General □; Epidural/Spinal □; Pudendal □; Other □

Date of delivery (dd-mm-yy)

Special Condition (No ○ Yes ○) If "Yes", please specify: Rupture of membrane > 24h □; Episiotomy □; Lacerations □; Hysterectomy < 48h □; Retained placenta □; Bleeding > 1000 ml □; Shoulder dystocia □; Other (give ICD-10 code) O

Infant

General: Infant number (multiple gestation) of; Sex Male ○ Female ○; Birth-weight g; Length cm; Head circum. cm; Cord-blood pH at delivery: Artery ○ Vein ○ Unknown ○

Apgar: at 1 minute; at 5 minutes

Feeding: Breastfeeding in delivery room No ○ Yes ○; Breast milk only ○; Infant formula ○; Formula and breast milk ○

Pathology (No ○ Yes ○) If "Yes", please specify: RDS/Hyaline membrane □; Other respiratory conditions □; Seizure within 7 days □; Congenital malformations (ICD-10 Code) Q; Breech presentation at delivery □; Transverse lie at delivery □; Hyperbilirubinaemia □; Sepsis □; Other (including infections) (ICD-10 Code) P

Cause of Death: Congenital malformations □; Pregnancy-related disorders □; Birth asphyxia/trauma □; Immaturity-related disorder □; Infection □; Other □

Discharge: Home ○; Transferred ○

Death: Prenatal ○ Intranatal ○ Postnatal ○; Days after delivery

Filled in by

Revision 1 Apr 1998

Figure 42.1. *OBSQID Basic information sheet.*

of active participation of clinicians and researchers in designing other databases is increasingly emphasized and is applied to ensure meaningfulness and usefulness for the quality measurement.

Evidence or lack of it?

The St Vincent Declaration integrates a commitment to continuous quality improvement through routine measure of outcomes, benchmarking and consolidation of processes in diabetic care.[17,18] Since its proclamation in 1989, different types of diabetes databases, national registries, subregional and regional databases or other types of information systems, have been developed to meet objectives set in the declaration.[19–22] The process of continuous quality improvement demands not only the gathering of reliable and validated data, but also acting upon this data. Many standardization, logistical and legal problems have been encountered, and have subsequently led to a better understanding of the successful implementation of these databases.[23–25]

Diabetes in pregnancy is not a rare condition and represents a specific area of diabetes population management. When a decision has to be made about measures or treatments in women or neonates from such pregnancies, physicians face a dearth of comparative evidence. However, reproducibility of results is often limited and most risk estimates are based on uncontrolled observational studies. According to the St Vincent Declaration, the ultimate goal for the management of pregnancies complicated by diabetes should be a maternal or neonatal outcome approaching that of the non-diabetic population. Some of previously set databases (e.g. DIABCARE) and national registries collected data on diabetes in pregnancy, primarily Type 1 diabetes.[21] Yet there seems to

be an appreciable gap between the obstetrical and perinatal information collected, and maternal diabetes-related data sets, preventing the necessary outcome of monitoring, benchmarking and clinical auditing to monitor changes. The situation is particularly complex with respect to gestational diabetes.

Several multicentre studies have been undertaken in recent years to provide baseline data on the outcomes of diabetic pregnancies with respect to obstetrical interventions, dietary and treatment alternatives, subsequent short- and long-term effects on offsprings' morbidity and mortality, as well as development and progression of long-term diabetes complications during the course of pregnancy. Systematic review of the literature in order to find evidence of best practice reveals a scarcity of adequate information on obstetrical outcomes, decision-making, guidelines and protocols in relation to diabetes in pregnancy. To implement changes in the clinical practice an audit mechanism should be initiated to continuously re-evaluate outcomes and practices. Strengthening epidemiological assessment has become an imperative strategy of diabetes surveillance and it is considered essential for quality management of diabetes in pregnancy too. The annual rate of pregnancies complicated by diabetes at an average maternity hospital is usually too small to be informative, making average data from several years necessary for analysis. Therefore, adverse effects may reflect performance in the past rather than the present.[14] Variations may be substantial to such a degree that it is impossible to assess its influence on real differences of an intervention or outcome. Because of small numbers or rare outcomes, the sample size is inadequate for statistical analysis, usually making compari-sons between subgroups impossible.

Large patient samples and a broad origin of data is a clear benefit of multicentre study, however, great care should be taken in harmonization of methodology. Examples of national and international data collection tools of WHO Pan European Database on Diabetes in Pregnancy are presented in Fig. 42.2 (aggregated data) and Fig. 42.3 (case-based data). Case-based data can be merged with basic information related to obstetrical history, diagnoses and interventions (Fig. 42.1) for detailed analysis of perinatal outcomes or with other databases containing data on metabolic control, dietary measures, diabetic complications, etc. Data and conclusions derived in such a way should be of a quality relevant for the institutions and applicable to the patients.[26]

Some cautions and concerns

Administrative and clinical databases are valuable assets which should be considered as evidence. However, the challenge remains to identify means by which various data can be collated from disparate sources into a single structure and used effectively. Frequently, diabetes- and pregnancy-related data are stored in several databases of unequal design. Attempts to successfully merge data sets, avoiding unrealistic assumptions and oversimplifications, should be done in a systematic fashion, with special consideration to consistency and validity of underlying data.

Databases are technologically sophisticated, complex and fascinating objects. When creating a database the objective of establishing it should be clear and not affected by architecture or functional characteristics. Limitations and potentially negative consequences of database use for quality improvement should be questioned early in the process. Dealing with these challenges will probably turn out to be at least as important to the implementation and full effectiveness of databases as the technical side

of the effort.[1] New statistical methods are required to analyse raw data from large databases, as traditional statistical methods using models that adjust for covariates do not eliminate biases. In fact, inherent biases are magnified, not minimized, by large databases.[10,27] Furthermore, an overlooked problem is that an overwhelming number of feasible comparisons show some results to be statistically significant simply by chance.[2,28]

Databases will not help directly any individual patient with the management of his or her condition. Rather, they will be tools in the development of new or improved methods of achieving better health, prediction, diagnoses and treatment of disease, and in establishing more cost-efficient ways of operating health services.[29] However, the results are often of uncertain generalizability, as they tend to be carried out in atypical settings. It is difficult to make adjustments in complex case-mix conditions, as databases usually contain minimal set of variables.

Once a database is established it should be run for an extended period of time to provide an overview of the epidemiological situation. Although some flexibility is beneficial, a basic variable set should be kept fixed to allow for comparisons and a minimal data set should be defined. Funding to run the service should be secured, feedback to the contributors must occur at regular intervals and, if on-line access is granted, the database should be updated regularly. Contributions to the database should be seen as part of ongoing work and so considered as highly beneficial.

Due to dangers inherent in modern technology, every care should be taken to improve the security of data, control of its dissemination and the potential for abuse minimized. Legal and ethical issues are clearly important, and are relevant to international conventions and policies concerned with human rights.[30,31]

Draft

OBSQID Perinatal Aggregated Data - Diabetes (DPAD)

WHO ID number or country acronym

Year
- ○ 1999
- ○ 2000
- ○ 2001

Data Level
○ National ○ Regional ○ Local
Location (if regional/local)

Women who gave birth (all deliveries)
Infants born (all births)

A

Women with pre-gestational diabetes mellitus
IDDM NIDDM
IGT MODY

Women with vascular complications
Retinopathy Nephropathy
Deterioration
Retinopathy Nephropathy

Pre-pregnancy counselling/care
HbA1C >8%
1 trimester
3 trimester

B

Women with
... GDM
... persisting DM post delivery
... persisting IGT post delivery

Treated with insulin
Post partum evaluation

	A: Pre-GDM			B: GDM
	Induced	Spontaneous	Total	
1. *Abortions				
2. Intrauterine deaths (22–27 completed weeks)				
3. Antenatal deaths (>27 completed weeks)				
Total antenatal deaths if 2/3 not available				
4. Fetal deaths during delivery				

Figure 42.2. *OBSQID Aggregated data sheet for pregnancies complicated by diabetes.*

Draft

	A: Pre-GDM	B: GDM
5. Preterm births (<32 completed weeks)		
6. Preterm birth (32–36 completed weeks)		
7. Labour induced		
8. Caesarean sections		
9. Forceps/vacuum extractions		
11. Early neonatal death (0–6 days)		
12. Late neonatal death (7–27 days)		
Total neonatal deaths if 11/12 not available		
13. Maternal PIH/PET		
14. Eclampsia (during pregnancy – 10 days after delivery)		
15. Macrosomia (>4000 g)		
16. Shoulder dystocia		
17. Apgar <=6 @ 5 minutes (>31 completed weeks)		
18. Major congenital malformations		
19. Infants with RDS		
22. Neonatal admissions to NICU		

Enter all data as absolute numbers.
Avoid leading zeros.
Where data are unavailable please leave the field blank.

Filled in by

Date

Name

Address

Revision 17 Sep 1999

Figure 42.2. *Continued.*

Draft

Basic Information Sheet for Diabetes and Pregnancy

Basic personal data

Local ID

Date of birth (day - month - year)

Previous
- Deliveries (>22 weeks)
- Caesarean sections

Classification of diabetes

Type of diabetes
- IDDM O
- NIDDM O
- IGT O
- Pre-GDM O
- GDM O
- G-IGT O

Diagnosis based on
- Blood glucose O
- GCT (50g) O
- oGTT (75g) O
- oGTT (100g) O
- Test meal O
- Unknown O

Date of diagnosis (day - month - year)

Booking

Date of first visit to specialist (day - month - year)

Proteinuria (g/24h)

HbA1c (%)

Agreed date of delivery (day - month - year)

Date of first HbA1c (day - month - year)

Retinopathy	Yes	No
Background	O	O
Profilerative	O	O

	Yes	No
Hypertension	O	O

Mother

Therapy
- Insulin O
- Diet O
- None O

Progress of	Yes	No
Retinopathy	O	O
Nephropathy	O	O

HbA1c (Third trimester)

Date of HbA1c (day - month - year)

	Yes	No
PIH	O	O

Maternal Discharge
- Alive O
- Dead O

Pregnancy outcome/delivery

Date of delivery (day - month - year)

Abortion
- Induced O
- Spontaneous O

Labour	Yes	No
Induced	O	O

Delivery	Yes	No
Spontaneous	O	O
Instrumental	O	O
Caesarean	O	O

Infant I

- Male O
- Female O

Weight

- Live born O
- Stillborn O

Pathologies	Yes	No
Shoulder dystocia	O	O
Erb's palsy	O	O

Apgar @ 5 min.

Congenital malformations	Yes	No
Cardiovascular	O	O
NTD	O	O
Other	O	O

Discharge
- Healthy O
- Ill O
- Dead O

Date of discharge/death (day - month - year)

Infant II

- Male O
- Female O

Weight

- Live born O
- Stillborn O

Pathologies	Yes	No
Shoulder dystocia	O	O
Erb's palsy	O	O

Apgar @ 5 min.

Congenital malformations	Yes	No
Cardiovascular	O	O
NTD	O	O
Other	O	O

Discharge
- Healthy O
- Ill O
- Dead O

Date of discharge/death (day - month - year)

Reclassification

New classification
- IDDM O
- NIDDM O
- Normal blood glucose O
- Type unknown O
- No reclassification O

If reclassified →

Based on
- Elevated blood glucose O
- oGTT (75g) O
- Other O

Figure 42.3. *OBSQID Case based data collection sheet for pregnancies complicated by diabetes.*

European legislation is not entirely clear on the issues of keeping case-based data in registers, the need for consent and how to consider aggregated databases.[23]

According to European Directive 95/46,[32] informed consent is necessary if personal data are to be used for purposes other than those for which they were originally gathered, but consent is not required if the data are not personal.[31] The public is sensitized to the potential for breaches of privacy. Many acknowledge the fundamental need for privacy, but only a few recognize that there may be circumstances under which the benefits to the public outweigh the cost of some limited loss of privacy. To get a pertinent snapshot of an epidemiological situation, data collection needs to be universal, i.e. population based. If patients refuse consent to their details being stored in registries then the epidemiological picture of the disease would be distorted.

Conclusions

It may seem difficult and cumbersome to establish an epidemiological surveillance system for diabetes in pregnancy. In fact, it is a matter of organizing available data rather than searching for new data-collection mechanisms, and extending use of the database to the epidemiological dimension. An epidemiological surveillance system could be attained by provision of routinely collected and aggregated data by centres providing obstetrical and neonatal care for pregnant diabetics and their infants. If diabetes and pregnancy is considered a public health issue, it is strongly recommended that epidemiological models should be further developed and implemented at various levels of services to provide data for the dimensioning of the current and future diabetes care systems.[33] Benefits of the surveillance system

should be clearly articulated: (a) utilization of perinatal performance indicators related to a subset of diabetic pregnancies in situation analysis, and for comparison with the general population; (b) benchmarking to aid target setting; (c) identification of areas of particular concern in terms of the need for improved management; (d) forecasting of trends in gestational diabetes prevalence; (e) implementation of the St Vincent Declaration. Critical attention should be given to database design, data sources and their validity, methodologies and interpretation of findings, and the implications for clinical practice.

References

1. Davidoff F. Databases in the next millennium. *Ann Intern Med* 1997; **127**:770–4.
2. Egberts J. Databases and the statistical usage of (perinatal) results. *Am J Obstet Gynecol* 1998; **178**:192.
3. Moher D, Cook DJ, Eastwood S et al. Improving the quality of reports of meta-analyses of randomised controlled trials: the QUOROM statement. QUOROM Group. *Br J Surg* 2000; **87**:1448–54.
4. Stroup DF, Berlin JA, Morton SC et al. Meta-analysis of observational studies in epidemiology: a proposal for reporting. Meta-analysis of observational studies in epidemiology (MOOSE) group. *J Am Med Assoc* 2000; **283**:2008–12.
5. Olkin I. Meta-analysis: reconciling the results of independent studies. *Stat Med* 1995; **14**:457–72.
6. Smith DM. Database research: is happiness a humongous database? *Ann Intern Med* 1997; **127**:725.
7. Imamura K, McKinnon M, Middleton R, Black N. Reliability of a comorbidity measure: the Index of Co-Existent Disease (ICED) *J Clin Epidemiol* 1997; **50**:1011–16.
8. Black N. Developing high quality clinical databases. *Br Med J* 1997; **315**:381–2.
9. Iezzoni LI. Assessing quality using administrative data. *Ann Intern Med* 1997; **127**:666–74.
10. Katz BP. Biostatistics to improve the power of large databases. *Ann Intern Med* 1997; **127**:769.
11. Beck JS, Brown RA. *Medical Statistics on Personal Computers*, 2nd edn. (BMJ Publishing Group: London, 1995).
12. Knottnerus JA, Dinant GJ. Medicine based evidence, a prerequisite for evidence based medicine. *Br Med J* 1997; **315**: 1109–10.

13. Olatunbosun OA, Edouard L. The teaching of evidence-based reproductive health in developing countries. *Int J Gynaecol Obstet* 1997; **56**:171–6.

14. Sheldon T. Promoting health care quality: what role performance indicators? *Qual Assur Health Care* 1998; **7** (**Suppl**):S45 6–S50.

15. Black N. A regional computerised surgical audit project. *Qual Assur Health Care* 1990; **2**:263–70.

16. World Health Organization, Regional Office for Europe, Quality of Care and Technologies. *http://qct.who.dk* (WHO: Copenhagen, 2000).

17. World Health Organization and International Diabetes Federation. Diabetes care and research in Europe: the Saint Vincent declaration. *Diabet Med* 1990; **7**:360.

18. Dunne F, Brydon P, Proffitt M et al. Approaching St Vincent. Working toward the St Vincent targets. *Diabet Med* 2001; **18**:333–4.

19. Piwernetz K, Benedetti MM, Johansen KS. Advanced health care initiatives in Europe on quality development, epidemiology and medical documentation. *Diabete et Metabolisme* 1993; **19**:213–17.

20. Palmer AJ, Brandt A, Gozzoli V et al. Outline of a diabetes disease management model: principles and applications. *Diabetes Res Clin Pract* 2000; **50** (**Suppl 3**): S47–S56.

21. Alexander W, Bradshaw C, Gadsby R et al. An approach to manageable datasets in diabetes care. *Br Diabetic Assoc Diabet Med* 1994; **11**:806–10.

22. Henrichs HR, Piwernetz K, Sonksen PH et al. The feedback between monitoring and improvement of quality of diabetes care. *Diabete et Metabolisme* 1993; **19**:70–3.

23. Vaughan NJ, Massi Benedetti M. A review of European experience with aggregated diabetes databases in the delivery of quality care to establish a future vision of their structure and role. *Diabetes Nutr Metab – Clin Exp* 2001; **14**:86–7.

24. Bloomgarden ZT. Computers in diabetes. *Diabetes Care* 1997; **20**:457–9.

25. Buxton C, Gibby O, Hall M et al. Diabetes information systems: a key to improving the quality of diabetes care. *Diabet Med* 1996; **13** (**Suppl 4**):S122–S128.

26. Johansen KS, Hod M. Quality development in perinatal care – the OBSQID project. *Int J Obstet Gynecol* 1999; **64**:167–72.

27. Byar DP. Problems with using observational databases to compare treatments. *Stat Med* 1991; **10**:663–6.

28. Bland JM, Altman DG. Multiple significance tests: the Bonferroni method. *Br Med J* 1995; **310**:170.

29. Council of Europe Steering Committee on Bioethics. *The Icelandic Act on a Health Sector Database and Council of Europe Conventions.* (Ministry of Health and Social Security: Strasbourg, 1999).

30. Lazaridis EN. Database standardization, linkage, and the protection of privacy. *Ann Intern Med* 1997; **127**:696.

31. Morrow JI. Data protection and patients' consent. Informed consent should be sought before data are used by registries. *Br Med J* 2001; **322**:549–50.

32. European Parliament. *Directive on the Protection of Individuals with Regard to the Processing of Personal Data.* (European Parliament: Brussels, 1995).

33. Glasgow RE, Wagner EH, Kaplan RM et al. If diabetes is a public health problem, why not treat it as one? A population-based approach to chronic illness. *Ann Behav Med* 1999; **21**:159–70.

43

Cost analysis of diabetes and pregnancy

Michael Brandle, William H Herman

Costs of pregnancy care and adverse outcomes of pregnancy

During the adult reproductive years, women have higher medical expenditures than men.[1] The difference in medical expenditures between women and men is related in large part to pregnancy care, childbirth and its complications. The costs of pregnancy and childbirth include the cost of outpatient prenatal care, hospitalizations and care of the newborn. Costs increase with higher frequencies of hospitalization,[2] alternative modes of delivery[3,4] and longer stays in hospital.[5] Costs also increase with multiple gestations[6] and with maternal obesity.[7]

Median hospital costs for preterm labor without delivery have been estimated to be US $2200; median hospital costs for preterm labor with early delivery are US $6600. The total annual expenditures for preterm-labor hospitalization in the United States (US) are in excess of $820 million.[2] A recent systematic review of the literature revealed that the range of costs are £600–1300 (US $1000–2200) for an uncomplicated vaginal delivery and £1200–£3600 (US $2100–$5900) for a Cesarean delivery.[3] In a large Scottish observational study, the health care costs of alternative modes of delivery were estimated to be £1700 for a spontaneous vaginal delivery, £2300 for an instrumental vaginal delivery and £3200 for a Cesarean delivery ($P < 0.001$).[4]

In 1991, the predicted charges for the family (mother and neonate) for a singleton pregnancy was $9800, as compared to $38,000 for twins ($19,000 per baby) and $110,000 for triplets ($36,600 per baby). Hospital charges for a 29-year-old white mother with a singleton pregnancy were $4800, as compared with $8000 for a mother of twins and $15,400 for a mother with a higher order multiple-gestation pregnancy. Daily charges increased from $600 for a singleton neonate to $1000 for each twin and to $1700 for each infant born of a higher order multiple pregnancy.[6]

The average costs of hospital prenatal care are approximately five times higher for mothers who are overweight before pregnancy than for normal-weight mothers.[7] In addition, obesity leads to significantly longer postpartum hospital stays as a result of more frequent Cesarean deliveries and endometritis. The percentage of infants of obese mothers requiring care in a neonatal intensive care unit is *c.* 3.5 times higher than that of infants of non-obese mothers.[8,9]

Adverse outcomes of pregnancy also contribute to substantially higher costs.[10,11] The inpatient and outpatient treatment costs for very-low-birthweight (VLBW) (birthweight < 1500 grams) infants during the first year of life was $59,700 (1987 US dollars).[12] Because of the greater mortality in the smallest infants, the average cost was lowest for infants with birthweights < 750 grams ($49,900) and highest among infants between 750 and 999 grams ($79,200).[12] The lifetime costs of major congenital anomalies are also high (Fig. 43.1): $393,000 for an infant with a major cardiac defect, $294,000 for spina bifida, $250,000 for diaphragmatic hernia, renal agenesis or dysgenesis, $199,000 for lower limb reduction, $176,000 for omphalocele, $108,000 for gastroschisis, $101,000 for cleft lip or palate, and $84,000 for urinary obstruction. The lifetime cost for one infant with cerebral palsy is estimated to be c. $503,000.

Cost-effectiveness of interventions in pregnancy

Cost-effectiveness analyses (CEA) explicitly compare the costs and outcomes of new treatments with alternative treatments so that the treatments can be ordered on the basis of how much benefit is gained relative to the expense.[13] CEA are being reported more frequently in medicine and specifically in obstetrics.[14] Recent CEA in obstetrics have studied the value of fortifying grain with folic acid to prevent neural tube defects (NTD), prenatal HIV screening, smoking cessation programs and vaginal birth after Cesarean delivery. In general, these interventions have proven to be cost-effective or even cost saving because the treatments are effective and often inexpensive, the risk of adverse outcomes is high, the time to the outcomes is short and the cost of the outcomes is large.

In one study, the economic benefit of fortifying grain with folic acid was assessed as the cost savings from NTD averted minus the costs of folic acid supplementation. In the US, the annual cost savings were estimated to be $94 million with low-level fortification (140 µg/100 gram grain) and $252 million with high-level fortification (350 µg/100 gram grain). The cost–benefit ratio was 4.3 for low-

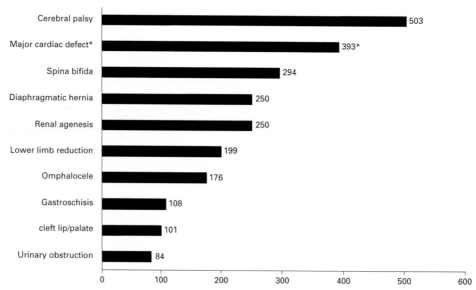

Figure 43.1. *Lifetime costs per new case of major congenital anomalies and cerebral palsy in thousands of US dollars (1992 US $). *Weighted average of the lifetime costs of truncus arteriosus, single ventricle, transposition and tetralogy of Fallot. Adapted from[10].*

level and 6.1 for high-level fortification, suggesting that $4–6 would be saved for each $1 spent on folic acid fortification.[15] Separate CEA performed in the US and the United Kingdom (UK) demonstrated that voluntary HIV screening would cost c. $10,600 per life-year gained in the US,[16] and less than £4000 for each life-year gained in high-HIV-prevalence areas and less than £20,000 for each life-year gained in low-HIV-prevalence areas of the UK.[17] Another CEA demonstrated that if a smoking cessation program decreased the prevalence of cigarette smoking by 1% per year in the US population, it would prevent 1300 low birthweight live births and save $21 million in direct medical costs in the first year and $473 million during the 7 years of the program.[18] Two recent CEA compared elective repeat Cesarean delivery with a trial of labor (vaginal delivery).[19,20] One study found that follow-up routine elective Cesarean delivery cost c. $179 million during the reproductive life of 100,000 women.[19] The prevention of one major adverse neonatal outcome would require c. 1600 Cesarean deliveries and would cost $2.4 million. Another study found that if the probability of successful vaginal delivery exceeded 0.74, a trial of labor was cost-effective.[20]

Cost-effectiveness of preconception care for women with pregestational diabetes

Preconception care for women with established diabetes reduces the incidence of fetal malformations and spontaneous abortions.[21] Three groups have assessed the costs of preconception care relative to the savings resulting from adverse maternal and neonatal outcomes averted. All demonstrated that preconception care for women with established diabetes is cost saving (Table 43.1).[22–24]

A case–control study of women with Type 1 diabetes mellitus was conducted by Scheffler et al to assess the cost–benefit of preconception care.[22] The study estimated the costs of a preconception care program using a time–motion methodology, and analyzed actual hospital charges and length of stay for women enrolled in the California Diabetes and Pregnancy Program (CDAPP). These included 102 women with Type 1 diabetes who participated in the preconception care program and subsequently received standard prenatal care: a group of 218 women with Type 1 diabetes who did not participate in the program but who received

Authors (reference)	Net savings (US $)	Savings on early versus no intervention (US $)	Savings on late versus no intervention (US $)	Cost–benefit ratio
Scheffler et al (22)	6000	7300	5700	5.19
Elixhauser et al (23)	1700	–	–	1.86
Herman et al (24)	34,000	–	–	NR

NR, Not reported.

Table 43.1. Net savings per pregnancy and cost–benefit ratios of preconception care.

standard prenatal care served as controls. Each CDAPP participant was randomly matched with an individual from the control group. The matching criteria were the mother's age, race, and severity and duration of diabetes according the White classification system. This procedure yielded 90 cases from the CDAPP group and 90 controls drawn from hospitals outside the program's catchment area. The researchers examined two groups of cases – those enrolled before 8 weeks of gestation and those enrolled after 8 weeks of gestation – and compared them with women who did not enroll in the program. The analysis adopted the perspective of a third-party payer and considered only direct medical costs. For each mother, charges were included through to delivery; for each infant, charges were included from birth through to discharge. Longer term medical costs due to adverse birth outcomes, which are potential savings of the CDAPP, and any potential health benefits to the mother were not included. Costs were expressed in 1988 US dollars; an 8% discount rate was applied to costs but not benefits. Not unexpectedly, the costs of preconception care were greatest for early enrollees ($1300), lower for late enrollees ($800) and lowest for non-enrollees ($0). In contrast, both maternal and neonatal charges increased from early enrollees to late enrollees to non-enrollees: the charges for maternal care increased from $8900 for early enrollees to $9500 for late enrollees to $11,000 for non-enrollees. The charges for neonatal care increased dramatically from $2300 for infants of early enrollees to $6600 for infants of late enrollees to $10,700 for infants of non-enrollees. Compared to non-enrollees, early enrollees experienced savings of $7300 per enrollee and late enrollees experienced savings of $5700 per enrollee. The cost–benefit ratio of the CDAPP was 5.19; thus, for every $1 spent on the program, $5.19 was recovered in charges averted.

A second cost–benefit study by Elixhauser et al[23] used consensus development, surveys of medical care personnel and a literature review to develop a model to determine whether the additional costs of preconception care are offset by the savings from complications averted. The analyses adopted the perspective of a third-party payer and considered direct medical costs. Costs were calculated in 1989 US dollars; discounting was not performed. Preconception care cost $2600 per enrollee and $4900 per delivery (recognizing that more women receive preconception care than go on to deliver.) The additional cost associated with preconception care was offset by the cost savings associated with adverse maternal outcomes averted ($2000 for women who received preconception care versus $3200 for those who received prenatal care only, a cost saving of $1200) and adverse neonatal outcomes averted ($7700 for infants of mothers who received preconception care versus $10,200 for infants of mothers who received prenatal care only, a cost saving of $2500). When the costs of care for the child were recalculated to include medical care for 3 years after discharge from the neonatal intensive care unit, lifetime medical care, residential care and community services associated with severe congenital malformations, the benefits of preconception care for women with established diabetes were $1700 per enrollee. The cost–benefit ratio was 1.86; thus, for every $1 spent on the preconception care program, $1.86 was gained. When the costs associated with postneonatal intensive care and long-term care were excluded, preconception care saved $480 per enrollee, and the cost–benefit ratio was 1.24.[25]

A third study by Herman et al[24] assessed pregnancy outcomes, resource utilization and costs among women with Type 1 diabetes who received preconception care (PC) and women who did not receive preconception care [prenatal care only (PN)]. The study found a small increase in outpatient visits (two visits) and a substantial, 20-day decrease in inpatient util- ization for women and infants who received PC compared to PN. This consistent and substantial reduction in resource utilization among PC women and their infants as compared to PN women and their infants translated into substantial cost savings. The net cost saving was c. $34,000 per patient (direct medical costs, undiscounted, 1992 US dollars), suggesting that the savings, measured as direct medical costs, may be several times greater than reported by the first two studies.

Cost-effectiveness of interventions in gestational diabetes mellitus

Investigators have studied both the costs of alternative approaches to diagnosing GDM, and the cost-effectiveness of alternative approaches to diagnosing and treating GDM.[26]

Costs of alternative approaches to diagnosing GDM

Over the past two decades, screening for GDM in the US has been performed according to the recommendations of the National Diabetes Data Group (NDDG), the American Diabetes Association (ADA), and the American College of Obstetricians and Gynecologists. Screening has been recommended for all pregnant women and has involved a two-tiered approach: a 1 hour 50 gram glucose challenge test (GCT) and for women with plasma glucose levels ≥ 140 mg/dl (7.8 mmol/l) on the GCT a 3 hour 100 gram oral glucose tolerance test (OGTT).[27]

Many studies have investigated alternative approaches to increase the efficiency and reduce the cost of screening for GDM. Lavin et al[28] estimated the costs incurred by the hospital laboratory in screening and diagnosing GDM in pregnant women with and without historical and clinical risk factors. They estimated that it cost $5 per patient screened with the 1 hour GCT and $329 per case of GDM diagnosed (1980 US dollars). Reed[29] estimated that the laboratory charges per patient screened and per case of GDM detected were $14 and $684, respectively (1984 US dollars) (Table 43.2). Performing a GCT in pregnant women > 25 years of age decreased the cost per patient screened to $7 and the cost per case of GDM detected to $386, but missed 24% of women with GDM.

Coustan et al[30] performed a cost analysis of a population-based study in 6214 universally screened pregnant women using Lavin et al's[29] unit costs for the GCT and OGTT (Table 43.3). A GCT screening threshold of 140 mg/dl (7.8 mmol/l) and NDDG criteria for the OGTT were used. If women < 30 years of age with risk factors and all pregnant women ≥ 30 years of age were screened, the cost per case of GDM diagnosed was $190. However, nearly one-third of women were missed with this protocol because many women with GDM < 30 years of age had no other risk factors or had GCT results between 130 and 139 mg/dl. Sensitivity of detection of GDM increased to 95% by screening women < 25 years of age with risk factors and all women ≥ 25 years of age, and by using a threshold of 130 mg/dl (7.2 mmol/l) for the GCT. The cost per case of GDM diagnosed increased from $195 to $215. If universal screening was performed and a GCT threshold of 130 mg/dl was used, the sensitivity was 100% but the cost per case of GDM increased to $249. Coustan et al[30] noted that if a protocol uses universal screening at ≥ 25 years of age, 78% of individuals will require screening:

Screening protocol	Cost per GDM case diagnosed (1984 US $)	Cases missed (%)
GCT* in all women, if positive OGTT†	684	20
GCT* in women > 25 years of age, if positive OGTT†	386	24
GCT* only in women with risk factors,‡ if positive OGTT†	683	60
OGTT† in all women with risk factors	938	48
OGTT† in all women	976	0

* GCT, 1 hour 50 gram glucose challenge test.
† OGTT, 3 hour 100 gram oral glucose tolerance test.
‡ Risk factors: birth of a baby weighing ≥ 4000 grams (c.) (≥ 9 lb); a history of two or more pregnancies of fetal death, neonatal death, congenital anomaly, prematurity, excessive weight gain, hypertension or proteinuria; family history of diabetes mellitus.

Table 43.2. *Cost per case of gestational diabetes mellitus (GDM) diagnosed using various screening protocols (adapted from Reed[29]).*

Screening protocol	Cost per GDM diagnosed (1980 US $)	Cases missed (%)
GCT* in women > 30 years of age or if risk factors† present, if positive (threshold > 140 mg/dl) OGTT‡	190	35
GCT* in all women ≥ 25 years of age or if risk factors† present, if positive (threshold > 140 mg/dl) OGTT‡	192	15
GCT* in all women ≥ 25 years of age or if risk factors† present, if positive (threshold > 130 mg/dl) OGTT‡	215	5
GCT* in all women, if positive (threshold > 140 mg/dl) OGTT‡	222	10
GCT* in all women, if positive (threshold > 130 mg/dl) OGTT‡	249	0

* GCT, 1 hour 50 gram glucose challenge test.
† Risk factors: previous GDM; previous macrosomic infant [baby weighing ≥ 4000 grams (c. ≥ 9 lb)]; obesity; previous stillborn or neonatal death; family history of diabetes mellitus.
‡ GTT, 3 hour 100 gram oral glucose tolerance test.

Table 43.3. *Cost per case of gestational diabetes mellitus (GDM) diagnosed using various screening protocols (adapted from Coustan et al[30]).*

the small (22%) decrement in cost that accrues as a result of selective screening must be weighed against the more complex logistics and increased probability of failing to screen high-risk women.

The Fourth International Workshop–Conference on Gestational Diabetes Mellitus[31] suggested that two techniques – the two-tiered protocol with Carpenter–Coustan modifications and the one-tiered protocol (2 hour 75 gram OGTT) – are both acceptable methods to screen for GDM. Lavin et al[32] compared the costs and the patient time associated with the two-tiered protocol and the one-tiered modification employing the 2 hour OGTT. The two-tiered protocol had lower costs than the one-tiered protocol: low-range and high-range costs for the two-tiered protocol were $3 and $8 per woman; low-range and high-range costs for the one-tiered protocol were $6 and $11 per woman. Test times were 1.4–1.5 hours for the two-tiered protocol and 2 hours for the one-tiered protocol. Travel time was lower in the one-tiered protocol than in the two-tiered protocol (2 versus 2.3 hours). The authors concluded that the two-tiered protocol appears to be associated with lower costs and less patient time than the one-tiered protocol.

Cost-effectiveness of alternative approaches to diagnosing and treating GDM

CEA are predicated on the demonstration of clinical effectiveness. If an intervention is not effective then it cannot be cost-effective. Ultimately, to determine if the costs of diagnosing GDM are worth paying, studies of cost-effectiveness must include the costs of diagnosing GDM, the costs of providing treatment for GDM, and the costs of the outcomes for the mothers and babies.[26]

Kitzmiller et al[33] performed a cost-identification analysis of a GDM program in Northern California (Santa Clara Valley). Program costs were defined as the cost of all health resources required to diagnose GDM, monitor blood glucose, maintain blood glucose levels within the target range, and monitor the pregnant women and their fetuses to ensure good outcome. Outcome costs included the costs of all health care resources used for inpatient antepartum care, delivery, postdelivery care and newborn care. Average reimbursed charges were used to establish direct medical costs (1996 US dollars). The analysis was performed from the perspective of managed care. The average total program costs per case of GDM were $1100. Program costs were higher for women requiring insulin treatment ($1800) than for women with diet therapy only ($800). The total costs of outcomes per case of GDM were $6000: outcome costs per patient were slightly higher in insulin-requiring GDM cases ($6500) than in those treated with diet therapy alone ($5800).

The costs from the Northern California program were also applied to prospectively collected data from a diabetes and pregnancy program at a large teaching hospital in New England.[33] The diagnostic strategy was the same as in the Northern California program, but more patients required insulin therapy in the New England program. Total program costs per case of GDM were $1800. In spite of good program outcomes, the outcome costs per case of GDM were $8900, substantially higher than in the Northern California program ($6000). The authors concluded that the analyses were potentially biased by the selection of complicated cases of GDM referred to the New England program.

Three studies have assessed the cost-effectiveness or cost–benefit of interventions in GDM. In one, the Northern California program, reimbursed charges were applied to the clinical outcomes of a prospective randomized trial of preprandial or postprandial blood glucose monitoring in GDM.[33,34] GDM was treated with insulin in all 66 women. Although mean gestational ages at delivery were similar, the postprandial monitoring group had lower glycohemoglobin levels, significantly lower birthweights, less macrosomia, less neonatal hypoglycemia and fewer Cesarean deliveries.[34] The program costs per case of GDM were slightly higher in the postprandial blood glucose monitoring group ($3800) than in the preprandial blood glucose monitoring group ($3600), but outcome costs per case of GDM were lower in the postprandial monitoring group ($7500) compared to the preprandial monitoring group ($8000).[33] The incremental cost-effectiveness of the postprandial blood glucose monitoring was $35 per Cesarean delivery averted and $25 per neonatal intensive care unit day prevented. Comparing input and outcome costs for the two blood glucose monitoring groups, the cost–benefit ratio was 2.98 in favor of postprandial blood glucose monitoring; thus, for every $1 spent on postprandial blood glucose monitoring, c. $3 would be saved in averted adverse outcome costs.[33]

Langer et al[35] performed a prospective population-based study of conventional versus intensified therapy in women with GDM and conducted a cost-benefit analysis. Intensified therapy was defined as self-blood glucose monitoring (SBGM) seven times daily with early institution of insulin therapy. Conventional therapy was defined as four times daily SBGM and weekly assessment of fasting and 2 hour postprandial venous plasma glucose.[36] Program costs included the costs of diagnosis, blood glucose evaluation, medication and supplies, and physician, nursing, social worker and dietitian care, and the costs of fetal surveillance. Outcome costs included antepartum and postpartum hospital stay, hospital and physician fees for vaginal or Cesarean deliveries, and neonatal intensive care unit and nursery admissions. Total program costs for the conventional therapy group were $1900 per woman with GDM compared to $2100 per woman with GDM in the intensified therapy group. The total outcome costs for the conventional therapy group were $4600 per woman versus $3900 per woman in the intensified therapy group. There was a 4.37 cost–benefit ratio in favor of the intensified therapy.[35]

Bienstock et al[37] conducted a retrospective cohort study to compare the costs of prenatal care and subsequent maternal and neonatal outcomes in women with GDM cared for in an inner-city university hospital house-staff clinic versus an inner-city managed-care organization. GDM was defined according to NDDG criteria. There were no differences between groups with respect to baseline maternal demographic factors. The cost of providing care to a patient with GDM by the managed-care organization was $10,000 versus $11,000 for the house-staff fee-for-service clinic setting (P = 0.20). A larger percentage of women had > 12 visits with their physician and more sonograms were performed in the house-staff clinic compared to the managed-care organization. In contrast, more fetal surveillance tests were performed in the managed-care organization group. The groups had similar rates of insulin treatment, antepartum admissions, Cesarean delivery, and maternal and infant lengths of stay. In the house-staff clinic group, there was a trend toward a lower frequency of preterm delivery (8.9 versus 13.3%) and significantly less macrosomia (15 versus 29%). The authors concluded that managed care does not decrease the cost of caring for patients with GDM but does lead to a greater rate of neonatal macrosomia, which may reflect poorer glucose control.

Conclusions

During the adult reproductive years, women have higher medical expenditures than men. The difference in medical expenditures between women and men is largely related to pregnancy care, childbirth and its complications. The costs of preterm and postpartum maternal hospitalization and the costs of hospital care for infants with adverse outcomes are major sources of increased cost. Because the cost of outcomes is large and the time to outcomes is short, treatments that are effective in preventing adverse outcomes of pregnancy are often cost-effective or even cost saving. Such interventions include folic acid fortification of grain to prevent NTD and smoking cessation programs to prevent low birthweight infants.

Preconception care for women with established diabetes reduces the incidence of fetal malformations and spontaneous abortions. Three groups have assessed the costs of preconception care relative to the savings resulting from adverse maternal and neonatal outcomes averted. All demonstrated that preconception care for women with established diabetes is cost saving. A number of investigators have also assessed the costs of alternative approaches to diagnosing GDM. Although selective screening for GDM is marginally less expensive than universal screening per case of GDM detected, most women require screening and the more complex logistics and increased probability of failing to screen high-risk women may offset any potential cost savings. It appears that a two-tiered approach to screening for GDM (involving a 1 hour 50 gram GCT followed by a 3 hour 100 gram OGTT) is more cost-effective than a one-tiered modification (employing a 2 hour 75 gram OGTT), with respect to both cost of laboratory testing and patient time.

Studies of the cost-effectiveness of alternative approaches to the treatment of GDM have been hampered by the lack of data demonstrating the clinical effectiveness of diagnosis and intervention. To date, cost-effectiveness and cost–benefit analyses of selected interventions have suggested that postprandial blood glucose monitoring is more cost-effective that preprandial monitoring, and that intensified monitoring and insulin treatment is more cost-effective than conventional monitoring.

Because of the high cost of hospitalization for mothers and infants, and the relatively short time course of pregnancy, many prenatal interventions, and particularly those that are relatively inexpensive, are cost-effective or even cost saving from the perspective of a health system. These interventions, like preconception care for women with established diabetes, should be rigorously implemented, as they both improve health outcomes and reduce costs of care. In the area of GDM, either universal screening or selective screening would appear to be cost-effective, depending upon the health system's ability to risk stratify and track pregnant women. Although perhaps counterintuitive, two-tiered screening appears to be more cost-effective than one-tiered screening, particularly in populations of low diabetes prevalence. Definitive analyses of the cost-effectiveness of alternative approaches to the treatment of GDM will ultimately require more clear-cut demonstration of the clinical effectiveness of those interventions.

References

1. Mustard CA, Kaufert P, Kozyrskyj A, Mayer T. Sex differences in the use of health care services. *N Engl J Med* 1998; **338**:1678–83.
2. Nicholson WK, Frick KD, Powe NR. Economic burden of hospitalizations for preterm labor in the United States. *Obstet Gynecol* 2000; **96**:95–101.
3. Henderson J, McCandlish R, Kumiega L, Petrou S. Systematic review of economic aspects of alternative

modes of delivery. *Br J Obstet Gynecol* 2001; **108:** 149–57.

4. Petrou S, Glazener C. The economic costs of alternative modes of delivery during the first two months postpartum: results from a Scottish observational study. *Br J Obstet Gynecol* 2002; **109:**214–17.

5. Johnson TR, Zettelmaier MA, Warner PA et al. A competency based approach to comprehensive pregnancy care. *Womens Health Issues* 2000; **10:**240–7.

6. Callahan TL, Hall JE, Ettner SL et al. The economic impact of multiple-gestation pregnancies and the contribution of assisted reproduction techniques to their incidence. *N Engl J Med* 1994; **331:**244–9.

7. Galtier-Dereure F, Boegner C, Bringer J. Obesity and pregnancy: complications and cost. *Am J Clin Nutr* 2000; **71 (Suppl 5):**S1242S–S1248.

8. Galtier-Dereure F, Montpeyroux F, Boulot P et al. Weight excess before pregnancy: complications and cost. *Int J Obes Relat Metab Disord* 1995; **19:**443–8.

9. Isaacs JD, Magann EF, Martin RW. Obstetric challenges of massive obesity complicating pregnancy. *J Perinatol* 1994; **14:**10–14.

10. Waitzman NJ, Romano PS, Scheffler RM, Harris JA. Economic costs of birth defects and cerebral palsy – United States, 1992. *MMWR Morb Mortal Wkly Rep* 1995; **44:**694–9.

11. Vintzileos AM, Ananth CV, Smulian JC et al. Routine second-trimester ultrasonography in the United States: a cost–benefit analysis. *Am J Obstet Gynecol* 2000; **182:** 655–60.

12. Rogowski J. Cost-effectiveness of care for very low birth weight infants. *Pediatrics* 1998; **102:**35–43.

13. Weinstein MC, Siegel JE, Gold MR et al. Recommendations of the Panel on Cost-effectiveness in Health and Medicine. *J Am Med Assoc* 1996; **276:**1253–8.

14. November MT. Cost analysis of vaginal birth after cesarean. *Clin Obstet Gynecol* 2001; **44:**571–87.

15. Romano PS, Waitzman NJ, Scheffler RM, Pi RD. Folic acid fortification of grain: an economic analysis. *Am J Public Health* 1995; **85:**667–76.

16. Zaric GS, Bayoumi AM, Brandeau ML, Owens DK. The cost effectiveness of voluntary prenatal and routine newborn HIV screening in the United States. *J Acquir Immune Defic Syndr* 2000; **25:**403–16.

17. Postma MJ, Beck EJ, Mandalia S et al. Universal HIV screening of pregnant women in England: cost effectiveness analysis. *Br Med J* 1999; **318:**1656–60.

18. Lightwood JM, Phibbs CS, Glantz SA. Short-term health and economic benefits of smoking cessation: low birth weight. *Pediatrics* 1999; **104:**1312–20.

19. Grobman WA, Peaceman AM, Socol ML. Cost-effectiveness of elective cesarean delivery after one prior low transverse cesarean. *Obstet Gynecol* 2000; **95:**745–51.

20. Chung A, Macario A, El-Sayed YY et al. Cost effectiveness of a trial of labor after previous cesarean. *Obstet Gynecol* 2001; **97:**932–41.

21. Kitzmiller JL, Buchanan TA, Kjos S et al. Pre-conception care of diabetes, congenital malformations, and spontaneous abortions. *Diabetes Care* 1996; **19:**514–41.

22. Scheffler RM, Feuchtbaum LB, Phibbs CS. Prevention: the cost-effectiveness of the California Diabetes and Pregnancy Program. *Am J Public Health* 1992; **82:** 168–75.

23. Elixhauser A, Weschler JM, Kitzmiller JL et al. Cost–benefit analysis of preconception care for women with established diabetes mellitus. *Diabetes Care* 1993; **16:**1146–57.

24. Herman WH, Janz NK, Becker MP, Charron-Prochownik D. Diabetes and pregnancy. Preconception care, pregnancy outcomes, resource utilization and costs. *J Reprod Med* 1999; **44:**33–8.

25. Elixhauser A, Kitzmiller JL, Weschler JM. Short-term cost benefit of pre-conception care for diabetes. *Diabetes Care* 1996; **19:**384.

26. Kitzmiller JL. Cost analysis of diagnosis and treatment of gestational diabetes mellitus. *Clin Obstet Gynecol* 2000; **43:**140–53.

27. National Diabetes Data Group (NDDG). Classification and diagnosis of diabetes mellitus and other categories of glucose intolerance. *Diabetes* 1979; **28:**1039–57.

28. Lavin JP, Barden TP, Miodovnik M. Clinical experience with a screening program for gestational diabetes. *Am J Obstet Gynecol* 1981; **141:**491–4.

29. Reed BD. Screening for gestational diabetes – analysis by screening criteria. *J Fam Pract* 1984; **19:**751–5.

30. Coustan DR, Nelson C, Carpenter MW et al. Maternal age and screening for gestational diabetes: a population-based study. *Obstet Gynecol* 1989; **73:**557–61.

31. Metzger BE, Coustan DR. Summary and recommendations of the Fourth International Workshop–Conference on Gestational Diabetes Mellitus. The Organizing Committee. *Diabetes Care* 1998; **21 (Suppl 2):** B161–B167.

32. Lavin Jr JP, Lavin B, O'Donnell N. A comparison of costs associated with screening for gestational diabetes with two-tiered and one-tiered testing protocols. *Am J Obstet Gynecol* 2001; **184:**363–7.

33. Kitzmiller JL, Elixhauser A, Carr S et al. Assessment of costs and benefits of management of gestational diabetes mellitus. *Diabetes Care* 1998; **21 (Suppl 2):**B123–B130.

34. de Veciana M, Major CA, Morgan MA et al. Postprandial versus preprandial blood glucose monitoring in women with gestational diabetes mellitus requiring insulin therapy. *N Engl J Med* 1995; **333:**1237–41.

35. Langer O, Conway D, Berkus MD, Xenakis EM. Conventional versus intensified management: cost/benefit analysis. *Am J Obstet Gynecol* 1998; **178 (Suppl 1):**S58.

36. Langer O, Rodriguez DA, Xenakis EM et al. Intensified versus conventional management of gestational diabetes. *Am J Obstet Gynecol* 1994; **170:**1036–46.

37. Bienstock JL, Blakemore KJ, Wang E et al. Managed care does not lower costs but may result in poorer outcomes for patients with gestational diabetes. *Am J Obstet Gynecol* 1997; **177:**1035–7.

44

Quality of care for the woman with diabetes in pregnancy

Alberto de Leiva, Rosa Corcoy, Eulalia Brugués

Quality assessment and improvement in diabetes care

The aim of health care is to achieve the best health outcomes in the most efficient manner, and the challenge for today's health delivery systems is to increase productivity and quality of care without increasing the economic costs.

Assessment of the quality of health care needs complex measures of **the structure** (staff, equipment, organization), **the process** (technical quality) and **the outcomes** (effectiveness, satisfaction, functional status, quality of life).

Health care delivery depends on efficient communication and cooperation amongst patients, health care services and professionals; this matter is particularly critical regarding chronic disorders in which **effective shared-care** is pursued by multiple health care providers and professionals, enabling the patient to become actively involved in the process of their care. The effective share of related information is highly facilitated by the operation of an electronic patient record and a telematic infrastructure.

Health care delivery is moving towards disease management, focused on a patient-oriented approach, illness prevention promoting good health and managing long-term care, all of which require integrated activities from generalists, specialists and other health care professionals. This type of care requires effective coordination and an interrelated, multidisciplinary approach.

In addition, the implementation of effective strategies for **continuous quality improvement** takes advantage of four main areas: (1) efficient use of health care resources (e.g. eliminating practices that are clearly harmful, or without known benefits); (2) linking clinical research to clinical practice (evidence-based care); (3) application of new concepts for improvement of care (the process of care must comply with the 'best practice', including solid methods to monitor and assess the outcomes); and (4) changing clinical practice (design of appropriate models for the management of health care services, based in valid, scientific information).

At a meeting held in St Vincent, Italy, in October 1989, representatives of government health departments and patients' organizations from all European countries met diabetes experts to discuss a set of recommendations – **the St Vincent Declaration,**[1] a joint initiative of the World Health Organization–Europe and the International Diabetes Federation–Europe (WHO/IDF) – with the intention of creating conditions allowing major reductions in deaths and the burden caused by diabetes mellitus. The declaration meant an important step forward in the general improvement in the quality of delivery of diabetes health care.

One of the main targets of the declaration was to establish monitoring and control systems using state-of-the-art **information technology (IT) for quality assurance** of diabetes health care provision. A European group of experts was established to design and implement mechanisms for the continuous improvement of the quality of diabetes care in Europe. The term 'continuous quality improvement' was accepted to emphasize the progressive nature of the never-ending process after reaching a determined standard. The assessment requires the comparison of care with standards that are derived from scientific evidence, consensus, good practice and clinical experience.

The St Vincent Declaration pointed out that **self-monitoring** results in very effective control of treatment. Later in this chapter, the quality assessment of the procedures for self-monitoring glycemic control will be reviewed in some detail.

European DiabCare quality network

A subgroup of the St Vincent Declaration Steering Committee was established to develop instruments and mechanisms for quality assurance in diabetes care. The first initiative of the DiabCare Program was the development of the St Vincent Diabetes Dataset from three main sources: (1) EuroDiabeta, a research project on modeling health care and the implementation of IT in diabetes;[2] (2) the specific recommendations provided by the different working groups of the St Vincent Declaration Steering Committee;[3] (3) the advice provided by more than 130 expert diabetologists from 21 European countries.

DiabCare Basic Information Sheet (BIS) contains 141 fields that include all the necessary data for the analysis of the quality of diabetes care (Fig. 44.1). The pertinent analysis provides the performance of care in both aspects of process and outcomes (intermediate and final). Demographic data (age, sex, etc.) are required for a number of purposes. True patient outcomes include the burden of the medical end points of the St Vincent Declaration (such as amputation, blindness, etc.). Symptoms of diabetes-related problems (e.g. painful neuropathy, angina pectoris, etc.) are also recorded. Specific outcomes regarding pregnancies are also included. For the measurement of quality of life, the DiabCare data sets only include information related to duration of hospital admissions and the number of days without the ability to perform normal activities. Assessment of diabetic complications (retinopathy, nephropathy, neuropathy), cardiovascular risk factors, pharmacological treatment and metabolic outcomes [glycated hemoglobin (HbA1c), lipid profile] were considered essential.[4] The computer database (Fig. 44.2) contains all the data items of the BIS and additional information with easy access by a single key stroke.

Once a year, at least, the data of all patients under care must be collected in the DiabCare BIS. The performance of the diabetes team is compared with the gold standards of the St Vincent Declaration program. The evaluation of the level of quality should cover the structure (housing, human resources, equipment, logistics), the process (the way the care is organized – from the first call to treatment plan; the annual measurements of indicators – HbA1c, blood pressure, etc; the way the treatment is initiated – use of antihypertensive drugs, cholesterol lowering agents, etc).

The **DiabCare Program** was designed for those services not having a computer database but having access to computers. In 1991, the feasibility phase, integrating the information from 4000 patients of 29 centers in 19 European countries, was completed. After some minor modifications it gained widespread adoption by

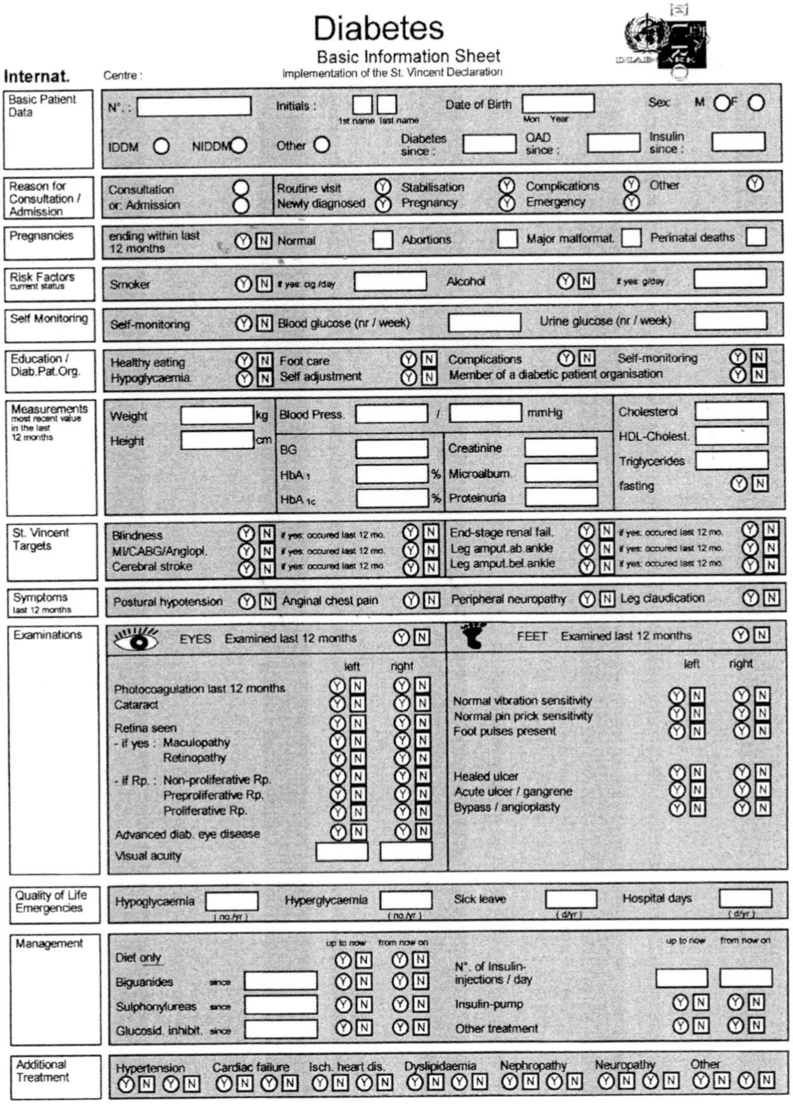
Diabetes
Basic Information Sheet
Implementation of the St. Vincent Declaration

Internat. Centre:

Basic Patient Data: N°.: Initials: 1st name last name; Date of Birth Mon Year; Sex: M F; IDDM; NIDDM; Other; Diabetes since:; OAD since:; Insulin since:

Reason for Consultation / Admission: Consultation or: Admission; Routine visit; Newly diagnosed; Stabilisation; Pregnancy; Complications; Emergency; Other

Pregnancies: ending within last 12 months Y N; Normal; Abortions; Major malformat.; Perinatal deaths

Risk Factors current status: Smoker Y N if yes: cig /day; Alcohol Y N if yes: g/day

Self Monitoring: Self-monitoring Y N; Blood glucose (nr / week); Urine glucose (nr / week)

Education / Diab.Pat.Org.: Healthy eating Y N; Hypoglycaemia Y N; Foot care Y N; Self adjustment Y N; Complications Y N; Self-monitoring Y N; Member of a diabetic patient organisation Y N

Measurements most recent value in the last 12 months: Weight kg; Height cm; Blood Press. / mmHg; BG; HbA_1 %; HbA_{1c} %; Creatinine; Microalbum.; Proteinuria; Cholesterol; HDL-Cholest.; Triglycerides; fasting Y N

St. Vincent Targets: Blindness Y N if yes: occured last 12 mo. Y N; MI/CABG/Angiopl. Y N if yes: occured last 12 mo. Y N; Cerebral stroke Y N if yes: occured last 12 mo. Y N; End-stage renal fail. Y N if yes: occured last 12 mo. Y N; Leg amput.ab.ankle Y N if yes: occured last 12 mo. Y N; Leg amput.bel.ankle Y N if yes: occured last 12 mo. Y N

Symptoms last 12 months: Postural hypotension Y N; Anginal chest pain Y N; Peripheral neuropathy Y N; Leg claudication Y N

Examinations: EYES Examined last 12 months Y N; left right; Photocoagulation last 12 months; Cataract; Retina seen; - if yes: Maculopathy; Retinopathy; - if Rp.: Non-proliferative Rp.; Preproliferative Rp.; Proliferative Rp.; Advanced diab. eye disease; Visual acuity
FEET Examined last 12 months Y N; left right; Normal vibration sensitivity; Normal pin prick sensitivity; Foot pulses present; Healed ulcer; Acute ulcer / gangrene; Bypass / angioplasty

Quality of Life Emergencies: Hypoglycaemia (no./yr); Hyperglycaemia (no./yr); Sick leave (d/yr); Hospital days (d/yr)

Management: up to now, from now on; Diet only Y N Y N; Biguanides since; Sulphonylureas since; Glucosid. inhibit. since; N°. of Insulin-injections / day; Insulin-pump Y N Y N; Other treatment Y N Y N

Additional Treatment: Hypertension; Cardiac failure; Isch. heart dis.; Dyslipidaemia; Nephropathy; Neuropathy; Other

Figure 44.1. *Basic Information Sheet, DiabCare.*

centers, and local, regional and national diabetes task forces all over Europe.[5–7]

The DiabCare Feasibility Study[5] demonstrated the achievements obtained by the implementation of local documentation compatible to the DiabCare Diabetes Data Set. It made possible the assessment of the quality of care and to install regional/national quality networks, along with establishing a standard documentation to be used in various health care settings in different countries.

A **quality circle** is a group of motivated and committed people acting as a structured forum to solve on-the-job problems affecting the quality of their work. Prerequisites for the constitution of the circle are the political awareness and the involvement of the decision-makers to get things going. The implementation of pilots

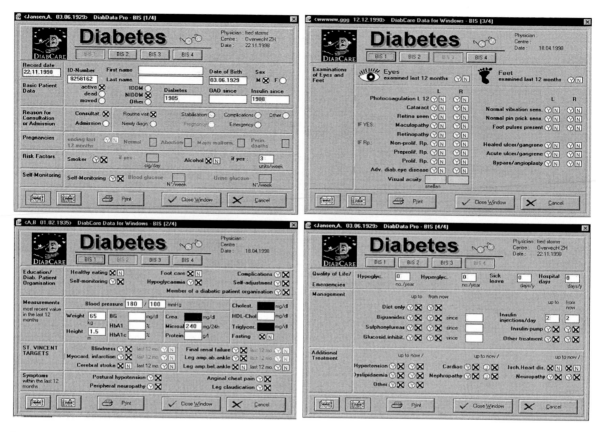

Figure 44.2. *DiabCare data for Windows.*

or demonstration projects make clear what the benefits are and the economic cost.

The quality circle must select targets according to the local health requirements. The information gathered after data collection, data aggregation and analysis (Figure 44.3) of proper indicators (clinical, analytical, etc.), allows a local evaluation (internal comparison); then, sending the aggregated data in anonymous fashion to a server, the comparison with all the other teams sharing the network is possible (external comparison). After all of this, the members of the local quality circle are in the situation to propose and debate measures for quality improvement. These measures are implemented in the following period and the evaluation of their effects will be then

analyzed, following the scheme of continuous assurance and improvement (Fig. 44.4).[7]

The present authors' use of DiabCare program, adapted to a net environment in a hospital-based outpatient consultation, has provided a variety of benefits, including Diabetes Data Set exploitation as a registry, diabetes-type characterization, assessment of self blood glucose monitoring (SBGM) status, St Vincent Declaration targets, treatment characterization, outcome for diabetic pregnancies, completeness assessment of medical records, cardiovascular risk factors, identification of groups of patients at risk, etc.[8] On the basis of this information, a quality assurance circle on diabetes care has been operating in the present authors' center since then, following the

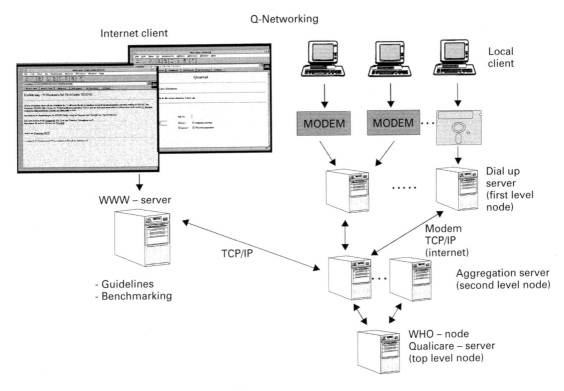

Figure 44.3. *DiabCare Q-Net, system architecture.*

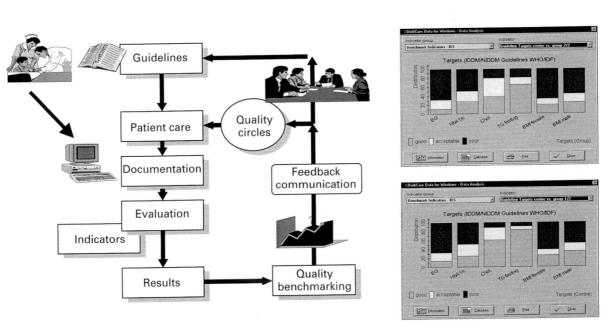

Figure 44.4. *Operation of the DiabCare quality circle.*

protocol proposed by the EU Consortium DiabCare Quality Network, integrated in a comprehensive disease management program (the Optidiab System). A recent report about the information provided by the annual evaluation (the 141 parameters of the DiabCare BIS) of > 1000 subjects confirmed the burden of Type 2 diabetes patients compared to Type 1 diabetes patients undergoing intensive and specialized care on regular basis.[9]

Interestingly, aggregated and compared data from the central server, integrating national centers from the European DiabCare Quality Network (> 22,000 patients), lead to the conclusion that the long-term metabolic outcome of patients under intensive management in European specialized centers are far short of achieving their desired goal [HbA1c < mean + four standard deviations (4 SD) of the nondiabetic population]; aggregated HbA1c levels [Diabetes Control and Complication Trial (DCCT) adjusted] recorded at the annual evaluation were optimal for only 26.9% of cases, acceptable for 23.2% and poor in the remaining 49.9% of subjects.[10]

The DiabCare program allows a simple registration procedure for collecting basic data from diabetic pregnant women; the system has also been demonstrated to be useful for limited evaluation of quality assurance in the broad field of diabetes and pregnancy.[11–13]

DiabCare BIS for diabetes and pregnancy

One of the main recommendations of the St Vincent Declaration was the following: 'Achieve pregnancy outcome in diabetic women that approximates to that of nondiabetic women'. In consequence, WHO/IDF guidelines for care and management of pregnant diabetic women have been proposed by an invited group of international experts in the field.[14] The document brought attention to the important differences in the provision of diabetes and obstetrical care in different European countries. Specifically, the relevance of intensive metabolic care before conception, during pregnancy and parturition, as well as the needs of special training and education of the diabetic women contemplating pregnancy, were addressed. For the purpose of developing the quality assurance program, a DiabCare BIS for diabetes and pregnancy was proposed by members of the WHO/IDF Working Group on Pregnancy Outcomes in the Diabetic Woman (Fig. 44.5), with data fields addressing diabetes diagnosis, past obstetrical history, prepregnancy counseling, status at entering the specialized interdisciplinary clinic, maternal and newborn outcomes, and reclassification after pregnancy. The OBSQID (OBStetrical Quality Indicators and Data) Perinatal Aggregated Data (PAD) protocol, mainly focused on outcomes, represents a valid alternative proposed by the Quality of Care and Technologies Program, WHO–Europe being exploited for epidemiologic studies.

DiabCard as an instrument for quality assurance

The DiabCard project (EU-AIM 2051) developed the specifications for a chip-card-based medical information system and the requirements for Europewide collection of data about diabetes for clinical and managerial purposes. A common diabetes data set based on EuroDiabeta was produced and validated in ambulatory and hospital care. An open architecture allowed a bandwidth of different security levels, covered by standards defined by the International Standard Organization (ISO) and the European Telecommunications Standards Institute (ETSI). Security and privacy of the information was provided with the addition of the health professional card for identification and access to the

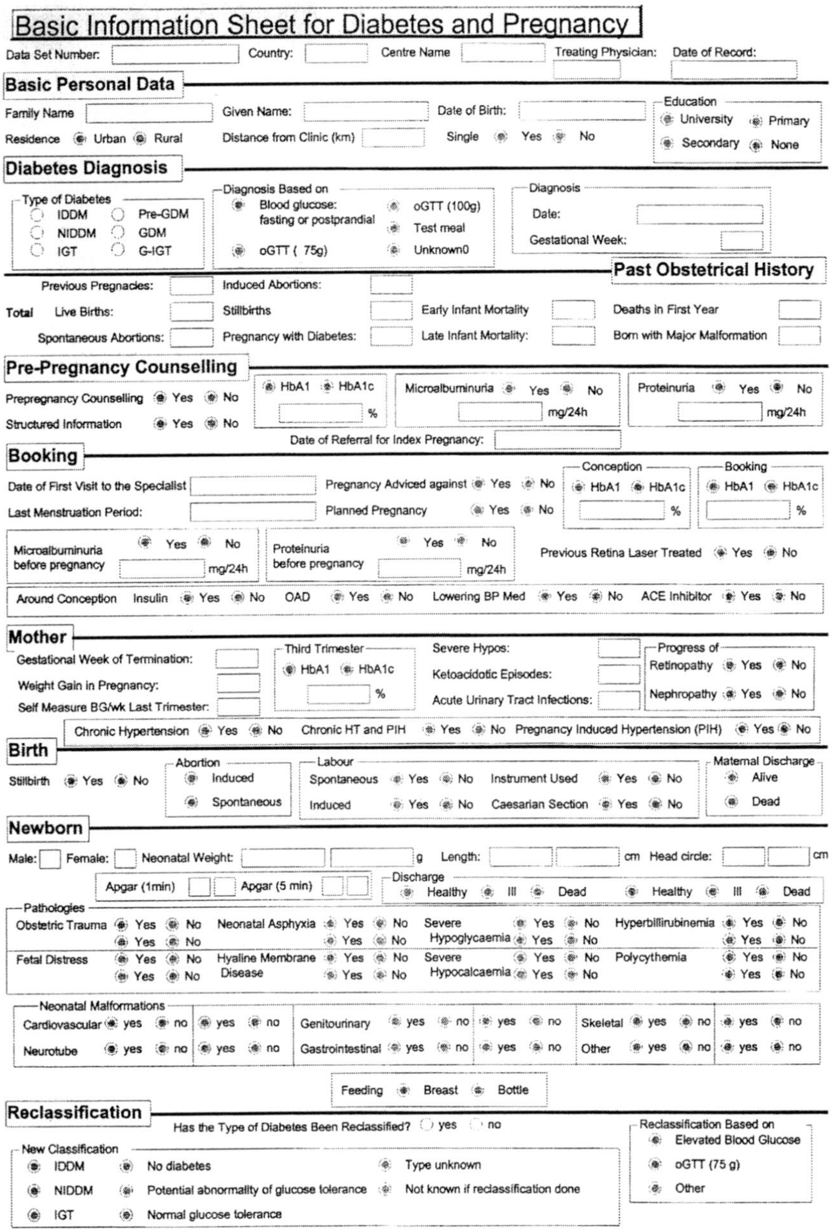

Basic Information Sheet for Diabetes and Pregnancy

Data Set Number: Country: Centre Name Treating Physician: Date of Record:

Basic Personal Data

Family Name Given Name: Date of Birth: Education: University Primary Secondary None

Residence Urban Rural Distance from Clinic (km) Single Yes No

Diabetes Diagnosis

Type of Diabetes: IDDM Pre-GDM NIDDM GDM IGT G-IGT

Diagnosis Based on: Blood glucose: fasting or postprandial oGTT (100g) Test meal oGTT (75g) Unknown0

Diagnosis: Date: Gestational Week:

Past Obstetrical History

Total: Previous Pregnacies: Live Births: Spontaneous Abortions: Induced Abortions: Stillbirths Pregnancy with Diabetes: Early Infant Mortality Late Infant Mortality: Deaths in First Year Born with Major Malformation

Pre-Pregnancy Counselling

Prepregnancy Counselling Yes No Structured Information Yes No HbA1 HbA1c % Microalbuminuria Yes No mg/24h Proteinuria Yes No mg/24h

Date of Referral for Index Pregnancy:

Booking

Date of First Visit to the Specialist Last Menstruation Period: Pregnancy Adviced against Yes No Planned Pregnancy Yes No Conception: HbA1 HbA1c % Booking: HbA1 HbA1c %

Microalbuminuria before pregnancy Yes No mg/24h Proteinuria before pregnancy Yes No mg/24h Previous Retina Laser Treated Yes No

Around Conception Insulin Yes No OAD Yes No Lowering BP Med Yes No ACE Inhibitor Yes No

Mother

Gestational Week of Termination: Weight Gain in Pregnancy: Self Measure BG/wk Last Trimester: Third Trimester: HbA1 HbA1c % Severe Hypos: Ketoacidotic Episodes: Acute Urinary Tract Infections: Progress of: Retinopathy Yes No Nephropathy Yes No

Chronic Hypertension Yes No Chronic HT and PIH Yes No Pregnancy Induced Hypertension (PIH) Yes No

Birth

Stillbirth Yes No Abortion: Induced Spontaneous Labour: Spontaneous Yes No Induced Yes No Instrument Used Yes No Caesarian Section Yes No Maternal Discharge: Alive Dead

Newborn

Male: Female: Neonatal Weight: g Length: cm Head circle: cm

Apgar (1min) Apgar (5 min) Discharge: Healthy Ill Dead Healthy Ill Dead

Pathologies: Obstetric Trauma Yes No Yes No Neonatal Asphyxia Yes No Yes No Severe Hypoglycaemia Yes No Yes No Hyperbillirubinemia Yes No Yes No

Fetal Distress Yes No Yes No Hyaline Membrane Disease Yes No Yes No Severe Hypocalcaemia Yes No Yes No Polycythemia Yes No Yes No

Neonatal Malformations: Cardiovascular yes no yes no Genitourinary yes no yes no Skeletal yes no yes no Neurotube yes no yes no Gastrointestinal yes no yes no Other yes no yes no

Feeding Breast Bottle

Reclassification

Has the Type of Diabetes Been Reclassified? yes no

New Classification: IDDM No diabetes Type unknown NIDDM Potential abnormality of glucose tolerance Not known if reclassification done IGT Normal glucose tolerance

Reclassification Based on: Elevated Blood Glucose oGTT (75 g) Other

Figure 44.5. *Basic Information Sheet for Diabetes and Pregnancy (DiabCare).*

system; the patient card contains most clinically relevant data.[15]

The randomized trial performed in the clinical scenario demonstrated the functionality of DiabCard as a patient record, and the main consequences in facilitating the effective communication between the patient and all levels of health care, and among health care providers as well. DiabCard was equally useful, as DiabCare, for quality assessment, and

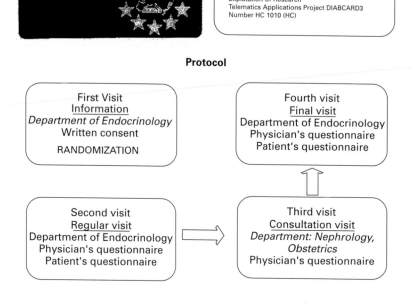

Protocol

First Visit
Information
Department of Endocrinology
Written consent

RANDOMIZATION

Second visit
Regular visit
Department of Endocrinology
Physician's questionnaire
Patient's questionnaire

Third visit
Consultation visit
Department: Nephrology, Obstetrics
Physician's questionnaire

Fourth visit
Final visit
Department of Endocrinology
Physician's questionnaire
Patient's questionnaire

Euopean Commission
Directorate-General XIII
Telecommunications, Information Market and
Explatation of Research
Telematics Applications Project DIABCARD3
Number HC 1010 (HC)

Diabcard data set

- General
- Basic Information Sheet (BIS)
- Education
- Monitoring
- Measurements
- Diet plan
- Ophthalmology
- Nephrology
- Autonomous nervous system
- Peripheral nervous system
- Cardiology
- Cerebrovascular system
- Foot
- Pregnancy
- Treatment
- Optional data

Figure 44.6. *DiabCard system and the clinical scenario.*

deserved its high acceptance by patients, promoting their empowerment and active involvement in the health care process (Fig. 44.6).[16]

Monitoring glycemic control in diabetes mellitus and during pregnancy in the woman with pregestational or gestational diabetes mellitus

The primary metabolic abnormality in diabetes mellitus (DM) is hyperglycemia, which is mainly responsible for acute and chronic complications of the disease, including feto-maternal mortality and morbidity.

The results of the DCCT showed that in Type 1 DM strict glycemic control resulted in a significant reduction in the rate of onset and progression of retinopathy, nephropathy and neuropathy.[17] In the United Kingdom Prospective Diabetes Study (UKPDS), the difference of 0.9% in HbA1c between the intensively treated group and the control group was associated with a 25% reduction in risk of microvascular end points;[18] intensive blood glucose control did not reduce the risk of myocardial infarction or stroke, but the control of hypertension was very important in this respect.[19]

Diabetes in pregnancy carries multiple risks to the mother and the fetus/newborn. For this reason, it is recommended to maintain blood glucose levels of 3.5–5.5 mmol/l at fasting and 5.0–8.0 mmol/l postprandially.[20] Although there is still some controversy concerning the implications of a mild degree of glucose intolerance for GDM, the same targets have been recommended in these pregnancies, in spite of arguments of insufficient evidence for therapeutic interventions in this condition.[21]

Blood glucose monitoring devices

Portable meters are used for health care workers and by patients. Because of their imprecision and variability, they should not be used for diagnosing diabetes and their value in screening must be limited.

SBGM is recommended for all insulin-treated patients. Glucose can be measured in whole blood, serum or plasma, but plasma is recommended for diagnosis. Although red blood cells are freely permeable to glucose, the concentration of water in plasma is *c.* 11% higher than that of whole blood; as a consequence, the glucose concentration in plasma is higher than in whole blood (being the hematocrit normal). The glucose concentration decreases with time in the assay tube because of *in vitro* glycolysis (on average by 5–7%, or 0.6 mmol/l or 10 mg/dl/hour), which can be attenuated by inhibition of enolase with sodium fluoride used in combination with anticoagulants. Therefore, when plasma glucose is going to be analyzed, plasma should be separated from cells within 1 hour. Glucose is almost exclusively measured by enzymatic methods (hexokinase, glucose oxidase). For plasma glucose, a coefficient of variation < 2.2% is recommended as a target for imprecision.

There is no standard protocol available for the evaluation of blood glucose meters. The evaluation of a single device may be misleading; in general, several units should be tested to explore interdevice variability. The evaluation should include the analysis of the mean difference of the device reading, with respect to a reference procedure at low, medium and high blood glucose concentrations. Other items of the evaluation will include customer acceptability (size, weight, portability, calibration, duration of a test performance, economic cost). Then, a validation protocol using an adequate sample size of recruited patients will follow, covering a wide range of blood glucose levels from the hypoglycemic range to extreme hyperglycemia.

The utilization of memory meters have shown that patients often make incomplete recordings of their daily blood glucose profiles (inaccurate readings, omission of outliers, false reports not recorded in the memory of the meter), usually depicting a trend towards correcting results of readings.[22,23] Of course, adequate training, visual acuity, hypoxia, altitude, hemolysis, hematocrit, hypertriglyceridemia, adequate sample volume,[24] and other technical elements, can influence the results. Reinforcing patient education at regular clinic visits, evaluating his/her technique and frequent comparison of SBGM profiles with concurrent laboratory blood glucose analysis, will assess the reliability of patient reports.

About 30 different brands of meters are commercially available. They use strips containing glucose-oxidase or hexokinase; some meters contain a porous membrane that separates erythrocytes, the analysis being carried out in plasma. The meters provide a digital read-out, using reflectance photometry or electrochemistry for the measurements of glucose concentration. There is a wide variability in the performance of the different meters and the level of imprecision remains high. No published reports of glucose meters have achieved the American Diabetes Association (ADA) goal of analytical deviation < 5% from reference values.[25,26]

SBGM should be performed at least four times per day in patients with Type 1 DM. It has been demonstrated that monitoring with lower frequency than this is associated with deterioration of glycemic control.[27–29]

Non-invasive or minimally invasive continuous monitoring of blood glucose is a high priority (both to detect unsuspected hypoglycemia and as a further step in the development of an artificial pancreas), allowing automatic measurement of blood glucose and adjustment of insulin administration (Fig. 44.7). Transcutaneous sensors and implanted sensors use multiple detection systems [enzymatic (e.g. glucose oxidase), electrode, fluorescence). The method for sampling in minimally invasive systems takes advantage of the correlation between the concentration of glucose in the interstitial fluid and in blood.[30,31]

Whereas microdialysis systems are inserted subcutaneously, reverse iontophoresis uses a low-level electrical current, which by electroosmosis moves glucose across the skin, being the glucose concentration measured with a glucose-oxidase detector.[32,33]

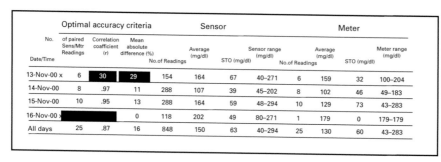

	No. of paired Sens/Mtr Readings	Optimal accuracy criteria		Sensor				Meter			
Date/Time		Correlation coafficient (r)	Mean absolute difference (%)	No. of Readings	Average (mg/dl)	STO (mg/dl)	Sensor range (mg/dl)	No. of Readings	Average (mg/dl)	STO (mg/dl)	Meter range (mg/dl)
13-Nov-00 x	6	30	29	154	164	67	40–271	6	159	32	100–204
14-Nov-00	8	.97	11	288	107	39	45–202	8	102	46	49–183
15-Nov-00	10	.95	13	288	164	59	48–294	10	129	73	43–283
16-Nov-00 x			0	118	202	49	80–271	1	179	0	179–179
All days	25	.87	16	848	150	63	40–294	25	130	60	43–283

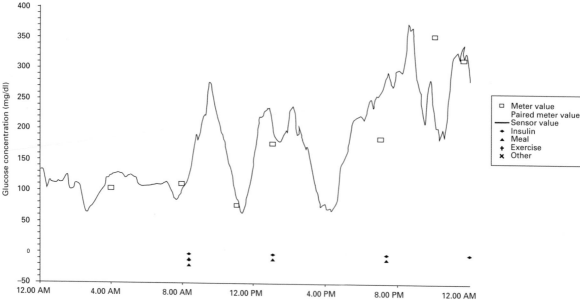

Figure 44.7. *Registry of continuous glucose monitoring in interstitial subcutaneous tissue.*

Total non-invasive technology for glucose sensing, including techniques of near-infrared spectroscopy, light scattering and photoacoustic spectroscopy, are in progress. The Gluco Watch Biographer and the Continuous Monitoring System (CMS) received a Food and Drug Administration (FDA) license. The Gluco Watch System can analyze glucose three times per hour for up 12 hours, and it is best indicated for detection of hypoglycemia. It has provided excellent correlation with SBGM. The CMS includes a subcutaneous glucose sensor connected to an external monitor; it allows glucose measurements every 5 minutes for 72 hours; values are not displayed until being downloaded into a computer at the end of the recorded interval.

It is anticipated that important progress in these methods for non-invasive or minimally invasive glucose monitoring will be made in the near future.

HbA1c

More than 40 years ago, it was observed that normal adult hemoglobin could be separated by chromatographic procedures into a major and various minor components. In one of the minor components – HbA1c – glucose was attached, non-enzymatically, to the terminal N-valine of the beta chain of HbA0. In the following years, numerous assays were developed to measure HbA1c levels.

The average lifespan of erythrocytes is 100–120 days. Measuring HbA1c offers an accurate estimation of the average blood glucose concentration of the past 2–3 months. HbA1c is used as an integrated estimation of mean glycemia and as a marker of risk for the development of diabetes complications. At present, there are > 30 HbA1c assay methods available. Certain methods quantify HbA1c based on charge differences of the glycated components (cation exchange chromatography, agar gel electrophoresis). Other methods analyze structural differences between glycated and non-glycated components (affinity chromatography, immunoassay). Certain methods quantify total glycated hemoglobin, including HbA1c and other hemoglobin–glucose adducts.

In 1996, the American Association of Clinical Chemists (AACC), in collaboration with the ADA established the National Glycohemoglobin Standardization Program. It was decided to adopt the high-performance liquid chromotography (HPLC) reference method used in the DCCT (Bio-Rex 70; between run CV < 3%), as the designated comparison method. The UKPDS incorporated the same standardization method; therefore, its HbA1c reports were compatible with those of DCCT. More than 90% of USA laboratories, and many others worldwide, are using this standardization program.[34]

Any condition that shortens erythrocyte survival (hemolytic anemia, acute blood loss) falsely lowers HbA1c test results; on the contrary, iron-deficiency anemia increases the value.[35] Glycation may also vary between patients with similar capillary blood glucose levels, and glycation appears to be lower in subjects with a higher body mass index (BMI).[36]

Several hemoglobinopathies interfere with some assay methods; the results can be falsely increased or decreased; non-hemoglobin-based methods for assessing long-term glycemic control may represent useful alternatives in these circumstances.

European guidelines have recommended the classification of blood glucose control by the number of SD the experimental value is from the non-diabetic mean for the particular assay.[37]

The International Federation of Clinical Chemistry (IFCC) has organized a working party to develop a scientifically based method of the production of a primary reference. Electrospray ionization mass spectrometry (ESIMS) has been demonstrated to be a precise measurement of HbA1c, in particular glycation of the beta chain, which has been proposed as a robust procedure for calibration purposes. In a protocol performed with 1022 patients, the comparison of the ESIMS with the ion-exchange chromatographic procedure showed excellent agreement, with values, on average, 0.7% lower with ESIMS. The comparison with DCCT-corrected ion-exchange values gave good agreement, with ESIMS showing an overall lower value of mean 0.4%.[38]

There is a general agreement that the new mass-spectroscopy-based method appears to be more accurate and to reflect 'true' HbA1c. It yields normal (non-diabetic) values that are significantly lower than those used by the National Glycohemoglobin Standardization Program, DCCT and UKPDS (3–5 versus 4–6%).

The Ames DCA 2000 Analyzer measures HbA1c by an agglutination inhibition immunoassay, allowing results in 6 minutes with 1 µl of blood. The Ames DCA 2000 analyzer offers reliable results, although showing a trend to lightly underestimate the results in comparison with HPLC.[39] This analyzer gave valid and reliable results when operated by non-medical personnel.

The Primus CLC330 provides an HPLC near-patient HbA1c method, comparable in precision and accuracy to the Ames DCA 2000 Analyzer.[40] Near-patient testing for HbA1c has practical clinical use in the diabetes clinic, avoiding the need for a second appointment and allowing immediate changes in therapy.

Glycated serum proteins

Mostly albumin, and other serum proteins, undergo the process of glycation. The turnover of serum albumin depicts a half-life of 25 days; it provides an index of a mean glycemic level of a shorter interval than HbA1c. The **fructosamine assay** is the most widely method being used for estimating glycated serum proteins. Nevertheless, although fructosamine levels correlate with HbA1c levels within a population, transference cannot apply for individual values.[41] Also, changes in serum proteins affect the readings of fructosamine;[42] the technique is unreliable in diabetic patients with renal failure,[43] liver cirrhosis and nephrotic syndrome.[44]

Assessment of the effectiveness of self blood glucose monitoring in diabetes in pregnancy

Various randomized controlled trials (RCT)[45–49] and case series studies,[50–55] carried out either in diabetes or obstetrics departments of university hospitals, have evaluated the clinical effectiveness of SBGM in women with GDM or diabetic pregnancies. Blood glucose and HbA1c determinations, as well as maternal and fetal outcomes, were recorded. Some studies examined the costs of hospital care and home monitoring, and the compared costs for a control group receiving standard care.[47,48] The largest of all protocols included a population of 153 women with GDM in the experimental group and 2153 non-diabetics in the control group. The main goal of the case series studies was to assess the feasibility of managing pregnant women with Type 1 DM/GDM at home using SBGM. There was general agreement that women were able to achieve satisfactory blood glucose profiles at home using SBGM; hospital utilization was lower, and infant birthweights and indicators of macrosomia were also more favorable in those women.

Main findings from the RCT demonstrated that patients with Type 1 DM managed by SBGM at home obtained similar results regarding glycemic control to those patients under intensive control in the hospital. Maternal and fetal outcomes were also similar in both groups. Women preferred lower use of the hospital and home management with SBGM. Particularly for GDM, monitoring blood glucose after meals, rather than before, contributed to better metabolic control and better fetal outcomes (there were fewer Cesarean sections for cephalopelvic disproportion, fewer cases of macrosomia and large-for-gestational-age infants, and fewer episodes of neonatal hypoglycemia).[49] In addition, women who utilized SBGM were less likely to require hospital admission, leading to a substantial cost saving.

References

1. World Health Organization (Europe) and International Diabetes Federation (Europe). Diabetes care and research in Europe: the St Vincent Declaration. *Diabet Med* 1990; 7:360.

2. Eurodiabeta. Information Technology for Diabetes Care in Europe: the Eurodiabeta initiative. *Diabet Med* 1990; 7:639–50.

3. Krans HMJ, Porta M, Kee H. Diabetes care and research in Europe. The St Vincent Declaration action programme. *G Ital Diabetologia* 1992; 12(Suppl 2):1–56.

4. Piwernetz K, Home PD, Snorgaard O et al. for the DiabCare Monitoring Group of the St Vincent Declaration Steering Committee. Monitoring the targets of the St Vincent Declaration and the implementation of Quality Managemant in Diabetes Care: the DiabCare Initiative. *Diabet Med* 1993; 10:371–7.

5. World Health Organization (WHO). *Diabetes care and research in Europe: implementation of the St Vincent Declaration.* Report on a joint WHO/IDF Meeting, Budapest 9–11 March 1992. (WHO Regional Office for Europe: Copenhagen, 1992) 1–25, (EUR/ICP/CLR0550235 g).

6. World Health Organization (WHO). *Recommendations to facilitate the implementation of the St Vincent Declaration initiatives by national, regional, and local diabetes task forces.* Report on the Consensus Workshop, Oslo, 26–27 June 1992. (WHO Regional Office for Europe: Copenhagen, 1992) EUR/ICPCLR0550279 g.

7. Piwernetz K, Massi Benedetti M, Vermeij D et al. DiabCare Thinkshop, 'Quality Network Diabetes'. *Diabetes Nutr Metab* 1993; 6:107–22.

8. Corcoy R, Muntaner F, Pou JM et al. DiabCare data set collection: benefits and warnings. *Diabetes Nutr Metab* 1993; 6:389–92.

9. Gallo G, Cermeño J, Brugués E et al. The burden of type 2 diabetes compared to the burden of type 1 diabetes in patients undergoing intensive and specialized care. *Diabetologia* 2001; 44 (Suppl 1):16-A.

10. Cubero JM, Hernández M, Brugués E et al. Metabolic outcome achieved by intensive management in European Diabetes Center are far from desirable targets. *Diabetologia* 2001; 44 (Suppl 1):17-A.

11. Kerényi Zs, Tamás Gy, Piwernetz K. Pregnancy complicated by diabetes: baseline data. *Diabetes Nutr Metab* 1993; 6:365–8.

12. Józwicka E, Krzymierí J, Tracz M et al. Implementation of the DiabCare program in registration of pregnant diabetic women. *Diabetes Nutr Metab* 1993; 6:369–71.

13. Thaisz E, Rappai A, Fövényi J, Závodi E. Screening and care of gestational and insulin-dependent diabtic pregnancies: the first four years experience. *Diabetes Nutr Metab* 1993; 6:373–5.

14. Tamás Gy, Hadden DR, Molsted-Pedersen L et al. WHO/IDF Guidelines for care and management of the pregnant diabetic women. *Av Diabetologia* 1992; 5:137–40.

15. Engelbrecht R, Hildebrand C, Kühnel E et al. A chip card for patients with diabetes. *Comput Meth Prog Biomed* 1994; 45:33–5.

16. Engelbrecht R, Hildebrand C, Brugués E et al. DIAB-CARD – an application of a portable medical record for persons with diabetes. *Med Inform* 1996; 21:273–82.

17. The Diabetes Control and Complications Trial Research Group. The effect of intensive treatment of diabetes on the development and progression of retinopathy in the Diabetes Control and Complications. *New Engl J Med* 1993; 329:977–86.

18. UK Prospective Diabetes Study (UKPDS) Group. Intensive blood glucose control with sulphonylureas or insulin compared with conventional treatment and risk of complications in patients with type 2 diabetes (UKPDS 33). *Lancet* 1998; 352:837–53.

19. UK Prospective Diabetes Study Group. Tight blood pressure control and risk of macrovascular and microvascular complications in type 2 diabetes: UKPDS 38. *Br Med J* 1998; 317:703–13.

20. European Diabetes Policy Group 1998. A desktop guide to type 1 (insulin-dependent) diabetes mellitus. *Diabet Med* 1999; 16:253–66.

21. Walkinshaw SA. Dietary regulation for 'gestational diabetes' (Cochrane Review). In: (Anonymous, ed.) *The Cochrane Library*, Issue 2. (Update Software: Oxford, 1999).

22. Ziegler O, Kolopp M, Got I et al. Reliability of self-monitoring of blood glucose by CSII treated patients with type 1 diabetes. *Diabetes Care* 1989; **12**:184–8.

23. Strowig SM, Raskin P. Improved glycaemic control in intensively treated type 1 diabetic patients using blood glucose meters with storage capability and computer assisted analysis. *Diabetes Care* 1998; **21**:1694–9.

24. Devreese K, Leroux-Roels G. Laboratory assesment of five blood glucose meters designed for self-monitoring of blood glucose concentration. *Eur J Clin Chem Clin Biochem* 1993; **31**:829–37.

25. Weitgasser R, Gappmayer B, Pichler M. Newer portable glucose meters – analytical improvement compared with previous generation devices? *Clin Chem* 1999; **45**: 1821–25.

26. Brunner GA, Ellmere M, Sendlfofer G et al. Validation of home blood glucose meters with respect to clinical and analytical approaches. *Diabetes Care* 1998; **122**:495–502.

27. American Diabetes Association. Self-monitoring of blood glucose. *Diabetes Care* 1996; **19 (Suppl 1)**:S62–S66.

28. Schiffrin A, Belmonte M. Multiple daily self-glucose monitoring: it is essential role in long-term glucose control in insulin-dependent diabetic patients treated with pump and multiple subcutaneous injections. *Diabetes Care* 1982; **5**:479–84.

29. Nathan DS. The importance of intensive supervision in determining the efficacy of insulin pump therapy. *Diabetes Care* 1983; **6**:295–7.

30. Bolinder J, Ungerstedt U, Arner P. Microdialysis measurement of the absolute glucose concentration in subcutaneous adipose tissue allowing glucose monitoring in diabetic patients. *Diabetologia* 1992; **35**:1177–80.

31. Hashiguchi Y, Sakakida M, Nishida K et al. Development of a miniaturized glucose monitoring system by combining a needle-type glucose sensor with microdialysis sampling method. Long-term subcutaneous tissue glucose monitoring in ambulatory diabetic patients. *Diabetes Care* 1994; **17**:387–96.

32. Tamada JA, Garg J, Jovanovic L et al. Noninvasive glucose monitoring: comprehensive clinical results. Cygnus Research Team. *J Am Med Assoc* 1999; **282**:1839–44.

33. Garg SK, Potts RO, Ackerman NR et al. Correlation of fingerstick blood glucose measurements with Gluco Watch Biographer glucose results in young subjects with type 1 diabetes. *Diabetes Care* 1999; **22**:1708–14.

34. Little RR, Rohlfing CL, Wiedmayer H-M et al. The National Glycohemoglobin Standardization Program (NGSP): a five-year progress report. *Clin Chem* 2001; **47**:1985–92.

35. Guerci B, Durain D, Leblanc H. Multicentre evaluation of the DCA 2000 system for measuring glycated haemoglobin. DCA 2000 Study Group. *Diabetes Metab* 1997; **23**:195–201.

36. Courturier M, Anman H, Des Rosiers C, Comtois R. Variable glycation of serum proteins in patiens with diabetes mellitus. *Clin Invest Med* 1997; **20**:103–9.

37. European IDDM Policy Group. Consensus guidelines for the management of insulin-dependent (type 1) diabetes. *Diabet Med* 1999; **10**:990–1005.

38. Roberts NB, Amara AB, Morris M, Green BN. Long-term evaluation of electrospray ionization mass spectrometric analysis of glycated hemoglobin. *Clin Chem* 2001; **47**:316–21.

39. Tarim O, Kucukerdogan A, Gunay U et al. Effects of iron deficiency anemia on hemoglobin A1c in type 1 diabetes mellitus. *Pediatr Int* 1999; **41**:357–62.

40. Phillipov G, Charles P, Beng C, Philips PJ. Alternate site testing for HbA_{1c} using Primus CLC330 GHb analyzer. *Diabetes Care* 1997; **20**:607–9.

41. Braadvedt GD, Drury PL, Cundy T. Assessing glycaemic control in disbetes: relationships between fructosamine and HbA_{1c}. *NZ Med J* 1997; **110**:459–62.

42. Kruseman AC, Mercelina L, Degenaar CP. Value of fasting blood glucose and serum fructosamine as a measure of diabetic control in non-insulin-dependent diabetes mellitus. *Horm Metab Res* 1992; **26 (Suppl)**: 59–62.

43. Morgan LJ, Marenah CB, Morgan AG et al. Glycated haemoglobin and fructosamine in non-diabetic subjects with chronic renal failure. *Nephrol Dial Transplant* 1990; **5**:868–73.

44. Kilpatrick ES. Problems in the assessment of glycaemic control in dibetes mellitus. *Diabet Med* 1997; **14**: 819–31.

45. Stubbs SM, Brudenell JM, Pyke DA et al. Management of the pregnant diabetic: home or hospital, with or without glucose meters? *Lancet* 1980; i:1122–4.

46. Goldstein A, Elliot J, Lederman S. Economic effects of self-monitoring of blood glucose concentrations by women with insulin dependent diabetes during pregnancy. *J Reprod Med* 1982; **27**:449–50.

47. Varner NW. Efficacy of home glucose monitoring in diabetic pregnancy. *Am J Med* 1983; **75**:592–6.

48. Hanson U, Person B, Enochsson E et al. Self-monitoring of blood glucose by diabetic women during the third trimester of pregnancy. *Am J Obset Gynecol* 1984; **150**: 817–21.

49. De Veciana M, Major CA, Morgan M et al. Postprandial versus prepandial blood glucose monitoring in women with gestational diabetes mellitus requiring insulin therapy. *N Engl J Med* 1995; **19**:1237–41.

50. Peacock M, Chunter JC, Walford S. Self-monitoring of blood glucose in diabetic pregnancy. *Br Med J* 1979; ii: 1333–6.

51. Jovanovic L, Peterson CM, Saxena BB et al. Feasibility of maintaining normal glucose profiles in insulin-dependent pregnant diabetic women. *Am J Med* 1980; **68**: 105–12.

52. Jovanovic L, Druzin ML, Peterson CM. Impact of euglycaemia on the outcome of pregnancy in insulin-dependent diabetic women compared with normal control subjects. *Am J Med* 1981; **71**:921–8.

53. Espersen T, Klebe JG. Self-monitoring of blood glucose in pregnant diabetics. A comparative study of the blood glucose level and course of pregnancy in pregnant diabetics on an out-patient regime before and after the introduction of methods for home analysis of blood glucose. *Acta Obstet Gynecol Scand* 1985; **64**:11–14.

54. Goldberg JD, Franklin B, Lasser D et al. Gestational diabetes: impact of home glucose monitoring on neonatal birth weight. *Am J Obstet Gynecol* 1986; **154**:546–50.

55. Wecher DJ, Kaufmann RC, Amankwah KS et al. Prevention of neonatal macrosomia in gestational diabetes by the use of intensive dietary therapy and home glucose monitoring. *Am J Perinatol* 1991; **8**:131–4.

45

Ethical issues in management of pregnancy complicated by diabetes

Frank A Chervenak, Laurence B McCullough

Introduction

Physicians caring for pregnant women with diabetes can confront ethical concerns and issues that arise when the physician's judgments about what is in her clinical interest and/or the fetus's interests differs from her judgment about what is in her or her fetus's interest.[1-6] One way to manage such differences would be to assert the primacy of the physician's judgment. This strategy has been discredited because it leads to paternalism in the care of patients.[7] Paternalism occurs when the physician's clinical judgments fail to take account of the patient's values and beliefs regarding her own health and medical care.[8] To avoid paternalism the physician could opt for the alternative of the primacy of the patient's judgment.[9] This approach, however, can reduce the physician's role to that of mere technician and may also require the physician to act in ways that contradict reasonable medical judgment.

In this chapter the methods of ethics are applied to the problem of differences between the obstetrician and the diabetic pregnant woman about what is in her interest and the fetal patient's interest in a way that avoids these two extremes. Our goal is to identify a framework for clinical judgment and decision-making about the ethical dimensions of the obstetrician–patient relationship. To achieve this goal ethics, medical ethics, and the fundamental ethical principles of medical ethics, beneficence and respect for autonomy will be defined. Secondly, the concept of the fetus as a patient will be identified, emphasizing counseling for a pregnancy complicated by a fetal anomaly. Thirdly, the implications of this concept for the role of Cesarean delivery in the care of pregnant women with diabetes will be discussed. A preventive ethics approach that appreciates the potential for ethical conflict and adopts ethically justified strategies to prevent those conflicts from occuring will be emphasized.[5,10] Preventive ethics helps to build and sustain a strong physician–patient relationship.

A framework for obstetric ethics

Ethics and medical ethics

Ethics can be usefully defined as the disciplined study of morality and draws on the disciplines of the humanities, especially philosophy. Medical ethics can therefore be defined as the disciplined study of morality in medicine and concerns the mutual obligations of physicians and their patients to health care organizations and society.

Ethics should not be confused with the many sources of morality in a pluralistic society.[11] In most countries, these include law, American political heritage as a free people, the world's religions (most of which now exist in the USA), ethnic and cultural traditions, families, the traditions and practices of medicine (including medical education and training), and personal experience. These sources of morality can be useful reference points for ethical inquiry.

The traditions and practices of medicine, including education and training, constitute an influential, and therefore important, source of morality for physicians. A basic obligation that has emerged from medical traditions and practices is the obligation to protect and promote the interests of the patient.[5,12] This obligation tells physicians what morality in medicine ought to be in very general abstract terms. Providing a more concrete, clinically applicable account of that obligation is the central task of medical ethics.

To undertake this task, medical ethics focuses on the question of: how *ought* the physician to conduct himself or herself with patients? Major tools of ethics for answering this question include ethical principles, because they help the physician to interpret and implement his or her general moral obligation to protect and promote the interests of the patient.[5,12]

Ethical principles

Principle of beneficence

The principle of beneficence requires each of us to act in a way that is expected reliably to produce the greater balance of goods over harms in the lives of others.[5,8,12] To put this principle into clinical practice requires a reliable account of the goods and harms pertinent to the care of the patient, and of how those goods and harms should be reasonably balanced against each other when not all of them can be achieved in a particular situation. In medical ethics, the principle of beneficence requires the physician to act in ways that are reliably expected to produce the greater balance of clinical goods over harms for the patient.

Beneficence-based clinical judgment possesses an ancient pedigree: its first expression is found in the Hippocratic Oath and accompanying texts.[5,8] Beneficence-based clinical judgment makes an important claim: to interpret reliably the interests of the patient from medicine's perspective.[5,12] This perspective is provided by accumulated scientific research, clinical experience and reasoned responses to uncertainty. It is not the function of the individual clinical perspective of a particular physician and therefore should not be based merely on clinical impression or intuition of an individual physician. On the basis of this rigorous, clinical perspective, beneficence-based clinical judgment identifies the goods that can be achieved for the patient in clinical practice based on the competencies of medicine. The goods that medicine is competent to seek for patients are the prevention and management of disease, injury, handicap, unnecessary pain and suffering, and the prevention of premature or unnecessary death.[5] Pain and suffering become unnecessary when they do not result in achieving the other goods of medical care.

It is important to note that there is an inherent risk of paternalism in beneficence-based clinical judgment. This means that beneficence-based clinical judgment, if it is, mistakenly, considered to be the sole source of moral responsibility, and therefore moral authority in medical care, invites the unwary physician to conclude that beneficence-based judgments can be imposed on the patient in violation of his or her autonomy.[5,8,12] Paternalism can be a dehumanizing response to the patient and therefore should be avoided in the practice of obstetrics.

The preventive ethics response to this inherent paternalism is for the physician to explain the diagnostic, therapeutic and prognostic reasoning that leads to his or her clinical judgment about what is in the interest of the patient, so that the patient can assess that judgment for him/herself. This strategy becomes important in the management of pregnancy in diabetic patients as a means to educating the pregnant woman about the implications of diabetes for pregnancy. These include informing her that meticulous outpatient care and even hospitalization may be necessary to optimize outcome. This process of explaining beneficence-based clinical judgment should enhance the patient's ability to understand and deal effectively with the technical aspects of managing a pregnancy complicated by diabetes, and help prepare her for decisions that may need to be made during the course of her pregnancy, e.g. ultrasound examination to detect diabetes-related fetal anomalies or Cesarean delivery to avoid the birth trauma associated with macrosomia.

A major advantage of sharing such beneficence-based clinical judgment for the physician in carrying out this approach is that it promotes compliance with the obstetrician's recommendations, especially those intended to prevent or minimize the complications of pregnancy. Another advantage would be to provide the patient with a better-informed opportunity to make a decision about whether to seek a second opinion. The approach outlined above should make such a decision less threatening to her physician, who has already shared with the patient the limitations on clinical judgment. A final advantage may be a reduction of the percentage (20%) of physicians who reportedly dismiss patients who disagree with them and the high percentage (36%) of patients who report that they have changed physicians who disagree with them.[13]

Principle of respect for autonomy

There has been increasing emphasis in the literature of medical ethics on the principle of respect for autonomy.[8,11] This principle requires one always to acknowledge and carry out the value-based preferences of others, irrespective of what one might think the consequences for them of so doing might be.

The pregnant patient, including pregnant diabetic patients, increasingly brings to her medical care her own perspective on what is in her interests. The principle of respect for autonomy translates this fact into autonomy-based clinical judgment. Autonomy-based clinical judgment has roots in the law of malpractice, dating from the second decade of the twentieth century, and then in ethics, dating from three decades ago.[8,14] Because each patient's perspective on her interests is a function of her values and beliefs, it is impossible to specify the goods and harms of autonomy-based clinical judgment in advance. Indeed, it would be inappropriate to do so, because the definition of her goods and harms, and their balancing, are the prerogative of the pregnant patient. Not surprisingly, autonomy-based clinical judgment is strongly antipaternalistic in nature.

To understand the moral demands of this principle, an operationalized concept of autonomy is needed, to make it relevant to clinical practice. To do so, three sequential autonomy-related behaviors on the part of the patient are identified: (a) absorbing and retaining information about her condition, and alternative diagnostic and therapeutic responses to it; (b) understanding that information, i.e. evaluating and rank-ordering those responses; and (c) expressing a value-based preference for a particular response. The physician has a role to play in each of these. They are, respectively: (a) to recognize (and not underestimate) the capacity of each patient to deal with medical information about pregnancy, especially diabetes and pregnancy, to provide information, i.e. disclosure and explanations of all alternatives supported in beneficence-based clinical judgment, and to recognize the validity of the values and beliefs of the patient; (b) not to interfere with but, when necessary, to assist the diabetic pregnant patient in her evaluation and ranking of diagnostic and therapeutic alternative responses to her condition; and (c) to elicit and implement the patient's value-based preference.[5]

Interaction of beneficence and respect for autonomy in obstetric clinical judgment and practice

The ethical principles of beneficence and respect for autonomy play a complex role in obstetric clinical judgment and practice (Box 45.1). There are obviously beneficence-based and autonomy-based obligations to the diabetic pregnant patient.[5] The physician's perspective on the pregnant woman's health-related interests provides the basis for the physician's beneficence-based obligations to her. Her own perspective on her health-related and other interests provides the basis for the physician's autonomy-based obligations to her. Because of an insufficiently developed central nervous system, the fetus cannot meaningfully be said to possess values and beliefs. Thus, there is no

basis for saying that a fetus has a perspective on its interests. There can therefore be no autonomy-based obligations to any fetus.[5] Hence, the language of fetal rights has no meaning and therefore no application to the fetus in obstetric clinical judgment and practice, despite its popularity in public and political discourse in the United States and other countries. Obviously, the physician has a perspective on the fetus's health-related interests and the physician can have beneficence-based obligations to the fetus, but only when the fetus is a patient. Because of its importance for obstetric clinical judgment and practice, the topic of the fetus as a patient requires detailed consideration.

The concept of the fetus as a patient

The concept of the fetus as a patient is essential to obstetric clinical judgment and practice. This concept has considerable clinical significance because, when the fetus is a patient, directive counseling, i.e. recommending a form of management, for fetal benefit is appropriate and, when the fetus is not a patient, non-directive counseling, i.e. offering but not recommending a form of management, is appropriate. However, these apparently straightforward roles for directive and non-directive counseling

---

Interests of the pregnant woman

Maternal autonomy-based obligations of physician

Maternal beneficence-based obligations of physician

Interests of the fetal patient

Fetal beneficence-based obligations of pregnant woman

Fetal beneficence-based obligations of physician

Box 45.1.   Ethical obligations of the physician in obstetric care.

are often difficult to apply in actual perinatal practice because of uncertainty about when the fetus is a patient.

Independent moral status of the fetus

One approach to resolving this uncertainty would be to argue that the fetus is or is not a patient in virtue of personhood, or some other form of independent moral status.[6,9,11,15–17] It will now be shown that this approach fails to resolve the uncertainty and we therefore defend an alternative approach that does resolve the uncertainty.[5]

Independent moral status for the fetus means that one or more characteristics that the fetus possesses in and of itself, and, therefore, independently of the pregnant woman or any other factor, generate and therefore ground obligations to the fetus on the part of the pregnant woman and her physician. Many characteristics have been nominated for this role.[15–17] Given the variability of proposed characteristics, there is considerable variation among ethical arguments about when the fetus acquires independent moral status. Some take the view that the fetus has independent moral status from the moment of conception or implantation.[15–17] Others believe that independent moral status is acquired in degrees, thus resulting in 'graded' moral status.[6,18] Still others hold, at least by implication, that the fetus never has independent moral status so long as it is *in utero*.[9]

Despite an ever-expanding theological and philosophical literature on this subject, there has been no closure on a single authoritative account of the independent moral status of the fetus.[5,17,19] This is an unsurprising outcome because, given the absence of a single method that would be authoritative for all of the markedly diverse theological and philosophical schools of thought involved in this endless debate, closure is impossible. For closure ever to be possible, debates about such a final authority within and between theological and philosophical traditions would have to be resolved in a way satisfactory to all, an inconceivable intellectual and cultural event. Therefore, it is proposed that these futile attempts to understand the fetus as a patient in terms of its independent moral status are abandoned and turn instead to an alternative approach that makes it possible to identify ethically distinct senses of the fetus as a patient, and their clinical implications for directive and non-directive counseling.

Dependent moral status of the fetus

Analysis of the dependent moral status of the fetus as a patient begins with the recognition that being a patient does not require that one possesses independent moral status.[20] Rather, being a patient means that one can benefit from the applications of the clinical skills of the physician. Put more precisely, a human being without independent moral status is properly regarded as a patient when two conditions are met: (a) a human being is presented to the physician and (b) there exist clinical interventions that are reliably expected to be efficacious, in that they are reliably expected to result in a greater balance of goods over harms for the human being in question.[21] This is the second sense of the concept of the fetus as a patient, termed the dependent moral status of the fetus.[5]

The present authors have argued elsewhere that beneficence-based obligations to the fetus exist when the fetus is reliably presented for medical interventions, whether diagnostic or therapeutic, that can reasonably be expected to result in a greater balance of goods over harms for the child or person the fetus can later become during early childhood. Whether the fetus is a patient depends on links that can be established between the fetus and its later achieving independent moral status.[5]

Viable fetal patient

One such link is viability. Viability is not, however, an intrinsic property of the fetus because viability must be understood in terms of both biological and technological factors.[19,22] These two factors do not exist as a function of the autonomy of the pregnant woman. When a fetus is viable, i.e. when it is of sufficient maturity so that it can survive into the neonatal period and achieve independent moral status given the availability of the requisite technological support, and when it is presented to the physician, the fetus is a patient.

Viability exists as a function of biomedical and technological capacities, which are different in different parts of the world. As a consequence there is, at the present time, no worldwide, uniform gestational age to define viability. In the United States, the present authors believe, viability presently occurs at c. 24 weeks of gestational age.[23–25]

When the fetus is a patient, directive counseling for fetal benefit is ethically justified. In clinical practice, directive counseling for fetal benefit involves one or more of the following: recommending against termination of pregnancy; recommending for or against aggressive management. Aggressive obstetric management includes interventions such as fetal surveillance, tocolysis, Cesarean delivery or delivery in a tertiary care center when indicated. Non-aggressive obstetric management excludes such interventions. Directive counseling for fetal benefit, however, must take account of the presence and severity of fetal anomalies, extreme prematurity and obligations to the pregnant woman.[5]

It is important to appreciate in obstetric clinical judgment and practice that the strength of directive counseling for fetal benefit varies according to the presence and severity of anomalies. As a rule, the more severe the fetal anomaly, the less directive counseling should be for fetal benefit.[5,26–29] In particular, when there is a very high probability of a correct diagnosis and either a very high probability of death as an outcome of the anomaly diagnosed or a very high probability of severe irreversible deficit of cognitive developmental capacity as a result of the anomaly diagnosed, counseling should be non-directive in recommending between aggressive and non-aggressive management as options.[30] In contrast, when lethal anomalies can be diagnosed with certainty then there are no beneficence-based obligations to provide aggressive management.[5,31] Such fetuses are not patients; they are appropriately regarded as dying fetuses and the counseling should be non-directive in recommending between non-aggressive management and termination of pregnancy, but directive in recommending against aggressive management for the sake of maternal benefit.[26]

The strength of directive counseling for fetal benefit in cases of extreme prematurity of viable fetuses does not vary. In particular, this is the case for what are termed just-viable fetuses,[5] i.e. those with a gestational age of 24–26 weeks for which there are significant rates of survival but high rates of mortality and morbidity.[23–25] These rates of morbidity and mortality can be increased by non-aggressive obstetric management, while aggressive obstetric management may favorably influence outcome. Thus, it would appear that there are substantial beneficence-based obligations to just-viable fetuses to provide aggressive obstetric management. This is all the more the case in pregnancies beyond 26 weeks gestational age.[23–25] Therefore, directive counseling for fetal benefit is justified in all cases of extreme prematurity of viable fetuses considered by itself. Of course, such directive counseling is only appropriate when it is based on documented efficacy of aggressive obstetric management for each fetal indication.

Any directive counseling for fetal benefit must occur in the context of balancing beneficence-based obligations to the fetus against beneficence- and autonomy-based obligations to the pregnant woman (Box 45.1).[5,32] Any such balancing must recognize that a pregnant woman is obligated only to take reasonable risks of medical interventions that are reliably expected to benefit the viable fetus or child later. The unique feature of obstetric ethics is that whether, in a particular case, the viable fetus ought to be regarded as presented to the physician is, in part, a function of the pregnant woman's autonomy.

Obviously, any strategy for directive counseling for fetal benefit that takes account of obligations to the pregnant woman must be open to the possibility of conflict between the physician's recommendation and a pregnant woman's autonomous decision to the contrary. Such conflict is best managed preventively through informed consent as an ongoing dialog throughout the pregnancy, augmented as necessary by negotiation and respectful persuasion.[5,10]

Previable fetal patient

The only possible link between the previable fetus and the child it can become is the pregnant woman's autonomy. This is because technological factors cannot result in the previable fetus becoming a child. This is simply what previable means. The link, therefore, between a fetus and the child it can become, when the fetus is previable, can be established only by the pregnant woman's decision to confer the status of being a patient on her previable fetus. The previable fetus, therefore, has no claim to

the status of being a patient independently of the pregnant woman's autonomy. The pregnant woman is free to withhold, confer or, having once conferred, withdraw the status of being a patient on or from her previable fetus according to her own values and beliefs. The previable fetus is presented to the physician solely as a function of the pregnant woman's autonomy.[5]

Counseling the pregnant woman regarding the management of her pregnancy when the fetus is previable should be non-directive in terms of continuing the pregnancy or having an abortion, if she refuses to confer the status of being a patient on her fetus. If she does confer such status in a settled way, at that point beneficence-based obligations to her fetus come into existence and directive counseling for fetal benefit becomes appropriate for these previable fetuses. Just as for viable fetuses, such counseling must take account of the presence and severity of fetal anomalies, extreme prematurity and obligations owed to the pregnant woman.

For pregnancies in which the woman is uncertain about whether to confer such status, the present authors propose that the fetus be provisionally regarded as a patient.[5] This justifies directive counseling against behavior that can harm a fetus in significant and irreversible ways, e.g. poorly controlled hyperglycemia, until the woman settles on whether to confer the status of being a patient on the fetus. This also justifies directive counseling about diagnostic surveillance, e.g. ultrasound examination to detect anomalies. When anomalies are detected, counseling about the disposition of the woman's pregnancy should be non-directive, as explained above.

Non-directive counseling is appropriate in cases of what is termed near-viable fetuses,[5] i.e. those which are 22–23 weeks gestational age for which there are anecdotal reports of survival.[25] In the present authors' view, aggressive obstetric and neonatal management should be regarded as clinical investigation, i.e. a form of medical experimentation, and not standard of care.[25] There is no obligation on the part of a pregnant woman to confer the status of being a patient on a near-viable fetus, because the efficacy of aggressive obstetric and neonatal management has yet to be proven.

When to offer, recommend and perform a Cesarean section

When to offer, recommend and perform Cesarean delivery is a clinical ethical challenge in the management of a pregnancy complicated by diabetes. In this section an ethically justified approach to offering and recommending Cesarean delivery is provided, based on the ethical principles of beneficence and respect for autonomy, and the concept of a fiduciary.[33] This approach is designed to prevent conflict between the physician and the pregnant woman about intrapartum management.

This approach begins by asking: Is Cesarean delivery substantively supported and vaginal delivery not supported in beneficence-based clinical judgment? Such cases occur with diabetic pregnancies based on clinical factors such as estimation of fetal weight, the maternal pelvis, the degree of control of diabetes in the pregnancy and previous obstetric history (these clinical factors are discussed in detail elsewhere in this book). When evidence or reliable clinical judgment support the view that the fetus' interests are best protected by Cesarean delivery, and there are no maternal contraindications, then such a delivery should be offered and recommended.

In some clinical circumstances, there is scientific controversy as to whether Cesarean delivery is the better alternative. Competing well-founded beneficence-based clinical judgments regarding how to balance the fetal benefit of preventing harm of Cesarean delivery generate these controversies, which are discussed elsewhere in this book. Whenever there is legitimate scientific disagreement about the benefits and risks of Cesarean versus vaginal delivery, both options should be offered to the pregnant woman and discussed with her so that she can exercise her autonomy meaningfully. Such disclosure empowers the woman to emphasize her own perspective in balancing maternal and fetal risks. It is appropriate for the physician to assist the woman's decision-making about both options in the form of a recommendation

In clinical circumstances when Cesarean delivery is substantively supported in beneficence-based clinical judgment but vaginal delivery is more substantively supported, vaginal delivery is the better alternative, but not the only one, e.g. a pregnant diabetic patient whose sugars have been well-controlled during pregnancy and in whom there is no macrosomia. Although Cesarean delivery is supported in beneficence-based clinical judgment, trial of labor is more substantively supported, and therefore should be offered and recommended.

Conclusions

Ethics is an essential dimension of obstetric practice, especially in the care of pregnant diabetic patients. In this chapter a framework for obstetric ethics based on ethical principles and the concept of the fetus as a patient are described. On this basis, two dimensions of the care of diabetes in pregnancy with important clinical dimensions are presented: counseling about fetal anomalies; when to offer and recommend Cesarean delivery. The present authors believe that the clinical application of ethical concepts will strengthen the doctor–patient relationship and therefore enhance the quality of care for pregnant diabetic patients.

References

1. Cain J, Stacy L, Jusenius K, Figge D. The quality of dying: financial, psychological, and ethical dilemmas. *Obstet Gynecol* 1990; 76:149–52.
2. Park RC. Old bedfellows: ethics and obstetrics and gynecology. *Obstet Gynecol* 1989; 73:1–3.
3. Jennings JC. Ethics in obstetrics and gynecology: a practitioner's review and opinion. *Obstet Gynecol Surv* 1989; 44:656–61.
4. Skrzydelwski WB. Gynæcology and ethics. *Eur J Obstet Gynecol Reprod Biol* 1990; 36:274–82.
5. McCullough LB, Chervenak FA. *Ethics in Obstetrics and Gynecology*. (Oxford University Press: New York, 1994).
6. Strong C. *Ethics in Reproductive Medicine: A New Framework*. (Yale University Press: New Haven, 1997).
7. Veath R. *A Theory of Medical Ethics*. (Basic Books: New York, 1981).
8. Beauchamp TL, Childress JF. *Principles of Biomedical Ethics*, 4th edn. (Oxford University Press: New York, 1994).
9. Annas GJ. Protecting the liberty of pregnant patient. *N Engl J Med* 1988; 316:1213–14.
10. Chervenak FA, McCullough LB. Clinical guides to preventing ethical conflicts between pregnant women and their physicians. *Am J Obstet Gynecol* 1990; 162:303–7.
11. Engelhardt Jr HT. *The Foundations of Bioethics*, 2nd edn. (Oxford University Press: New York, 1996).
12. Beauchamp TL, McCullough LB. *Medical Ethics: The Moral Responsibilities of Physicians*. (Prentice-Hall: Englewood Cliffs, 1984).
13. Louis Harris and Associates. Views on informed consent and decision making: parallel surveys of physicians and the public. In: *President's Commission for the Study of Ethical Problems in Medicine and Biomedical and Behavior Research, Making Health Care Decisions, Volume 2, Appendices: Empirical Studies of Informed Consent*. (US Government Printing Office: Washington, DC, 1982).
14. Faden RR, Beauchamp TL. *A History and Theory of Informed Consent*. (Oxford University Press: New York, 1986).
15. Noonan JT, ed. *The Morality of Abortion*. (Harvard University Press: Cambridge, 1970).
16. Noonan JT. *A Private Choice. Abortion in America in the Seventies*. (The Free Press: New York, 1979).
17. Callahan S, Callahan D, eds. *Abortion: Understanding Differences*. (Plenum Press: New York, 1984).
18. Evans MI, Fletcher JC, Zador IE et al. Selective first-trimester termination in octuplet and quadruplet pregnancies: clinical and ethical issues. *Obstet Gynecol* 1988; 71:289–96.
19. Roe versus Wade, 410 US 113 (1973).
20. Ruddick W, Wilcox W. Operating on the fetus. *Hastings Cent Rep* 1982; 12:10–14.
21. Chervenak FA, McCullough LB. What is obstetric ethics? *J Perinat Med* 1996; 23:331–41.
22. Mahowald M. Beyond abortion: refusal of cesarean section. *Bioethics* 1989; 3:106–21.
23. Hack M, Fanaroff AA. Outcomes of extremely-low-birth-weight infants between 1982 and 1988. *N Engl J Med* 1989; 321:1642–7.
24. Whyte HE, Fitzhardinge PM et al. External immaturity: outline of 568 pregnancies of 23–26 weeks' gestation. *Obstet Gynecol* 1993; 82:1–7.
25. Chervenak FA, McCullough LB. The limits of viability. *J Perinat Med* 1997; 25:418–20.
26. Chervenak FA, McCullough LB. An ethically justified, clinically comprehensive management strategy for third-trimester pregnancies complicated by fetal anomalies. *Obstet Gynecol* 1990; 75:311–16.
27. Chervenak FA, McCullough LB. Does obstetric ethics have any role in the obstetrician's response to the abortion controversy? *Am J Obstet Gynecol* 1990; 163:1425–9.
28. Chervenak FA, McCullough LB. Is third trimester abortion justified? *Br J Obstet Gynaecol* 1995; 102:434–5.
29. Chervenak FA, McCullough LB. Third trimester abortion: is compassion enough? *Br J Obstet Gynaecol* 1999; 106:293–6.
30. Chervenak FA, McCullough LB. Nonaggressive obstetric management: an option for some fetal anomalies during the third trimester. *J Am Med Assoc* 1989; 261:3429–30.
31. Chervenak FA, Farley MA, Walters L et al. When is termination of pregnancy during the third trimester morally justifiable? *N Engl J Med* 1984; 310:501–4.
32. Chervenak FA, McCullough LB. Perinatal ethics: a practical method of analysis of obligations to mother and fetus. *Obstet Gynecol* 1985; 66:442–6.
33. Chervenak FA, McCullough LB. An ethically justified algorithm for offering, recommending, and performing cesarean delivery and its application in managed care practice. *Obstet Gynecol* 1996; 87:302–5.

46

Legal aspects of diabetic pregnancy
Kevin J Dalton

Introduction – the law and medicine

Legal problems relating to diabetic pregnancy may be considered from three aspects:

(1) legal problems specific to pregnancy in a woman who is diabetic;
(2) legal problems specific to diabetes in a woman who is pregnant;
(3) legal problems specific to diabetic pregnancy.

When an obstetrician or diabetologist hears that the law may be relevant to medicine, immediately he/she will think of medical malpractice and of litigation for alleged negligence. But the law applies to medicine in many other ways. Thus, when considering the legal aspects of diabetic pregnancy, one must look not only at matters arising under civil law, but also those arising under criminal law, administrative law and forensic medicine.

Few obstetricians or diabetologists are trained in medical law, and so concepts that are considered mainstream in law may appear utterly alien to them. A few of these concepts will be explained very briefly here because unless they are understood then the law set out relating to diabetic pregnancy may not be fully understood. For doctors, difficulties often arise with the following legal concepts: the doctrine of precedent, standard of proof, case and statute law, and law in different jurisdictions.

Doctrine of legal precedent

When considering the law relating to any field of medicine, it is essential to recognize that the doctrine of **binding precedent** is of prime importance in the common-law environment that covers most of the English-speaking world. Briefly, the doctrine of **binding precedent** states that whenever: (1) a legal case is being tried **and** (2) a higher court (i.e. an appellate court) has already decided a case that is similar to the present case, then the lower court **must** follow (i.e. uphold) the previous decision of the higher court. By extension, a court should usually follow the decisions of courts of equal standing within the same jurisdiction. They may even follow decisions made by courts in foreign jurisdictions if they find their decisions helpful.

Sometimes the previous decision of relevance may have been made many decades or even centuries previously. For example, whenever English courts consider the question of consent to surgery, even today, they will frequently cite a New York court's decision made in 1914.[1]

It is also important to recognize that, in the common-law environment, court decisions that are made in one field of human activity may be readily applicable to other fields. For example, a decision made regarding the liability of an engineer may be highly relevant in deciding a case involving the liability of an architect or a medical doctor. Similarly, a decision made on a case involving only the single disease of hypertension may be relevant to a case involving only diabetes.

It follows from this that when an individual obstetrician or diabetologist discusses a medical case with his/her lawyer, the lawyer has no professional choice other than to accept and follow previous rulings of courts in the same jurisdiction, unless he/she can somehow distinguish the instant case from a related case that the court has already decided.

Standard of proof

In medicine, the level of proof is expected to be *c.* 95–99% before stating belief in a proposition. This high level of proof, i.e. that one is sure beyond reasonable doubt, is almost identical to the level which the court uses to decide criminal matters that are in dispute.

However, in legal disputes on civil matters, the court requires a level of proof of only 51%. In other words, the court will make its decision on the balance of probability, i.e. when it believes that the proposition in dispute is more likely than not. In medical negligence cases, only this lower level of proof is needed for a decision to be made.

This distinction between making medical decisions or legal decisions is most important.

Case law

From the above, it follows that, in deciding legal cases that arise under point (1) (i.e. problems specific to pregnancy), then previously decided cases relating to any pregnancy, even in non-diabetics, may be highly relevant. Similarly, in deciding cases that arise under

point (2) (i.e. problems specific to diabetes), previously decided cases relating to diabetes, even if the diabetic is a man, may be highly relevant. In deciding cases under points (1)–(3), even cases from quite different fields of human activity may be relevant. Thus, in any given jurisdiction in the common-law world, there is a very wide range of case law that may be relevant when considering diabetic pregnancies.

In the common-law jurisdictions there have been many cases litigated that refer to diabetic pregnancy,[2] but in this chapter only the briefest details of just a few of them can be given. For a fuller understanding of each case, and of the rationale for each individual decision that was made, clearly it will be necessary to read the full text of the decision that was handed down by the court – nowadays, such full texts are often available on the World Wide Web.

Statute law

As with case law, in any given jurisdiction there is a considerable amount of statute law that may be relevant when considering diabetic pregnancies.

The law in different jurisdictions

The law relating to health care, and so the law relating to diabetic pregnancy, will differ from one jurisdiction to another. Within the United States the 56 (*sic*) separate jurisdictions have a different body of law, one from another. Even within the British Isles, the four separate jurisdictions each have a different body (and system) of law.

Covering all aspects of the law that relate to diabetic pregnancy in all jurisdictions is beyond the scope of this chapter. Instead, a limited series of topics from different jurisdictions will be considered to illustrate the diversity of the law that may apply to diabetic pregnancy.

Antenatal care

Menopause or pregnancy?

A 47-year-old insulin-dependent diabetic mentioned to her doctor that she had missed her last period and was having hot flushes. He offered no advice on this, nor did he take any action. When he saw her on later occasions, he did not ask about her periods. Subsequently, and unexpectedly, she delivered a 28-week stillborn fetus. She had not realized that she was pregnant. She took legal action against her doctor and claimed for wrongful death of her fetus, who might have survived with better medical care. She also sought damages for 'physical pain, mental anguish, medical expenses and lost wages'. Even though the Virginia court[3] held (on appeal) that no cause of action lies for the wrongful death of a stillborn child, as it is part of its mother until birth, nevertheless it awarded damages to the mother for her emotional distress.

Fetal macrosomia

In 1988, the Supreme Court of Alabama tried a case[4] in which a diabetic mother who weighed 143 kg delivered a fetus of 5.2 kg. There was shoulder dystocia and the child suffered Erb's palsy. Expert evidence was given relating to two schools of thought on whether a Caesarean section should have been performed. Although the court acknowledged the two schools, it gave greater weight to the breach of a guideline previously issued by the American College of Obstetricians and Gynecologists, which said that there should be an elective Caesarean section when a fetus is believed to weigh > 4 kg particularly in a diabetic pregnancy. The court therefore ruled that it was open to the jury to find the obstetrician negligent, despite the two schools of thought.

Other cases where there was fetal macrosomia will be referred to below.

Screening for diabetes in pregnancy

In 1994, a court in Alberta tried a 1988 case[5] in which a macrosomic baby suffered Erb's palsy after shoulder dystocia. During pregnancy the family doctor had failed to implement the universal screening policy for gestational diabetes that had been recommended by the Alberta Medical Association and the Society of Obstetricians of Canada. He also overlooked maternal glycosuria and significant maternal weight gain. He then failed to recognize fetal macrosomia on manual palpation and failed to request an ultrasound scan. The court found that his care was negligent in that he failed to follow guideline recommendations and that he failed to recognize clinical signs.

This Canadian case contrasts with a similar English case decided shortly afterwards. In 1998 the English Court of Appeal decided a 1990 case[6] relating to the screening for diabetes in pregnancy. At 30 weeks gestation a woman exhibited glycosuria ++. Her family doctor carried out a random blood glucose test, which was normal at 4.6 mmol/l. [A glucose tolerance test (GTT) at 30 weeks in her previous pregnancy had also been normal.] Nevertheless, the family doctor referred her to an obstetrician, at a hospital whose policy was to screen selectively rather than universally. The obstetrician saw her at 34 weeks, on which occasion she exhibited no glycosuria. She was considered to be at a low risk of diabetes and was told that no GTT was needed. This followed the screening policy set out in the leading English obstetrical textbook of the time (*Dewhurst's Obstetrics*).[7] The baby delivered at 39 weeks and weighed 5.8 kg. There was insuperable shoulder dystocia and so an emergency

Caesarean section had to be carried out. The baby suffered both hypoxic damage to his brain (cerebral palsy) and traction damage to his brachial plexus (Erb's palsy). A claim for clinical negligence was made on the grounds that: (1) a GTT should have been organized at 34 weeks; (2) this would have revealed gestational diabetes; (3) she would then have been delivered by Caesarean section; and (4) the baby would have had no serious injury.

The case was first heard in the High Court, but then it went to appeal. The Court of Appeal held that the obstetrician was entitled to be reassured by the random blood glucose at 30 weeks, i.e. the single episode of glycosuria did not put her in a high-risk group that needed a GTT. When she saw her at 34 weeks there was now no glycosuria and so there was no reason for a GTT. The claim for negligence (along the lines that had been argued) was therefore dismissed, on the grounds that it was both reasonable and not negligent to decide not to carry out a GTT.

These two cases illustrate the fact that different courts in different jurisdictions, when trying similar cases relating to the screening for, and the management of, diabetic pregnancy, may arrive at decisions that on the face of it seem contradictory. Such a situation is by no means unusual in comparative international law.

In English law, the importance of this case is that the Court of Appeal has recognized that universal screening for gestational diabetes is not a legal requirement and that selective screening is sufficient. Furthermore, it accepts that a policy of selective screening may fail to recognize complicated cases. American readers will note that the American Diabetic Association has only recently moved away from recommending universal screening for gestational diabetes and now recommends selective screening.[8]

Hypoglycaemic attacks

In pregnancy, diabetic women become more liable to hypoglycaemic attacks than before pregnancy. If they are under tighter glycaemic control than before pregnancy, then they may even become less aware of their hypoglycaemic attacks than they were previously. It may therefore be thought reasonable to discriminate against such women in terms of the activities in which they are allowed to participate. However, an English court has recently ruled as illegal, under the Disability Discrimination Act 1995, a high school's attempt to ban a diabetic student from a watersports holiday in France, on the grounds that there had been hypoglycaemic attacks when the student was on an earlier skiing trip.[9]

In England, if a pregnant woman commits a crime when she is hypoglycaemic, this fact may provide a valid and sufficient defence in law, although not for all offences (see later). In the case of *R v. Padmore*,[10] a diabetic committed the crime of homicide when in a state of hypoglycaemic automatism. The jury cleared him on the grounds that he was unaware of his condition and therefore had no control over his actions.

Dietary control

In gestational diabetes, there is no unambiguous scientific literature to demonstrate that good dietary control, or a special diet, will result in the birth of a smaller infant. Nevertheless, legal cases are often argued on the basis that better diabetic control would have resulted in a smaller baby and in fewer problems at the time of delivery.

One such case was heard in Ontario in 1982.[11] The mother claimed that her doctor's failure to test for, and to diagnose, gestational diabetes led to birth injuries. She had had three vaginal deliveries. Her first child weighed 3.65 kg, and he did well. Her second child weighed 4.4 kg; his delivery was complicated by shoulder dystocia, and he suffered numerous bruises and a fractured clavicle. She requested a Caesarean section for the delivery of her third child, but she was told that this was not necessary, and so again she delivered vaginally. This third child weighed 5.26 kg. His delivery was complicated by shoulder dystocia, and he suffered brachial plexus palsy and a skull fracture.

The mother brought a legal action, on the grounds that she should have been tested for gestational diabetes and a special diet should have been started in order to minimize the risk of fetal macrosomia.

The court held that the diagnosis of gestational diabetes had never been established during her pregnancy and that it could not be determined retrospectively. Moreover, even if she did have gestational diabetes, there was no convincing evidence that dietary management or insulin would have affected the size of the baby. The expert medical evidence in this case was contradictory, but the judge said that:

> The evidence of Dr Allen [the defence expert] is preferable because his opinion was carefully documented by an assessment of forty studies done by learned researchers. There is no strong body of medical opinion to support the proposition that controlled diet of the mother would have produced a smaller baby.

The case was dismissed.

Although this case was heard in 1982, many would argue that scientific evidence on the benefits of dietary control in gestational diabetes has changed little since then.

Bank robbery

A bank teller who was 28 weeks pregnant came face to face with an armed robber. He pointed a sawn-off shotgun at her and demanded money. She was terrified and feared for her life. Eventually, the robber was arrested and convicted. Later in the pregnancy the woman went on to develop gestational diabetes. She also developed depression and a profound fear of returning to the work at the counter, and needed psychological counselling. She claimed that stress from the robbery had caused her gestational diabetes and that this increased her chance of developing diabetes in later life. At trial, the court took her allegations into account, and so it enhanced the severity of the custodial sentence that was passed.[12]

Labour and delivery

Amniocentesis and delivery

Until recently, it was common to plan the timing of delivery on the basis of testing the amniotic fluid for evidence of fetal lung maturity. In a diabetic pregnancy in South Carolina, the expected date of delivery was only 4 days away. The mother noticed a reduction in fetal movements. A fetal heart rate recording was made, which suggested an active and healthy fetus. Nevertheless, the obstetrician decided upon an amniocentesis with a view to delivery. She admitted that several times during the procedure she stuck the fetus with the amniocentesis needle. Blood was aspirated but no amniotic fluid was obtained. At birth the child had puncture sites on the left and right sides of his face. Right-sided facial paralysis was immediately apparent. As he has grown, his facial appearance has become distorted and his speech is impaired. He cannot close his right eye, and has had several operations on it. His right visual field is restricted. When the case came to trial, evidence was presented of an emotional impact, and of an increased risk of depression and of suicide as he grows older.[13]

Dead or alive?

In New Jersey, an insulin-dependent diabetic became pregnant for the third time. During the pregnancy her diabetes proved difficult to control. At 26 weeks gestation she developed both ketoacidosis and intermittent contractions. She was admitted to hospital but no fetal heart beat could be detected. Fetal death was diagnosed, and the patient and her husband were told the sad news. Labour started spontaneously and so no attempt was made to prevent delivery. Intermittent auscultation during the labour failed to reveal a fetal heart beat: no more accurate a method of detection of fetal heart beat was used. Eventually the baby delivered by the breech, with no one assisting in the birth. Quickly, the baby was taken away and placed in another room. There it became apparent that the baby was in fact alive and pink. He gasped for air and a heart beat was detected. He was rushed to the intensive care nursery. A nurse met the husband on the corridor. She told him the baby was alive, but would soon die, and so it would be best if he did not tell his wife that the baby was still alive. Eventually, a paediatrician arrived and he told everyone that the baby was still alive.

Unfortunately, the baby died 10 days later. With a better quality of medical care, the child may have survived and been born healthy. Not surprisingly, a successful legal action followed, brought on behalf of the parents and the (estate of the) child.[14]

Stillbirth

In obstetrical cases, it is unusual for three of the four principal actors to die before a legal action comes to trial. But fetus, father and obstetrician all died in a recent (2002) Ontario case; only the mother survived.[15]

She had a stillbirth at 33 weeks gestation. The fetus was normal in weight and in structure. Autopsy failed to reveal a cause of death. Gestational diabetes was never proven medically in this case, but its possibility was contended in argument, and the case revolved around this point. The mother and her partner (who died during the case) brought a legal action on the grounds that the obstetrician (who died a year after the stillbirth) had been negligent in his care. At trial (where the obstetrician's estate and the hospital were co-defendants), the issues in dispute were as follows: (1) gestational diabetes should have been diagnosed; (2) it had not been treated appropriately; (3) it contributed to the stillbirth; and (4) appropriate treatment would have avoided stillbirth.

The expert evidence given to the judge by eminent physicians was contradictory. It well illustrated the considerable confusion and disagreement that abound in the literature concerning screening, diagnosis and management of gestational diabetes.

After hearing the evidence, the judge decided that on the balance of probabilities: (1) the mother did not have gestational diabetes; (2) even if she did have it, then it did not contribute to the stillbirth; (3) even if she did have it, and even if it did contribute to the stillbirth, appropriate treatment of the gestational diabetes would not have prevented the stillbirth; and (4) she was treated appropriately. The case was therefore dismissed.

However, it illustrates the complexity of medical issues where a judge sitting alone may be required to reach a decision that is potentially worth many millions of dollars. It also demonstrates how an obstetrician may be sued even when he/she is in his/her grave, on grounds that might seem implausible, as gestational diabetes was never diagnosed.

The baby

Congenital disability

In British Columbia, a mother developed gestational diabetes during her pregnancy, but this was not diagnosed until late. She developed polyhydramnios. Eventually, labour was induced, but it was prolonged and so a Caesarean section was performed. The child was born with numerous defects (these were not specified in the judgment).

The mother started a legal action. She alleged poor medical care, both during the antenatal period and in labour, and so she claimed damages. Her claim on behalf of the child was dismissed because there was no causative link between the standard of care and the child's congenital abnormalities. Only part of the mother's claim for damages was upheld: that for pain and suffering. However, the court held that there was no basis in tort law for her claim of emotional distress for the delivery of a disabled child.[16] Furthermore, it would be wrong in principle to award the mother compensation for lost earnings for devoting herself to the care of her disabled child.

Respiratory distress syndrome

In a South Carolina case from 2000,[17] a woman in her third pregnancy developed gestational diabetes for the first time. Her obstetrician consulted with a diabetologist and her condition was managed by diet alone. Her due date of delivery was known. However, at 36 weeks of gestation the obstetrician attempted an amniocentesis under ultrasound control in order to determine fetal lung maturity. The attempt failed owing to the position of the placenta. However, he told her that the baby was 'big enough' and he delivered her by Caesarean section the next day: the birthweight was 3.75 kg. They parents recollect that the obstetrician was 'enormously happy' during the Caesarean operation, but the baby developed respiratory distress syndrome and was admitted to the neonatal intensive care. In the longer term he went on to have breathing difficulties.

The parents started a legal action against the obstetrician. They alleged that he was negligent in delivering the baby 4 weeks early without medical justification and in violation of accepted medical standards. They also asserted that the doctor was:

> ... addicted to the use of drugs and narcotics to the extent that he was not mentally, emotionally or physically able to have provided competent medical care and attention.

They had discovered that the doctor had been treated for alcohol dependency and that he had returned for inpatient treatment < 1 month after the Caesarean section: a few days later his partners ousted him from the partnership. At trial the parents asked the court to order release of the doctor's alcohol treatment records, but their motion was refused because it would violate federal and state confidentiality statutes. However, the court rejected the doctor's motion that all reference to his alcohol addiction should be excluded as this could not establish his alcohol status at the time in question and it would only serve to prejudice him in the eyes of the jury. The court took the view that 'the probative value is not substantially outweighed by any prejudicial effect'.

Forensic matters

Detainees

Occasionally, a diabetic pregnant woman may be held in custody, either in jail, or in police detention pending investigations or awaiting trial. Under Britain's Police and Criminal Evidence Act 1984 (PACE), a forensic medical examiner must be called to attend each prisoner who is taking medication for a chronic illness, such as diabetes, and so he/she must therefore be called to attend any diabetic pregnant prisoner. He/she must take an appropriate medical and social history, paying particular attention to whether other drugs (prescribed or not) have been taken recently. Then he/she will carry out an appropriate general and antenatal examination. He/she must then check the patient's blood glucose level at least once during a brief period of custody. Following this, he/she must (at least) discuss the case with a specialist in the management of diabetic pregnancy. If the patient is to remain in brief custody, it is important for him/her to ensure that an appropriate regime of feeding and insulin therapy is in place. However, a diabetic pregnant woman destined for a longer episode of custody will need personal attention and careful ongoing management by a specialist.

In any episode of custody, if a pregnant diabetic becomes unstable, with either hypoglycaemia or hyperglycaemia, she must be transferred immediately to hospital for appropriate assessment and stabilization. (Clearly, hypoglycaemia should be managed by giving glucose or sugar before transfer, if this is possible.) After she has been stabilized in hospital, a decision can then be taken as to when, or whether, she may safely be returned to custody. Clearly, the prison cell is not the safest of places to manage a diabetic pregnancy.

It is important to remember that a pregnant woman will be unfit for interview by the police if her diabetes is in any way unstable at the time of the proposed interview. If an interview takes place when she is (or should be) considered as medically unfit, then any information or confession she gives will be considered unreliable,

and so the circumstances of the interview may provide legal grounds for appeal.

Post-mortem examination

Occasionally, a diabetic pregnant woman may die unexpectedly, e.g. in a road traffic accident or suddenly whilst alone. Hypoglycaemia may be the root cause of death. However, at autopsy it is generally not possible to make a firm diagnosis of either hypoglycaemia or hyperglycaemia. The pathologist will therefore need to take circumstantial evidence into account in determining whether unstable diabetes has played a part in the death.

Administrative and related issues

Public assistance grants

The US Federal Aid for Families with Dependent Children (AFDC) programme is a cash-assistance programme designed to provide ongoing aid to poor families where at least one minor child has been deprived of parental support by reason (*inter alia*) of a parent's physical incapacity. A number of disadvantaged people started a class action against the Mayor of New York (et al) in regard to alleged misadministration of AFDC.

One of them was a 30-year-old woman who had developed gestational diabetes. She needed a 2200 calorie-a-day diet, which she could not afford without the monthly special-needs grant of $50 that should have been made available to her. She had first requested the grant when she was at 13 weeks gestation, but she did not receive it until 36 weeks. Although her money was then paid retrospectively, she claimed that she had suffered irreparable injury to herself and her child through deprivation of funds necessary to buy medically required nutrition during a substantial part of her pregnancy.

The District Court agreed to her claim and it certified her as a member of the class action.[18] It also granted (to all the class members) the preliminary injunction that they had requested against the Mayor of New York, relating to the future administration of AFDC.

Employment

Sometimes employers are not sympathetic to women's requests for time off work to attend medical appointments relating to pregnancy. This problem may be worse for pregnant diabetics, as they need more frequent appointments than most women.

There have been many cases where legal action has been taken against an employer, with allegations of discrimination, but the claimants rarely win. The reason for this may be that most cases turn on the intent of one party or the other, and this is difficult to prove after the event, particularly as there is usually no direct evidence of discriminatory intent on the part of the employer. Sometimes claims are brought under the Americans with Disabilities Act. However, temporary, non-chronic impairments of short duration, with little or no long-term impact, are not usually considered in law as disabilities.[19]

Driving

Most countries impose driving regulations on diabetics. Under British regulations, diabetics on treatment with insulin (including gestational diabetics on insulin) are barred from driving heavy goods vehicles and public services vehicles, no matter how good their diabetic control.[20] However, they may drive private cars, provided that they can recognize the symptoms of hypoglycaemia. If they cannot recognize hypoglycaemia, then they must stop driving. Diabetics on long-term insulin must also meet required visual standards. For those taking insulin, any licence to drive will be limited to 1, 2 or 3 years. Gestational diabetics who are not taking insulin have no driving restrictions. However, if they start insulin therapy in pregnancy, then they must report this fact to the Driver and Vehicle Licensing Authority in Swansea if they wish to continue driving.

Insulin-dependent diabetics who become pregnant often find that their diabetes becomes more difficult to control. Hypoglycaemic attacks become more frequent and are more difficult to recognize. Clearly, this presents a danger in terms of driving a car.

In an English case,[21] an insulin-dependent diabetic became pregnant. Her diabetic control had been good but it deteriorated in pregnancy, although she had taken specialist advice about this. One day she drove her car at high speed round a bend, on the wrong side of the road, where she collided with a tractor. She was charged with dangerous driving. Although she pleaded guilty, she claimed that she was unexpectedly hypoglycaemic at the time of the accident and so had committed the offence through no fault of her own. The magistrates rejected her claim. They fined her, and they disqualified her from driving for 12 months and until she had passed an extended driving test. She appealed on the grounds that her diabetes provided a special reason entitling the court not to impose a mandatory disqualification for the minimum period under s34 (1) of the Road Traffic Offenders Act (RTA) 1988. At appeal, the court recognized that she was not personally culpable for her offence. Nevertheless, it held that the test to establish the offence of dangerous driving is an objective test, in that the offence lies in the mode of driving, whatever the reason for it. In her case, her temporary condition (of hypoglycaemia) was special to her personally and it formed no part of the content of the offence. Thus, these circumstances did not amount to a special reason to avoid an automatic penalty of disqualification, as laid down in s34 of RTA 1988. Her appeal against disqualification was therefore dismissed. Although this decision may seem unfair to the woman, there are clear grounds of public policy as to why she should be disqualified, i.e. the protection of the public and of herself.

Note how the legal consideration of hypoglycaemia in this driving case contrasts with that in the case of that of *R v. Padmore*[10] mentioned above. In *R v. Padmore* the initial charge of murder was dismissed, as a conviction for murder requires proof of intention to kill and this was not present during that episode of hypoglycaemia. By contrast, a conviction for dangerous driving does not require any specific intention to drive dangerously.

Certification of diabetics

In England, diabetics who wish to drive must ask their doctor to complete a certificate to confirm that they have not had evidence of blackouts or loss of consciousness within the past 5 years, and have not had any significant episodes of hypoglycaemia. The present author has recently been involved in one such case. A family doctor had signed this certificate for a diabetic patient, but he signed negative answers to these two questions. He failed to mention that 5 years previously the patient had caused a motoring accident in which a heavy truck was driven through the central reservation of a major motorway, and that the episode was attributed to hypoglycaemia. Thus, the doctor had signed false entries on the driving licence application, which misled the Driving and Vehicle Licensing Authority into issuing

another heavy goods vehicle licence. A few months later the driver had a more serious trucking accident in which three people were killed: two adults and one child. Again, this accident was attributed to hypoglycaemia. On this occasion the driver was imprisoned for causing death by dangerous driving.

The family doctor was called before the Professional Conduct Committee of the General Medical Council to face charges that included making false and misleading entries on a patient's driving licence application form. He was found guilty of serious professional misconduct and the General Medical Council reprimanded him.[22]

The cost of diabetes care

Looking after diabetic women in pregnancy is expensive and so those who are ineligible for care provided by the state or by their insurance may be tempted to run their pregnancies without appropriate diabetic care. Sometimes insurers will deny funding to their insurees. But this will bring increased morbidity for mother and fetus.

For these reasons, and for longer term reasons of cost reduction, most American states have now enacted measures to require comprehensive insurance reimbursement for diabetes care, e.g. Massachusetts has its Diabetes Cost Reduction Act 2000.

The Americans with Disability Act may also be invoked in such cases. Under the Americans with Disabilities Act, in 2000 a Maine court awarded $60,000 in both compensatory and discriminatorial damages against a health maintenance organization HMO that had refused to fund a sign-language interpreter for the antenatal visits of a pregnant diabetic who was deaf, and whose husband was deaf too.[23] The couple were unable fully to communicate with their physician about dietary concerns or about complications that arose in the pregnancy.

Examination fraud

Two lawyers were married. She was an insulin-dependent diabetic; he had a history of professional setbacks, including loss of employment and bar exam failures in both Texas and California. She then became pregnant: he reacted with violent rage and depression, and the marriage deteriorated. Her diabetic pregnancy suffered a series of complications. In an attempt to save her own health, the marriage and also the future for their unborn baby, she agreed to her husband's request that she should take the state bar examination in his place. She did so, and she obtained the ninth highest mark in the state. She then went on to deliver a healthy child. However, the examination fraud was later discovered, and they were both prosecuted and disbarred.[24] They lost their jobs and now they are now divorced.

Excuse for non-performance

A diabetic solicitor was pregnant, but she continued in her law practice throughout the pregnancy, which ended in a Caesarean section. In the final few days of her pregnancy, when she was preparing for her imminent delivery, she missed an important court deadline for submission of certain papers relating to the case of a client. The court therefore struck out her client's case. She did not become aware of this problem until a few days after delivery. She therefore apologized to the court and to her client, and she made an application to court for a reversal of its decision, on the grounds that she was unable to conduct her affairs properly under the circumstances of her health. The court rejected her submission on the grounds that she knew she was to deliver soon and should have submitted the papers earlier, or made alternative arrangements by handing the case over to a colleague.[25] Her client's case therefore remained struck out.

Related medical matters

Involvement of other specialists in the care

Nowadays, reputable doctors would agree that diabetic pregnancy must be managed by an obstetrician with significant experience of such cases, but it has not always been so. In an Ontario case from 1982,[26] a pregnant woman at 37 weeks gestation was found to have glucose and ketones in her urine. Her family doctor admitted her to hospital for investigation of suspected diabetes. This diagnosis was confirmed the following day, but she was not referred to a diabetologist or an obstetrician, and no special treatment was started. Instead, she was allowed home. A few days later she went into diabetic ketoacidosis and fetal death occurred: her stillborn child was delivered 2 days later. She brought a legal action. The court held that the family doctor's failure to start insulin therapy on the evening she was first admitted to hospital was 'merely error in judgement'. However, the doctor's failure to act positively once the diagnosis of diabetes was confirmed constituted professional negligence, as also did his decision to discharge her from hospital at a time when her diabetes was not under control. The court held that damages could not be awarded for loss of the fetus or grief. However, it did award general damages to the mother for her physical pain and suffering.

By contrast, another pregnant diabetic (who also had epilepsy) sued her obstetrician because he *did* refer her on to another specialist for ongoing care. Her obstetrician had looked after her in two previous pregnancies, but early in her third pregnancy he discovered that she was

HIV positive and so he referred to another hospital for care. She took legal action against him on the grounds that he had denied her treatment solely because she was HIV positive, in violation of various disability discrimination laws. In his defence, the obstetrician explained to the court that he had never used AZT, which is recommended for such patients, and that this is why he referred her to another hospital. The court accepted his explanation, and the case was dismissed.[27]

In a Californian case from 1992,[28] Dr Klvana (a licensed doctor who practised obstetrics) was convicted of: nine counts of second degree murder, five counts of aiding and abetting the practice of medicine without a licence, one count of conspiracy to practise medicine without a licence, 19 counts of preparing a fraudulent insurance claim, 10 counts of presenting a false insurance claim, two counts of grand theft, and two counts of perjury. One of these cases involved a diabetic pregnancy. The patient concerned was an insulin-dependent diabetic, and he saw her throughout the pregnancy. At 30 weeks gestation she found glucose in her urine and so she consulted a diabetologist. He advised her that her diabetes was out of control and so he increased her insulin dosage. She told Dr Klvana about this consultation and about the increase of insulin dosage. At 34 weeks she experienced uterine contractions. Dr Klvana examined her in his office (i.e. not at the hospital) and he found that her cervix was already 3 cm dilated. He told her she would deliver that afternoon. Later he found that her cervix was 5 cm dilated and so he ruptured the membranes. At his next examination he found the cervix to be 9 cm dilated; she had not yet been transferred to hospital. Soon, the premature infant was delivered in the office. The baby was bluish purple in colour and wheezing, and he would not cry. Dr Klvana advised the mother that the baby would be all right within 24 hours. He sent them both home,

with instructions for her to give the baby sugar water, and to return within 1–2 days. He did not consult or refer to a paediatrician. The mother went home and slept, but when she awoke her baby was dead. At autopsy the baby's cause of death was given as perinatal complications associated with a diabetic mother and prematurity.

The case came to trial. At trial, the following further facts emerged:

> Klvana visited [the patient] later that morning. He told her that the police would accuse them both of killing the baby if she told them that she had planned a hospital delivery but did not know the name of the hospital. Klvana indicated that he would insert the name of a hospital in her medical records. Klvana stated that the baby would have died anyway even if hospitalized immediately.

Mental illness

Sometimes a diabetic woman may be mentally ill. She may then become pregnant. If so, she may not receive the care necessary for her health and safety, nor for that of her fetus. In Oregon, a 25-year-old woman of 32 weeks gestation had a schizoaffective disorder and severe social problems. Management of her diabetic pregnancy proved problematic, as she was a regular defaulter from health care. An application to commit her to the care of the Mental Health Division was made, but she opposed it. At the civil commitment hearing, no expert testimony was presented on the dangers generally posed by diabetes in pregnancy, nor about the specific risks to the patient or her fetus. Moreover, her attorney argued that she was not a danger to herself or others. The commitment hearing agreed that she was not a danger to herself, but it considered that her mental illness (through her diabetes being incorrectly managed) presented a danger to the fetus, and so a committal order was made. She appealed the decision. Although the Court of Appeals heard general evidence about diabetes and pregnancy, it did not hear any evidence relating to the patient's specific circumstances, which would have needed expert medical testimony. The court therefore reversed the committal order, on the ground that insufficient evidence had been presented to prove that her diabetes presented a specific threat to herself and her fetus.[29]

This case illustrates the importance of thorough preparation before a medical case is taken to court, as otherwise a decision that is medically undesirable, even though legally sound, may be handed down.

Consent to sterilization

In Colorado in 1976, a schizophrenic woman had badly controlled diabetes and she defaulted from care. Her mother wanted this diabetic daughter to be sterilized, on the grounds that any future pregnancy would be dangerous to both mother and baby. Moreover, the daughter had already had a preterm delivery at 34 weeks gestation. The mother argued that her daughter did not have the capacity to understand the risks of pregnancy in the face of unstable diabetes and she had a history of preterm delivery. However, the daughter refused to be sterilized and so the matter was taken to court. The Supreme Court ruled in favour of the mentally ill daughter, on the basis that the legal case turned on her understanding of the concept of sterilization, and not on her understanding of the risks of diabetic pregnancy and pre-term delivery.[30] Thus, the mentally ill daughter could not be sterilized unless she herself consented to surgery.

Congenital abnormality following failed sterilization

It is well known that cardiac defects are more common in children born of diabetic mothers.

A Missouri case involved a woman who had a previous history of difficult pregnancy complicated by gestational diabetes. Her husband had a vasectomy and this was followed by negative semen analysis. But she fell pregnant again, this time with twins. A repeat semen analysis was positive, and so the vasectomy had failed. Eventually the babies delivered, but one had a severely defective heart condition. Despite multiple operations and a prolonged period of hospitalization, he died at 7 months of age.

A legal action followed, on the grounds that the vasectomy must have been performed incorrectly. At that time in Missouri, claims for damages arising from birth defects were not in themselves actionable. Nevertheless, the claim was for medical expenses associated with the birth defects, lost income and emotional distress.

The Court of Appeals[31] held that, as a matter of law, a negligent vasectomy alone will not normally be the cause of a child's birth defects; it is too far removed from the damage and it is not the cause of the damage. Furthermore, it follows that negligent performance of a vasectomy was not the proximate cause of the medical expense resulting from the child's birth defects. Thus, the claim for damages was dismissed.

Involuntary participation in research

In 1976 an insulin-dependent diabetic was delivered by Caesarean section at the Boston Hospital for Women. She became infected afterwards and then she became sterile. Later she discovered that her obstetrician had curetted her uterus after the operation. She claimed that she was thus unknowingly the subject of an experiment, in that her obstetrician wanted to obtain tissue for a research study on maternal infant health problems in diabetic pregnancy, which was being funded at the hospital by the National Institute for Neurological Disease and Blindness.

The obstetrician denied this. He claimed that performing curettage was part of his standard treatment of diabetic women in childbirth, so that he could study the uterine decidua to determine the effect of diabetes on the vascular system, and to determine if future pregnancies were desirable.

She brought a legal action against the hospital. However, the court determined that the hospital could not be held liable, as she was the obstetrician's private patient.[32]

Expert witnesses

A diabetic woman from Michigan died in early pregnancy due to the complications of undiagnosed diabetes (these were not detailed in the judgment). The (husband and estate of the) plaintiff took legal action and they brought a claim against the specialist in internal medicine who had last treated her. They also put forward supportive evidence from a doctor whose principal work was that of a pathologist and a coroner. However, under cross-examination he had to acknowledge that he only practised internal medicine on a limited 'moonlight basis'. Following a review by the Court of Appeals,[32] his evidence was not admitted, on the grounds that he was not an appropriate expert to comment on the actions of a specialist in internal medicine. The case was therefore dismissed.

This case illustrates that if the management of a medical case is to be criticized, this can only reasonably be done by a doctor who is expert in the relevant area of medicine.

Conclusions

From the legal point of view, the topic of diabetic pregnancy is a very wide one. But most legal issues or disputes that arise in relation to diabetic pregnancy will already have arisen in health fields outside of diabetic pregnancy, or even in fields well outside of medicine, and a court will take such external references into account. Very few cases will arise in diabetic pregnancies that have not already been addressed previously, at least in a related fashion, by one jurisdiction or another.

Finally, it is important to remember that, just like medicine, the field of medical law is changing continuously and more rapidly than hitherto. What a court may have decided last year may not be valid next year, if the law or our medical understanding changes in the interim. An example here lies in the American Diabetic Association's recent change in the guidelines relating to universal or selective screening for gestational diabetes.[8]

These are but two of the reasons why it is so important in the field of legal medicine to keep up to date, not only with changes in medical understanding but also with changes in medical law, both locally and in other jurisdictions.

References and notes

1. *Schloendorff v. Society of New York Hospital* [1914] 105 NE 92 MLC 0678.
2. In researching this paper, > 100 decided legal cases relating to diabetic pregnancy were found by the present author.
3. *Shoemaker v. Hotchkiss* [1984] 4 Va Cir 166: 6684.
4. *James v. Wooley* [1998] a/a 523 So 2d 110.
5. *Pierre v. Marshall* [1994] 8 WWR 478.
6. *Hallatt v. North West Anglia Health Authority* [1998] 4ML 2; [1998] Lloyd's Rep Med 197 (CA).
7. Dewhurst CJ (ed). Integrated obstetrics and gynaecology for postgraduates, 4th Edn. Oxford: Blackwell, 1986.
8. American Diabetic Association. Gestational diabetes mellitus: a position statement. *Diabetes Care* 2002; **25**: S94–S96.
9. *White v. Clitheroe Royal Grammer School* [2002], reported on *www.diabetes.org.uk/news* on 30.04.02.
10. *R v. Padmore*, reported in *The Times*, 17 December 1999.

11. *Quiroz v. Austrup, Simpson and Kitchener-Waterloo Hospital* [1982] ACWSJ 538408; 17 ACWS (2d) 245.

12. *USA v. Murray* [1999] US Court of Appeals Fourth Circuit: 97–6735.

13. *Rush v. Blanchard* [1993] 310 SC 375; 426 SE 2d 802: 23794.

14. *Careys v. Lovett and others* [1993] 132 NJ 44; 622 A.2d 1279: A-8.

15. *Wereszczakowski and Darrock v. Swales and St Joseph's Health Centre*, [2002] Ont Sup CJ, 98-CV–140516.

16. *Oliver v. Ellison, Mitchell and the Salvation Army Grace Hospital* [2001] BC CA; 2001 BCD Civ J 2079 – CA 024495.

17. *Watson v. Chapman* [2000] SC CA Op 3272.

18. *Brown, Corredor et al v. Giuliani et al* [1994] USDC Eastern District of New York, 158 FRD 251; CV-94–2842 (CPS).

19. *LaCoparra v. Pargament Home Ctrs Inc* [1997] 982 F Supp 213, 228 (SDNY).

20. Drivers' Medical Group, Driver and Vehicle Licensing Authority. *For Medical Practitioners: At a Glance Guide to the Current Medical Standards of Fitness to Drive.* (Driver and Vehicle Licensing Authority: Swansea, 2002).

21. *Jarvis v. Director of Public Prosecutions* [2000] Queen's Bench Division 164 JP 15.

22. *General Medical Council v. Krishnamurthy*, Hearing of the GMC's Professional Conduct Committee in Manchester on 29 August 2002. (The present author sat on the panel at this hearing, which was in public and before the national press.)

23. *US v. York Women's Care Associates* [2000] US District Court for the District of Maine.

24. *re Lamb on Disbarment* [1989] 49 Cal 3d 239; 776 P.2d 765; 260 Cal Rptr 856–S007499.

25. *Florida Municipal Liability Self Insurers Program v. Mead Reinsurance Corporation, and the Town of Pembroke Park* [1993] US Dist. LEXIS 7501; 7 Fla. L. Weekly Fed. D. 191.

26. *MacRae v. MacKenzie and West Lincoln Memorial Hospital* [1984] Ontario High Court of Justice, ACWSJ 446604; 24 ACWS (2d) 514.

27. *Lesley v. Chie* [2001] 250 F.3d 47 (1st Cir).

28. *People v. Klvana* [1992] 11 Cal App 4th 1679; 15 Cal Rptr 2d 512.

29. *State of Oregon v. Ayala* [1999] 164 Ore App 399; 991 P.2d 100; A101430.

30. *re Romero (Incapacitated Person)* [1990] 790 P.2d 819; 1990 Colo. LEXIS 306; 14 BTR 541.

31. *Williams and Williams v. van Biber* [1994] 886 SW.2d 10: WD 47567.

32. *Schwartz v. Boston Hospital for Women* [1976] USDC Southern District of New York, 422 F Supp 53; 71 Civ 1562.

33. *McDougall v. Schanz and others* [1999] 461 Mich 15; 597 NW.2d 148.

47

Diabetologic education in pregnancy

Luis Cabero Roura

Introduction

All complications of pregnancy in diabetic patients are directly or indirectly related to the degree of metabolic control, as much as to other factors that affect the course of gestation, e.g. embryonic or fetal lesions. This is true for pregestational diabetics, insulin dependent or not, and for gestational diabetics. The only way to reduce complications to a minimum, comparable with the normal population, is for woman to stay as near as possible to normoglycemia during pregnancy. To achieve this objective requires a major effort, not only on the part of the therapeutic team but also by the patient herself.

Maybe more than in any other illness, during pregnancy it is true to say that treatment is only possible with the patient's direct and active participation. Treatment is not prescription of a certain medication, but involves a change of habits from the first hospital visit until childbirth, with the patient's rhythm of life revolving around the need for metabolic control. The patient's participation is therefore indispensable, and can only be achieved when she understands what is required and why. Secondly, once the patient has the necessary knowledge, she must go on incorporating changes in a progressive and continuous way, so that her effort is effective, resulting in a better evolution of her gestation.

Transmitting sufficient motivation, knowledge and skill to the patient is called **diabetologic education**. This is a cornerstone of the management of patients with diabetes because they are the ones who actually put into practice and follow the therapeutic regime recommended by the help group.

The recognition of a diabetic patient's need to be involved in their own treatment dates back to the discovery of insulin. This is a drug with a very small therapeutic margin and potentially serious secondary effects, which cannot be taken orally nor can it be administered exclusively in hospitals because the patient needs it every day. The insulin-dependent diabetic needs to know how to administer it, how to recognize the effects produced by too much or too little, and how to compensate for this. The Joslin Clinic in Boston was one of the first centers to establish formal education for diabetics; this can now be considered the general approach, at least as far as the theoretical definition of overall care for diabetics is concerned. The efficacy of structured diabetologic education in achieving better glycemic profiles and in reducing complications in patients with access to such education has been shown in many studies. However, we are a long way from achieving a generalized easy access to diabetologic education programs, and it is true to say that even in highly developed

	Gestational diabetes	Pregestational diabetes

Short term	Diabetes awareness
	Mutual interference between diabetes and gestation
	Basic management skills
		Identification
		    Degree of previous training
		    Degree of independence achieved
		    Family support
		Knowledge
		    Interrelation between diabetes and gestation
		Increase
		    Level of awareness and skills
		    Degree of independence

Medium to long term	Healthy habits and diabetes
	Prevention/detection of diabetes:
	    Diabetes Type 2
	    Gestational diabetes in another pregnancy
		Promote healthy attitudes
		Promote positive and proactive attitudes to the disease
		Prevention of complications in a new pregnancy

Table 47.1. *Objectives of diabetology education in pregnancy.*

countries there is a notable difference between the recommended standards and everyday reality.[1]

Reaction to the disease

The reaction to the diagnosis of a chronic disease is similar to the process of grieving: in fact, it is a grieving process brought about by the loss of health. It involves a number of phases, from initial denial to final acceptance, which are normal provided that their duration and intensity do not exceed certain limits (Box 47.1). In any case, medical staff dealing with the chronically ill should be familiar with these phases in order to understand certain

- Shock phase or initial denial. The patient rejects the diagnosis, believing that it is due to laboratory error or result interpretation and that it is not actually happening to them. A second opinion or repeat tests may be requested, and the patient may argue about the reliability of the tests.
- Protest phase. This involves rebellious or angry reactions. Not complying with medical instructions, or deception and evasiveness in response to compliance, may be seen in this phase.
- Anxiety phase. Melancholic or inhibited reactions.
- Negotiation phase. The disease is accepted, but the patient tries to set limits on the impact that this will have on their life. One characteristic may be a partial acceptance of the proposed instructions, e.g. 'Okay, I'll do the controls but only twice a day' or 'I'll follow the diet but I'm not injecting myself with insulin'.
- Adaptation phase, i.e. 'If there is no way back, I'd better do as best I can'.

Box 47.1. Phases of reaction to diagnosis of chronic disease.

types of behavior or attitudes, and to be able to respond in the most effective way at any given time.

During pregnancy, it is slightly different.[2] Women with Type 1 or Type 2 diabetes already have a known disease at the start of the gestation period and, therefore, it might be expected that they would be in the adaptation phase. However, this is not always the case. Furthermore, one of the educator's first interventions should be to identify exactly which phase the patient is in. Sometimes, the patient can remain in the anxiety or negotiation phase for years, while at other times the patient can be in a hidden denial phase. Identifying which phase the patient is in is fundamental in order to focus the situation effectively and to reinforce or begin, if appropriate, the education process efficaciously. Getting over the initial phases, especially if they are prolonged, is more difficult in these patients than in gestating patients, because their experiences are more prolonged and intense, and because sometimes elaborate schemes are created (excessive family or work problems, supposed difficulty in response or negative effects of the disease, etc.) to justify an evasive attitude to diabetes.

Gestational diabetics scarcely have time to progress through the different phases. They could easily stay in the first phase because they do not perceive any inconvenience as a consequence of the disease. However, frequently, this is not the case as the fetus is presented as being the most affected in the process, making the mother advance quickly to the negotiation or adaptation phase. As the inconvenience is perceived as transitory, and the effect on lifestyle is of low intensity this also adds to a quick acceptance. However, in some cases, the initial denial phase is strongly manifest.[3] Continuation of pregnancy without the relief of specific problems or without the detection of fetal anomalies can reinforce this attitude of distrust of

the diagnosis or its relevance, and convert it into a definitive attitude. Sometimes, it is difficult to overcome this response which is theoretically reinforced by events, or rather by the absence of events, and the best that can be obtained is to control the patient's evolution and to hope that she is in the group of patients who do not spontaneously develop complications. Fortunately, this is not a normal response.

In both types of diabetes, the presence of the fetus and the knowledge that it will be the main beneficiary of the correct treatment provide the patient with a stimulus.[4] The concept of the fetus as a patient is a key factor in the transmission of information and it is undoubtedly helpful in making the pregnant patient's attitude, in most cases, a collaborative one.

Diabetologic education

The objective of medical care for diabetic patients is to normalize glycemia levels and to minimize the complications of the disease. Achieving near-normal glycemia levels delays the onset of chronic complications, reduces the number of medical visits and hospital stays, and lowers health costs. During pregnancy, the effects of normoglycemia are not so manifest in the mother, given that it is a very limited period of disease, as in the gestation period itself and during fetal development. Normoglycemia is associated with reduced perinatal mortality and morbidity.[5]

To obtain normal or near-normal glycemic controls, it is necessary for the diabetic patient to become sufficiently skilled in choosing, distributing and preparing foods conveniently; to be able to self-administer insulin; and to periodically check glycemia levels. The objective of diabetologic education is to give the patient the knowledge and skills to be able to attend to their own daily care. Medical care that does not enable diabetics to gain a good degree of independence in the control of their disease is insufficient care, which will, in the medium to long term, struggle to reflect satisfactory results. In the case of pregnant women, medical control without active participation of the patient creates a serious obstacle to obtaining normal perinatal results. Without an adequate diabetic education and with a minimum of instructions, serious imbalances may be avoided; however, it is practically impossible to achieve euglycemia in many cases, especially in previously diagnosed diabetics.[6]

Diabetologic education is a collaborative and interactive process which is established between the diabetic patient and the educator.[7] The process includes:

- knowledge of the specific individual educational needs;
- identification of the objectives of specific individual self-controls;
- education and direct follow-up to help the diabetic meet the objectives set;
- evaluation of the achievement of the objectives set.

In diabetes, an educator can be defined as a health care professional with thorough knowledge and skills in physiology, pathology, social relations, communication and education, and with experience in the care of diabetic patients. This role can be undertaken by nurses, doctors, psychologists, dieticians, etc., since the function is neither specific nor exclusive to any one group. In multidisciplinary teams, all the members should possess knowledge and sufficient training for the role, even although the role is assumed and led by a certain member of the team.[8]

Education in self-management should be aimed at diabetics and, as far as possible, at their family and friends, so that they can offer the diabetic the necessary support and be able to act appropriately in a crisis. The content of the information and training given to patients should include topics such as the physiopathology of diabetes mellitus, its short- and long-term consequences, appropriate kinds of food, physical activity, drug therapy, self-control of glycemia, the prevention and management of acute and chronic complications, how to act in situations of conflict, psychosocial adaptation, and the use of the health service.[9] Pregnant women or those of child-bearing age considering pregnancy should also be made aware of how the disease can influence gestation and fetal development, how the pregnancy affects the metabolic balance, to what extent the disease could influence the aggravation or appearance of chronic complications, and which are the general treatment principles during this period.[10]

The information and the method of education should be adapted to the personal characteristics of each individual, taking into account the level of education, knowledge and prior preparation, capacity of understanding and learning, existence of concomitant diseases, social or cultural differences, lifestyle and predisposition or capacity to collaborate.[11]

Although the final objective of getting a healthy newborn baby with the minimum possible interference to health or discomfort to the mother is similar for all patients, individual objectives may vary greatly. With each individual patient, it is necessary to establish learning objectives which are both reasonable and achievable. During the first visit the educator should identify the needs and the specific objectives of each gestating or non-gestating patient, and, thus, establish a learning calendar which will enable each patient to participate fully.[12] Furthermore, the educator should set down a number of indicators which can be evaluated to determine the success of the process. Depending on the degree of independence that the patient manages to obtain, the rhythm of the gestation follow-up schedule can be established with either more or fewer visits. The ideal situation is one in which the pregnant patient has sufficient resources to make small adjustments to correct glycemic deviations, and to be able to identify when to go to the hospital or call the doctor when warning signs appear.

Despite the obvious needs to instill diabetic patients with autonomy in the daily control of the disease, the existence of inadequate education programs or the failure to implement such programs is a general problem. More than half of the diabetic population receive little or no diabetology education. A national survey carried out in the USA in patients with Type 1 diabetes, insulin-dependent Type 2 diabetes and non-insulin-dependent Type 2 diabetes, it was revealed that 41, 51 and 76%, respectively, had never taken a class, course or any other diabetology education-related program.[13]

It is not simply an issue of gestational diabetics not having sufficient resources to manage their metabolic changes, because this would be a limited problem moderated by the dysfunction and the short period of duration. A good number of diabetic adults clearly lack the skills associated with management of the disease, such as preparation of an adequate diet, adjusting their insulin dose, or making adequate compensation for occasional glycemic deviations. Hospitalization of patients with poor metabolic control is frequently attributed to their insufficient awareness of self-control. It is also more likely that such patients end up developing complications or requiring emergency services.

Deficits in training are not solely due to lack of awareness and skills; often, an incomplete first educational stage has led the patient to make supposed 'deductions' or 'misunderstandings' and, over the passage of time, these have

been assumed by the patient to be correct. Detection of these suppositions can be complex: they do not arise during the interview but, based on the suspicion that they do exist, the interviewer has to review in great detail all the knowledge that the patient should have. The types of errors that the patient has incorporated into daily control can be wide-ranging, affecting the diet, such as its distribution and preparation, types of food containing carbohydrates and their approximate proportion, choosing food when eating out, as well as insulin-administering techniques and their effect, dosage errors, effects of exercise, etc. The task of correcting skills and knowledge is as difficult as that of identifying them, given that the patient is usually reluctant to accept that, often over a prolonged period of time, they have habits which were not only incorrect but also, at times, counterproductive. The educator should have sufficient communication and educational skills not only to explain the error(s) but also to convince the patient that the analysis being carried out is appropriate and that the resulting change in attitude will have a positive effect on their own control.

An educational model will be effective depending on the extent of independence it gives the patient to participate effectively in the management of their disease. The time required for a complete educational process is usually greater than the gestational period, however, if it is a basic issue for an existing diabetic, then its importance is more relative for gestational diabetes. The specific objective for pregnancy should be clear. For gestational diabetics: make them aware of the disease; give basic knowledge so that interference with fetal development is minimal; over the medium to long term, encourage healthy eating and lifestyle habits; persuade a preventative and proactive approach towards a new pregnancy. For existing diabetics: detect deficits or errors in the educational process to date; identify the patient's degree of independence; evaluate the degree of family support; increase the patient's awareness and skills; facilitate the maximum degree of independence possible during pregnancy; in the medium to long term, promote healthy attitudes; adopt a stance of prevention of complications in a new pregnancy.

Protocol of the Vall d'Hebron Hospital

The acquisition of knowledge and abilities on the part of the patient can be subdivided into three stages that are continuous and superimposed:

* Informative stage;
* Training stage;
* Support stage.

Informative stage

All patients who go to a diabetes and gestation clinic should receive complete, clear and comprehensible information of the basic aspects related their illness. They should understand:

* what is happening;
* what dangers they and the fetus run;
* why complications can arise;
* what treatment is proposed and why.

This means that the following should be explained:

* What diabetes is and the relationship it has with pregnancy.
* The influence of diabetes on the course of the pregnancy, and on the development of the fetus and neonate.
* The long-term repercussions of diabetes on the mother and her offspring.
* The fundamental cause of the complications, in particular the relationship with glycemia levels.
* Why and how diabetes must be treated during pregnancy.
* The importance of diet:
  * what are carbohydrates and what purpose do they serve;
  * what types of carbohydrates are there, and which are forbidden and which are not;
  * what are the fundamental rules that should be followed in a suitable diet;
  * the proportion of carbohydrates required;
  * the number of meals required per day;
  * the preparation of food.
* The purpose of exercise.
* What is metabolic autocontrol and why it is important.
* How glycemia levels can be determined.
* What insulin is and when it is used.

If, after the stage of information, the patient is clear about the above points, then half of the treatment will have been achieved. A faithful collaborator who feels an active part of the therapeutic team will have been gained. But to transmit this knowledge requires special abilities: the information given should be:

* *Important*
  The patient cannot be expected to assimilate the entire knowledge about diabetes in half an hour, nor in 3 days! Only key points should be chosen for transmission, bearing in mind that the objective is to motivate the patient to follow her treatment. She should receive enough information so that she considers it important to undertake treatment but not so much as to worry her unnecessarily,

thus magnifying the perceived risks, nor should she be disconcerted with a great number of figures or secondary details.

- **Clear**

  The information must be made accesible for the patient, thus appropriate to her language and level of education. It serves no purpose to choose the fundamental points of the illness correctly if later an excessively scientific language is used, with terms that are not comprehensible for those without any scientific training, or with tortuous rhetorical constructions, so that when concluding a sentence nobody can remember how it began. The chosen level should be the lowest in the group. Nobody is offended when simple words and short sentences are used, nor when they are spoken slowly stressing those words that need to be highlighted. The educator should never forget that he/she speaks for the patients and not for a committee of experts.

- **Concise**

  The patient is not an expert in perinatology and her notions of medicine can be very limited. It is very probable that most of what is said, is for her, unknown and whilst it is relatively easy to remember three sentences it is very difficult to retain 30. The educator should be able to synthesize and to extract, from the extent of his/her knowledge, those basic points that are important for the patient to know.

- **Sufficient**

  The information cannot be broken into fragments, as this causes it to lose value. If how to follow a diet is well explained, but the justification is omitted, then most likely the patient will not follow it. What is the point in changing her actions if she has no clear reason for doing so? The objective of the information is not omission but receipt and assimilation. Thus, it may be necessary

to repeat the same arguments, or the same concepts with different arguments, many times until the patient understands what is being explained.

Although the information can be transmitted in an individualized way, the present author prefers the interactive group method, in which all patients in gestation who go to the clinic for the first time in their present pregnancy, whether diabetic or not, meet together. The group offers several advantages.

- **Acceptance**

  The patient is, from the first moment, with women in her situation. This allows better acceptance of the process as she does not feel alone or of being a 'strange' case, but rather there is a reference group who can share their problems. This normalizes the diabetes.

- **Participation**

  The group grants a certain degree of freedom and stimulus. A comment from one can suggest a question to another which spontaneously would not have occurred to her. What we would not sometimes think about because it is considered banal or inadequate, is verbalized with more freedom if somebody has said something similar. It is easier to request a repetition of an explanation if it is seen that there is another person who has not understood, rather than when the patient is alone in which case there are times she remains silent so as not to appear dumb. Individual embarrassment is diluted in the group situation.

- **Collaboration**

  The use of the knowledge and experience of the patients themselves, whether pregestational diabetics or women who have had gestational diabetes in previous pregnancies, allows reinforcement of the information that is given. If one knows how to channel their participation they also become educators and their previous experience is a 'guarantee' that what is being said is true and what is requested is possible.

The inclusion of pregestational diabetics in the group offers another possibility: to assess, without their having the sensation of being examined, the degree of previous diabetic education and to know which are the areas that need to be reinforced in future.

The reactions and the difficulties of the patients before the situation are sometimes linked to the diabetes type. The pregestational diabetic already has an idea about what diabetes involves and also regarding what is normal or abnormal for glycemia, but her concepts do not always correspond to the needs of pregnancy. The fact that slightly high glycemia is frequently tolerated in the general diabetic population causes certain patients to consider themselves to be normal and so to refuse acceptance of the normoglycemia concept.

When gestation begins, not only is the illness distorted in a way that frequently surprises the patient herself, but she comes to understand that what she had considered normal has ceased to be, so that levels of glucose that before were considered good are now unacceptable. That she understands that the euglycemia is fundamental during pregnancy is indispensable in the treatment process. In this sense, the concept of the fetus as patient is basic. The pregnant patient should understand that the increased attention to adjustment of metabolic control is designed to safeguard her fetus from feeling any consequences of the illness.

The gestational diabetic patient, on the other hand, is a woman who may not have had any previous contact with diabetes, who feels well (she does not have indisposition, nor pain, nor any negative symptoms), and whom the doctor tells that she has a metabolic 'upset', although only for the duration of pregnancy. The first effort that must be made is for the patient to believe what is being said and later to accept that to treat the illness that she is unaware of having she has to change her daily habits. This acceptance supposes an effort that the therapeutic team should facilitate and value. Also, as she will receive a great quantity of information which needs to be assimilated in a short period of time, she will require support from the medical personnel who assist her.

In general, the gestational diabetic patient needs to receive a greater quantity of new information than the pregestational one, but this is easier to transmit, because it is made on clean slate. An effort may be required in persuading acceptance of metabolic dysfunction, but once this is made the patient rarely offers further resistance. While the pregestational diabetic patient can have ample prior knowledge this should be reassessed and corrected if necessary. It is, on occasions, difficult to change an erroneous idea, and it requires greater effort and skill on the part of the educator to do so rather than to establish a new one.

Training stage

The general ideas that have been expounded in the information stage should be transferred to each patient and adapted to her characteristics. If it has been explained to her how to treat her diabetes, now the necessary instruments should be provided so that she can undertake the task.

- *Diet*
  - to check the degree of understanding of the written diet;
  - how to calculate the quantity of foods;
  - how to cook the foods;

- how to carry out simple dietary substitutions;
- how to calculate the diet if she eats out;
- how to adjust the diet if activities different to the habitual ones are carried out (e.g. night outings, holiday periods, etc).
- *Metabolic control*
  - technique for obtaining capillary blood;
  - reading of reactive ribbons of blood and urine;
  - functioning of the reflectometer: (1) management and conservation; (2) most usual errors;
  - registry of the values obtained in the diabetes notebook;
  - other data that should be registered down: diet excesses (transgressions), decrease in night rest, infections, etc.
  - in which situations patients should go to the doctor's surgery without a previous appointment.
- *Administration of insulin*
  - places for the administration of insulin;
  - administration technique;
  - types of insulin with which work and the fundamental differences between them;
  - metabolic objectives, i.e. the glycemic margins taken as normal;
  - how to proceed if the wrong dosage is administered;
  - precautions to take if insulin is administered (hypoglycemia prevention);
  - how to act faced with a hypoglycemic attack.

The information from each of the above sections should be given according to patient needs. The first two are general, while the third is reserved for the gestational diabetic patients who require insulin. In the case of the pregestational diabetics, this stage may not be training as much as confirmation that she has acquired the necessary skills.

Although giving general information in a group situation facilitates understanding and acceptance of the process, training should be carried out in a personalized way. Each pregnant patient has her own characteristics: e.g. habit schedules, family relations, work type, way of cooking, etc. The diet recommended should adapt to these peculiarities, so that it accomplishes the objective but does not become an uncomfortable straitjacket that distorts the daily activities of the patient.

The time that each woman requires to incorporate this knowledge is variable, depending on her learning capacity, previous notions, stress levels and, of course, the competence of the person who is training her. The patient always feels at a certain disadvantage with respect to the health personnel: they speak to her of her illness, about which they know more, and they know more about her than she does about herself. If the personnel is not capable of creating a relaxed and pleasant atmosphere of mutual trust from the beginning, and if the patient perceives, by means of the language used or the educator's attitude, that he/she finds her slow, or simply that he/she is in a hurry or indifferent because they must attend to another patient, the most likely thing is that the patient will say that she has understood everything perfectly only to please the trainer or for shame that her ineptitude will be discovered. The time that each patient requires does not matter. The fundamental thing is that in the end she has acquired the necessary capacity to manage her condition and that she perceives that she has progressed.

Also, if possible complications have been talked of, it must be explained when they can be expected and how to identify them at an early stage, so that she can go to the doctor's surgery before the situation is serious. A final aspect of training is:

- *Obstetric self-control*
  - Control of fetal well-being – fetal movements: (1) what they mean and how they are controlled; (2) why they can diminish; (3) how to act in the case of (2).
  - Alarm signs – (1) how to identify contractions and which are those that could be worrying; (2) what other symptoms should receive attention and when should the patient consult a doctor or go to an emergency department.

Each of these sections of information should be given when they will be useful to the patient or when she enters a specific risk situation.

Support stage

Care of the patient must be personalized and mantained at different intensities if necessary throughout the whole gestation. During each visit the following should be checked:

- suitability of the diet, solving possible errors;
- correction in the reflectometer technique and in the collection of results;
- correct handling and administration of insulin;
- appropriate control of fetal movements.

The patient's management does not conclude until the moment of delivery because new situations can appear daily (e.g. a different food causing an unexpected glycemic response, changes in the rhythm of fetal movements, etc.) that require explanation so that the patient understands that what has happened and how to act in that situation. If during the two previous stages of management an empathetic bond

has been established between educator and patient, then communication will be fluid and the patient will not only detect quickly possible situations of risk, but she will also feel she participates in the treatment. At this stage, depending on the degree of autonomy that has been reached, the patient can be delegated to manage modifications in her diet and adjustments in the dosage of her insulin.

It is an appropriate and effective policy to try to implicate the patient to the maximum in her own control, making her perceive the importance of her role as part of the therapeutic team. This will diminish the degree of restlessness concerning the illness, it will make her feel useful and in control of the situation, and it will reduce the perception of discomfort from the treatment. The degree of delegation will depend on each patient, on her previous preparation, on the speed of understanding and of learning, and on the family and social support upon which she can count, etc. The assistance team should be willing to go as far as the patient can and wants. For example, in women with a good level of knowledge and an appropriate capacity for decision-making, it is not in the hospital visits that the doses of insulin are adjusted, but rather at home, and in the visits, or by means of phone contact, the patient receives confirmation that her decisions have been the right ones. Changes in dosage or substantial variations in the diet are not the doctor's exclusive decisions, but can be reasoned and shared with the patient as her level of autonomy increases.

The assistance team must have sufficient preparation to be able to accept a relationship of collaboration and dialogue with the patient, which is much more difficult than the traditional doctor–patient or nurse–patient relationship. They should be able to listen to her and to respond appropriately to her needs. If the patient completes the treatment because she is ordered, she will do it only during the period in which she perceives the doctor's authority, but if she does it because she understands its function and agrees on its utility, she will prolong it. The time that is invested in education will be saved later, when the metabolic situation remains stable, and the incidence and seriousness of complications, diminishes.

References

1. American Diabates Association. Third-party reimbursement for diabetes care, self-management education and supplies. *Diabetes Care* 2002; **25 (Suppl 1)**:S134–S135.
2. American Diabetes Association. National standards for diabetes self-management education. *Diabetes Care* 2002; **25 (Suppl 1)**:S140–S147.
3. American Association of Diabetes Educators. The scope of practice for diabetes educators and the standards of practice for diabetes educators. *Diabetes Educ* 2000; **26**:25–31.
4. Brown SL, Pope JF, Hunt AE, Tolman NM. Motivational strategies used by dietitians to counsel individuals with diabetes. *Diabetes Educ* 1998; **24**:313–18.
5. Clements S. Diabetes self-management education (technical review). *Diabetes Care* 1995; **18**:1204–14.
6. Glasgow RE. A practical model of diabetes management and education. *Diabetes Care* 1995; **18**:117–26.
7. Peyrot M, Rubon RR. Modeling the effect of diabetes education on glycemic control. *Diabetes Educ* 1994; **20**:143–8.
8. Heins JM, Nord WR, Cameron M. Establishing and sustaining state-of-the-art diabetes education programs: research and recommendations. *Diabetes Educ* 1992; **18**:501–8.
9. Greene DS, Beaudin BP, Bryan JM. Addressing attitudes during diabetes education: suggestions from adult education. *Diabetes Educ* 1993; **19**:497–502.
10. Armstrong CL, Brown LP, York R et al. From diagnosis to home management: nutritional considerations for women with gestational diabetes. *Diabetes Educ* 1991; **17**:455–9.
11. Rubin RR, Peyrot M, Saudek CD. Effect of diabetes education on self-care, metabolic control and emotional well-being. *Diabetes Care* 1989; **12**:673–9.
12. Padgett D, Mumford E, Hynes M, Carter R. Meta-analysis of the effects of educational and psychosocial interventions on the management of diabetes mellitus. *J Clin Epidemiol* 1988; **41**:1007–30.
13. Greenfield S, Kaplan SH, Ware Jr JE et al. Patients' participation in medical care: effects on blood sugar control and quality of life in diabetes. *J Gen Intern Med* 1988; **3**:448–57.

48

Optimal contraception for the diabetic woman
Siri L Kjos

Introduction

For a woman with diabetes to decide whether and when she desires to become pregnant is not simply a question of choice. A planned or unplanned pregnancy can have lifelong implications for her own health and most importantly for the health of her future child. Whether she has Type 1, Type 2 or prior gestational diabetes mellitus (GDM), optimizing her health prior to pregnancy should be a primary educational and medical goal promoted by her health care providers. Pregnancy planning can reduce her risk for elective abortion by offering her reliable methods to prevent conception or for spontaneous abortion by enabling her to plan a pregnancy in good glycemic control. Her own risk of developing serious medical complications such as ketoacidosis, accelerated retinopathy or proteinuria can similarly be reduced by controlling her medical problems prior to conception. Lastly, her risk of giving birth to an anomalous infant can be reduced by achieving euglycemia at conception and during embryogenesis. The risk of major congenital anomalies in offspring of women with Type 1[1] and Type 2[2] diabetes has been shown to be increased by up to 20–25%, and to be more than doubled (> 5.5%) in GDM[3] when initial fasting glucose levels were > 120 mg/dl. Achieving euglyemic control prior to and early in pregnancy has been shown to normalize rates of congenital malformations in women with Type 1 diabetes.[4] In the woman with GDM, there may be an additional long-term health benefit in avoiding pregnancy: a subsequent pregnancy has been shown to increase their risk of subsequent diabetes c. threefold.[5] Periodic testing for diabetes, regardless of the contraceptive method used, is recommended in all women with prior GDM,[6] especially prior to a subsequent pregnancy.

This chapter will discuss methods with a low failure rate, specifically combination oral contraceptives, progestin-only oral contraceptives, longer acting (injectable and implantable) hormonal methods and the intrauterine devices (IUD), in women with diabetes. Barrier methods will not be addressed, as they are metabolically neutral and have no medical contraindication to their use except for their significantly higher failure rates.

Hormonal contraceptives

The formulation, dosage and route of delivery all influence the various metabolic and endocrine effects of hormonal contraceptive methods in diabetic women. The first question to consider is whether estrogen-containing oral contraceptives should be prescribed. Estrogen is always prescribed in combination with progestins and most commonly as a combination oral contraceptive. More recently, it has become available in combination with progestins delivered via intramuscular or transvaginal routes. Estrogen beneficially decreases the rate of breakthrough bleeding, thus increasing patient continuation of oral contraceptives. However, estrogen stimulates hepatic globulin production in a dose-dependent fashion. It produces an increase in angiotensinogen II levels, which in turn produces a slight but significant increase in mean arterial blood pressure,[7] and an increase in coagulation factors which thereby increases thromboembolic risk.[8] Estrogen also increases high-density lipoprotein and triglyceride levels, while decreasing low-density lipoprotein levels.[9] Important for the care of diabetic women, estrogen does not have any significant effect on carbohydrate metabolism.[10] In the general population these metabolic effects of combination oral contraceptives are subclinical and have been minimized by a steady decrease in ethinyl estradiol dosage in pill preparations. Currently, the lowest combination oral contraceptive preparations contain 20 μg of ethinyl estradiol. In women with medical conditions, generally the lowest dose preparations should be prescribed to minimize metabolic side effects, unless other medical conditions dictate otherwise. Estrogen-containing oral contraceptives should be avoided in women with hypertension or a history of thromboembolic disease.

If estrogen prescription is contraindicated, a progestin-only method should be selected. Progestin-only methods can be delivered via the oral, intramuscular, subcutaneous or intrauterine route, each with advantages and disadvantages. While progestins have a neutral effect on blood pressure[7] and coagulation factors,[8] they adversely decrease glucose tolerance, increase insulin resistance and increase low-density

lipoprotein levels parallel to the dose and potency of the progestin formulation.[11] Thus, similar to estrogen, the lowest dose and least 'androgenic' progestin formulation should be selected in diabetic women.

Combination and progestin-only oral contraception

Type 1 and Type 2 diabetes

In diabetic women, formulations which contain the lowest dose and potency of progestin should be selected to minimize deterioration in glucose tolerance[11,12] and lipid metabolism.[9] These include the newer, less androgenic progestins or lower dose preparations containing the older progestins. Prospective studies with 1 year follow-up have shown combination preparations with low doses of older progestins, either norethindrone (≤ 0.75 mg mean daily dose) or triphasic levonorgestrel preparations, or newer progestins (gestodene, desogestrel) to have minimal effect on diabetic control, lipid metabolism[13–15] and cardiovascular risk factors.[16,17] All preparations examined in these studies also contained a low estrogen dosage (≤ 35 μg). The progestin-only oral contraceptive, containing 0.35 mg of norethindrone, has also been similarly studied in diabetic women and found to have no significant effect on carbohydrate or lipid metabolism.[15]

While recent short-term studies have shown oral contraceptive use to be safe in women with Type 1 diabetes, no long-term, prospective studies have been done which evaluate their effect on diabetic sequelae. While one older retrospective study suggested that thromboembolic disease may be accelerated by combination oral contraceptive use,[18] newer studies, which control for underlying risk factors, have not. Studies have not found any increased risk of or progression of diabetic sequelae (retinopathy, renal disease or hypertension) with past or current use of oral contraceptives.[19,20] In a case–control study, young women with Type 1 diabetes who either used or had never used oral contraception were followed for up to 7 years. There was no difference in the mean glycosylated hemoglobin levels (HbA1c), the mean albumin excretion rates or retinopathy scores.[20] Similarly, in a cross-sectional study of 384 women with Type 1 diabetes, no association was found between the use of oral contraceptives, either current, past or present, and the severity of retinopathy, hypertension or HbA1c levels when the known risk factors for diabetic sequelae were controlled for.[19]

The reluctance to prescribe oral contraceptives in diabetic women stems from the increase in cardiovascular complications and hypertension associated with both diabetes and older preparations of combination oral contraceptives. Current evidence from short-term trials in healthy women[9,21–24] have failed to find an association between cardiovascular risk markers and low-dose combination oral contraceptives. Furthermore, large, prospective cohort trials of healthy women have found no evidence for any excess risk of myocardial infarction with the use of low-dose oral contraceptives.[25–29] The increased risk for cardiovascular events appears to be related to their diabetes and not to oral contraceptive use. A recent multicenter, case–control study, examining acute myocardial infarction in women between the ages of 20 and 44, found that the use of combined oral contraceptives was associated with an increased risk of acute myocardial infarction in women with known cardiovascular risk factors, especially in those with hypertension.[29] Similarly, the risk of cerebral thromboembolism in young women has been related to known risk factors for stroke and not to combination oral contraceptive exposure. In a case–control study examining almost 500 women, aged 15–44, with documented cerebral thromboembolism, diabetes, prior thromboembolic disease, hypertension and migraine headaches were significantly associated with cerebral thromboembolism, but not the use of combination oral contraceptives.[30]

In summary, of the current available data, low-dose combination oral contraceptives can be used in diabetic women. The lowest dose/potency of both estrogen and progestins should be selected. In diabetic women with coexisting vascular disease, progestin-only oral contraceptives are preferred, because of the lack of effect of progestin on coagulation or blood pressure.

Currently, there are no studies examining either the retrospective use or the short-term prospective use of oral contraceptives in women with Type 2 diabetes. In the absence of studies, and given the generally safety of low-dose oral contraceptives, the guidelines suggested for prescription in women with Type 1 diabetes should be followed.

Women with Type 1 or Type 2 diabetes using oral contraceptives should be monitored more frequently than others for changes in blood pressure and weight. A baseline evaluation of weight, blood pressure and fasting lipids are recommended. Consultation between the woman's internist/primary care physician and her gynecologist should occur to establish a monitoring program which involves both specialists. Her gynecologist should be aware of her diabetic therapy, home glucose monitoring regimen and any vascular sequelae, while the internist should be aware of the type of birth control and specific metabolic side effects. Blood pressure, weight and glycemic parameters should be established. After 1 month and every 4–6 months thereafter the patient should return for blood pressure and weight measurements, as well as for evaluation of glycemic control. Lipids should be reassessed annually in diabetic women and more frequently if abnormal values are detected, following standard guidelines.[31]

Prior history of GDM

Over half of women with a history of GDM will develop diabetes, primarily Type 2, in their lifetime.[6,32] Their risk for subsequent diabetes varies and parallels the background rates for Type 2 diabetes for their ethnic group.[33,34] Periodic testing every 1–3 years for diabetes is recommended in women with prior GDM.[6] Testing should be done after delivery and prior to a subsequent pregnancy, as undiagnosed diabetes and untreated hyperglycemia,[2] which is often asymptomatic, has been associated with an increased risk for major congenital malformations. Additionally, recent evidence suggests that a subsequent pregnancy after a pregnancy complicated by GDM may be diabetogenic. In a cohort of Latino women, a second pregnancy following GDM was shown to triple the risk of subsequent diabetes.[35] Thus, women with prior GDM need effective contraception that does not accelerate their already increased risk of developing diabetes.

For the same reasons as in women with Type 1 and Type 2 diabetes, the lowest dose and potency progestin and estrogen combination oral contraceptive should be selected, in order to minimize adverse deterioration in glucose tolerance, lipid metabolism and blood pressure effects. Combination oral contraceptives with low-dose/potency progestins have been shown, in short-term studies, to have no adverse effect of on glucose and lipid metabolism.[36–38] Recently, in a longer retrospective follow-up of 904 women with prior GDM, the

long-term use of low-dose/potency progestin combination oral contraceptives had no effect on cumulative incidence rates of diabetes. After 3 years of uninterrupted use of the combination oral contraceptive, the diabetes rate (25.4%) was almost identical to non-hormonal forms of contraception (26.5%).[39] However, breastfeeding women who were using the progestin-only oral contraceptive had an almost a threefold increase in the risk of development of diabetes, which was further increased with the duration of uninterrupted use.[29] Thus, the progestin-only oral contraceptive should not be given to women with prior GDM who are breastfeeding. In breastfeeding women either a non-hormonal method or a low-dose combination oral contraceptive can be initiated 6–8 weeks postpartum, after the establishment of lactation. It is not clear whether the use of progestin-only oral contraceptives in non-breastfeeding women with prior GDM has any adverse effect.

Evidence supports the use of low-dose/potency progestin combination oral contraceptive use in women with prior GDM. As these preparations do not accelerate the development of diabetes, routine testing for diabetes using fasting plasma glucose levels should be performed every 1–3 years, regardless of the contraceptive method used.[6] A confirmed fasting plasma glucose level ≥ 126 mg/dl is diagnostic of diabetes, and a fasting plasma glucose level ≥ 110 mg/dl and < 126 mg/dl is diagnostic of impaired fasting glucose.[40]

Long-acting hormonal methods

The two long-acting preparations that have been in use for some time contain progestational agents only; one, depomedroxyprorgesterone acetate (DMPA), is delivered via injection and the other as a subdermal implant containing levonorgestrel (Norplant; recently withdrawn from the US market). Currently, no studies address the use of either DMPA or levonorgestrel implants (Norplant) in women with diabetes or prior GDM. However, data regarding thier effect on carbohydrate metabolism in healthy women are available. Norplant has been shown to have no significant effect on carbohydrate metabolism during its 5-year insertion period in healthy women.[41] In contrast, DMPA injections significantly increase fasting and post-glucose challenge levels of both insulin and glucose.[42,43] Recently, in Navajo women, who as an ethnic group are at high risk for diabetes, the use of DMPA contraception for ≥ 1 year was associated with an eightfold increased risk in the development of Type 2 diabetes compared to combination or progestin-only oral contraceptives.[44] DMPA contraception has also been associated with increased weight gain,[45] which is undesirable in women with Type 2 diabetes or with prior GDM. Thus, if contraindications to estrogens exist, a progestin-only oral contraceptive would be preferable, based on their demonstrated safety in women with Type 1 diabetes.[15] In select patients where compliance is a problem, strong consideration should be given to the IUD.

New progestin-only implant products, one containing levonorgestrel (Norplant II)[46] and another containing 3-ketodesogestrel (Implanon),[47] may provide alternative choices as studies become available. Also, long-acting combination hormonal methods will offer new alternatives. A monthly combination contraceptive injection containing estradiol cypionate and MPA has recently become available, but information regarding its effect on carbohydrate metabolism is lacking.[48] Similarly,

hormone-releasing vaginal rings deliver sustained release of etonogestrel and ethinyl estradiol in lower dosage and serum concentrations than when taken orally.[49] Again, in the absence of data, these methods remain second-line choices. They should only be presribed if similar guidelines for periodic monitoring of glycemia and lipids are followed.

Intrauterine devices

The legacy of the Dalkon Shield intrauterine device (IUD) was to associate IUD use with pelvic inflammatory disease (PID), a complication that in diabetic women could precipitate life-threatening ketoacidosis. Physicians caring for diabetic women have since been reluctant to prescribe the IUD. This misconception is being slowly reversed. Studies have shown that the development of pelvic inflammatory disease and subsequent tubal infertility were not related to the use of the IUD, *per se*, but the exposure risk for sexually transmitted disease.[50–52] Newer copper-medicated IUD, currently on the market, have not been associated with any increase in risk of PID after the post-insertion period. In a large meta-analysis involving almost 60,000 women-years of copper-medicated IUD use, the overall incidence of PID associated with IUD use was 1.6/1000 women-years of IUD use.[53]

Similarly, none of the studies examining copper-medicated IUD use in diabetic women with either Type 1[54,55] or Type 2[56] diabetes have found any support for an increased risk of PID. In two controlled trials examining copper-medicated IUD use in healthy and Type 1 diabetic women, followed for 1[54] or 3[55] years, there were no cases of PID. The rates of perforations, failure, expulsion, pain and discontinuation were not different between diabetic and healthy control women. Similarly, in a 3-year uncontrolled study in women with Type 2 diabetes, no cases of PID were found.[56] In fact, no study which has examined IUD use in diabetic women,[54–59] has found any demonstrable increase in PID. However, caution must be exercised. The risk of PID is extremely low with use of medicated IUDs in the general population, making it highly unlikely that large enough studies can ever be conducted in diabetic women to demonstrate the absence of any increase in risk.[60]

In addition to the copper-medicated IUD, a levonorgestrel-releasing IUD provides an excellent alternative. It can be considered a hybrid of a long-acting hormonal method and an IUD. The levonorgestrel-releasing IUD has been extensively used during the past decade and provides extremely effective contraception with a 5-year cumulative failure rate of 0.71/100 women.[61] The IUD provides sustained low-dose (20 µg daily) release of levonorgestrel, which inhibits pregnancy by thickening the cervical mucus,[62] and by inhibiting motility and function of sperm,[63] rather than by inhibiting ovulation. The high levels of levonorgestrel released into the endometrium decreases menstrual bleeding and atrophies the uterine lining.[64,65] This effect would be a desirable benefit in obese, Type 2 diabetic women, who tend to be parous, older and at higher risk of endometrial cancer.

In summary, either the copper-medicated or levonorgestrel-releasing IUD provide excellent long-term pregnancy protection, and their use should be encouraged in women with overt diabetes and prior GDM. General gynecological principles should be followed for proper patient selection, insertion and monitoring of IUD use. Ideal candidates are parous, without a history of PID and at low risk for sexually transmitted disease. General prophylaxis with insertion or removal has not been shown to provide any benefit and is not indicated.

Conclusions

Women with either Type 1 or Type 2 diabetes or prior GDM can be offered several contraceptive options, which when properly selected and closely monitored do not accelerate their disease process or affect their medical therapy. Their contraceptive choice should address their individual lifestyle preferences as well as their state of health and possible pregnancy plans. Consultation and coordinated medical care between their internists and gynecologists should occur. Most importantly, each diabetic or potentially diabetic woman needs to be educated and be an active participant in her pregnancy planning, which allows her to choose either to avoid conceiving or to time her pregnancy to meet personal and health reasons. This can only happen when she is provided with an effective contraceptive method.

References

1. Mills JL, Baker L, Goldman AS. Malformations in infants of diabetic mothers occur before the seventh gestational week. *Diabetes* 1979; 28:292–3.
2. Towner D, Kjos SL, Leung B et al. Congenital malformations in pregnancies complicated by NIDDM. *Diabetes Care* 1995; 18:1446–51.
3. Schaefer UM, Songster G, Xiang A et al. Congenital malformations in offspring of women with hyperglycemia first detected during pregnancy. *Am J Obstet Gynecol* 1997; 177:1165–71.
4. Fuhrmann K, Reiher H, Seemler K et al. The effect of intensified conventional insulin therapy before and during pregnancy on malformation rate in offspring of diabetic mothers. *Exp Clin Endocrinol* 1984; 83:173–7.
5. Peters RK, Kjos SL, Xiang A, Buchanan TA. Long-term diabetogenic effect of a single pregnancy in women with prior gestational diabetes mellitus. *Lancet* 1996; 347: 227–30.
6. Metzger BE, Coustan DM and the Organizing Committee. Summary and recommendations of the Fourth International Workshop–Conference on Gestational Diabetes Mellitus. *Diabetes Care* 1998; 21 (**Suppl 2**):B161–B167.
7. Wilson ES, Cruickshank J, McMaster M et al. A prospective controlled study of the effect on blood pressure of

contraceptive preparations containing different types of dosages and progestogen. *Br J Obstet Gynaecol* 1984; **91**:1254–60.

8. Meade TW. Oral contraceptives, clotting factors and thrombosis. *Am J Obstet Gynecol* 1982; **142**:758–61.

9. Godsland IF, Crook D, Simpson R et al. The effects of different formulations of oral contraceptive agents on lipid and carbohydrate metabolism. *N Engl J Med* 1990; **323**:1375–81.

10. Spellacy WN, Buhi WC, Birk SA. The effect of estrogens on carbohydrate metabolism: glucose, insulin and growth hormone studies on one hundred seventy-one women ingesting premarin, mestranol and ethinyl estradiol for six months. *Am J Obstet Gynecol* 1971; **114**:388–92.

11. Perlman JA, Russell-Briefel R, Ezzati T et al. Oral glucose tolerance and the potency of contraceptive progestins. *J Chronic Dis* 1985; **338**:857.

12. Spellacy W. Carbohydrate metabolism during treatment with estrogen, progestogen and low-dose oral contraceptive preparations on carbohydrate metabolism. *Am J Obstet Gynecol* 1982; **142**:732.

13. Skouby SO, Jensen BM, Kuhl C et al. Hormonal contraception in diabetic women: acceptability and influence on diabetes control of a nonalkylated estrogen/progestogen compound. *Contraception* 1985; **32**:23.

14. Skouby SO, Molsted-Pedersen L, Kuhl C et al. Oral contraceptives in diabetic women: metabolic effects of four compounds with different estrogen/progestogen profiles. *Fertil Steril* 1986; **46**:858.

15. Radberg T, Gustafson A, Skryten A et al. Oral contraception in diabetic women. Diabetes control, serum and high density lipoprotein lipids during low-dose progestogen, combined oestrogen/progestogen and non-hormonal contraception. *Acta Endocrinol* 1981; **98**:246.

16. Peterson KR, Skouby SO, Sidelmann J et al. Effects of contraceptive steroids on cardiovascular risk factors in women with insulin-dependent diabetes mellitus. *Am J Obstet Gynecol* 1994; **171**:400–5.

17. Peterson KR, Skouby SO, Vedel P, Haaber AB. Hormonal contraception in women with IDDM. *Diabetes Care* 1995; **18**:800–6.

18. Steel JM, Duncan LJP. Serious complications of oral contraception in insulin-dependent diabetics. *Contraception* 1978; **17**:291.

19. Klein BEK, Moss SE, Klein R. Oral contraceptives in women with diabetes. *Diabetes Care* 1990; **13**:895.

20. Garg SK, Chase HP, Marshal G et al. Oral contraceptives and renal and retinal complications in young women with insulin-dependent diabetes mellitus. *J Am Med Assoc* 1994; **271**:1099–102.

21. Loke DFM, Ng CSA, Samsioe G et al. A comparative study of the effects of a monophasic and a triphasic oral contraceptive containing ethinyl estradiol and levonorgestrel on lipid and lipoprotein metabolism. *Contraception* 1990; **42**:535–54.

22. Petersen KR, SKouby SO, Pederson RG. Desogestrel and gestodene in oral contraceptives: 12 months' assessment of carbohydrate and lipoprotein metabolism. *Obstet Gynecol* 1991; **78**:666–72.

23. Runnebaum B, Grunwald K, Rabe T. The efficacy and tolerability of norgestimate/ethinyl estradiol (250 µg of norgestimate/35 µg of ethinyl estradiol): results of a open, multicenter study of 59,701 women. *Am J Obstet Gynecol* 1992; **166**:1963–8.

24. van der Vange N, Kloosterboer HJ, Haspels AA. Effect of seven low-dose combined oral contraceptive preparations on carbohydrate metabolism. *Am J Obstet Gynecol* 1987; **156**:918–22.

25. Stampfer MJ, Willet WC, Colditz GA et al. A prospective study of past use of oral contraceptive agents and risk of cardiovascular disease. *N Engl J Med* 1988; **319**:1313.

26. Porter JB, Hunter JR, Jick H et al. Oral contraceptives and nonfatal vascular disease. *Obstet Gynecol* 1985; **66**:1.

27. Porter JB, Jick H, Walker AM. Mortality among oral contraceptive users. *Obstet Gynecol* 1987; **70**:29.

28. Rosenberg L, Palmer JR, Lesko SM et al. Oral contraceptive use and the risk of myocardial infarction. *Am J Epidemiol* 1990; **131**:1009.

29. WHO Collaborative Study of Cardiovascular Disease and Steroid Hormone Contraception. Acute myocardial infarction and combined oral contraceptives; Results of an international multicenter case-control study. *Lancet* 1997; **349**:1202–9.

30. Lidegaard Ø. Oral contraceptives, pregnancy and the risk of cerebral thromboembolism: the influence of diabetes, hypertension, migraine and previous thrombotic disease. *Br J Obstet Gynaecol* 1995; **102**:153–9.

31. National Cholesterol Education Project. *Second Report of the Expert Panel on Detection, Evaluation and Treatment of High Blood Cholesterol in Adults.*

32. O'Sullivan JB. Diabetes after GDM. *Diabetes* 1991; **40** (**Suppl 2**):131–5.

33. Kjos SL, Peters RK, Xiang A et al. Predicting future diabetes in Latino women with gestational diabetes: utility of early postpartum glucose tolerance. *Diabetes* 1995; **44**:586–91.

34. Pettitt DJ, Knowler WC, Baird HR, Bennet PH. Gestational diabetes: infant and maternal complications of pregnancy in relation to third-trimester glucose tolerance in Pima Indians. *Diabetes Care* 1979; **3**:458–64.

35. Peters RK, Kjos SL, Xiang A, Buchanan TA. Long-term diabetogenic effect of a single pregnancy in women with prior gestational diabetes mellitus. *Lancet* 1996; **347**:227–30.

36. Skouby SO, Kuhl C, Molsted-Pedersen L et al. Triphasic oral contraception: metabolic effects in normal women and those with previous gestational diabetes. *Am J Obstet Gynecol* 1985; **153**:495.

37. Skouby SO, Anderson O, Saurbrey N et al. Oral contraception and insulin sensitivity: in vivo assessment in

normal women and women with previous gestational diabetes. *J Clin Endocrinol Metab* 1987; **64**:519.

38. Kjos SL, Shoupe D, Douyan S et al. Effect of low-dose oral contraceptives on carbohydrate and lipid metabolism in women with recent gestational diabetes: results of a controlled, randomized, prospective study. *Am J Obstet Gynecol* 1990; **163**:1822.

39. Kjos SL, Peters RK, Xiang A et al. Contraception and the risk of type 2 diabetes mellitus in Latina women with prior gestational diabetes mellitus. *J Am Med Assoc* 1998; **280**:533–8.

40. The Expert Committee on the Diagnosis and Classification of Diabetes Mellitus. Report of the Expert Committee on the Diagnosis and Classification of Diabetes Mellitus. *Diabetes Care* 1997; **20**:1183–97.

41. Konje JC, Otolorin EO, Ladipo AO. The effect of continuous subdermal levonorgestrel (Norplant) on carbohydrate metabolism. *Am J Obstet Gynecol* 1992; **166**: 15–19.

42. Liew DFM, Ng CSA, Yong YM et al. Long term effects of depo-provera on carbohydrate and lipid metabolism. *Contraception* 1985; **31**:51.

43. Fahmy K, Abdel-Razik, Shaaraway M et al. Effect of long-acting progestaten-only injectable contraceptives on carbohydrate metabolism and its hormonal profile. *Contraception* 1991; **44**:419–29.

44. Kim C, Seidel KW, Degier EA, Kwok YS. Diabetes and depot medroxyprogesterone contraception in Navajo women. *Arch Intern Med* 2001; **1616**:1766–71.

45. World Health Organization. Special programme of research, development, and research training in human reprodcution: a multi-centered phase III comparative clinical trial of depot medroxyprogesterone acetate given 3-monthly at doses of 100 mg, or 150 mg. *Contraception* 1986; **34**:223–35.

46. Sivin I, Viegas O, Campodonico I et al. Clinical performance of a new two-rod levonorgestrel contraceptive implant: a three-year randomized study with Norplant implants as controls. *Contraception* 1997; **55**:73–80.

47. Zheng SR, Zheng HM, Qian SZ et al. A long-term study of the efficacy and accetability of a single-rod hormonal contraceptive implant (Implanon) in healthy women in China. *Eur J Contracept Reprod Health Care* 1999; **4**:85–93.

48. Kaunitz AM, Garceau RJ, Cromie MA. Comparative safety, efficacy and cycle control of Lunelle monthly contraceptive injection (medroxyprogesterone acetate and estradiol cypionate injectable suspension) and Ortho-Novum 7/7/7 oral contraceptive (norethindrone/ethinyl estradiol triphasic). Lunelle Study Group. *Contraception* 1999; **60**:179.

49. Timmer CJ, Mulders TM. Pharmacokinetics of etonogestrel and ethinylestradiol released from a combined contraceptive vaginal ring. *Clin Pharmacokinet* 2000; **39**:233.

50. Cramer DW, Schiff I, Schoenbaum SC et al. Tubal infertility and the intrauterine device. *N Engl J Med* 1985; **312**:941.

51. Lee NC, Rubin GL, Ory HW et al. Type of intrauterine device and the risk of pelvic inflammatory disease. *Obstet Gynecol* 1983; **62**:1.

52. Lee NC, Rubin GL. The intrauterine device and pelvic inflammatory disease revisited: new results form the Women's Health Study. *Obstet Gynecol* 1988; **72**:1.

53. Farley TMM, Rosenberg MJ, Rowe PJ et al. Intrauterine devices and pelvic inflammatory disease: an international perspective. *Lancet* 1992; **339**:785–8.

54. Skouby SO, Molsted-Pedersen L, Kosonen A. Consequences of intrauterine contraception in diabetic women. *Fertil Steril* 1984; **42**:568.

55. Kimmerle R, Weiss R, Berger M, Kurz K-H. Effectiveness, safety and acceptablilty of a copper intrauterine device (CU Safe 300) in type I diabetic women. *Diabetes Care* 1993; **16**:1227–30.

56. Kjos SL, Ballagh SA, La Cour M et al. The copper T380A intrauterine device in women with type II diabetes mellitus. *Obstet Gynecol* 1994; **84**:1006–9.

57. Gosen C, Steel J, Ross A et al. Intrauterine contraception in diabetic women. *Lancet* 1982; **1**:530–5.

58. Lawless M, Vessey MP. Intrauterine device use by diabetic women. *Br J Fam Plan* 1982; **7**:110–11.

59. Wiese J. Intrauterine contraception in diabetic women. *Fertil Steril* 1977; **28**:422.

60. Kjos SL. Contraception in diabetic women. *Obstet Gynecol Clin N Am* 1996; **23**:243.

61. Andersson K, Odlind V, Rybo G. Levonorgestrel-releasing and copper-releasing (Nova T) IUDs during five years of use: a randomized comparative trial. *Contraception* 1994; **49**:56.

62. Jonsson B, Landgren B-M, Eneroth O. Effects of various IUDs on the composition of cervical mucus. *Contraception* 1991; **43**:447.

63. Rivera R, Yacobson I, Grimes D. The mechanism of action of hormonal contraceptives and intrauterine contraceptive devices. *Am J Obstet Gynecol* 1999; **181**: 1263.

64. Andersson K. Levonorgestrel releasing IUD – more than a contraceptive. *Acta Obstet Gynecol Scand* 1994; **73** (**Suppl 161**):55.

65. Lahteenmake P, Haukkamaa M, Puolakka J et al. Open randomized study of the use of levonorgestrel releasing intrauterine system as an alternative to hysterectomy. *Br Med J* 1998; **316**:1122.

49

Hormone replacement therapy and diabetes

Bari Kaplan, Michael Hirsch, Dov Feldberg

Introduction

After the onset of menopause, the average woman in developed countries lives for nearly 30 years in an estrogen-deficient state. Unfortunately, only 20% of these women receive any form of treatment.[1]

The use of postmenopausal hormone replacement therapy (HRT) poses one of the most difficult health care decisions women face today. HRT offers well-established benefits, including alleviation of vasomotor symptoms, management of urogenital atrophy and libido decline, and prevention of osteoporosis and fractures. It may also provide a cardiovascular protective effect, reduce the risk of colorectal cancer[2] and lower overall mortality rates.[3,4] However, concerns regarding the safety of HRT have recently been raised concerning the cardioprotective effect of HRT (see effect on cardiovascular risk below).

HRT is prescribed less often for women with diabetes than for non-diabetic women.[5-9] The reasons for this are unclear, although fear of adverse effects among both patients and physicians may play an important role. Many cautions are included in the product literature and, until recently, both diabetes and hypertension were listed as contraindications in the *British National Formulary*.[10] In addition, studies have shown that women 65 years of age or older with chronic medical disease tend to be under-treated for other, unrelated, disorders.[11]

Carbohydrate metabolism and aging

The prevalence of Type 2, or non-insulin-dependent, diabetes increases with age,[11-13] affecting *c.* 20% of individuals more than 65 years old. Older individuals with Type 2 diabetes tend to be leaner than younger ones. Most studies demonstrate an age-related increase per decade of 10–20 mg/l in fasting glucose concentrations and *c.* 150 mg/l in postprandial glucose concentrations.[11-14] This is accompanied, on average, by a small increase in fasting hepatic glucose output, impaired non-insulin-dependent glucose disposal,[11,12] and less insulin release in the early and late phase after glucose challenge.[15] The distribution of insulin moieties also appear to shift with age.[16] Other endocrine changes, particularly in adrenal function, may contribute to this process.[11]

Obesity, fat distribution and body composition also alter with age. Generally, fat mass increases until about the age of 65 and then it begins to decrease.[17] Lean body mass decreases steadily from the fifth or sixth decade onward. In women, adiposity tends to concentrate in the abdomen (central obesity). Obesity itself increases insulin resistance, and the emerging dyslipidemia and disturbances in the coagulation system.

The weight gain and altered body composition are, in turn, affected by changing habits in dietary intake and physical activity with aging, which alone may play a role in increasing insulin resistance. Individuals with leaner body mass have lower skeletal muscle volume, the main target tissue that lowers plasma glucose concentrations in reaction to insulin.

Effects of menopause on carbohydrate metabolism

Type 2 diabetes occurs more often in women than men in the older age group. Whether menopause contributes to this difference remains unclear because the discrimination of changes associated with menopause from those due to aging is difficult. Any changes observed in individual women followed through menopause will be influenced by aging and, given the extended duration of the perimenopause, such studies are extremely difficult to undertake.

No effect of menopause on fasting plasma glucose levels was found in women who became postmenopausal during the course of the Framingham Study.[18] Similarly, there was no effect of menopause on fasting or on the 2 hour oral glucose tolerance test (OGTT) glucose or insulin levels in the prospective study of Matthews et al.[19]

Nevertheless, menopause is associated with many characteristics of the insulin resistance syndrome, including increased cardiovascular morbidity and mortality, and accretion of generalized and visceral adiposity. Reduced lean body mass, sedentary lifestyle and, possibly, reduced estrogen-dependent blood flow to skeletal muscles may result in decreased peripheral glucose uptake, impaired insulin secretion and increased insulin resistance.

Some insight into whether menopause affects insulin and glucose metabolism may be gained from experimental studies of the effects of estrogen and progesterone. Early studies consistently demonstrated increased pancreatic insulin secretion in response to glucose in animals treated with estrogens;[20–22] similar observations were subsequently made in islet cells isolated from estrogen-treated animals.[23–25]

Estrogen and progesterone may augment the pancreatic insulin response to glucose. However, estrogen apparently increases the sensitivity of insulin-dependent metabolic processes, such as tissue glucose uptake and lipid synthesis, to insulin,[26–28] whereas progesterone has the opposite effect.[29–31] Therefore, menopause might be expected to result in some reduction in pancreatic insulin output and deterioration in glucose tolerance, but the effects on insulin sensitivity are likely to depend on the relative contributions of the two hormones. It is conceivable that insulin sensitivity might increase with the reduction in progesterone concentrations at menopause.

Effects of diabetes mellitus on postmenopausal women

Diabetes mellitus (DM) was found to be associated with an increase in uterine size in postmenopausal women.[32] In addition, the relative risk of endometrial cancer in diabetic women is fourfold higher than in non-diabetic women.[26,33] The risk of endometrial cancer also increases with the use of unopposed estrogen in non-hysterectomized women[34] and is reduced with the use of cyclical or continuous progestogen.[35–37]

According to most studies, Type 2 diabetes is associated with high bone mineral densities (BMD)[38,39] and Type 1, or insulin-dependent, diabetes with decreased BMD. The prospective Iowa Women's Health Study of > 30,000 women revealed that women with Type 1 diabetes were 12.25 times more likely to have an incident hip fracture than non-diabetic women; the relative rate for women with Type 2 diabetes was only 1.7.[40] Most studies have reported no consistent relationship between metabolic control of diabetes and BMD.

Possible mediators of the osteopenia are microangiopathy at the bone tissue, and changes in insulin, insulin-related growth factors (IGF) and other cytokines involved in bone metabolism.[41] Recent studies have also tentatively attributed the higher incidence of hip fractures in Type 1 diabetics to the absence of amylin, a 37-amino-acid polypeptide normally secreted by the pancreatic beta cells. Amylin binds to calcitonin receptors, lowers plasma calcium concentrations, inhibits osteoclasts and stimulates osteoblasts.[42] Leptin may play a role in bone regulation in Type 2 diabetes.

Effect of hormone replacement therapy on carbohydrate metabolism

HRT reportedly contributes to the control of glucose levels. One study reported lower glycosylated hemoglobin (HbA1c) levels (i.e. greater glycemic control) in 14 overweight diabetic women treated by HRT [2 months of conjugated equine estrogen (CEE) 0.625 mg, followed by combined CEE 0.625 mg and medroxyprogesterone acetate (MPA) 5 mg] than in an equal number of age- and weight-matched untreated women.[43] The treated women also showed a reduction in total cholesterol, but no change in triglyceride (TG), fasting glucose or insulin concentrations. These findings were confirmed in another study wherein short-term (6 weeks) oral estradiol was administered to women with Type 2 diabetes.[44] In a retrospective study of c. 15,000 women with Type 2 diabetes in northern California, glycemic control improved to an equal degree with either estrogen or estrogen–progesterone replacement therapy.[45]

In non-diabetic postmenopausal women, HRT seems to have no increased effect on future diabetic risk. Gabal et al[46] reported no change in the age-adjusted relative risk of developing Type 2 diabetes in postmenopausal women followed for 11.5 years. Similarly, in a prospective follow-up study of 12 years, Manson et al[47] noted no increase in the incidence of Type 2 diabetes among past users of HRT; the relative risk (RR) in current users was 0.8 (RR 0.67–0.96). These findings did not change significantly after multivariate adjustment for age, body mass index (BMI), family history of diabetes and coronary risk factors. Accordingly, one 10-year literature review found no compelling evidence for a reduced risk of diabetes in women treated by HRT.[48]

Contrary findings were reported in studies conducted with HRT in American Indians, who have a particularly high prevalence and incidence of the disease. The Strong Heart Study (SHS), which investigated 13 tribes in three geographic areas, noted a 40–70% prevalence of Type 2 diabetes in women aged 45–74.[49] Postmenopausal estrogen therapy led to a reduction in fasting glucose but was associated with a deterioration in glucose tolerance. The authors concluded that long-term use of estrogen use may increase the risk of Type 2 diabetes.

Hormone replacement therapy in the diabetic patient

Traditionally, the prevention of severe renal disease and retinopathy has been the primary target in the long-term management of diabetes. In a 10 year follow-up of women with late-onset diabetes, HRT use was found to be unrelated to the severity of retinopathy or the incidence of macular edema.[50]

Effect of HRT on cardiovascular risk

Diabetes is a major risk factor for coronary heart disease (CHD) in women and event rates increase substantially after menopause. Older individuals with diabetes are more prone to cardiovascular and peripheral vascular complications than older individuals without diabetes, and they have a poorer prognosis in the presence of these complications.[12]

This risk is greater in women than in men. Many observational studies have shown that HRT reduces mortality due to CHD by c. 50%; however, this has not been confirmed in randomized controlled trials (RCT). Two recent long-term prospective randomized studies, the Heart and Estrogen/progestin Replacement Study (HERS)[51] and the Women's Health Initiative (WHI), suggested that HRT may actually increase the risk of coronary vascular disease. Therefore, HRT is not currently indicated for the primary or secondary prevention of CHD. In diabetic women specifically, there are, at present, no long-term studies. The many short-term studies infer that HRT may have beneficial effects on glucose homeostasis, the lipid profile and fibrinolytic activity, all compatible with the prevention of CHD. A recent study suggests that women with Type 2 diabetes may stand to benefit more from any HRT cardioprotection than their non-diabetic counterparts because of their higher absolute baseline risk.[53] Nevertheless, the unknown effect of HRT on endometrial cancer and venous thromboembolism, which occur more often in diabetic women than in the general population, need to be considered.

Effect of HRT on atherosclerosis

One case–control study reported an absence of adverse effects of HRT on the risk of fatal and non-fatal myocardial infarctions in diabetic women,[54] and another 27 month observational follow-up study reported a positive impact of HRT, with fewer myocardial infarctions in estrogen-treated compared to untreated patients after percutaneous transluminal coronary balloon angioplasty (PTCA).[55] A larger cross-sectional study on 623 postmenopausal women with diabetes showed that atherosclerosis, as determined by the intimal–medial wall thickness of the common and internal carotid arteries, was reduced in the internal carotid in both current and former users of HRT.[56]

Effect of HRT on vascular reactivity

Menopause and diabetes have independent and adverse impacts on microvascular reactivity, as measured by forearm cutaneous vasodilation in response to acetylcholine and nitroprusside. HRT was found to improve this relaxation response in both healthy and diabetic subjects.[57] Other *in vitro* studies conducted in patients with Type 2 diabetes given HRT for 6 months yielded similar results, demonstrating an effect of HRT on both endothelium-dependent and -independent mechanisms of vascular relaxation.[58] There was no effect on clinic or ambulatory blood pressure, arterial load indexes or circadian blood pressure variations in the diabetic group, as was anticipated according to such improvements noted in non-diabetic women treated by HRT.[59] HRT also failed to reduce elevated levels of endothelin-1, a natural vasoconstrictor, which is characteristic of Type 2 diabetes.[60]

Effect of HRT on the coagulation system

Short-term (3 month) treatment with oral estradiol in diabetic women led to a significant increase in tissue plasminogen activator activity and, thereby, an improvement in fibrinolytic activity.[27] As observed by others, the increase in tissue plasminogen activator activity was noted only when TG levels were within the normal range.[12] Other effects on the coagulation system included a small reduction in antithrombin level. There was no change in the levels of fibrinogen, the von Willebrand factor, prothrombin, protein S or protein C, or in resistance to activated protein C.[61]

Effect of HRT on blood lipids

Apolipoprotein A1V levels are increased by c. 20% in diabetic subjects and can be reduced by HRT.[62] In one study, short-term oral estradiol treatment of postmenopausal diabetic women increased high-density lipoprotein (HDL) cholesterol and its subfraction HDL2 and apolipoprotein A1, whereas low-density lipoprotein (LDL) cholesterol and apolipoprotein B levels decreased.[44,63] Andersson et al,[63] using a double-blind crossover placebo-controlled design, investigated 25 postmenopausal women with Type 2 diabetes treated with oral estradiol. Blood tests performed after 68 days yielded an increase in sex-hormone-binding globulin and a decrease in free testosterone compared to controls. Blood glucose, HbA1c, total cholesterol and LDL cholesterol

decreased, and HDL cholesterol increased.[63] Another cross-sectional study of 694 diabetic patients showed that HRT (type and length of treatment not specified) caused an increase in HDL cholesterol, but to a lesser degree than in the non-diabetic control women, resulting in proportionally lower levels of HDL, HDL2 and HDL3 cholesterol. TG increased to a greater extent than in controls. LDL cholesterol and apolipoprotein B decreased, and apolipoprotein A increased to a similar degree in both groups.[64]

Effect of HRT on miscellaneous cardiovascular risk factors

C-reactive protein (CRP), a marker of inflammation, is associated with increased cardiovascular risk; levels are increased in diabetes. Both HRT and ERT, regardless of specific type of preparation, caused a significant increase in the CRP concentration.[65] However, in diabetic women, transdermal estradiol with continuous oral norethisterone acetate (NETA) significantly reduced CRP concentrations.[66]

Effect of type and mode of delivery of hormone replacement therapy

Most studies report that oral estradiol and transdermal estrogen have no adverse effect on insulin resistance.[67] A few trials have actually shown a positive effect of oral estrogen, which the authors suggested was mediated by a reduction in fasting glucose and insulin levels, and an increase in the glucose metabolism rate.

In women with diabetes, one recent work suggested that HRT regimens based on 17β-estradiol and progestogen (norethisterone) may be more appropriate than those based on synthetic conjugated estrogens.[66]

Various synthetic progestogens are currently available, such as medroxyprogesterone acetate, dydrogesterone, levonorgestrel and NETA, and they may have differing effects on glucose and insulin metabolism.[67,68] Luotola et al[69] examined the effects of orally administered cyclical NETA given with continuous 17β-estradiol in 30 postmenopausal women followed over 6 months. The combination had little effect, although in women who commenced the study with impaired glucose tolerance, there was some improvement in glucose response. This is in agreement with another study showing that the addition of a progestogen does not appear to reverse the observed benefit of estrogen.[70] DeCleyn et al[71] studied 20 postmenopausal women before and 2 months after taking conjugated equine estrogens, and then after 6 months of cyclically administered dydrogesterone (20 mg for 12 days). The lack of change in glucose and the reduction in insulin concentrations suggested that combined therapy improves insulin sensitivity and elimination in postmenopausal women. It was reported that medroxyprogesterone acetate given together with oral estrogen may abolish any beneficial effect on carbohydrate metabolism.[67]

Comparison of oral and transdermal combined hormonal treatment yielded no effect of transdermal treatment on glucose tolerance or insulin concentrations. Both routes were associated with increased hepatic insulin uptake, but with transdermal therapy this was compensated for by an increase in first-phase pancreatic insulin secretion. Neither treatment caused significant insulin resistance compared with baseline levels, but with the oral treatment insulin resistance was significantly greater during the combined phase than the estrogen-only phase.[72]

Thus, some combined regimens appear to better sustain the improvements in glucose and insulin metabolism seen with the native hormone.

Effects of hormone replacement therapy on obesity and body composition

The effect of HRT on accretion of visceral adiposity remains unclear. While short-term studies have shown that it is preventive, longer term studies fail to support this finding.[67] In a study of young postmenopausal women of normal range body weights, previous use of HRT was associated with reduced intra-abdominal fat, but not reduced abdominal subcutaneous fat, sagittal diameter, fat-free mass, total fat, insulin sensitivity or body weight.[73] In overweight postmenopausal women with Type 2 diabetes, HRT reduced the waist-to-hip ratio but not the total fat mass.[43]

Conclusions

Diabetes is apparently not a contraindication for HRT. HRT does not have adverse effects on glycemic control in women with diabetes and certain preparations may even have a positive effect. Some forms also improve the lipid profile in this population. It seems that transdermal hormonal therapy, containing natural estrogens combined with natural progesterones or NETA, may be the preferable regimen recommended for the diabetic patient, interfering less with an already deranged metabolism.

At present, the use of HRT for the prevention or treatment of cardiovascular disease is unclear, and women should be informed about these data before starting therapy for other reasons. This should not prevent clinicians from prescribing HRT in diabetic women mainly for menopausal symptom control and maybe for the prevention of osteoporosis. Women with diabetes should also not be denied interventions proven to reduce cardio-vascular events. However, since there are no long-term studies in women with diabetes who have received HRT, definitive conclusions cannot be reached. On the basis of the data collected so far, however, it is suggested that the risk–benefit ratio is similar to that for the non-diabetic population. Both the decision to prescribe HRT and the specific preparation used should always be tailored to the individual. Individual assessment of the potential benefits and risks of long-term HRT should be performed in women with diabetes as it is for all women when HRT is considered.

References

1. Ravnikar VA. Barriers for taking long-term hormone replacement therapy: why do women not adhere to therapy? *Eur Menopause J* 1996; 3:90–3.
2. Lester S, Moore V. Oral oestrogen replacement therapy versus placebo for hot flushes (Cochrane Review). *The Cochrane Library* 1, 2002.
3. Cauley JA, Seeley DG, Browner WS et al. Estrogen replacement therapy and mortality among older women: the study of osteoporotic fractures. *Arch Intern Med* 1997; 157:2181–7.
4. Henderson BE, Paganini-Hill A, Ross RK. Decreased mortality in users of estrogen replacement therapy. *Arch Intern Med* 1991; 151:75–8.
5. Feher MD, Issacs AJ. Is hormone replacement therapy prescribed for post-menopausal diabetic women? *Br J Clin Pract* 1996; 50:431–2.
6. Moorhead T, Hannaford P, Warskyj M. Prevalence and characteristics associated with use of hormone replacement therapy in Britain. *Br J Obstet Gynaecol* 1997; 104:290–7.
7. Lawrenson RA, Newson RB, Feher MD. Do women with diabetes receive hormone replacement therapy? *Pract Diabetes Int* 1998; 15:71–2.
8. Keating NL, Cleary PD, Rossi AS et al. Use of hormone replacement therapy by post-menopausal women in the United States. *Ann Intern Med* 1999; 130:545–53.
9. Troici RJ, Cowie CC, Harris MI. Hormone replacement therapy and glucose metabolism. *Obstet Gynecol* 2000; 96:665–70.
10. British Medical Association (BMA) and Royal Pharmaceutical Society of Great Britain. *British National Formulary*. (BMA/Royal Pharmaceutical Society of Great Britain: London, 1999) 38.
11. Carey VJ, Walters EE, Colditz G et al. Body fat distribution and risk of non-insulin-dependent diabetes mellitus in women. The Nurses' Health Study. *Am J Epidemiol* 1997; 145:614–19.
12. Morrow LA, Halter JB. Treatment of the elderly with diabetes. In: (Kahn CR, Weir GC, eds) *Joslin's Diabetes Mellitus*, 13th edn. (Lea & Febiger: Malvern, PA, 1994) 552–9.
13. Meneilly GS, Tessier D. Diabetes in the elderly. *Diabet Med* 1995; 12:949–60.
14. Meneilly GS, Dawson K, Tessier D. Alterations in glucose metabolism in the elderly patient with diabetes. *Diabetes Care* 1993; 16:1241–7.
15. Shimizu M, Kawazu S et al. Age-related alteration of pancreatic β-cell function: increased proinsulin and proinsulin-to-insulin molar ratio in elderly, but not in obese, subjects without glucose intolerance. *Diabetes Care* 1996; 19:8–11.
16. Perry III HM, Morley JE, Horowitz M et al. Body composition and age in African-American and Caucasian women: relationship to plasma leptin levels. *Metabolism* 1997; 46:1399–405.
17. Silver AJ, Guillen CP, Kahl MJ et al. Effect of aging on body fat. *J Am Geriatr Soc* 1995; 41:211–13.
18. Hjortland MC, McNamara PM, Kannel WB. Some atherogenic concomitants of the menopause: the Framingham Study. *Am J Epidemiol* 1976; 103:304–11.
19. Matthews KA, Meilahn E, Kuller LH et al. Menopause and risk factors for coronary heart disease. *N Engl J Med* 1989; 321:641–6.
20. Barnes B, Regan J, Nelson W. Improvement in experimental diabetes following the administration of Amniotin. *Am Med Assoc* 1933; 101:926–7.
21. Nelson W, Overholser M. The effect of oestrogenic hormone on experimental pancreatic diabetes in the monkey. *Endocrinology* 1936; 20:473–80.
22. Griffiths M, Young F. Does the hypophysis secrete a pancreotropic hormone? *Nature* 1940; 146:266–7.
23. Costrini N, Kalkhoff R. Relative effects of pregnancy, estradiol and progesterone on plasma insulin and pancreatic islet insulin secretion. *Clin Invest* 1971; 50:992–9.
24. Howell S, Tyhurst M, Green I. Direct effects of progesterone on rat islets of Langerhans in vivo and in tissue culture. *Diabetologia* 1977; 13:579–83.
25. Faure A, Sutter-Dub M-T. Insulin secretion from isolated pancreatic islets in the female rat. Short and long term estradiol influence. *J Physiol* 1979; 75:289–95.
26. Hager D, Georg J, Leitner J, Beck P. Insulin secretion and content in isolated rat pancreatic islets following

treatment with gestational hormones. *Endocrinology* 1972; **91**:977–81.

27. Ashby J, Shirling D, Baird J. Effects of progesterone on insulin secretion in the rat. *J Endocrinol* 1978; **76**:479–86.

28. Bailey C, Ahmed-Sorour H. Role of ovarian hormones in the long-term control of glucose homeostasis. *Diabetologia* 1980; **19**:475–81.

29. Neilsen J. Direct effect of gonadal and contraceptive steroids on insulin release from mouse pancreatic islets in organ culture. *Acta Endocrinol* 1984; **105**:245–50.

30. McKerns K, Coulomb B, Kaleita E, DeRenzo E. Some effects of in vivo administered oestrogens on glucose metabolism and adrenal cortical secretion in vitro. *Endocrinology* 1958; **63**:709–22.

31. Samos LF, Roos BA. Diabetes mellitus in older persons. *Med Clin N Am* 1998; **82**:791–803.

32. Gull B, Karlsson B, Milsom I, Granberg S. Factors associated with endometrial thickness and uterine size in a random sample of postmenopausal women. *Am J Obstet Gynecol* 2001; **185**:386.

33. Purdie DM, Green AC. Epidemiology of endometrial cancer. *Best Pract Res Clin Obstet Gynaecol* 2001; **15**:341–54.

34. Grady D, Gebretsadik J, Kerlikowske K et al. Hormone replacement therapy and endometrial cancer risk: a meta-analysis. *Obstet Gynecol* 1995; **85**:304–13.

35. Sturdee DW, Wade-Evans T, Paterson ME et al. Relations between bleeding pattern, endometrial biopsy and oestrogen treatment in post-menopausal women. *Br Med J* 1978; **1**:1575–7.

36. The Writing Group for the PEPI Trial. Effects of hormone replacement therapy on endometrial histology in post-menopausal women. *J Am Med Assoc* 1996; **275**:370–5.

37. Sturdee DW, Ulrich LG, Barlow DH et al. The endometrial response to sequential and continuous combined oestrogen progestogen replacement therapy. *Br J Obstet Gynaecol* 2000; **107**:1392–400.

38. Barrett-Connor E, Holbrook TL. Sex differences in osteoporosis in older adults with non-insulin-dependent diabetes mellitus. *J Am Med Assoc* 1992; **268**:3333–7.

39. Lunt M, Masaryk P, Scheidt-Nave C et al. The effect of lifestyle, dietary dairy intake and diabetes on bone density and vertebral deformity prevalance: The EVOS Study. *Osteoporos Int* 2001; **12**:688–98.

40. Nicodemus KK, Folsom AR, Iowa Women's Health Study. Type 1 and type 2 diabetes and incident hip fractures in postmenopausal women. *Diabetes Care* 2001; **24**:1192–7.

41. Leidig-Bruckner G, Ziegler R. Diabetes mellitus a risk for osteoporosis? *Exp Clin Endocrinol Diabetes* 2001; **109** (**Suppl 2**):S493–S514.

42. Horcajada-Molteni MN, Chanteranne JB, Lebecque P et al. Amylin and bone metabolism in streptozotocin-induced diabetic rats. *Bone Miner Res* 2001; **16**: 958–65.

43. Samaras K, Hayward CS, Sullivan D et al. Effects of postmenopausal hormone replacement therapy on central abdominal fat, glycemic control, lipid metabolism and vascular factors in type 2 diabetes: a prospective study. *Diabetes Care* 1999; **22**:1401–7.

44. Brussaard HE, Gevers LJ, Frolich M et al. Short-term oestrogen replacement therapy improves insulin resistance, lipids and fibrinolysis in postmenopausal women with NIDDM. *Diabetologia* 1997; **40**:843–9.

45. Ferrara A, Karter AJ, Ackerson LM et al. Hormone replacement therapy is associated with better glycemic control in women with type 2 diabetes: The Northern California Kaiser Permanente Diabetes Registry. *Diabetes Care* 2001; **24**:1144–50.

46. Gabal LL, Goodman-Gruen D, Barrett-Connor E. The effect of postmenopausal estrogen therapy on the risk of non-insulin-dependent diabetes mellitus. *Am J Public Health* 1997; **87**:443–5.

47. Manson JE, Rimm EB, Colditz GA et al. A prospective study of postmenopausal estrogen therapy and subsequent incidence of non-insulin-dependent diabetes mellitus. *Ann Epidemiol* 1992; **2**:665–73.

48. Barrett-Connor E. Postmenopausal estrogen therapy and selected (less-often-considered) disease outcomes. *Menopause* 1999; **6**:14–20.

49. Zhang Y, Howard BV, Cowan LD et al. The effect of estrogen use on levels of glucose and insulin and the risk of type 2 diabetes in American Indian postmenopausal women: the strong Heart Study. *Diabetes Care.*

50. Klein BE, Klein R, Moss SE. Exogenous estrogen exposures and changes in diabetic retinopathy. The Wisconsin Epidemiologic Study of Diabetic Retinopathy. *Diabetes Care* 1999; **22**:1984–7.

51. Hulley SB, Grady D, Bush TL et al. Randomized trial of estrogen plus progestin for secondary prevention of coronary heart disease in postmenopausal women. Heart and Estrogen/Progestin Replacement Study (HERS) Research Group. *J Am Med Assoc* 1998; **280**:605–13.

52. Writing Group for the Women's Health Initiative Investigators. Risks and benefits of estrogen plus progestin in healthy postmenopausal women. *J Am Med Assoc* 2002; **288**:321–33.

53. Sattar N, McKenzie J, MacCuish AC, Jaap AJ. Hormone replacement therapy in type 2 diabetes mellitus: a cardiovascular perspective. *Diabet Med* 1998; **15**:631–3.

54. Abu-Halawa SA, Thompson K, Kirkeeide RL et al. Estrogen replacement therapy and outcome of coronary balloon angioplasty in postmenopausal women. *Am J Cardiol* 1998; **82**:475.

55. Kaplan RC, Heckbert SR, Weiss NS et al. Postmenopausal estrogens and risk of myocardial infraction in diabetic women. *Diabetes Care* 1998; **21**:1117–21.

56. Dubuisson JT, Wagenknecht LE, D'Agostino Jr RB, et al. Association of hormone replacement therapy and carotid wall thickness in women with and without diabetes. *Diabetes Care* 1998; **21**:1790–6.

57. Lim SC, Caballero AE, Arora S et al. The effect of hormonal replacement therapy on the vascular reactivity and endothelial function of healthy individuals and individuals with type 2 diabetes. *J Clin Endocrinol Metab* 1999; **84**:4159–64.

58. Perera M, Petrie JR, Hillier C et al. Hormone replacement therapy can augment vascular relaxation in postmenopausal women with type 2 diabetes. *Hum Reprod* 2000; **17**:497–502.

59. Hayward CS, Samaras K, Campbell L, Kelly RP. Effect of combination hormone replacement therapy on ambulatory blood pressure and arterial stiffness in diabetic postmenopausal women. *Am J Hypertens* 2000; **14**:699–703.

60. Saltervo J, Puolakka J, Ylikorkala O. Plasma endothelin in postmenopausal women with type 2 diabetes mellitus and metabolic syndrome: a comparison of oral combined and transdermal oestrogen-only replacement therapy. *Diabetes Obesity Metab* 2000; **2**:293–8.

61. Hahn L, Mattsson LA, Andersson B, Tengborn L. The effects of oestrogen replacement therapy on haemostatic variables in postmenopausal women with non-insulin-dependent diabetes mellitus. *Blood Coagul Fibrinolysis* 1999; **10**:81–6.

62. Sun Z, Larson IA, Ordovas JM et al. Effects of age, gender and lifestyle factors on plasma apolipoprotein A-IV concentrations. *Atherosclerosis* 2000; **15**:381–8.

63. Andersson B, Mattsson LA, Hahn L et al. Estrogen replacement therapy decreases hyperandrogenicity and improves glucose homeostasis and plasma lipids in postmenopausal women with noninsulin-dependent diabetes mellitus. *J Clin Endocrinol Metab* 1997; **82**:638–43.

64. Robinson JC, Folsom AR, Nabulsi AA et al. Can postmenopausal hormone replacement improve plasma lipids in women with diabetes? The Atherosclerosis Risk in Communities Study Investigators. *Diabetes Care* 1996; **19**:480–5.

65. Ridker PM, Hennekens CH, Rifai N et al. Hormone replacement therapy and increased plasma concentration of C-reactive protein. *Circulation* 1999; **100**: 713–16.

66. Sattar N, Perera M, Small M, Lumsden MA. Hormone replacement therapy and sensitive C-reactive protein concentrations in women with type-2 diabetes. *Lancet* 1999; **354**:1908.

67. Fineberg SE. Glycaemic control and hormone replacement therapy: implications of the Postmenopausal Estrogen Progestogen Intervention (PEPI) study. *Drugs Aging* 2000; **17**:453–61.

68. Godsland I, Crook D, Simpson R et al. The effects of different formulations of oral contraceptive agents on lipid and carbohydrate metabolism. *N Engl J Med* 1990; **323**:1375–81.

69. Luotola H, Pyorala T, Loikkanen M. Effects of natural oestrogen/progestogen substitution therapy on carbohydrate and lipid metabolism in post-menopausal women. *Maturitas* 1986; **8**:245–53.

70. Grodstein F, Stampfer MJ, Manson JE et al. Postmenopausal estrogen use and progestin use and the risk of cardiovascular disease. *N Engl J Med* 1996; **335**:453–61.

71. DeCleyn K, Buytaert P, Coppens M. Carbohydrate metabolism during hormonal substitution therapy. *Maturitas* 1989; **11**:235–42.

72. Spencer CP, Godsland IF, Cooper AJ et al. Effects of oral and transdermal 17beta-estradiol with cyclical oral norethindrone acetate on insulin sensitivity, secretion, and elimination in postmenopausal women. *Metabolism* 2000; **49**:742–7.

73. Sites CK, L'Hommediew GD, Brochu M, Poehlman ET. Previous exposure to hormone replacement therapy and confounders in metabolic studies. *Menopause* 2000; **8**:281–5.

50

Diabetes and infertility
Avi Ben-Haroush, Raoul Orvieto, Benjamin Fisch

Introduction

Patients with diabetes mellitus often have reproductive disturbances. For women these include delayed menarche, menstrual irregularities, subfertility, early onset of menopause and increased incidence of spontaneous abortions, and for men impotence, hypospermia and impaired spermatogenesis. The exact mechanisms underlying diabetes-related infertility remain unknown. Studies have implicated a central effect on the pituitary–gonadal axis, abnormal antral follicle development, as in polycystic ovary syndrome (PCOS), and microangiopathy or other tissue-damaging factors.

This chapter reviews the known data on the association between diabetes and infertility, including the cumulative information on the pivotal role of insulin resistance in the pathogenesis of prediabetic states such as PCOS, and the effect of insulin-sensitizing drugs, such as metformin. The risks of spontaneous abortion and male infertility are discussed as well.

Type 1 diabetes and reproductive disturbances

Delayed menarche and menstrual irregularities

Prior to the identification and isolation of insulin in 1921, diabetic females rarely underwent secondary sexual development.[1] Today, menarche is usually delayed if the disease develops in the prepubertal years, and early if it precedes the onset of the disease.[2,3] Almost one third of diabetic women of reproductive age have some form of menstrual dysfunction.[4] In a study of 337 women with Type 1 diabetes, Burkart et al[5] noted an inverse correlation between age at menarche and patient age, with age at menarche being 0.8–2 years higher in diabetic patients than in the patients in whom diabetes developed after menarche, and 0.4–1.3 years higher than in non-diabetics. The increase was most pronounced if the diabetes was diagnosed between 3 and 8 years of age. A delay in menarche was also noted in a later retrospective study of 100 diabetic women when the disease was diagnosed before the age of menarche and before 10 years of age:[6] the average age at menarche in this series was 13.5. In addition, there was a significant correlation between menstrual disturbances and both late menarche and diabetic complications.[6] The authors suggested that one possible explanation for the delayed menarche in Type 1 diabetes is the characteristic weight loss that occurs at the time of diagnosis.

Burkart et al[5] found that the prevalence of primary amenorrhea was 3.6% in women with Type 1 diabetes, compared to 1.5% in healthy controls and in women with late-onset diabetes. The rates of oligomenorrhea and secondary amenorrhea were 14 and 7%, compared to 12% in the patients with late-onset diabetes. Menstrual irregularities were more frequent at the time of diabetes onset, although 76% of the patients had not complained of any change in menstrual bleeding and it normalized with time. Over 70% of patients < 35 years of age had spontaneous conceptions and only 2.1% were infertile; both these rates are similar to those in the control group.

Yeshaya et al[6] also noted a 32% rate of oligomenorrhea, amenorrhea and polymenorrhea, which was in agreement with the study of Bergquist[7] but higher than the 21.6% reported by Kjaer et al.[8]

Infertility

A questionnaire survey of an unselected population of 18–49-year-old diabetic women (*n* = 245) and a comparable control group (*n* = 253) failed to yield differences in the cumulative rates of pregnancies and involuntary infertility (17%).[9,10] However, the diabetic women had significantly fewer pregnancies (1.4 versus 1.7) and fewer births per pregnancy than controls, and more were nulliparous (48 versus 38%). Half of all the diabetic pregnancies were planned. The women reported that their diabetes had a negative influence on their attitude toward having children.

Briese and Muller,[11] in a study of 672 diabetic women between the ages of 17 and 42, of whom 72% were taking insulin, found that one third had successful pregnancies, but only one in 10 delivered more than once after the diabetes became manifest. At the time of the study, 126 patients (19.1%) were attempting pregnancy, about one fifth of them for > 2 years. Manifestations of diabetes occurred significantly earlier in the patients who did not achieve pregnancy. Infertility was correlated with daily insulin dose but was unrelated to duration of diabetes.

Euglycemia at the time of conception is crucial for the success of the pregnancy. Considering the difficulties in achieving and maintaining tight glycemic control for long periods, clomiphene citrate (CC) may be used to enhance fecundability in diabetic patients with good glycemic control.[12] This new 'sweet' indication for the use of CC is probably debatable. Nevertheless, fertility, like all other health issues in diabetic patients, depends on good metabolic control.

It may be concluded that although diabetic patients tend to have a negative attitude towards pregnancy and motherhood, their fertility potential is usually not substantially impaired when in good glycemic control.

Mechanisms for infertility

Hypothalamic–pituitary–gonadal dysfunction

Uncontrolled Type 1 diabetes is thought to disrupt normal hypothalamic–pituitary–gonadal function, and animal studies have suggested that poorly controlled Type 1 diabetes may adversely affect the uterovaginal outflow tract and/or ovarian function. However, clinical studies do not relate this factor to menstrual dysfunction.[4] Similarly, pituitary function, as assessed by basal gonadotropins and gonadotropin-releasing hormone (GnRH)-stimulated gonadotropin release, appears to be normal in young women with Type 1 diabetes. Although there is some evidence that pituitary function declines with increasing duration of diabetes, this issue has not been thoroughly investigated. Therefore, the oligo/amenorrhea in Type 1 diabetes appears to be principally hypothalamic in origin and may represent intermittent (and perhaps reversible) failure of the GnRH pulse generator. This is similar to the mechanism in anorexia nervosa or in women who engage in endurance training.[4] The exact pathophysiology of the GnRH neuronal system dysfunction is still not well understood, but attention is currently focused on increased central opioidergic activity, increased central dopaminergic activity and central glucose deprivation.

Role of insulin

The role of insulin in folliculogenesis has been studied extensively. Insulin receptors have been localized in the ovary, within the stromal cells, granulose and theca cells of developing follicles.[13] Studies that specifically examined primordial follicles localized insulin receptors primarily to the oocyte.[14] Some growth factors promote the primordial to primary follicle transition to a greater degree in the presence of insulin.[15] Direct ovarian organ culture studies have demonstrated that high concentrations of insulin stimulate primordial follicle development in the hamster.[16] Insulin also stimulates androgen production by cultured theca cells,[17] as well as estrogen and progesterone production by cultured granulosa cells.[18]

Kezele et al[19] suggested that insulin's site of action is likely the oocyte and that its activity is mediated via the insulin receptor, not the insulin-like growth factor (IGF)-I receptor. Thus, insulin helps to coordinate the primordial to primary follicle transition at the level of the oocyte. Abnormal insulin levels may alter or inhibit early follicular development.

Role of catecholamines

Impaired hypothalamic regulation of gonadotropin secretion may be caused by disrupted noradrenergic feedback. Monoamines and opioids are involved in the regulation of luteinizing hormone (LH) secretion.[20] Substances that block hypothalamic adrenergic receptors or activate opioid receptors suppress the release of GnRH and the preovulatory LH surge. The actions of opioids appear to involve noradrenergic mechanisms.[21] Thus, increased norepinephrine turnover in the preoptic areas may be a prerequisite for the LH surge, and the noradrenergic control of LH secretion is regulated by an opioid pathway.[22] Bitar[23] suggested that the endocrine abnormalities in diabetes are due, at least in part, to a functional deficit in noradrenergic neurons within the hypothalamus. Therefore, diabetes could suppress the cyclic reproduction function by disrupting these regulatory mechanisms.

Microangiopathy and decreased ovarian superoxide dismutase activity

Microangiopathy is the major cause of tissue damage in Type 1 diabetes[24] and may therefore be a mechanism for ovulatory dysfunction as well. The risk of microangiopathic abnormalities does not appear to increase linearly with the duration of diabetes, nor can it be prevented by good glycemic control.[24] Nitric oxide (NO), an important mediator in the regulation of the blood–follicle barrier and ovulation, is inactivated in the presence of clinical and experimental diabetes, leading to impaired endothelial-dependent vascular activity.[25] This state can be reversed by administration of insulin or free-radical scavengers, such as superoxide dismutase (SOD).[26] Powers et al[27] localized endothelial NO synthase (NOS), inducible NOS, SOD and the LH receptor to the same population of endothelial cells surrounding the preovulatory follicle. They suggested that short periods of hyperglycemia may cause a decrease in activity of ovarian SOD, thereby increasing the production of superoxide anion and disrupting the homeostatic vascular activity of NO. Specifically, the loss of the protective activity of SOD in diabetes may compromise the signaling of NO within the ovarian microvasculature at the time of ovulation.

Insulin resistance and polycystic ovary syndrome

PCOS is a heterogeneous disorder affecting 5–10% of women of reproductive age.[28] It is characterized by chronic anovulation with oligo/amenorrhea, infertility, typical sonographic appearance of the ovaries, i.e. multiple small follicles distributed around the ovarian periphery or throughout the echodense stroma[29] and clinical or biochemical hyperandrogenism. As anovulation accounts for an estimated 40% of all cases of female infertility, PCOS, being the most common cause of anovulation, is the most important cause of this type of infertility.[30]

Insulin resistance is present in 40–50% of patients, especially in obese women,[31] making PCOS a prediabetic state. The prevalence of impaired glucose tolerance (IGT) in PCOS is 31–35%, and the prevalence of Type 2 diabetes mellitus is 7.5–10%.[32] The conversion rate from IGT to overt Type 2 diabetes is increased 5–10-fold in women with PCOS.[33]

Hyperinsulinemic insulin resistance

Insulin resistance is defined as the decreased ability of insulin to stimulate glucose disposal into target tissues, or a reduced glucose response to a given amount of insulin. Chronic hyperinsulinemia is a compensatory response to this target tissue resistance. Several mechanisms have been suggested to explain insulin resistance, including peripheral target tissue resistance, decreased hepatic clearance, or increased pancreatic sensitivity. Studies with the euglycemic clamp technique indicate that hyperandrogenic woman with hyperinsulinemia have peripheral insulin resistance and a reduced insulin clearance rate due to decreased hepatic insulin extraction.[34,35]

The peripheral insulin resistance in PCOS is uniquely due to a defect beyond the activation of the receptor kinase, namely, reduced tyrosine autophosphorylation of the insulin receptor.[36,37] The reduced signal transmission caused by excessive phosphorylation of serine residues on the insulin receptor also explains the hyperandrogenism caused by the concomitant serine phosphorylation of P450c17, the key enzyme in ovarian and adrenal androgen biosynthesis, which increases the 17,20-lyase activity and androgen production.[37,38] Thus, insulin resistance may be causally related to overactivity of cytochrome P450c17.[39] Insulin, by acting via its own receptors, appears to promote ovarian and adrenal androgen biosynthesis,[40,41] amplifying LH-induced androgen production by theca cells and resulting in hyperandrogenemia.[42,43] Amelioration of the hyperinsulinemia leads to a dramatic decline in circulating androgens to normal levels.[44] Hyperinsulinemia may also upregulate IGF-I receptors, which are potent stimulators of LH-induced androgen synthesis, and increase the bioavailability of IGF-I secondary to the suppression of IGF binding protein (BP) I (IGF-BPI) production by the liver.[45,46] Additionally, insulin may potentiate the response of adrenal steroidogenesis to adrenocorticotropic hormone (ACTH),[47] and enhance the expression of hyperandrogenism by its inhibitory effect on hepatic sex hormone binding globulin (SHBG) production,[48] thereby increasing the bioavailability of androgens. Fig. 50.1 presents the potential mechanisms of insulin resistance in PCOS.

Although some studies indicate that androgens can induce hyperinsulinemia, most of the evidence supports hyperinsulinemia as the primary factor leading to hyperandrogenism.[49,50]

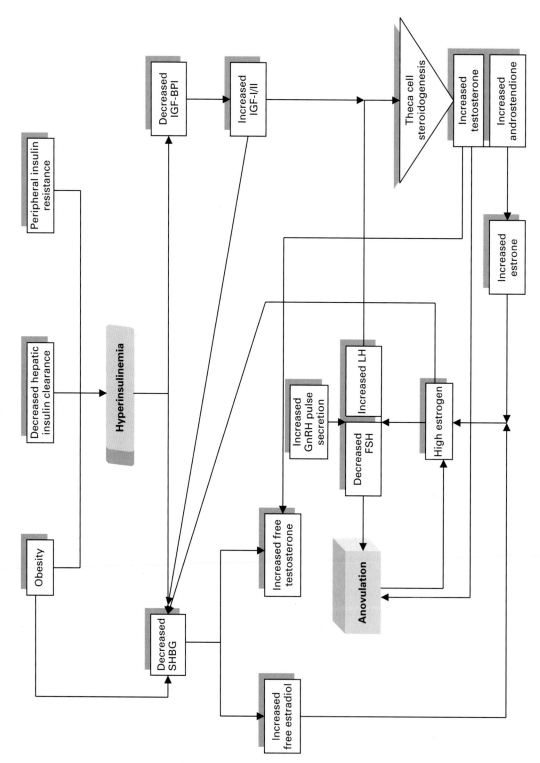

Figure 50.1. *Potential mechanisms of insulin resistance in polycystic ovary syndrome. FSH, Follice-stimulating hormone; GnRH, gonadotropin-releasing hormone; IGF, insulin-like growth factor; IGF-BPI, IGF binding protein I; LH, luteinizing hormone; SHBG, sex hormone binding globulin.*

Both lean and obese women with PCOS may be insulin resistant.[51–54] Affected lean women appear to have an intrinsic and still poorly understood form of insulin resistance,[36,37] and obese women probably have this form in addition to insulin resistance due to overweight.

Clinical findings that suggest the presence of insulin resistance and hyperinsulinemia include body mass index (BMI) > 27 kg/m^2, waist-to-hip ratio > 0.85, waist > 100 cm, acanthosis nigricans and numerous achrochordons (skin tags).[55] However, according to the American Diabetes Association (ADA) Consensus Conference,[56] there is still no satisfactory method for determining insulin resistance in the clinical practice setting. None of the tests, such as fasting insulin, glucose or glucose-to-insulin ratio, has been shown to be a useful predictor of the ovulatory response to insulin-sensitizing drugs. Although the fasting glucose-to-insulin ratio (< 4.5) correlates with insulin sensitivity as determined by the insulin–glucose clamp,[57] it has never been tested as a predictor of response to insulin-sensitizing therapy.[33]

Hyperinsulinemia and impaired ovulation

Dale et al[58] examined the correlation between insulin metabolism and outcome of gonadotropin stimulation in 42 infertile, CC-resistant women with PCOS. Using continuous infusion of glucose with the model assessment test, they identified 17 patients with insulin resistance who required higher doses of gonadotropins and a longer duration of treatment to achieve follicular maturation. In this group, 35% of the cycles were cancelled due to a multifollicular response compared to 2.5% in the non-insulin-resistant PCOS group. Moreover, although the ovulation rate in completed cycles was similar

between the groups, the conception rate was significantly better in the women with non-insulin-resistant PCOS.

Hyperinsulinemia and obesity correlate directly with the failure to ovulate in response to CC, or with the need for multiple repeated courses and increasing doses of CC.[59,60] Thus, women with PCOS and severe insulin resistance are more likely to fail to respond to CC.[61] BMI is a major determinant of insulin resistance and hyperinsulinemia. Insulin resistance is unlikely in women with BMI < 22 kg/m^2, common in women with BMI > 27 kg/m^2 and almost always present in women with BMI > 30 kg/m^2.[62] In obese women, weight reduction can reduce circulating androgen, LH and insulin concentrations, and, thereby, may induce ovulation and even improve the pregnancy rate.[63–65] The difficulty obese women have in losing weight, coupled with the fact that 10–30% of women with PCOS are lean, led to the introduction of insulin-sensitizing drugs to improve peripheral insulin sensitivity and reduce plasma insulin concentrations.[33,66,67]

Metformin

Metformin is an oral biguanide, category B drug for pregnant women, which has been approved for the treatment of Type 2 diabetes mellitus. It is thought to affect multiple metabolic pathways, decreasing glucose absorption, and suppressing hepatic glucose output and gluconeogenesis.[68,69] Metformin also improves the action of insulin at the cellular level by enhancing glucose uptake by fat and muscle cells,[70,71] and by increasing insulin receptor binding.[72] The reduction in free fatty acid release from adipose tissue further enhances insulin sensitivity.[73] Recently, Attia et al[74] showed that metformin directly inhibits androgen production in human thecal cells. Importantly, the actions of metformin are not associated with an increase in insulin secretion and, hence, with hypoglycemia. It is possible that the weight loss that often accompanies protracted metformin therapy may account for some of the beneficial effects observed in many studies.[75,76]

Metabolic and endocrine effects of metformin

Women with PCOS and fasting hyperinsulinemia who were treated with metformin showed a significant decrease in fasting insulin and total testosterone levels, and an increase in SHBG, leading to a decrease in the free testosterone index. In addition, there was a significant decline in mean BMI, the waist-to-hip ratio, hirsutism and acne, as well as an improvement in menstrual cyclicity. No changes in the LH level or in LH-to-follicle-stimulating hormone (FSH) ratio were observed. The greatest decline in testosterone and its free index occurred in the patients with the most pronounced hyperandrogenemia. Women with high levels of dehydroepianosterone sulfate (DHEAS) exhibited less improvement in menstrual cycle regularity, no change in hirsutism, and an increase in levels of IGF-I.[77] In addition, plasma 17-hydroxyprogesterone response to human chorionic gonadotropin (hCG) was significantly lower after treatment,[78] and the adrenal steroidogenesis response to ACTH was reduced, supporting the hypothesis that the high insulin levels associated with PCOS may cause an increase in plasma levels of adrenal androgens.[47] Accordingly, decreasing serum insulin concentrations with metformin also reduce ovarian cytochrome P450c17 alpha activity and ameliorate hyperandrogenism.[79] Thus, metformin apparently affects ovarian steroidogenesis, possibly via decreased insulin action.[80]

Spontaneous ovulation after metformin treatment

Vrbikova et al[81] showed that a 6-month course of metformin 1000 mg daily significantly improved the menstrual cycle pattern in 58% of the 24 women evaluated. In a study of 50 women with PCOS given metformin 1500 mg daily for 12 months, Baysal et al[82] found a statistically significant decrease in mean BMI, with no differences in fasting serum insulin and testosterone levels. Metformin improved menstrual patterns in 60% of cases. The authors speculated that the changes in menstrual cyclicity in response to metformin possibly occurred independent of insulin sensitivity or circulating insulin concentrations. A similar effect has also been reported by others.[76, 83–85]

Metformin treatment and ovulation induction with CC

CC-resistant and obese women have a high prevalence of insulin resistance. This subgroup may benefit more from treatment with metformin. In a large prospective trial, an oral glucose tolerance test (OGTT) was performed in 61 obese women with PCOS before and after administration of metformin 500 mg or placebo three times daily for 35 days.[86] Those who failed to ovulate spontaneously were given CC 50 mg daily for 5 days, concomitant with metformin or placebo. This regimen was successful in 19 of 21 women (90%) in the metformin group and two of 25 women (8 %) in the placebo group. Overall, 31 of the 35 women (89%) treated with metformin ovulated spontaneously or in response to CC, compared with only three of the 26 untreated women (12%). This finding agrees with other studies reporting an increase in pregnancy rate with combined metformin–CC treatment.[87–90] By contrast, however, Ng et al[87] noted no improvement in ovulation rate in CC-resistant women after metformin treatment, despite a significant reduction in BMI and serum testosterone and fasting leptin concentrations.

Metformin treatment and ovulation induction with FSH

De Leo et al[88] showed that cycles performed with metformin had significantly fewer follicles measuring > 15 mm in diameter on the day of hCG administration. In addition, hCG was withheld in a significantly lower percentage because of excessive follicular development. Plasma levels of E2 were significantly higher in cycles treated with FSH alone than in those treated with FSH and metformin. Recently, Yarali et al[89] concluded that in CC-resistant PCOS patients with normal glucose tolerance, metformin may restore ovulation with no improvement in insulin resistance. However, it has no significant effect on ovarian response during recombinant FSH treatment.

Metformin treatment and in vitro fertilization

Stadtmauer et al[90] hypothesized that metformin may improve the quality of oocytes retrieved from patients with PCOS by reducing hyperinsulinemia and by modulating the local insulin and IGF levels. They retrospectively analyzed 46 women with CC-resistant PCOS who underwent 60 cycles of *in vitro* fertilization (IVF) embryo transfer with intracytoplasmic sperm injection. In half the cycles, patients received metformin 1000–1500 mg daily, starting with the cycle prior to gonadotropin treatment. The authors found that the metformin cycles were associated with a decrease in the total number of follicles on the day of hCG treatment, with no change in mean follicular diameter. There was no effect on mean number

of oocytes retrieved, although the mean number of mature oocytes and embryos cleaved was higher. Fertilization rates (64 versus 43%) and clinical pregnancy rates (70 versus 30%) were also increased. Metformin led to a modulation of preovulatory follicular fluid IGF levels, with increases in IGF-I and decreases in IGF-BPI.

Contrary to these findings, however, Fedorcsak et al[91] reported that in woman with PCOS who received long-term downregulation and stimulation with recombinant FSH, insulin resistance was not related to either hormone levels or IVF outcome. Obesity was independently associated with relative gonadotropin resistance.

Metformin treatment in pregnancy

In addition to poor conception rates, pregnancy loss rates are high (30–50%) in the first trimester in women with PCOS. Hyperinsulinemia may contribute to the early pregnancy loss by adversely affecting endometrial function and environment. Serum glycodelin, a putative biomarker of endometrial function, is decreased in women with early pregnancy loss. IGF-BPI may also play an important role in pregnancy by facilitating adhesion processes at the feto-maternal interface. Jakubowicz et al[92] studied 48 women with PCOS before and after administration of metformin 500 mg ($n = 26$) or placebo ($n = 22$) three times daily for 4 weeks. OGTT were performed, and serum glycodelin and IGF-BPI were measured during the follicular and CC-induced luteal phases of menses. The authors found a decrease in mean area under the serum insulin curve after glucose administration. In the metformin group, follicular and luteal phase serum glycodelin and IGF-BPI concentrations were significantly increased, as was the luteal phase blood flow in the spiral arteries, as indicated by a 20% decrease in resistance index. Thus, metformin-induced changes may reflect an improved endometrial milieu for the establishment and maintenance of pregnancy.

In a later study, the same group studied 96 women with PCOS who became pregnant during a 4.5 year period, of whom 65 had taken metformin during pregnancy and 31 had not.[93] Early pregnancy loss rate was 8.8% in the metformin group compared with 41.9% in the control group. The authors concluded that metformin administration during pregnancy reduces first trimester pregnancy loss in women with PCOS.

Glueck et al[94] prospectively followed 33 non-diabetic women with PCOS who conceived while taking metformin and gave birth to live babies; 28 took metformin through delivery. These findings were compared with the file data of 39 non-diabetic women with PCOS giving birth to live babies who were not given metformin. One of the 33 pregnancies (3%) achieved during metformin therapy was associated with gestational diabetes mellitus (GDM), compared to eight of 12 (67%) previous pregnancies in the same group achieved without metformin and to 14 of 60 pregnancies (23%) in the control group (total non-metformin GDM rate, 31.9%). Thus, metformin was associated with a 10-fold reduction in GDM in women with PCOS. Importantly, these findings emphasize the possible role of metformin in preventing GDM and overt diabetes in these patients. Metformin does not appear to be teratogenic.[95]

Type 1 diabetes and spontaneous abortions

Epidemiology

Women with Type 1 diabetes are at increased risk of both first trimester spontaneous abortions and major congenital malformations. The magnitude of the risk depends on the degree of metabolic control in the first trimester.[96] Stricter control is necessary to avoid spontaneous abortions than major malformations. At the same time, the timely institution of intensive therapy yields excellent results with regard to spontaneous abortions, whereas the risk of major malformations remains elevated compared to non-diabetic pregnancy even when control is good.[97]

The multicenter Diabetes in Early Pregnancy (DIEP) study, which was designed to answer questions about causes of spontaneous abortion and malformations, found that the risk of spontaneous abortion increased from 9% with good glucose control to 45% when the glycemic level was markedly elevated.[98] Recently, Temple et al[99] showed that among 242 diabetic pregnancies, the poor control group [glycosylated hemoglobin (HbA1c) > 7.5%] had a fourfold higher spontaneous abortion rate than the fair-control group [relative risk (RR) 4.0, 1.2–13.1].

Dorman et al[100] found that improvement in maternal care over the past 30 years in the USA was accompanied by a significant temporal decline in the rates of spontaneous abortion for women with Type 1 diabetes as follows: up to 1969, 26.4%; 1970–1979, 31.0%; 1980–1989, 15.7%; $P < 0.05$. No differences were noted for the non-diabetic partners of Type 1 diabetic men (up to 1969, 4.2%; 1970–1979, 9.5%; 1980–1989, 5.7%; $P > 0.05$). Current rates in Denmark and the UK are about 17.5%.[101,102]

Etiology

Although some authors attribute spontaneous abortions in diabetic pregnancy to early fetal growth delay,[103] others suggest that this finding is probably an artifact of incorrectly estimated ovulation date.[104,105] To clarify this issue,

Ivanisevic et al[106] confirmed the pregnancy duration in their cohort by beta-human chorionic gonadotropin (hCG) measurements within a fortnight of the missed menstrual period. They found that the risk of spontaneous abortion in the Type 1 diabetic pregnancies with delayed embryonal growth was eight times higher than in the diabetic pregnancies with a normal growth pattern, which were matched for gestational age, prepregnancy weight, newborn birthweight and sex. Neither group had fetal malformations. Corresponding HbA1c levels were 9.39±2.37 and 7.3±1.5% (*P* = 0.006), confirming the relationship between embryonal growth, spontaneous abortions and abnormal metabolic control of diabetic pregnancy.

On the basis of *in vitro* findings of an association of high levels of beta-hydroxybutyrate (beta-HOB) and malformations and growth retardation, Jovanovic et al[107] studied these factors in diabetic and non-diabetic women. Although the first trimester beta-HOB levels were significantly higher in the diabetic group, they tended to be lower, not higher, in mothers in both groups who had a malformed infant or pregnancy loss. The biological significance of this trend remains unclear.

There is considerable amount of clinical and experimental evidence suggesting the involvement of free-radical-mediated oxidative processes in the pathogenesis of diabetic complications. These might be contributory factors to conceptus damage, leading to embryonic death and abortion or the appearance of fetal malformations.[108] Another hypothesis claims that the diabetic milieu causes a reduction in phosphatidylinositol turnover, leading to a disruption in the arachidonic acid cascade and resulting in a deficiency of prostaglandins, particularly prostaglandin E2 (PGE2). Accordingly, it was found that yolk sac prostaglandin levels were undetectable in diabetic women prior to elective abortion but high in normal controls.[109]

Other researchers introduced a mouse model of premature programmed cell death to explain adverse pregnancy outcomes in diabetes. In this model, raised glucose concentrations altered gene expression in developing tissues, leading to apoptosis in key progenitor cells of the mouse blastocyst or mouse postimplantation embryos, resulting in abnormal morphogenesis or miscarriage.[110] Although these findings are still preliminary and limited to mouse, the paradigm is supported by examples in other cell systems including human-derived cell lines.[110]

Diabetes and male infertility

Erectile dysfunction

Diabetic men have a higher prevalence of erectile dysfunction (ED) than non-diabetic men. Erectile function is primarily a vascular phenomenon, triggered by neurologic controls and facilitated by appropriate hormonal and psychological components. All of these factors are affected by diabetes. Recent advances in the understanding of the physiology of penile vasculature and its role in male sexual performance have influenced the clinical approach to ED. A thorough history and physical examination are an important aspect of ED management. It is also important to rule out secondary causes such as hypogonadism and thyroid abnormalities.[111]

A large cohort study of 31,027 men between the ages of 53 and 90[112] showed that the age-adjusted RR of ED was 1.32 [95% confidence interval (CI) 1.3–1.4) in those who had diabetes compared to those who did not. These findings remained significant in multivariate regression analyses (Type 1 diabetes: RR = 3.0, 95% CI 1.5–5.9; Type 2 diabetes: RR = 1.3,

1.1–1.5). In men with Type 2 diabetes, the risk of ED increases with increased duration of disease. Another study reported ED in 86.1% of diabetic males, varying in degree from mild in 7.7%, to moderate in 29.4%, to severe in 49.1%.[113] The prevalence of ED was three times higher in the group over 50 years of age compared those under 50 years of age, and was also higher in the group with a long (> 10 years) history of disease compared to those with a history of < 5 years. Men with poor metabolic control were 12.2 times more likely to report ED than men with good metabolic control. Over half the diabetic patients with ED had one or more diabetes-related complication compared with 20.5% of those without ED.

Various treatment modalities have been suggested for ED in diabetic patients. The development of oral medications that inhibit the action of phosphodiesterase in the penile vasculature has revolutionized the treatment of impotence in diabetic men. These drugs are currently the treatment of choice for most patients.[111,114] However, some authors claim that self-intracavernous injection of vasoactive substances is still the sole effective therapeutic modality when ED is severe, and that younger men with Type 2 diabetes treated with low doses of PGE1 are more likely to respond to oral sildenafil (Viagra) than men with Type 1 diabetes or men treated with mixtures of vasoactive drugs.[115]

Retrograde ejaculation

Retrograde ejaculation causes < 2% of all cases of male infertility but it is the leading cause of aspermia,[116] the incidence of which is increased in patients with diabetes because of the presence of diabetic neuropathy. Treatment approaches include drugs such as imipramine or ephedrine,[117] insemination with sperm-rich urine obtained after masturbation, bladder washing after masturbation for sperm retrieval and assisted reproduction technology using the intracytoplasmic sperm injection.

Impaired semen production

In adult rats, long-term diabetes with sustained hyperglycemia leads to significant testicular dysfunction associated with decreased fertility potential,[118] and this may also be true for humans. Garcia-Diez et al,[119] in a study of 80 patients with Type 1 diabetes, found significant alterations in semen parameters and levels of prolactin and testosterone. In all patients, seminal insulin concentrations were higher than serum concentrations. The authors speculated that the hormone freely crosses the blood–testis barrier. The levels of insulin in serum and seminal plasma did not correlate with semen parameters and were not suitable markers of seminal quality.

Padron et al[120] studied 32 adolescents with Type 1 diabetes and aged-matched controls. The Type 1 diabetes group had significantly lower semen volume, motility and morphology, non-significantly lower sperm count, and significantly higher seminal fructose and glucose levels. There were no differences in plasma testosterone levels. No correlation was detected between clinical parameters (age at onset and duration of diabetes and time since first ejaculation), semen parameters, plasma testosterone level, glycemia, or glycosuria.

In another study, subjects with Type 1 or Type 2 neuropathic diabetes showed a highly significant increase in total sperm output and sperm concentration compared to age-matched non-diabetic controls.[121] Sperm motility and semen volume were reduced by about 30 and 60%, respectively. Sperm morphology and quality of sperm motility remained unaffected. The authors suggested that the significant decrease in semen volume could be the result of Leydig cell hyperplasia, which in turn may stimulate spermatogenesis and atonia of the bladder and urethra, resulting in retrograde ejaculation.

Conclusions

Type 1 diabetes is associated with delayed menarche if diabetes is diagnosed prior to 11 or 12 years of age. Menstrual disturbances, such as oligomenorrhea, amenorrhea and polymenorrhea, occurr in 16–30% of women. Diabetes apparently does not affect the ability to conceive, but affected women have fewer pregnancies and fewer births per pregnancy than controls. Suggested mechanisms for infertility in diabetes are hypothalamic–pituitary dysfunction, impaired folliculogenesis, functional deficit in noradrenergic neurons within the hypothalamus, microangiopathy and decreased ovarian SOD activity.

PCOS is a metabolic disorder with widespread systemic effects. The accompanying insulin resistance and hyperinsulinemia mark this syndrome as a prediabetic state, with high incidence of IGT, GDM and overt diabetes. Fertility may also be impaired due to anovulation, impaired implantation and higher rates of spontaneous abortions. All of these effects may be related to the hyperinsulinemia. Lifestyle interventions, such as weight loss and exercise, should be the first line of treatment in women with PCOS. Those who cannot maintain weight loss and those who are not overweight but nevertheless hyperinsulinemic should be considered candidates for metformin treatment. Metformin, an insulin-sensitizing drug, is being evaluated for its potential long-term disease-modifying effect, such as prevention of GDM and diabetes. Its use may also help restore spontaneous ovulation and improve menstrual cyclicity, improve the success rate of induction of and decrease early pregnancy loss. Though not all of these benefits have been proven by evidence-based medicine, given the drug's relatively low rate of side effects and the growing experience with metformin in the treatment of women with PCOS receiving fertility treatment and even those in early pregnancy, we believe, in agreement with others, that metformin should be considered in women with PCOS and insulin resistance.

Although the risk of major malformations remains elevated, despite good to excellent metabolic control, the risk of spontaneous abortions is substantially lower in well-treated women and is comparable to that seen in non-diabetic women. Male diabetic patients may suffer from impotence, retrograde ejaculation and sexual dysfunction, as well as from impaired semen production.

References

1. Drash A. Diabetes mellitus in childhood. *J Pediatr* 1971; **78**:919–41.
2. Post RH. Early menarchial age of diabetic women. *Diabetes* 1962; **11**:287–90.
3. Tattersal RB, Pyke DA. Growth in diabetic children. *Lancet* 1973; **2**:1105–9.
4. Griffin ML, South SA, Yankov VI et al. Insulin-dependent diabetes mellitus and menstrual dysfunction. *Ann Med* 1994; **26**:331–40.
5. Burkart W, Fischer-Guntenhoner E, Standl E, Schneider HP. Menarche, menstrual cycle and fertility in diabetic patients. *Geburtshilfe Frauenheilkd* 1989; **49**:149–54.
6. Yeshaya A, Orvieto R, Dicker D et al. Menstrual characteristics of women suffering from insulin-dependent diabetes mellitus. *Int J Fert Menopausal Stud* 1995; **40**:269–73.
7. Bergquist N. The gonadal function in female diabetics. *Acta Endocrinol* 1954; **15**:3–20.
8. Kjaer K, Hagen C, Sando SH. Epidemiology of menarche and menstrual disturbances in an unselected group of women with insulin-dependent diabetes mellitus compared to controls. *J Clin Endocrinol Metab* 1992; **75**:524–9.
9. Kjaer K, Hagen C, Sando SH, Eshoj O. Infertility and pregnancy outcome in an unselected group of women

with insulin-dependent diabetes mellitus. *Am J Obstet Gynecol* 1992; **166**:1412–18.

10. Pedersen KK, Hagen C, Sando-Pedersen SH, Eshoj O. Infertility and pregnancy outcome in women with insulin-dependent diabetes. An epidemiological study. *Ugeskr Laeger* 1994; **156**:6196–200.

11. Briese V, Muller H. Diabetes mellitus – an epidemiologic study of fertility, contraception and sterility. *Geburtshilfe Frauenheilkd* 1995; **55**:270–4.

12. Peled Y, Rabinerson D, Kaplan B et al. A 'sweet' indication for ovulation induction. *Hum Reprod* 1996; **11**:1403–4.

13. El-Roeiy A, Chen X, Roberts VJ et al. Expression of the genes encoding the insulin-like growth factors (IGF-I and II), the IGF and insulin receptors, and IGF binding proteins 1–6 and the localization of their gene products in normal and polycystic ovary syndrome ovaries. *J Clin Endocrinol Metab* 1994; **78**:1488–96.

14. Samoto T, Maruo T, Ladines-llave C et al. Insulin receptor expression in the follicular and stromal compartments of the human ovary over the course of follicular growth, regression, and artesia. *Endocr J* 1993; **40**:715–26.

15. Nilsson E, Skinner MK. Cellular interactions that control primordial follicle evelopment and folliculogenesis. *J Soc Gynecol Invest* 2001; **8**:S17–S20.

16. Yu N, Roy S. Development of primordial and prenatal follicles from undifferentiated somatic cells in oocytes in the hamster prenatal ovary in vitro: effect of insulin. *Biol Reprod* 1999; **61**:1558–67.

17. McGee EA, Sawetawan C, Bird I et al. The effect of insulin and insulin-like growth factors on the expression of steroidogenic enzymes in a human ovarian thecal-like tumor cell model. *Fert Steril* 1996; **65**:87–93.

18. Willis D, Mason H, Gilling-Smith C, Franks S. Modulation by insulin of follicle stimulating hormone and luteinizing hormone actions in human granulosa cells of normal and polycystic ovaries. *J Clin Endocrinol Metab* 1996; **81**:302–9.

19. Kezele PR, Nilsson EE, Skinner MK. Insulin but not insulin-like growth factor-1 promotes the primordial to primary follicle transition. *Mol Cell Endocrinol* 2002; **192**:37–43.

20. Kalra SP. Mandatory neuropeptide-steroid signaling for the preovulatory luteinizing hormone-releasing hormone discharge. *Endocrinol Rev* 1993; **14**:507–38.

21. Nishihara M, Hiruma H, Kimura F. Interactions between the noradrenergic and opioid peptidergic systems in controlling the electrical activity of luteinizing hormone-releasing hormone pulse generator in ovariectomized rats. *Neuroendocrinology* 1991; **54**:321–4.

22. Dyer RG, Grossmann R, Mansfield S et al. Opioid peptides inhibit noradrenergic transmission in the preoptic area to block LH secretion: evidence from neonatally androgenised rats. *Brain Res Bull* 1988; **20**:721–7.

23. Bitar MS. The role of catecholamines in the etiology of infertility in diabetes mellitus. *Life Sci* 1997; **61**:65–73.

24. Chittenden SJ, Shami SK. Microangiopathy in diabetes mellitus. Causes and prevention and treatment. *Diabetes Res* 1991; **17**:105–14.

25. Mayhan WG. Impairment of endothelium dependent dilatation of the basilary artery during diabetes mellitus. *Brain Res* 1992; **580**:297–302.

26. Hattori Y, Kawasaki H, Kazuhiro A, Kanno M. Superoxide dismutase recovers altered endothelium-dependent relaxation in diabetic rat aorta. *Am J Physiol* 1991; **261**:H1086–H1094.

27. Powers RW, Chambers C, Larsen WJ. Diabetes-mediated decreases in ovarian superoxide dismutase activity are related to blood–follicle barrier and ovulation defects. *Endocrinology* 1996; **137**:3101–10.

28. Franks S. Polycystic ovary syndrome. *N Engl J Med* 1995; **333**:853–61.

29. Adams J, Polson DW, Franks S. Prevalence of polycystic ovaries in women with anovulation and idiopathic hirsutism. *Br Med J Clin Res Ed* 1986; **293**:355–9.

30. Nestler JE, Stovall D, Akhter N et al. Strategies for the use of insulin-sensitizing drugs to treat infertility in women with polycystic ovary syndrome. *Fert Steril* 2002; **77**:209–15.

31. Franks S, Gilling-Smith C, Waston H. Insulin action in the normal and polycystic ovary. *Metab Clin N Am* 1999; **28**:361–78.

32. Ehrmann DA, Barnes RB, Rosenfield RL et al. Prevalence of impaired glucose tolerance and diabetes in women with polycystic ovary syndrome. *Diabetes Care* 1999; **22**:141–6.

33. Nestler JE. Should patients with polycystic ovarian syndrome be treated with metformin? *Hum Reprod* 2002; **17**:1950–3.

34. Poretsky L. On the paradox of insulin-induced hyperandrogenism in insulin-resistant states. *Endocrinol Rev* 1991; **12**:3–13.

35. O'Meara NM, Blackman JD, Ehrman DA et al. Defects in beta-cell function in functional ovarian hyperandrogenism. *J Clin Endocrinol Metab* 1993; **76**:1241–7.

36. Ciaraldi TP, el Roeiy A, Madar Z et al. Cellular mechanisms of insulin resistance in polycystic ovarian syndrome. *J Clin Endocrinol Metab* 1992; **75**:577–83.

37. Dunaif A, Xia J, Book CB et al. Excessive insulin receptor serine phosphorylation in cultured fibroblasts and in skeletal muscle. A potential mechanism for insulin resistance in the polycystic ovary syndrome. *J Clin Invest* 1995; **96**:801–10.

38. Zhang L, Rodriguez H, Ohno S, Miller WL. Serine phosphorylation of human P450c17 increases 17,20-lyase activity: implications for adrenarche and the polycystic ovary syndrome. *Proc Natl Acad Sci USA* 1995; **92**:106–19.

39. Ehrmann DA, Rosenfield RL, Barnes RB. Detection of functional ovarian hyperandrogenism in women with androgen excess. *N Engl J Med* 1992; **327**:157–62.

40. Barbieri RL, Makris A, Randall RW. Insulin stimulates androgen accumulation in incubations of ovarian stroma obtained from women with hyperandrogenism. *J Clin Endocrinol Metab* 1986; **62**:904–10.

41. Barbieri RL, Smith S, Ryan KJ. The role of hyperinsulinemia in the pathogenesis of ovarian hyperandrogenism. *Fert Steril* 1988; **50**:197–212.

42. Nahum R, Thong KJ, Hillier SG. Metabolic regulation of androgen production by human thecal cells in vitro. *Hum Reprod* 1995; **10**:75–81.

43. Willis DS, Watson H, Mason HD et al. Premature response to luteinizing hormone of granulosa cells from anovulatory women with polycystic ovary syndrome: relevance to mechanism of anovulation. *J Clin Endocrinol Metab* 1998; **83**:3984–91.

44. Murray RD, Davison RM, Russell RC. Clinical presentation of PCOS following development of an insulinoma: case report. *Hum Reprod* 2000; **15**:86–8.

45. Suikkari AM, Koivisto VA, Rutanen EM. Insulin regulates the serum levels of low molecular weight insulin-like growth factor-binding protein. *J Clin Endocrinol Metab* 1988; **66**:266–72.

46. Suikkari AM, Koivisto VA, Koistinen R. Dose–response characteristics for suppression of low molecular weight plasma insulin-like growth factor-binding protein by insulin. *J Clin Endocrinol Metab* 1989; **68**:135–40.

47. La Marca A, Morgante G, Paglia T et al. Effects of metformin on adrenal steroidogenesis in women with polycystic ovary syndrome. *Fert Steril* 1999; **72**:985–9.

48. Botwood N, Hamilton-Fairley D, Kiddy D. Sex hormone-binding globulin and female reproductive function. *J Steroid Biochem Mol Biol* 1995; **53**:529–31.

49. Geffner ME, Kaplan SA, Bersch N et al. Persistence of insulin resistance in polycystic ovarian disease after inhibition of ovarian steroid secretion. *Fert Steril* 1986; **45**:327–33.

50. Dunaif A, Green G, Futterweit W, Dobrjansky A. Suppression of hyperandrogenism does not improve peripheral or hepatic insulin resistance in the polycystic ovary syndrome. *J Clin Endocrinol Metab* 1990; **70**:699–704.

51. Chang RJ, Nakamura RM, Judd HL, Kaplan SA. Insulin resistance in nonobese patients with polycystic ovarian disease. *J Clin Endocrinol Metab* 1983 **57**:356–9.

52. Dunaif A, Graf M, Mandeli J et al. Characterization of groups of hyperandrogenemic women with acanthosis nigricans, impaired glucose tolerance, and/or hyperinsulinemia. *J Clin Endocrinol Metab* 1987; **65**:499–507.

53. Dunaif A, Segal KR, Futterweit W, Dobrjansky A. Profound peripheral insulin resistance, independent of obesity, in polycystic ovary syndrome. *Diabetes* 1989; **38**:1165–74.

54. Dunaif A, Segal KR, Shelley DR et al. Evidence for distinctive and intrinsic defects in insulin action in polycystic ovary syndrome. *Diabetes* 1992; **41**:1257–66.

55. Barbieri RL. Induction of ovulation in infertile women with hyperandrogenism and insulin resistance. *Am J Obstet Gynecol* 2000; **183**:1412–18.

56. American Diabetes Association (ADA). Consensus Development Conference on Insulin Resistance. *Diabetes Care* 1998; **21**:310–14.

57. Legro RS, Finegood D, Dunaif A. A fasting glucose to insulin ratio is a useful measure of insulin sensitivity in women with polycystic ovary syndrome. *J Clin Endocrinol Metab* 1998; **83**:2694–8.

58. Dale PO, Tanbo T, Haug E, Abyholm T. The impact of insulin resistance on the outcome of ovulation induction with low-dose follicle stimulating hormone in women with polycystic ovary syndrome. *Hum Reprod* 1998; **13**:567–70.

59. Shepard MK, Balmaceda JP, Leija CG. Relationship of weight to successful induction of ovulation with clomiphene citrate. *Fert Steril* 1979; **32**:641–5.

60. Lobo RA, Gysler M, March CM et al. Clinical and laboratory predictors of clomiphene response. *Fert Steril* 1982; **37**:168–74.

61. Murakawa H, Hasegawa I, Kurabayashi T, Tanaka K. Polycystic ovary syndrome. Insulin resistance and ovulatory responses to clomiphene citrate. *J Reprod Med* 1999; **44**:23–7.

62. Weyer C, Bogardus C, Mott DM, Pratley RE. The natural history of insulin secretory dysfunction and insulin resistance in the pathogenesis of type 2 diabetes mellitus. *J Clin Invest* 1999; **104**:787–94.

63. Bates GW, Whitworth NS. Effects of obesity on sex steroid metabolism. *J Chronic Dis* 1982; **35**:893–6.

64. Pasquali R, Antenucci D, Casimirri F et al. Clinical and hormonal characteristics of obese amenorrheic hyperandrogenic women before and after weight loss. *J Clin Endocrinol Metab* 1989; **68**:173–9.

65. Clark AM, Thornley B, Tomlinson L et al. Weight loss in obese infertile women results in improvement in reproductive outcome for all forms of fertility treatment. *Hum Reprod* 1998; **13**:1502–5.

66. Homburg R. Should patients with polycystic ovarian syndrome be treated with metformin? *Hum Reprod* 2002; **17**:853–6.

67. Seli E, Duleba AJ. Should patients with polycystic ovarian syndrome be treated with metformin? *Hum Reprod* 2002; **17**:2230–6.

68. Meyer F, Ipaktchi M, Clauser H. Specific inhibition of gluconeogenesis by biguanides. *Nature* 1967; **213**:203–4.

69. Wollen N, Bailey CJ. Inhibition of hepatic gluconeogenesis by metformin. Synergism with insulin. *Biochem Pharmacol* 1988; **37**:4353–8.

70. Jacobs DB, Hayes GR, Truglia JA. Effects of metformin on insulin receptor tyrosine kinase activity in rat adipocytes. *Diabetologia* 1986; **29**:798–801.

71. Matthaei S, Hamann A, Klein HH. Association of metformin's effect to increase insulin-stimulated glucose transport with potentiation of insulin-induced translocation of glucose transporters from intracellular pool to plasma membrane in rat adipocytes. *Diabetes* 1991; **40**:850–7.

72. Bailey CJ. Metformin: an update. *Gen Pharmacol* 1993; 24:1299–309.

73. Abbasi F, Kamath V, Rizvi AA. Results of a placebo-controlled study of the metabolic effects of the addition of metformin to sulfonylurea-treated patients. Evidence for a central role of adipose tissue. *Diabetes Care* 1997; 20:1863–9.

74. Attia GR, Rainey WE, Carr BR. Metformin directly inhibits androgen production in human thecal cells. *Fert Steril* 2001; 76:517–24.

75. Crave C, Fimbel S, Lejeune H et al. Effects of diet and metformin administration on sex hormone-binding globulin, androgens, and insulin in hirsute and obese women. *J Clin Endocrinol Metab* 1995; 80:2057–62.

76. Glueck CJ, Wang P, Fontaine R et al. Metformin-induced resumption of normal menses in 39 of 43 (91%) previously amenorrheic women with the polycystic ovary syndrome. *Metabolism* 1999; 48:511–19.

77. Kolodziejczyk B, Duleba AJ, Spaczynski RZ, Pawelczyk L. Metformin therapy decreases hyperandrogenism and hyperinsulinemia in women with polycystic ovary syndrome. *Fert Steril* 2000; 73:1149–54.

78. La Marca A, Egbe TO, Morgante G et al. Metformin treatment reduces ovarian cytochrome P-450c17alpha response to human chorionic gonadotrophin in women with insulin resistance-related polycystic ovary syndrome. *Hum Reprod* 2000; 15:21–3.

79. Nestler JE, Jakubowicz DJ. Decreases in ovarian cytochrome P450c17 alpha activity and serum free testosterone after reduction of insulin secretion in polycystic ovary syndrome. *N Engl J Med* 1996; **335**:617–23.

80. Koivunen RM, Morin-Papunen LC, Ruokonen A et al. Ovarian steroidogenic response to human chorionic gonadotrophin in obese women with polycystic ovary syndrome: effect of metformin. *Hum Reprod* 2001; 16:2546–51.

81. Vrbikova J, Hill M, Starka L, Vondra K. Prediction of the effect of metformin treatment in patients with polycystic ovary syndrome. *Gynecol Obstet Invest* 2002; 53:100–4.

82. Baysal B, Batukan M, Batukan C. Biochemical and body weight changes with metformin in polycystic ovary syndrome. *Clin Exp Obstet Gynecol* 2001; 28:212–14.

83. Fleming R, Hopkinson ZE, Wallace AM et al. Ovarian function and metabolic factors in women with oligomenorrhea treated with metformin in a randomized double blind placebo-controlled trial. *J Clin Endocrinol Metab* 2002; 87:569–74.

84. Glueck CJ, Wang P, Fontaine R et al. Metformin to restore normal menses in oligo-amenorrheic teenage girls with polycystic ovary syndrome (PCOS). *J Adolesc Health* 2001; 29:160–9.

85. Velazquez E, Acosta A, Mendoza SG. Menstrual cyclicity after metformin therapy in polycystic ovary syndrome. *Obstet Gynecol* 1997; **90**:392–5.

86. Nestler JE, Jakubowicz DJ, Evans WS, Pasquali R. Effects of metformin on spontaneous and clomiphene-induced ovulation in the polycystic ovary syndrome. *N Engl J Med* 1998; **338**:1876–80.

87. Ng EH, Wat NM, Ho PC. Effects of metformin on ovulation rate, hormonal and metabolic profiles in women with clomiphene-resistant polycystic ovaries: a randomized, double-blinded placebo-controlled trial. *Hum Reprod* 2001; 16:1625–31.

88. De Leo V, la Marca A, Ditto A et al. Effects of metformin on gonadotropin-induced ovulation in women with polycystic ovary syndrome. *Fert Steril* 1999; 72:282–5.

89. Yarali H, Yildiz BO, Demirol A et al. Co-administration of metformin during rFSH treatment in patients with clomiphene citrate-resistant polycystic ovarian syndrome: a prospective randomized trial. *Hum Reprod* 2002; 17:289–94.

90. Stadtmauer LA, Toma SK, Riehl RM, Talbert LM. Metformin treatment of patients with polycystic ovary syndrome undergoing in vitro fertilization improves outcomes and is associated with modulation of the insulin-like growth factors. *Fert Steril* 2001; 75:505–9.

91. Fedorcsak P, Dale PO, Storeng R et al. The impact of obesity and insulin resistance on the outcome of IVF or ICSI in women with polycystic ovarian syndrome. *Hum Reprod* 2001; 16:1086–91.

92. Jakubowicz DJ, Seppala M, Jakubowicz S et al. Insulin reduction with metformin increases luteal phase serum glycodelin and insulin-like growth factor-binding protein 1 concentrations and enhances uterine vascularity and blood flow in the polycystic ovary syndrome. *J Clin Endocrinol Metab* 2001; 86:1126–33.

93. Jakubowicz DJ, Iuorno MJ, Jakubowicz S et al. Effects of metformin on early pregnancy loss in the polycystic ovary syndrome. *J Clin Endocrinol Metab* 2002; 87:524–29.

94. Glueck CJ, Wang P, Kobayashi S et al. Metformin therapy throughout pregnancy reduces the development of gestational diabetes in women with polycystic ovary syndrome. *Fert Steril* 2002; 77:520–5.

95. Glueck CJ, Phillips H, Cameron D et al. Continuing metformin throughout pregnancy in women with polycystic ovary syndrome appears to safely reduce first-trimester spontaneous abortion: a pilot study. *Fert Steril* 2001; 75:46–52.

96. Greene MF. Spontaneous abortions and major malformations in women with diabetes mellitus. *Semin Reprod Endocrinol* 1999; 17:127–36.

97. Pregnancy outcomes in the Diabetes Control and Complications Trial. *Am J Obstet Gynecol* 1996; **174**:1343–53.

98. Mills JL, Simpson JL, Driscoll SG et al, the National Institutes of Child Health and Human Development – Diabetes in Early Pregnancy Study: incidence of spontaneous abortion among normal and insulin-dependent diabetic women whose pregnancies were identified within 21 days of conception. *N Engl J Med* 1988; **319**:1617–23.

99. Temple R, Aldridge V, Greenwood R et al. Association between outcome of pregnancy and glycaemic control in early pregnancy in type 1 diabetes: population based study. *Br Med J* 2002; **325**:1275–6.

100. Dorman JS, Burke JP, McCarthy BJ et al. Temporal trends in spontaneous abortion associated with type 1 diabetes. *Diabetes Res Clin Pract* 1999; **43**:41–7.

101. Lorenzen T, Pociot F, Johannesen J et al. A population-based survey of frequencies of self-reported spontaneous and induced abortions in Danish women with type 1 diabetes mellitus. Danish IDDM Epidemiology and Genetics Group. *Diabet Med* 1999 **16**:472–6.

102. Casson IF, Clarke CA, Howard CV et al. Outcomes of pregnancy in insulin dependent diabetic women: results of a five-year population cohort study. *Br Med J* 1997; **315**:275–8.

103. Pedersen JF, Molsted-Pedersen L, Lebech PE. Is the early growth delay in the diabetic pregnancy accompanied by a delay in placental development? *Acta Obstet Gynecol Scand* 1986; **65**:675–7.

104. Steel JM, Wu PS, Johnstone FD et al. Does early growth delay occur in diabetic pregnancy? *Br J Obstet Gynaecol* 1995; **102**:224–7.

105. Hieta-Heikurainen H, Teramo K. Comparison of menstrual history and basal body temperature with early fetal growth by ultrasound in diabetic pregnancy. *Acta Obstet Gynecol Scand* 1989; **68**:457–9.

106. Ivanisevic M, Bukovic D, Starcevic V et al. Influence of hyperglycemia on early embryonal growth in IDDM pregnant women. *Coll Antropol* 1999; **23**:183–8.

107. Jovanovic L, Metzger BE, Knopp RH et al. The Diabetes in Early Pregnancy Study: beta-hydroxybutyrate levels in type 1 diabetic pregnancy compared with normal pregnancy. NICHD – Diabetes in Early Pregnancy Study Group (DIEP). National Institute of Child Health and Development. *Diabetes Care* 1998; **21**:1978–84.

108. Damasceno DC, Volpato GT, de Mattos Paranhos Calderon I, Cunha Rudge MV. Oxidative stress and diabetes in pregnant rats. *Anim Reprod Sci* 2002; **72**:235–44.

109. Schoenfeld A, Erman A, Warchaizer S et al. Yolk sac concentration of prostaglandin E2 in diabetic pregnancy: further clues to the etiology of diabetic embryopathy. *Prostaglandins* 1995; **50**:121–6.

110. Moley KH. Hyperglycemia and apoptosis: mechanisms for congenital malformations and pregnancy loss in diabetic women. *Trends Endocr Metab* 2001; **12**: 78–82.

111. Dey J, Shepherd MD. Evaluation and treatment of erectile dysfunction in men with diabetes mellitus. *Mayo Clin Proc* 2002; **77**:276–82.

112. Bacon CG, Hu FB, Giovannucci E et al. Association of type and duration of diabetes with erectile dysfunction in a large cohort of men. *Diabetes Care* 2002; **25**:1458–63.

113. el-Sakka AI, Tayeb KA. Erectile dysfunction risk factors in noninsulin dependent diabetic Saudi patients. *J Urol* 2003; **169**:1043–7.

114. Boulton AJ, Selam JL, Sweeney M, Ziegler D. Sildenafil citrate for the treatment of erectile dysfunction in men with type II diabetes mellitus. *Diabetologia* 2001; **44**:1296–301.

115. Perimenis P, Markou S, Gyftopoulos K et al. Switching from long-term treatment with self-injections to oral sildenafil in diabetic patients with severe erectile dysfunction. *Eur Urol* 2002; **41**:387–91.

116. Silva PD, Larson KM, Van Every MJ, Silva DE. Successful treatment of retrograde ejaculation with sperm recovered from bladder washings. A report of two cases. *J Reprod Med* 2000; **45**:957–60.

117. Gilja I, Parazajder J, Radej M et al. Retrograde ejaculation and loss of emission: possibilities of conservative treatment. *Eur Urol* 1994; **25**:226–8.

118. Cameron DF, Rountree J, Schultz RE et al. Sustained hyperglycemia results in testicular dysfunction and reduced fertility potential in BBWOR diabetic rats. *Am J Physiol* 1990; **259**:E881–E889.

119. Garcia-Diez LC, Corrales Hernandez JJ, Hernandez-Diaz J et al. Semen characteristics and diabetes mellitus: significance of insulin in male infertility. *Arch Androl* 1991; **26**:119–28.

120. Padron RS, Dambay A, Suarez R, Mas J. Semen analyses in adolescent diabetic patients. *Acta Diabetol Lat* 1984; **21**:115–21.

121. Ali ST, Shaikh RN, Siddiqi NA, Siddiqi PQ. Semen analysis in insulin-dependent/non-insulin-dependent diabetic men with/without neuropathy. *Arch Androl* 1993; **30**:47–54.

Index

abortions, spontaneous, type 1 diabetes 614–15
accelerated starvation   32
ADA *see* American Diabetes Association
administrative issues, legal aspects   570–3
adrenomedullin   43
AGA infants, follow-up studies   320
age, GDM risk factor   67–8, 75
aging, and carbohydrate metabolism 597–8
alcohol, GDM risk factor   76
aldose reductase inhibitors (ARI), embryopathy   269–70
algorithms
   CGM   400
   insulin   383–4
Allen, FM   2
alpha-glucosidase inhibitors   380, 383–4
alpha-thalassemia trait, GDM risk factor 71
alternative approaches, GDM   535–6
American Diabetes Association (ADA), classification   162–3
amino acid metabolism
   fetus   215–17
   metabolic adaptation, maternal   54
amino acid transfer, placenta   134–5
amino acid uptake
   fetus   214–15
   placenta   214–15
aminophylline, fetal lung maturity   283
amniocentesis, legal aspects   567
amniotic fluid   148–57
   C-peptide   151–5
   glucose intolerance   154–5
   insulin   151–5
   volume homeostasis   149–51
animal models, fetal growth manipulation 225–6
animals   90–112
   STZ(streptozotocin)-induced diabetes 90–101
   type 1 diabetes, genetically determined 102–3
   type 2 diabetes, genetically determined 103–7
antenatal care, legal aspects   565–7
antibody formation, anti-insulin, pregnancy 362, 363
antioxidants
   embryopathy   270–1
   nutritional management   352–3
apoptosis, pre-implantation embryopathy 244–5
arachidonic acid, embryopathy   269–70
ARI *see* aldose reductase inhibitors

atherosclerosis, HRT   600
autonomy, ethical principle   556–7

b-adrenergic agonists, fetal lung maturity 283
Banting, F   2
BB rats, type 1 diabetes, genetically determined   102
benificence, ethical principle   555–6, 557
Bennewitz, HG   5–7
beta-cell function   43–4
biguanides   380, 382–3, 386
   infertility   611–14
binding precedent, legal aspects   563–4
biphasic ST events   422–3
blood glucose, screening strategies   172–6
blood lipids, HRT   601
blood pressure
   GDM risk factor   75
   see also hypertensive disorders
BMI *see* body mass index
body composition, HRT   602
body mass index (BMI)
   GDM risk factor   69–70
   nutritional management   343–5
Brandstrup, E   10, 11
breastfeeding   302–3

C-peptide, amniotic fluid   151–5
C-reactive protein (CRP), cardiovascular risk 601
C57 BIKS lepr^{db+} heterozygotes, type 2 diabetes, genetically determined 103–4
C57BL/6J mice, type 2 diabetes, genetically determined   104–5
caesarian section, GDM risk factor   74
carbohydrate metabolism
   and aging   597–8
   HRT   597–8, 599
   menopause effects   598–9
   metabolic adaptation, maternal   50–4
carbohydrate supply and metabolism, fetus 203–12
carbohydrates, dietary
   fats, dietary   350–1
   high-fat/low-carbohydrate diet   347–8
cardiovascular risk
   CRP   601
   HRT   600, 601
care quality *see* quality of care
case law, legal aspects   564
catecholamines, infertility   608
caudal regression syndrome   405–8
CEA *see* cost-effectiveness analyses
certification of diabetes, legal aspects   572

Cesarean delivery
   benefits   436–9
   ethical issues   561
   vs. vaginal delivery   513
CGM *see* continuous glucose monitoring
chlorpropamide   382
chromium deficiency   295
chronic hyperinsulinemia   101
classification
   ADA   162–3
   diabetic pregnancy   158–67
   diabetic retinopathy   475–6
   GDM   183–4
   Japan Diabetes Society   163–6
   oral hypoglycemic agents   380–4
   Pedersen Classification   160–1
   simple   161
   White Classification   16–20, 158–60
   WHO   161–2
clinical research, monitoring   423–6
coagulation system, HRT   601
colon, small left   300–1
congenital abnormalities, ultrasound assessment   405–8
congenital disability, legal aspects   569
congenital malformations, GDM   73, 83–4
consent to sterilization, legal aspects   575
continuous glucose monitoring (CGM) 395–400
   preventing adverse fetal outcome   401
contraception   589–96
   combination   590–2
   GDM, prior history   592
   hormonal   589–93
   intrauterine devices   593–4
   long-acting hormonal   592–3
   progestin-only   590–2
Copenhagen Centre   23–8
   follow-up   193–4
coronary heart disease   460–2
cortisol   41
cost analysis   529–38
   CEA   530–1
   GDM   533–7
   preconception care   531–3
   pregnancy care   529–30
cost-effectiveness analyses (CEA)   530–1
cost of care, legal aspects   572
CRP *see* C-reactive protein
cytoplasmic islet cell autoantibodies, GDM 114–17

databases   519–28
   developments   519–20
   evidence-based medicine   520–2
   OBSQID   520–7

delivery
  cervical ripeness 448–9
  Cesarean benefits 436–9
  Cesarean ethical issues 561
  Cesarean vs. vaginal 513
  epidural analgesia 450
  GDM 334–5
  induction 447–54, 512–13
  labor management 448–9
  legal aspects 566–8
  macrosomia 447–54
  mode 430–41
  timing 430–41, 447–54, 457–8
  see also labor
depomedroxyprogesterone acetate (DMPA)
  592–3
detection strategies, GDM 168–82
developing countries, GDM 183–90
developmental studies, growth, children
  322–6
DiabCare 540–6
diabetes
  following GDM 191–200
  predictive factors 194–6
Diabetes in Pregnancy Center (DPC) 30–7
  IGM 311
  obesity 307–8
diabetic ketoacidosis (DKA) 495–501, 510
  biochemical changes 496–8
  diagnosis 498
  fatal effects 498–9
  pathogenesis 496–8
  precipitating factors 495–6
  prevalence 495–6
  prognosis 495–6
  treatment 499–500
diabetic nephropathy 486–94
  hypertension 487, 490
  pathophysiology 486–7
  pregnancy 487–90
  pregnancy outcome 490–2
diabetic retinopathy 165–6, 367–8, 475–85
  classification 475–6
  management recommendations 481–2
  pathogenesis 476–9
  pregnancy impact 479–81
  proliferative retinopathy 477–9
  treatment 481
diabetologic education 578–88
  informative stage 583–5
  objectives 579, 580–1
  process 581–2
  protocol, Vall d'Hebron Hospital 583–8
  reaction to diagnosis 579–80
  support stage 587–8
  training stage 585–7
diagnosis
  GDM 185–9, 330–1, 514–15, 533–7
  reaction to 579–80
diagnostic criteria
  GDM 163–6
  impact 179

diagnostic strategies, GDM 168–82
diet
  diabetologic education 585–6
  evidence-based medicine 511
  see also nutritional management
dietary control, legal aspects 566–7
DKA *see* diabetic ketoacidosis
DM-1A, GDM 120–2
DMPA *see* depomedroxyprogesterone
  acetate
DPC *see* Diabetes in Pregnancy Center
driving, legal aspects 571–2
Duncan, JM 8
dynamic assessment
  fetal well-being 410–13
  ultrasound assessment 410–13

ECG, fetal, monitoring 421–3
ED *see* erectile dysfunction
education, diabetologic *see* diabetologic
  education
EFM *see* electronic fetal monitoring
electronic fetal monitoring (EFM) 419
embryopathy
  advances 262–75
  antioxidants 270–1
  arachidonic acid 269–70
  ARI 269–70
  clinical advances 262–75
  clinical studies 263–6
  experimental advances 262–75
  experimental studies 267–70
  folic acid supplementation 266–7
  fuel-mediated teratogenesis 263–4
  implications 263–6
  and maternal diabetes 240–52
  myoinositol 268–9
  pathophysiology 262–3
  polyol pathway 268–9
  pre-implantation *see* pre-implantation
    embryopathy
  signal transduction 268
  STZ(streptozotocin)-induced diabetes
    95–6
  unifying theory 270, 271
employment, legal aspects 571
endocrine pancreas development, fetus
  226–7
energy expenditure, maternal 55–7
energy requirements, nutritional
  management 342
energy restriction, nutritional management
  343–5
epidemiology, GDM 64–89
epidural analgesia 450
Erb's palsy 457, 510
erectile dysfunction (ED) 615–16
erythremia, neonatal 295–6
essential hypertension 463–4
estrogen 40–1
ethical issues 554–62
  Cesarean delivery 561

ethical principles 555–7
ethics defined 554
fetus 557–61
framework 554–7
etiology
  hypomagnesemia 294
  neonatal hypocalcemia 293
evidence-based medicine 508–18
  databases 520–2
  diet 511
  exercise 513
  GDM 514–15
  glucose monitoring 513–14
  induction 512–13
  insulin 511–12
  screening practices 512
  ultrasound assessment 511
examination fraud, legal aspects 573
exercise, evidence-based medicine 513
expectant management, vs. induction
  451–2
expert witnesses, legal aspects 576

facilitated anabolism 32–4
family history, GDM risk factor 72–3
fasting plasma glucose (FPG), screening
  strategy 173–5
fat intake, GDM risk factor 72
fats, dietary
  carbohydrates, dietary 350–1
  high-fat/low-carbohydrate diet 347–8
  metabolic effects 348–50
  nutritional management 348–50
fatty acids transfer, placenta 135–6
FBS *see* fetal blood sampling
fertilization *see* infertility
fetal blood sampling (FBS) 420
fetal body composition 450–1
fetal ECG, monitoring 421–3
fetal effects, insulin lispro 364–5
fetal growth, maternal metabolism 57–60
fetal hyperinsulinemia, macrosomia 100–1
fetal-maternal transfer, placenta 131–7
fetal maturity 276–88
  confirmation 286
  lung maturity evaluation 278–82
  lung maturity induction 282–6
  lung maturity pathophysiology 277–8
fetal overgrowth 433–5
  ultrasound assessment 435–6
fetal well-being, ultrasound assessment
  410–13
fetus
  amino acid metabolism 215–17
  amino acid uptake 214–15
  carbohydrate supply and metabolism
    203–12
  CGM 401
  dependent moral status 558–61
  endocrine pancreas development 226–7
  ethical issues 557–61
  glucogenesis 211–12

fetus (*Contd*)
  glucose supply responses 209
  glucose transport 204–12
  glycemic exposure 346–7
  glycogen metabolism 209
  growth factors and islet development
    228–31
  growth regulation 222–39
  hypoxia 254–7
  IGF-1 209
  independent moral status 558
  insulin secretion 209–10
  islet development 227–31
  legal aspects 569
  lipid metabolism 212–14
  metabolic rate and nutrient supply
    202–3
  mineral metabolism 253–61
  moral status 558–61
  nutrient delivery 201–21
  nutrient metabolism 201–21
  oxygenation 253–61
  pancreas 231–5
  protein synthesis 216–17
  shoulder dystocia 436–9
  transcription factors and islet development
    227–8
  VEGF 229
fibroblast growth factor-4 (FGF-4),
  pre-implantation embryopathy 247–8
flow velocity waveforms (FVW) 411–13
fluorescence polarization, fetal lung maturity
  281
folic acid supplementation, embryopathy
  266–7
follow-up
  GDM 185–9, 191–200
  growth, children 320–2
  postpartum maternal 335
forensic matters, legal aspects 569–70
FPG *see* fasting plasma glucose
Freinkel concepts, metabolic regulation
  32–5
Freinkel, Professor Norbert 30–8
frequency, GDM 184
fuel-mediated teratogenesis, embryopathy
  263–4
FVW *see* flow velocity waveforms

GAD *see* glutamic acid decarboxylase
GDM *see* gestational diabetes mellitus
genetic markers, GDM 118–19
genetics
  GDM 44–5
  GDM risk factor 79–80
gestational diabetes mellitus (GDM) 4–5,
  19, 28
  adrenomedullin 43
  alternative approaches 535–6
  beta-cell function 43–4
  classification 183–4
  congenital malformations 73, 83–4

contraception 592
cost analysis 533–7
defined 64, 163–6, 183–4
delivery 334–5
detection strategies 168–82
developing countries 183–90
developmental studies 322–6
diabetes following 191–200
diagnosis 185–9, 330–1, 514–15, 533–7
diagnostic criteria 163–6
diagnostic strategies 168–82
DM-1A 120–2
epidemiology 64–89
evidence-based medicine 514–15
follow-up 185–9, 191–200
frequency 184
genetic factors 79–80
genetic markers 118–19
genetics 44–5
glycemic control 546–50
hormonal effect 40–3
hypertensive disorders 84
and hypertensive disorders 466–7
IAA 114–17
IGM 80–3
immunology 44–5, 113–25
insulin resistance 39–40
insulin sensitivity 39–40, 56–60
insulin signaling system 45–6
Japan Diabetes Society 163–6
management 330–9
monitoring 331–4
multiple pregnancies 75, 78–9, 502–3,
  505–6
NIDDM 85
pathogenesis 39–49
pathophysiology 184
PCOS 64, 71–2, 77–8
cf. PGDM 321–2
predictive factors 194–6
pregestational diabetes 335–8
prevalence 64–6
racial distribution 64–6
recurrence 80
risk factors 66–77, 184–5
screening strategies 169–76
therapy 331–4
TNF-a 43
glimeperide 382
glucogenesis, fetus 211–12
glucose
  fetal growth 318–19
  pre-implantation embryopathy 242–3,
    246–7
glucose control, intrapartum 511
glucose intolerance, amniotic fluid 154–5
glucose metabolism
  pre-implantation embryopathy 246–7
  STZ(streptozotocin)-induced diabetes
    91–2
glucose monitoring 394–403
  continuous 395–400

evidence-based medicine 513–14
  MiniMed CGM system 395–400
  postprandial 394–5
glucose requirements, postpartum 375
glucose screening tests 172–7
glucose toxicity, postprandial hyperglycemia
  359–60
glucose transport 53–4
  fetus 204–12
  gestational changes 206
  kinetics 205–6
  placenta 132–4, 204–12
glucose treatment, labor 374–5
glucose uptake 206–12
glucose utilization 206–12
  kinetics 207–9
GLUT *see* glucose transport
glutamic acid decarboxylase (GAD) 117–18
glyburide 382, 389–90
glycated serum proteins, glycemic control
  550
glycemia, normoglycemia 368–9
glycemic control
  monitoring 546–50
  nutritional management 345–6
  short-term neonatal complications
    301–2
glycemic exposure, fetus 346–7
glycemic response, factors influencing 347
glycogen metabolism
  fetus 209
  STZ(streptozotocin)-induced diabetes
    91–2
Goto-Kakizaki (GK) rats, type 2 diabetes,
  genetically determined 105–7
growth abnormalities, ultrasound assessment
  408–10
growth, children 317–29
  developmental studies 322–6
  follow-up studies 320–2
  postnatal development 320–2
growth factors and islet development, fetus
  228–31
growth, fetal overgrowth 433–5
growth, intrauterine 317–20
  low birthweight 319
growth regulation
  animal models 225–6
  fetus 222–39
  placenta 140–2
guidelines, fetal maturity
  National Institute of Health (NIH) 284
  Royal College of Obstetricians and
    Gynaecologists 285

HbA1c, glycemic control 549–50
HDL *see* high-density lipoprotein
height, GDM risk factor 70
hematologic disorders, other 297
high-density lipoprotein (HDL) 55
histocompatibility leukocytic antigen (HLA)
  79

history
  1940–1980; 24–6
  1980–present 26–8
  diabetic pregnancy 1–12
HLA *see* histocompatibility leukocytic
  antigen
hormonal contraception 589–93
hormonal effect, pregnancy 40–3
hormone replacement therapy (HRT)
  597–605
  atherosclerosis 600
  blood lipids 601
  body composition 602
  carbohydrate metabolism 597–8, 599
  cardiovascular risk 600, 601
  coagulation system 601
  delivery 601–2
  lipid metabolism 601
  obesity 602
  vascular reactivity 600–1
hPL *see* human placental lactogen
HRT *see* hormone replacement therapy
human placental lactogen (hPL) 42
  multiple pregnancies 503
hyperbilirubinemia, neonatal 296–7
hyperglycemia
  glucose toxicity 359–60
  placenta 131
  pregnancy 367
hyperinsulinemia, fetal *see* fetal
  hyperinsulinemia
hyperinsulinemic insulin resistance
  609–11
hypertension
  essential hypertension 463–4
  nephropathy 487, 490
hypertensive complications, pregestational
  diabetes 467–9
hypertensive disorders 460–74
  epidemiological studies 466
  fetal origin of adult disease 460–2
  GDM 84
  and GDM 466–7
  IGF-1 460–2
  IGM 460–2
  physiological studies 466–7
  see also blood pressure
hyperviscosity, neonatal 295–6
hyperzincuria 294–5
hypoglycemia
  detection 400–1
  maternal 510
  neonatal *see* neonatal hypoglycemia
hypoglycemic agents, oral *see* oral
  hypoglycemic agents
hypoglycemic attacks, legal aspects 566
hypomagnesemia, neonatal *see* neonatal
  hypomagnesemia
hypothalamic-pituitary-gonadal dysfunction,
  infertility 607–8
hypoxia
  consequences 255–7

fetus 254–7
  see also oxygenation

IAA *see* islet cell autoantibodies
iatrogenic prematurity 256
  lung maturity (fetal) 432–3
IDF *see* International Diabetes Federation
IFCC *see* International Federation of Clinical
  Chemistry
IGF-1 *see* insulin-like growth factor-1
IGM *see* impaired glucose tolerance
immunology
  cytoplasmic islet cell autoantibodies
    114–17
  GAD 117–18
  GDM 44–5, 113–25
  IAA 114
impaired glucose tolerance (IGM)
  and diabetes mellitus 309–13
  DPC 311
  following GDM 191–200
  GDM risk factor 80–3
  hypertensive disorders 460–2
  long-term implications 309–13
  implications
    long-term 305–16
    neonates 289–304
    short-term 289–304
in vitro fertilization, metformin 613
induction
  clinical trials 452
  confounders 448–51
  evidence-based medicine 512–13
  vs. expectant management 451–2
  labor 447–54, 512–13
infertility 606–21
  biguanides 611–14
  insulin resistance 609–14
  male 615–17
  mechanisms 607–8
  metformin 611–14
  PCOS 609–14
inositol, fetal lung maturity 283
insulin
  amniotic fluid 151–5
  discovery 2
  evidence-based medicine 511–12
  fetal growth 318
  infertility 608
  prior to discovery 2–4
  sensitivity 39–40, 56–60
  trophic actions 222–5
insulin administration, diabetologic
  education 586–7
insulin algorithms 383–4
insulin analogs
  risks, theoretical 364–8
  see also insulin lispro
insulin infusion pumps 372–4
insulin-like growth factor-1 (IGF-1) 140–2
  fetus 209
  hypertensive disorders 460–2

islet size 229–31
  trophic actions 222–5
insulin lispro
  effects on mother 365–8
  fetal effects 364–5
  pregnancy 362
  see also insulin analogs
insulin requirements
  postpartum 375
  pregnancy 360–1, 369–72
insulin resistance 39–40
  clinical consequences 465
  hyperinsulinemic 609–11
  infertility 609–14
  mechanisms of action 464–5
  PCOS 609–14
  and pregnancy 465–70
  syndrome 462–5
insulin secretion, fetus 209–10
insulin signaling system
  GDM 45–6
  PKC isoenzymes 105–7
insulin therapy
  glucose toxicity 359–60
  infusion pumps 372–4
  labor 374–5
  postprandial hyperglycemia 359–60
  pregnancy 359–78
intellectual development 320–2
International Diabetes Federation (IDF)
  31
International Federation of Clinical
  Chemistry (IFCC), glycemic control
  549–50
iron stores, GDM risk factor 75
iron transfer, placenta 131–2
islet cell autoantibodies (IAA) 114
islet development, fetus 227–31
islet size, IGF-1 229–31

Japan Diabetes Society, classification
  163–6
Joslin Clinic 13–21
Joslin, Dr Elliot 2, 9–10, 13
Joslin's Diabetes Mellitus 18–19
Juan A Fernández Hospital 187–9
jurisdictions, different, legal aspects 564

ketoacidosis *see* diabetic ketoacidosis

labor
  glucose treatment 374–5
  induction 447–54, 512–13
  insulin therapy 374–5
  legal aspects 566–8
  management 448–9
  monitoring in 418–29
  see also delivery
Laurence, Dr Robin 2
LDL *see* low-density lipoprotein
lecithin-sphingomyelin (LS) ratio, fetal lung
  maturity 278–80

legal aspects 563–77
  administrative issues 570–3
  amniocentesis 567
  antenatal care 565–7
  binding precedent 563–4
  case law 564
  certification of diabetes 572
  congenital disability 569
  consent to sterilization 575
  cost of care 572
  delivery 566–8
  dietary control 566–7
  driving 571–2
  employment 571
  examination fraud 573
  expert witnesses 576
  fetus 569
  forensic matters 569–70
  hypoglycemic attacks 566
  involvement, other specialists 573–4
  jurisdictions, different 564
  labor 566–8
  macrosomia 565
  mental illness 574–5
  post-mortem examinations 570
  precedent, legal 563–4
  public assistance grants 570–1
  related medical matters 573–6
  research, involuntary participation
    575–6
  respiratory distress syndrome 569
  screening 565–6
  standard of proof 564
  statute law 564
  sterilization 575
  stillbirth 568
leptin 42–3
  intrauterine growth 319
  molecular pathways 140
  placenta 138–42
  production regulation 139–40
  synthesis 138–9
lipid metabolism
  fetus 212–14
  HRT 601
  metabolic adaptation, maternal 54–5
  placenta 212–13
  STZ(streptozotocin)-induced diabetes
    92–3
lipids, fetal lung maturity 281
lipids transfer, placenta 135–6
long-term consequences
  intrauterine exposures 35–6
  nutritional management 353
long-term implications 305–16
  IGM 309–13
  neurodevelopment 313–14
  obesity 305–9
  psychological development 313–14
low-density lipoprotein (LDL) 55
LS ratio see lecithin-sphingomyelin ratio

lung maturity (fetal)
  evaluation 278–82
  iatrogenic prematurity 432–3
  induction 282–6
  macrosomia 457–8
  pathophysiology 277–8

Macleod, JJR 2
macrosomia 408–10
  defined 408
  defining 442–3
  delivery 447–54
  fetal hyperinsulinemia 100–1
  follow-up studies 320
  GDM risk factor 73
  legal aspects 565
  lung maturation 457–8
  management 455–9
  NOD mice 102–3
  obstetric management 455–8
  prevention 442–6
  risk 401
  shoulder dystocia 456–7
  sonographic criteria 410
  stillbirth 455–6
  types 442–3
magnesium see neonatal hypomagnesemia
management databases, pregnancy
  519–28
maternal-fetal transfer, placenta 131–7
maternal metabolic adaptation see metabolic
  adaptation, maternal
menarche, delayed 606–7
menopause effects, carbohydrate metabolism
  598–9
menstrual irregularities 606–7
mental illness, legal aspects 574–5
metabolic adaptation, maternal 50–63
  amino acid metabolism 54
  carbohydrate metabolism 50–4
  energy expenditure, maternal 55–7
  fetal growth 57–60
  lipid metabolism 54–5
  weight gain, maternal 55–7
metabolic control, diabetologic education
  586
metabolic monitoring, pregnancy 337–8
metabolic rate and nutrient supply, fetus
  202–3
metabolic regulation, Freinkel concepts
  32–5
metabolism, carbohydrates, fetus 203–12
metformin 382–3, 386, 389, 390
  endocrine effects 612
  infertility 611–14
  metabolic effects 612
  ovulation 612–13
  pregnancy 613–14
  in vitro fertilization 613
microalbuminaria 469–70, 490–2
microangiopathy, infertility 608

mineral metabolism
  chromium deficiency 295
  fetus 257–61
  hyperzincuria 294–5
  see also neonatal hypo…
MiniMed CGM system 395–400
Minkowski, Oscar 2
mitochondria, placenta 137–8
monitoring
  CGM 395–400
  clinical research 423–6
  fetal ECG 421–3
  GDM 331–4
  glucose 394–403
  glycemic control 546–50
  in labor 418–29
  metabolic monitoring 337–8
  Plymouth RCT 423
  postprandial glucose levels 394–5
  SBGM 331
  Swedish multicenter RCT 423–5, 426
multiple pregnancies 502–7
  conflicting data 504–5
  GDM risk factor 75, 78–9, 502–3,
    505–6
  hPL 503
myoinositol, embryopathy 268–9

National Institute of Health (NIH),
    guidelines, fetal maturity 284
neonatal erythremia 295–6
neonatal hyperbilirubinemia 296–7
neonatal hyperviscosity 295–6
neonatal hypocalcemia 256, 257–8, 292–4
  clinical manifestations 293
  defined 292–3
  etiology 293
  prevalence 292–3
  risk factors 293
  treatment 293–4
neonatal hypoglycemia 256, 289–92
  clinical manifestations 291–2
  complications 292
  defined 289
  etiology 291
  prevalence 289–91
  risk factors 291
  treatment 292
neonatal hypomagnesemia 257–8, 294
neonatal polycythemia 295–6
neonates, short-term implications 289–304
nephropathy see diabetic nephropathy
nestin-positive cells, pancreas 233–4
neural tube defects (NTD)
  folic acid supplementation 266–7
  ultrasound assessment 405–8
neurodevelopment 317–29
  long-term implications 313–14
NIDDM see non-insulin-dependent diabetes
  mellitus
NIH see National Institute of Health